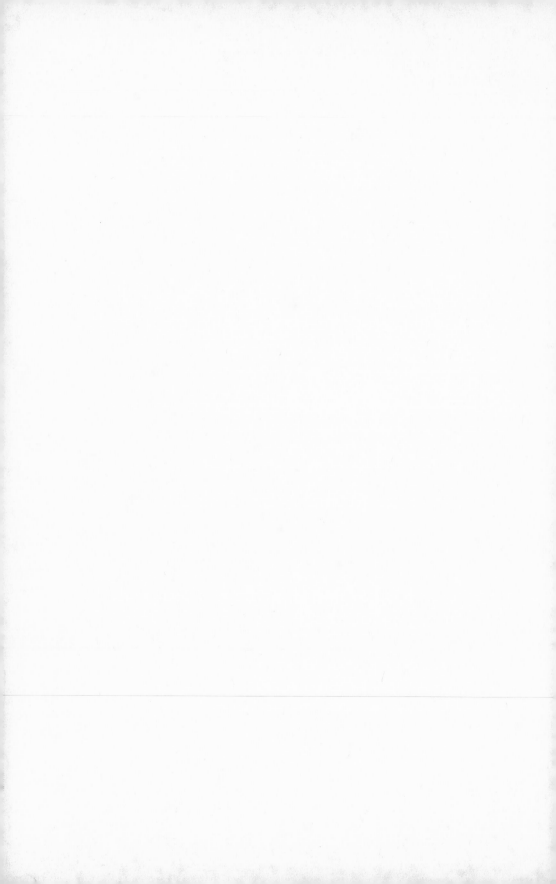

THE HYPERKINETIC CHILD

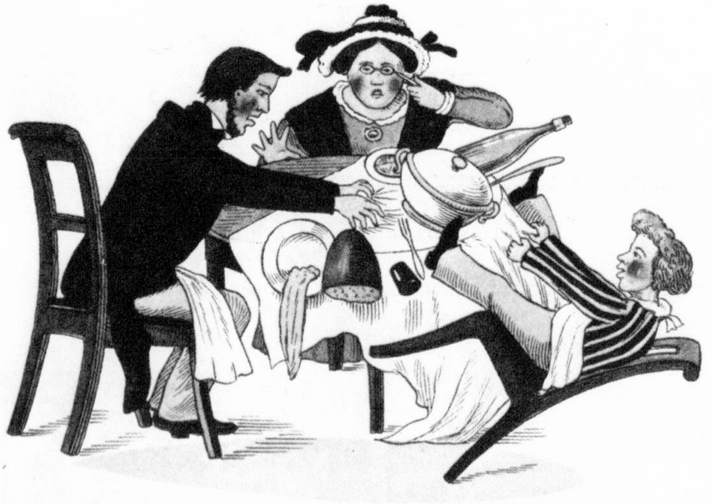

Among the earlier examples of a hyperactive child was Fidgety Philip, here portrayed in Heinrich Hoffmann-Donner's *Der Struwwelpeter*.

THE HYPERKINETIC CHILD

AN ANNOTATED BIBLIOGRAPHY 1974-1979

Carol Ann Winchell

Contemporary Problems of Childhood, Number 4

GP
GREENWOOD PRESS
Westport, Connecticut • London, England

Library of Congress Cataloging in Publication Data

Winchell, Carol Ann.
The hyperkinetic child.

(Contemporary problems of childhood, ISSN 0147-1082; no. 4)
Includes bibliographical references and indexes.
1. Hyperactive children—Bibliography. I. Title.
II. Series: Contemporary problems of childhood; no. 4.
Z5814.C52W53 1981 [LC4711] 305.2'3s 81-6200
ISBN 0-313-21452-2 (lib. bdg.) [016.61892'8589] AACR2

Library of Congress Catalog Card Number: 81-6200
ISBN: 0-313-21452-2
ISSN: 0147-1082

First published in 1981

Greenwood Press
A division of Congressional Information Service, Inc.
88 Post Road West
Westport, Connecticut 06881

Printed in the United States of America

10 9 8 7 6 5 4 3 2 1

In
memory
of
Jim

CONTENTS

PREFACE

PURPOSE

This volume, number four of the series *Contemporary Problems of Childhood*, identifies, collects, classifies, abstracts, and indexes relevant material on the topic of the hyperkinetic child.

A cursory perusal of the literature reveals a vast outpouring of publications pertaining to children's problems. These problems have not only been the subject of academe, but also the mass media: magazines, newspapers, and commercial and educational television specials have devoted considerable attention to them.

The plethora of publications, the strong and enduring interest in hyperactivity, and the multidisciplinary nature of the problem all suggest the utility of some form of bibliographic control. This volume has been prepared to aid in the retrieval of information for educators, psychologists, physicians, researchers, parents, and others interested in locating pertinent references in a rapidly expanding body of literature.

COVERAGE

This annotated supplement covers the years 1974 through 1979. An unannotated addendum contains some citations for 1980. The present bibliography updates the author's previous book, *The Hyperkinetic Child: A Bibliography of Medical, Educational, and Behavioral Studies* (Greenwood Press, 1975) which covers the literature up to 1974. More than 2,000 citations from widely scattered and diverse sources have been gathered for this supplement.

SCOPE

More than 2,000 citations have been culled from a five-year search of both manual and computerized information sources. The broadest possible investigation was made to incorporate all relevant literature from diverse fields of knowledge: medicine, education, psychology, child development, nursing, sociology, social work, rehabilitation, and law. Nearly 350 popular and professional journals are covered. The bibliography also cites books, chapters in books, conference proceedings, government documents, pamphlets, and doctoral dissertations. Excluded are animal studies (except those that use animals as models for the hyperkinetic syndrome in children), foreign language references, newspaper articles, personal correspondence, and masters' theses.

ARRANGEMENT

Entries are grouped according to the major categories in the Contents, which identifies the headings under which the references have been clustered. Exact categorization is difficult since a single article may deal with several aspects of a topic; generally, entries are placed according to the predominant focus of the article. Each reference is cited only once. The Selective Key Word Subject Index (see Indexes) provides an alternative method of access. Within each section, arrangement is alphabetical by author. Entry numbers preceding the author's name run consecutively throughout the text.

THE ENTRIES

For books and monographs the complete citation includes author(s), title, edition, place, publisher, date, pages, inclusive pages of sections appearing as parts of larger works, and presence of bibliography. Journal citations contain author (three are given; *et al.* is used to indicate additional names), title of the article, journal abbreviation, volume number, issue number (in parentheses), inclusive pages, month, year, the number of references, and ED (ERIC Document Numbers) where appropriate and available. ERIC Documents (for example ED 139 182) are available in microfiche at many research libraries or may be ordered from the ERIC Document Reproduction Service, P.O. Box 190, Arlington, Virginia 22210. Refer to the most recent issue of *Resources in Education* for current ordering information. For dissertations the user is referred to *Dissertation Abstracts International* with author, title, volume number, section, pages, and date given.

Books and conference proceedings have been verified and entered in the bibliography under the United States Library of Congress *National Union Catalog: Author List* entry to facilitate retrieval for the user. If a book has been catalogued under its title, cross references refer the user from the editor to the main entry.

Annotations have been provided for all available publications; dissertations and items in the addendum have not been abstracted. The full contents of several compilations have been included as an indication of the scope of the volume (item number 1043 is an example).

APPENDIXES

Appendix A alphabetically lists various terms found in the literature which have been applied to the syndrome.

Appendix B alphabetically lists some of the pharmacologic agents used to treat hyperkinesis. Information is provided about: generic name, trade name, therapeutic class, chemical class, manufacturer, and date.

Appendix C is a glossary of terms most commonly encountered in the literature.

Appendix D lists audiovisual materials by title.

Appendix E provides the names of selected organizations which serve the exceptional child.

Appendix F identifies the major manual and computerized bibliographical sources that were used to collect and verify citations in this bibliography.

INDEXES

The Author Index includes the names of all individuals cited as author, joint author, editor, or compiler, including up to three names per citation. Numbers following the names refer to item numbers in the text.

The Selective Key Word Subject Index alphabetically lists important words in entry titles. The user may find it convenient to use the broader subject arrangement under the categories in the Contents, or this index may be consulted for more specific aspects of the topic. In general only unique terms are given; phrases are used to put certain words in more meaningful contexts; and "see also" references are used to refer the reader to similar concepts. Numbers following the words refer to item numbers in the text.

The List of Journal Abbreviations lists alphabetically all journals cited in the text. Journal title abbreviations have been formulated according to the rules of the *American National Standard for the Abbreviation of Titles of Periodicals*, and the individual words of the title are abbreviated according to the forms given in the *International List of Periodical Title Word Abbreviations*.

ACKNOWLEDGMENTS

I would like to express my gratitude to the following Ohio State University faculty members for their assistance in the preparation of this volume: L.

Eugene Arnold, M.D., M.Ed., Professor of Psychiatry and Pediatrics, for writing the introduction; Hazel B. Benson, Director of Public Services, Health Sciences Library, for help in categorizing the entries; Beverly I. McDonald, Head, Authority Files Section, Cataloging Services, Main Library, for assisting with the finer points of filing and alphabetizing; Noelle Van Pulis, Information Specialist, Mechanized Information Center, Main Library, for help in developing the key word index; Linda Schamber, School of Journalism, for copy editing the manuscript; and James A. Visconti, Associate Professor of Pharmacy, for checking the drug table. I am also grateful to Jean Stouder for patiently typing the final manuscript, and to Dr. James Sabin, Vice-President, Editorial, Greenwood Press, for guidance and encouragement. Completion of the project was facilitated by the cooperation of the Ohio State University Libraries.

My son, Philip, whose happy face inspired my continued efforts, and my mother, Mrs. Helen French, deserve a special thank you.

INTRODUCTION

HYPERKINESIS BY ANY OTHER NAME PUZZLES THE SAME: PAST, PRESENT, AND FUTURE INVESTIGATIONS

The hyperkinetic literature explosion of the 1970s, so dramatically shown in the size of this six-year bibliography, reflects the amount of professional and popular interest focused on this many-named problem. Whether called hyperkinesis, hyperactivity, minimal brain dysfunction (MBD), impulse disorder, or most recently, attention deficit disorder (ADD), it has become one of the most popular diagnoses by both professional and lay persons. In fact, some of the publications, both professional and popular, focus on the dangers inherent in overdiagnosis. Some authors even deny that any child should be thus diagnosed, claiming that the diagnosis is a myth of convenience used to drug, control, or otherwise discriminate against normally energetic school children.

Regardless of one's political or philosophical position regarding the existence, etiology, or treatment of this syndrome, there is little doubt that it has increased dramatically in prominence and frequency of diagnosis. This leads to a question often asked by lay audiences: Why is there so much more hyperkinesis now than twenty or thirty years ago? We'll examine that question in detail after defining the term.

DEFINITION AND EVOLUTION OF THE TERMINOLOGY

One of the most obvious developments in the six years since the first volume of Winchell's *Hyperkinetic Child* bibliography is the evolution of terminology. The term *hyperkinesis* (or *hyperkinetic syndrome*) was not clearly favored until the 1960s when it was felt that this was the most accurate term because it was more descriptive than etiologic. It came to replace the term minimal brain damage because it was realized that not all children manifesting the "organic impulse disorder" were brain damaged. As it became clear that not all such affected children were overactive, the concept of a neurologic handicap was resurrected with such terms as psycho-neurologic integration deficit and minimal brain dysfunction, which implied that something was not working quite right in the brain but that it was not necessarily damaged.

The term minimal brain dysfunction was favored because it embraced the problems of impulsiveness, overactivity, inattentiveness, perceptual deficits, and other soft neurological signs and implied that there was something wrong with the child rather than that he was merely misbehaving. This term enjoyed a good deal of popularity in the early 1970s and Paul Wender's 1971 book, *Minimal Brain Dysfunction in Children*, was the first to be dedicated to this problem. Thus the term minimal brain dysfunction had gained increasing acceptance in place of hyperkinesis or hyperkinetic syndrome even as the first edition of Winchell's bibliography was published in 1975.

However, the MBD term did not remain in favor long enough to become official diagnostic terminology. During its heyday, hyperkinetic reaction, a term adopted in 1968 by the American Psychiatric Association in its *Diagnostic and Statistical Manual* (DSM-II),[2] was still the officially coded diagnostic term. By 1980, when DSM-II was replaced by DSM-III,[3] attention deficit disorder had gained favor based on the belief by many experts that the central phenomena in this disorder are the problems of attention and impulse control, with or without hyperactivity.

According to DSM-III, to warrant a diagnosis of attention deficit disorder with hyperactivity, the child must show:

1. at least three signs of inattention (such as failing to finish things, not seeming to listen, being easily distracted, difficulty concentrating, or difficulty sticking with a play activity)
2. at least three signs of impulsivity (such as acting before thinking, shifting excessively from one activity to another, difficulty in organizing work, needing a lot of supervision, frequently calling out in class, or difficulty in waiting turn in games)
3. at least two signs of hyperactivity (such as excessive running or climbing, difficulty sitting still or fidgeting, difficulty staying seated, restlessness during sleep, or always being on the go or driven by a motor).

The onset of these symptoms must be before the age of seven and of at least six months' duration and they must not be due to schizophrenia, affective disorder, or severe or profound mental retardation.

It is possible to diagnose attention deficit disorder without hyperactivity, but then the child would not by "hyperkinetic" in the usual sense. This is a good illustration of how the concept of the syndrome evolved over the past few decades. One of the first terms used was hyperkinetic because one of the more prominent symptoms of the most severely affected children was their overactivity. Gradually the literature began to reflect an increasingly sophisticated appreciation of other aspects of the disorder, including attention deficit, impulsiveness, and perceptual deficits and other "soft" neurological signs.

The validity of soft signs is even more controversial than the concept of hyperkinesis, and this may be one reason why DSM-III did not consider them in the operational diagnostic criteria. This is unfortunate because both clinical impression and voluminous literature attest to the disproportionately high association of this disorder with perceptual deficits, if not other soft signs.

Michael Rutter[4] has also criticized the DSM-III operational criteria, pointing out that there is no good research evidence to show that these particular criteria should have been chosen above others, though he admits they are commonly occurring signs of the disorder.

The words hyperkinetic and hyperactive deserve some comparative comment. They are often used as synonomous terms, even in the titles of professional journal articles. Some people, however, have made a distinction and consider hyperkinetic to be a diagnostic term referring to the syndrome, and hyperactive to be a descriptive term referring to one sign that is part of the syndrome, but does not in itself justify the diagnosis of hyperkinesis or attention deficit disorder. For example, manic patients are often described as hyperactive, which is an accurate description of their agitated, euphoric, pressured state during a manic psychosis, but does not imply that they have attention deficit disorder. DSM-III criteria seem to make a similar distinction between the syndrome and the symptom of hyperactivity. As used in DSM-II, hyperactivity refers only to symptoms directly related to quantity and quality of motor drivenness, with the other aspects of the hyperkinetic syndrome described under the rubrics of attention deficit and impulsivity, the latter two being considered the more essential elements.

WHY THE INCREASE IN HYPERKINESIS?

The first explanation that comes to mind for the increased hyperkinesis is that perhaps there has not really been any increase in hyperkinesis, but rather an increased awareness. As the syndrome became better known among physicians, educators, parents, relatives, and neighbors, diagnostic suspicion soared, and a national zeal for ferreting out and identifying cases has developed. Of course, cases are not counted for incidence or prevalence unless they have been identified or diagnosed in some way, so there could be an apparent increase without an actual increase. I do not believe, however, that increased awareness of the syndrome is the sole explanation for the apparent increase in incidence and prevalence.

I believe there is also an actual increase in occurrence of the syndrome for a variety of reasons. The diagnosable presence of the syndrome depends on a cluster of characteristic signs and symptoms. No matter how much potential the child may have for developing the syndrome, he does not really have the disorder unless he manifests the signs and symptoms in sufficient quantity and severity. Therefore, one possible reason for the apparent increase in hyperkinesis might be that some children with the potential for it who would previously have been protected by fortuitous circumstances from manifesting the signs and symptoms are now sufficiently stressed to show them.

There have been a number of changes in our educational, social-community, political, and other systems that could buttress this explanation. It is well known that hyperkinetic children function best in a highly structured situation with close supervision, in a small group, and among older people rather than age peers. The old one-room schoolhouse provided all this very well; a small group of children (usually smaller than the current age-homogeneous classes), and a mix of different ages, with the older ones often expected to tutor and supervise the younger ones. There was a very authoritarian social community network backing up a very firm teacher, and individualized educational plans were necessary because there were not enough children of a given age to provide an "average" Procrustean expectation. A tightly knit family with at least one parent at home, and often both, also provided a great deal of structure and supervision. Lower density of population provided less distraction and less opportunity for bumping into trouble when an occasional youngster did manifest some Brownian motion. Further, the agricultural economy of a hundred years ago provided more constructive outlets for activity. I have personally known of several youngsters who were constantly in trouble in the city because of their hyperkinetic problems, but who, on moving to a farm, were able to put their motor-driven characteristics to good use.

Most hyperkinetic children are action oriented and many have deficits in verbal and math skills. An agricultural society such as America's was a hundred years ago was action oriented in an individualistic manner; an urban society is machine oriented in a forced-affiliative manner; the society of the future as predicted by the social big thinkers is a communication society that will be word-and-number oriented in an intrusively affiliative manner. We might predict that the individual who has more trouble in the current forced-affiliative urban society than in the old individualistic agricultural society would have even more trouble in the word-oriented communication society of the future.

There is another side to our current industrial, technological society. Not only can it bring out these problems in vulnerable individuals, but it may actually produce the vulnerability, perhaps damaging individuals so they are more likely to become hyperkinetic. One major culprit seems to be widespread heavy metal pollution, particularly lead. Other possibilities are: cleaning compounds, solvents, insecticides, herbicides, and contaminants of these chemicals; dyes, flavorings and preservatives added to food; a relative deficiency of certain nutrients in highly processed foods; increased chronic radiation exposure; and even such things as antiseptics and antibiotics.

The mining and widespread use of lead, though predating the industrial revolution, has increased as more uses have been found for this toxic metal. Three million tons annually are mined and some finds its way into the dirt with which children contaminate their food by eating with dirty hands, as well as into the food that is canned in lead-soldered containers.[5] We know that a child does not have to eat lead-painted plaster chips to develop lead poisoning—at least the subclinical variety with serum levels from 20 to 70 micrograms percent. Tetraethyl lead is seven times as toxic as inorganic lead salts, can be absorbed through the skin, and has an affinity for nervous tissue. A child who eats with dirty hands after playing near a highway or street can ingest lead precipitated from gasoline exhausts. David and Associates[6] have reported an association of subclinical plumbism and hyperkinetic behavior and this seems to be supported by the work of Needelman and Associates.[7] However, this association has been questioned by Ernhart[8] in a well-controlled study.

A nonchemical pathogen to which increasing attention is directed is maternal deprivation with deficiency in such biological stimulants as tactile, auditory, vestibular, and visual stimulation of the developing infant. The work of numerous authors (for example Klaus and Kennell,[9] and Salk[10]) underscores the delicate, complex, and essential bonding mechanism between infant and mother. Prior to a hundred years ago, this bonding generally took place without notice and did its essential work for the normal development of the infant and young child without scientific scrutiny or help. Two modern "improvements" in childbearing and childrearing inadvertently disrupted the normal process that has evolved in our species over the preceding millenia.

One of these was changing the place of birth from home to hospital, with the resulting separation of mother and infant in the crucial first hours after birth. It was accepted as normal that the infant should lose a half a pound or so "physiologically" in the first day after birth. Salk[10] has now demonstrated that if the infant has access to a heart beat sound, he cries less and does not lose weight the first day. Henderson[11] reports that colic can be prevented by laying the infant on his mother skin-to-skin in the delivery room. Klaus and Kennell[9] have detected a critical period for bonding to the mother in the first half hour or so after birth when the infant is more alert and appealing than later. Modern obstetrical practices, in addition to posing risk to the newborn from maternal anesthetics, could impair the bonding process which would otherwise insure that the infant gets adequate mothering.

The other development is the nursing bottle, which became so popular that at one point over half the infants in America were not breast fed. Though the chemical intake through a nursing bottle formula may be adequate, it makes it easy to neglect the handling and stimulation of the baby that was previously insured by breast feeding.

Hyperactivity has been reported as a symptom of maternal deprivation. There is also a recent comparative psychiatry report that links maternal separation even more closely with the symdrome. This series of studies by Corson and associates[12] demonstrates an interaction between genetic predisposition and maternal deprivation in a dog model. Corson at Ohio State University[13] and Ginsberg[14] at Yale did experiments with a strain of naturally hyperkinetic dogs provided by Scott of Bowling Green. They found the majority of dogs to be hyperkinetic in a structured learning situation such as a Pavlovian conditioning stand or an obedience trial that involved sitting still for one minute, tasks that were relatively easy and quickly learned by normal dogs. Most of these hyperkinetic dogs responded well to amphetamine, as do hyperkinetic children. When Scott tried to replicate Corson's and Ginsberg's findings in dogs from the same colony in their home kennel, he found only a few to be hyperkinetic and those were not responsive to amphetamine. However, when he took the same dogs thirty miles away from their home and mothers, he found the majority of them to be hyperkinetic and most of these were responsive to amphetamine, similar to the results that Corson and Ginsberg found.

Aside from such pathological interferences in the normal psychosocial environment as maternal deprivation, it is possible that other human errors in the management of the psychosocial environment could contribute to an increased manifestation of hyperkinesis. Insofar as behavior is learned, the models of behavior that are offered on television, in movies, and through other media, and the expectations and reinforcement contingencies that interact with the child, could reinforce or otherwise accentuate certain patterns of behavior at the expense of others. Perhaps there is even a phenomenon of overstimulation with the steady diet of excitement offered by commercial panderers.

Besides human interference in the physical, chemical, and psychosocial environment, there could be an increase in the actual occurrence of hyperkinesis from natural causes. Intrauterine rubella, for example, in addition to causing hearing, vision, and intelligence deficits, has also been associated with learning and behavior disorders. Infectious agents evolve and wax and wane. Epidemics have occurred spontaneously throughout history and it is conceivable that an upsurge in viral or other microorganism virulence in the past few decades has contributed to an increased prevalence of neurologically-based behavior and learning problems that include hyperkinesis.

RESEARCH TRENDS

Some of the literature explosion of the last six years has been popularization, "rehash" journalism, and political polemic. However, the amount of good, rigorous scientific investigation has also multiplied. One benefit of the popular interest in hyperkinesis is the turning of scientific resources toward its investigation and the willingness of funding sources to underwrite research on the problem. I would like to elaborate on the following five trends in the literature that I consider particularly interesting or encouraging: (1) increased interest in follow-up studies; (2) finer distinctions among subgroups of hyperkinetic children; (3) careful investigations of etiological hypotheses that at first appear to be conjecture and/or demagoguery (for example, the work on dietary additives such as colorings, flavorings, and preservatives); (4) the laboratory study of drug effects on afflicted children and their parents and teachers; (5) the increasing awareness of the need to study the summation and synergism of several simultaneous or successive treatment modalities.

FOLLOW-UP STUDIES AND NATURAL HISTORY OF HYPERKINESIS

Prior to 1967 there were few published systematic follow-up studies of hyperkinesis. It was widely assumed that children outgrew the problem by age eighteen, and this statement appears in the literature.[15] It was further assumed in some quarters that merely giving hyperkinetic children a stimulant drug to tide them over was all the treatment they needed, even though some of the literature spoke of the need for a combined management plan of medication, parent guidance, and psychological treatment. Finally, it was tacitly assumed that the benefits and side effects noted in short-term controlled studies of drug treatment could be extrapolated to long-term effects.

Therefore, it came as a disappointment when follow-up studies[16,17] showed persistence of the problems into late adolescence and adulthood. Though the hyperactivity abated somewhat with age, the problems with attention span and impulsiveness seemed to persist, as well as the perceptual deficits that contributed to associated learning disabilities. Eventually publications appeared on minimal brain dysfunction in adults,[18,19,20] most of whom had a history of the same problem in childhood that was not always diagnosed. We were thus faced with the sad fact that the problem is not necessarily outgrown, but can be a life-long handicap when there is no treatment or when treated in the vogue of fifteen years ago. Further discouragement came from reports of mild height growth retardation at the one-to-two-year follow-up of stimulant treatment.[21] Fortunately, this concern has since been allayed by longer follow-up studies on larger samples showing return to the expected growth curve even when the stimulant is continued.[22] Another ray of hope is that most of the samples showing poor results over a period of ten years or more were children without consistent follow-up treatment. A typical child may have had one or two years of stimulant medication or a major tranquilizer with no further intervention until follow-up ten to twenty-five years later. Very few were given concomitant psychotherapy, family therapy, or perceptual training. More recent studies utilizing a multimodal approach show more promise.[23]

One sidelight that helped to focus interest on follow-up studies was the finding of a high incidence of sociopathy, hysterical personality, and alcoholism among the biological parents of hyperkinetic children.[24-27] This raised the interesting question whether such disorders in adulthood are a natural outcome of hyperkinetic disorders in childhood, or whether alcoholic, sociopathic, and hysterical parents do things to children that make them hyperkinetic, or whether there is some sort of pleomorphic genetic substrate that can result in either hyperkinesis, alcoholism, sociopathy, or hysterical personality. Adoptive and foster studies[26,27] suggest a genetic rather than parental-environmental explanation of the correlation of these parental disorders with hyperkinesis in childhood. The final word is not in, however; recently the methodology of studies that support the genetic etiology has been criticized. No studies have directly addressed the issue of whether these adult disorders are actually the outcome of previous childhood hyperkinesis.

Nevertheless, there is enough presumptive evidence[24-29] and clinical impression to stimulate speculation such as illustrated in Figure 1, which follows the possible progression of MBD and attention deficit disorder through several channels to various adult personality disorders and depression. This graph is a visual example of the kind of synthetic speculation easily provoked by the literature now available.

The possibilities of inputs other than those considered in the flow network are represented by arrows from question marks; progress to other than a diagnostic syndrome are represented by the outflows marked "OK." These do not necessarily imply sound mental health or normality but that the problems abate enough so they no longer warrant clinical recognition.

Some relationships are suggested by clinical observation supported by such as the shift from identity disorder to borderline personality after adolescence. Others are suggested by a reading of specific diagnostic criteria and knowledge of the research literature. We have already mentioned the suggested genetic link between attention deficit disorder in children and histrionic or antisocial personality in parents. Children with attention deficit disorder manifest many of the symptoms of these two personality disorders: impulsiveness, somatization, failure to learn from aversive ex-

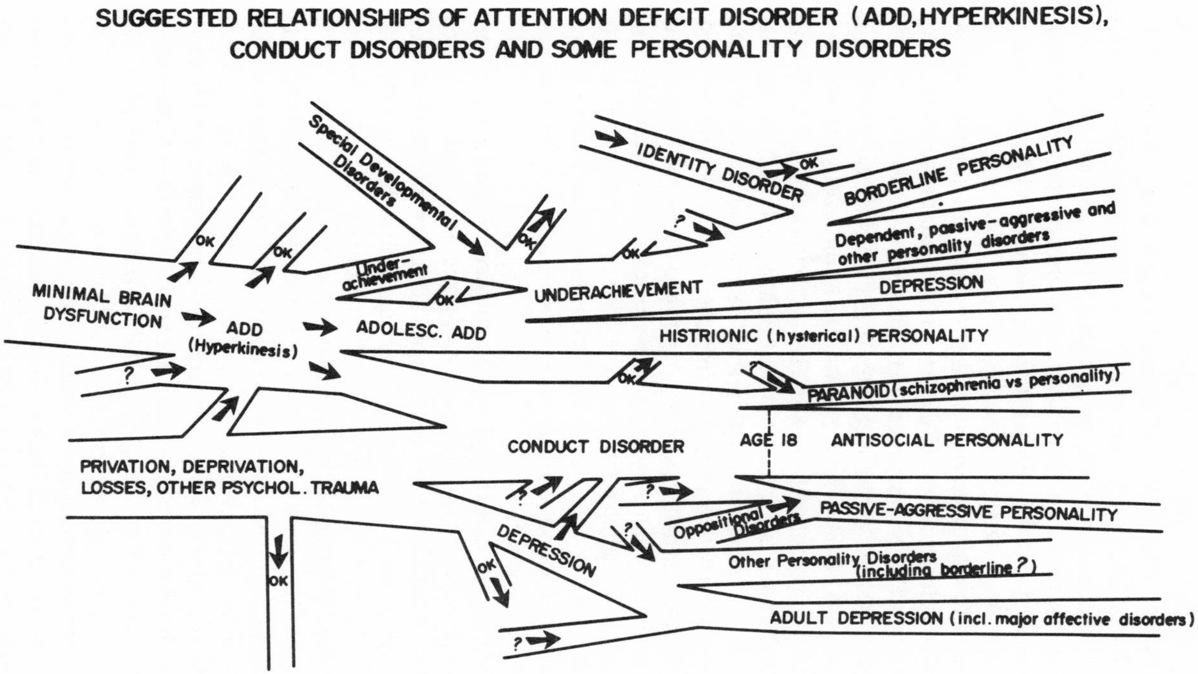

Figure 1. Longitudinal diagnostic flow network speculated from literature of the past decade and from clinical impression.

perience, superficiality, and poor peer relations. These facts suggest a flow from attention deficit disorder through two different tracks to histrionic and antisocial personalities.

Some relationships are suggested by clinical observation supported by specific DSM-III encouragement to make concomitant diagnoses. DSM-III states that conduct disorders may coexist with an attention deficit disorder, and in such cases both should be coded. My experience is that this does occur often and the history usually reveals that the attention deficit syndrome preceded the full-blown conduct disorder, which may result from the frustration engendered by the attention deficit. It seems reasonable to graph the flow from ADD to conduct disorder, which makes a logical intermediary step from ADD to antisocial personality.

Some of the relationships shown are supported only by common sense and clinical observation. One example is the paranoid adjustment I have observed in several adolescent and preadolescent youngsters with a history of attention deficit disorder and recent undersocialized conduct. A paranoid outcome should not be entirely unexpected if we consider the plight of a person who finds himself constantly "picked on" for unacceptable behavior that he cannot control, and who may sense that he is in some way damaged. Figure 1 is subject to continued revision as new data becomes available.

FINER DISTINCTIONS AMONG SUBGROUPS

Finer distinctions among subgroups of hyperkinetic children have been based on several criteria. The most impressive of these involve physiological studies, but there are also phenomenological subdivisions. One of the most prominent phenomenological distinctions is embodied in the DSM-III criteria, where it is possible to have attention deficit disorder with or without hyperactivity. This reflects the increased conviction among clinicians and authors that hyperactivity is not the most essential feature of the hyperkinetic syndrome, but merely characterizes an important subgroup. Other phenomenological distinctions that have been made are: the presence or absence of soft neurologic signs, the concomitant presence of specific learning disability, the amount of unsocialized aggressiveness, the degree of family pathology, and a history suggesting the presence or absence of certain hypothesized etiological considerations. These would include: intrauterine insult, genetic loading, early deprivation or privation (material, nutritional, or psychosocial), and the presence of chronic emotional stress.

Physiological distinctions that have been investigated are galvanic skin response,[30] evoked potentials on electroencephalogram,[31] pupillary light reaction on electropupillogram,[32] and serotonin levels.[33] Each of these physiological parameters has yielded a subgroup showing a deviation from both normal and other hyperkinetic children. Satterfield and Associates,[30] for example, showed a subgroup of about one-third that was hypoaroused; Knopp and associates[32] showed a subgroup of about one-fourth that was hypoaroused and another subgroup of about one-third that was hyperaroused. Responsiveness to stimulant drugs correlated somewhat with the hypoarousal. Coleman found that by selecting for low blood serotonin (less than half of normal), she was able to get a good response to pyridoxine in pharmacological doses.[34]

INVESTIGATIONS OF ETIOLOGICAL AND THERAPEUTIC HYPOTHESES

Careful scientific follow-up on new etiological and therapeutic hypotheses is a credit to the community of experts investigating this problem. Some of the hypotheses would have been easy to dismiss because of the unscientific way they were advocated. A good example of this is the concept that hyperkinesis can be caused by food additives (flavorings, colorings, and preservatives) as well as natural constituents of food such as salicylates. This is often called the Feingold hypothesis or Feingold diet. Benjamin Feingold was not the only one advocating such an approach but he was the best known and named the most additives and foods to be eliminated from the diet, implying that these were the reasons for all hyperkinesis. A further reason for his notoriety was that he chose political and popular press means to publicize his views rather than scientific literature, and had no controlled studies to document his claims. This engendered a good deal of skepticism among the experts, who then initiated studies of their own. The first studies seemed to confirm their doubts because significant group differences were not found and challenges with the suspected offending substances did not seem to confirm their pathogenicity.[35]

Even in those early studies, however, the investigators noticed that an occasional child seemed to benefit from the elimination diet and agreed that the hypothesis deserved further investigation. A major breakthrough resulted from focusing on the time between the elimination and the challenge, which had to be between four and ten days to show the expected deterioration. Apparently the child became desensitized to the substance if it was withheld for more than a few weeks. Another refinement was to increase the dose of the challenge substance to the range actually consumed by many children rather than using a national average. With such refinements, Kinsbourne and Swanson at Toronto have found significant group differences on double-blind challenge as well as on open dietary elimination. Informally they estimate that about one-third of the children in the sample showed definite dietary responsiveness.

Vitamin therapy is another area that has been met with some skepticism by more orthodox clinicians and investigators, and the only published controlled study of megavitamin combination therapy as advocated by some of the orthomolecular school did not show any significant benefits.[36] More sophisticated work using specific vitamins in response to specific biochemical abnormalities detected through blood and urine tests has shown more promising results. The best example of this is Coleman's treatment of the low-serotonin subgroup of hyperkinetic children with pyridoxine.[34]

Another line of inquiry related to ingestion is the previously mentioned work showing a correlation between hyperkinesis and lead levels that are higher than normal but below the amount traditonally accepted as threshold for frank plumbism.[6] Deleading with penicillamine has resulted in improvement of hyperkinetic ratings.

Another interesting line of investigation concerns the effectiveness of vestibular stimulation. Bhatara and Clark[37,38] have reported significant benefits from systematic eyes-open rotation in a swivel chair with the head cocked to stimulate in turn each of the pairs of semicircular canals. They felt that the benefit was confined mainly to children under the age of ten without unsocialized aggressive tendencies.

Though related more to prevention than to treatment, the studies of channel-specific perceptual training should be mentioned here. Silver and Hagin's work[39] was replicated in a controlled manner because of skepticism about their reports. The significant findings of the controlled replication[40] were met with further skepticism[41,42] but have not been disproven.

LABORATORY STUDIES OF DRUG EFFECTS

Laboratory studies of drug effects have become increasingly popular and have contributed to the scientific rigor of the investigative effort. They cannot stand alone but they supplement and complement clinical investigation. Sprague and Sleator's work on dosage effect[43,44] has been one contribution. They found that the methylphenidate benefit on a laboratory learning task was best at a dose less than half the optimum dose for behavioral control, which should alert clinicians to the need for titrating and balancing out the trade-off between the two effects. Rapoport and Associates[45] investigated amphetamine effects on normal and hyperkinetic boys and adult men, helping to clarify the mechanism of benefit. Barkley and Associates[46] have reported changes in mother-child social interactions with changes in the mother's behavior when a hyperkinetic child is medicated under controlled laboratory observation. Whalen and Associates[47] reported similar changes in teachers' behavior when a stimulant was administered to hyperkinetic children in small laboratory classes in a double-blind, placebo-controlled situation. Shekim and Associates[48] found that amphetamine reduced low urinary norepinephrine metabolites even further.

INTERACTION AND SUMMATION OF SIMULTANEOUS OR SUCCESSIVE TREATMENT MODALITIES

There seem to be as many different treatments for hyperkinesis as there are suggested etiologies. An old clinical axiom states that when there are many treatments for a given disorder, none of them is one hundred percent effective. Therefore, clinicians know there is a need for several treatment modalities. One of the encouraging research trends of the past few years is the study of the interactions of different treatments. Gittelman-Klein[49] looked at the interaction of methylphenidate and behavior modificiation. Satterfield and Cantwell[23] recently reported on the efficacy of multimodality treatment in which they include drug treatment (usually methylphenidate), psychotherapy, and parent guidance. Corson and Associates[50] have reported an interaction of drugs and tender loving care in a dog model.

SYNTHESIZING AND SPECULATING FROM THE LITERATURE

The challenge confronting the 1981 hyperkinesiologist is the comparing, integrating, and synthesizing of the mass of data available. The August 1980 issue of *Archives of General Psychiatry* contained three articles[23,45,51] relating to treatment of hyperkinetic children. They provoked the following thoughts:

In "Multimodality Treatment," Satterfield and Associates[23] found a sustained gain in academic achievement (on the Peabody). I suspected that this was intimately related to the behavioral improvement, and at my request they checked this by correlating behavioral and academic improvement across children, and did not find a significant correlation.

They attributed the academic benefit to the use of methylphenidate in a dosage of .32 mg/kg B.I.D., which was consonant with Sprague and Sleator's[43,44] recommendation of .3 mg/kg/dose. It is possible that the concomitant psychosocial treatment also effected achievement or that the two may have acted synergistically. Possibly the psychosocial treatment allowed behavioral control to occur at a lower dose of stimulant than reported by other authors.

In their comparison of pemoline and methylphenidate, Conners and Taylor[51] used only slightly higher doses of methylphenidate (.82 mg/kg/-day) and found no changes on the Wide Range Achievement Test at eight weeks. Thus we have related reports, one showing significant achievement effects at the end of two years and the other showing no effects at eight weeks. How can these findings be reconciled? One possibility is that the Conners and Taylor sample might have shown significant achievement effects if the treatment had continued long enough. Another possibility is that concomitant psychosocial therapy made the difference for Satterfield's group. A third factor is the different instruments used and the possibility that the Wide Range might not be as sensitive as the Peabody. Could the small difference in dosage (.64 mg/kg/day for Satterfield vs. .82 mg/kg/-day for Conners) be enough to make the difference? If this were true it would support Sprague and Sleator's hypothesized therapeutic window for learning effect with a vengeance, and would corroborate the critical .3 mg/kg/dose that they suggest and which Satterfield's group used B.I.D. Perhaps the difference between the two reports could merely be a matter of sample differences. Though the ages of the children are not remarkably different, the racial and socioeconomic composition differ somewhat, with Conners and Taylor's sample more white middle class. The failure of Conners and Taylor's sample to show a significant achievement effect supports Satterfield and Cantwell's contention that their achievement effects were not simply the result of better test-taking performance during medication.

Rapoport and Associates[45] studied the cognitive and behavioral effect of dextroamphetamine in normals. They found that amphetamine does not work like aspirin, which in moderate therapeutic doses lowers a high temperature but does not affect a normal temperature; instead, it acts more like an ice pack, which lowers the temperature of hyperpyrexics and normals alike, or a laxative, which purges one and all without distinction. Thus, in using stimulants on children we are using cruder tools than we would like to believe. Nevertheless, ice packs and laxatives are sometimes indicated, and this finding need not discredit judicious stimulant therapy.

Rapoport's low-dose condition for normal men (.25 mg/kg dextroamphetamine) is higher than that used by either of the other two studies, if we accept a 2:1 potency ratio for amphetamine and methylphenidate. The high-dose men and both the normal and hyperkinetic boys were given twice that dosage. Yet all four groups showed improvement on laboratory tests of verbal learning and memory. If we assume that improved laboratory learning results in improved academic achievement, this finding seems at odds with the therapeutic window hypothesis and with Conners and Taylor's achievement data. Possible explanations are:

1. the traditional 2:1 potency ratio for amphetamine and methylphenidate may be invalid
2. dextroamphetamine may have a higher therapeutic window (or perhaps no upper limit at all for learning)
3. the first few days the stimulant enhances learning but then the benefit decays unless the patient is also receiving psychosocial therapy.

PHILOSOPHICAL CONSOLATIONS

The hyperkinetic literature reflects in a microcosm and microchronism what has happened with human knowledge in the past thousand years. In

1970 it was possible for one person to know everything that had been written about hyperkinesis: the references, the authors, their research designs, and all the treatment approaches. It is still possible to be aware of all areas of this rapidly expanding field of knowledge, but it is no longer possible to know everything in detail. Another decade may see the amount of knowledge expanded to the extent that there will be subspecialities within the study of hyperkinesis and its treatment, or at least subspecialities within the experts' ranks. Possible areas for subspecializing might be: nutritional and other dietary considerations; constitutional, enzymatic, immunological, and other physiological substrate; perceptual deficits and their remediation; psychosocial treatments (psychotherapy, behavior modification, parent guidance, family therapy, hypnotherapy, biofeedback, etc.); toxicology and drug treatment; and prevention.

Though I mourn the passing of the renaissance hyperkinesiologist, I welcome the challenges and opportunities that new investigations will bring. The handicap of partial knowledge of the field can, I am sure, be overcome by teamwork analogous to that used in other fields with greatly expanded knowledge. Annotated bibliographies such as this will undoubtedly be one of the important means of communication among the subspecializing experts.

L. Eugene Arnold, M.D., M.Ed.
Professor of Psychiatry and Pediatrics
The Ohio State University
Columbus, Ohio

NOTES

1. Wender, P. *Minimal brain dysfunction in children*, New York, New York: Wiley-Interscience, 1971. 242 p. (Wiley Series on Psychological Disorders).

2. American Psychiatric Association. Committee on Nomenclature and Statistics. *Diagnostic and statistical manual of mental disorders (DSM-II).* 2d ed. Washington, D.C.: American Pyschiatric Association, 1968. 134 p.

3. American Psychiatric Association. Task Force on Nomenclature and Statistics. *Diagnostic and statistical manual of mental disorders* (*DSM-III*). 3rd ed. Washington, D.C.: American Psychiatric Association, 1980. 494 p.

4. Rutter, M., and Shaffer, D. DSM-III: a step forward or backward in terms of classification of child psychiatric disorders?'' *J Am Acad Child Psychiatry* 19 (3): 371-84, Summer, 1980.

5. Settle, D. M., and Patterson, C. C. ''Lead in albacore: guide to lead pollution in Americans.'' *Science* 207: 1167-76, March 14, 1980.

6. David, O.; Clark, J.; Voeller, K. "Lead and hyperactivity." *Lancet* 2: 900–903, October 28, 1972.

7. Needelman, H. L., et al. "Deficits in psychologic and classroom performance of children with elevated dentine lead levels." *N Engl J Med* 300 (13): 689-94, March 29, 1979.

8. Ernhart, C. B.; Landa, B.; Schell, N. B. "Subclinical levels of lead and developmental deficit: a multivariate follow-up reassessment." *Pediatrics,* 1981, in press.

9. Klaus, M. H., and Kennell, J. H. *Maternal-infant bonding: the impact of early separation or loss on family development*. St. Louis, Missouri: Mosby, 1976. 257 p.

10. Salk, L. "The role of the heartbeat in the relations between mother and infant." *Sci Am* 228: 12, 24-29, May, 1973.

11. Henderson, A. T. Statement at Minimal Brain Dysfunction Symposium, Ohio State University, 1975.

12. Corson, S. A.; Corson, E. O'L.; Becker, R. E. "Interaction of genetics and separation in canine hyperkinesis and in differential responses to amphetamine." *Pav J Biol* 15 (1): 5-11, 1980.

13. Corson, S. A.; Corson, E. O'L.; Arnold, L. E., et al. "Animal models of violence and hyperkinesis." In Serban, G., and King, A., eds. *Animal models in human psychobiology*. New York, New York: Plenum Press, 1976.

14. Ginsburg, B. E., et al. "Genetic variation in drug responses in hybrid dogs: a possible model for the hyperkinetic syndrome." *Behav Genet* 6: 107, 1976.

15. Laufer, M. W., Denhoff, E. "Hyperkinetic behavior syndrome in children." *J. Pediatr* 50 (1): 463–73, January, 1967.

16. Menkes, M. H.; Rowe, J. S.; Menkes, J. H. "A 25-year follow-up study on the hyperkinetic child with MBD." *Pediatrics* 39 (3): 393-99, March, 1967.

17. Mendelson, W.; Johnson, N.; Stewart, M. A. "Hyperactive children as teenagers: a follow-up study." *J Nerv Ment Dis* 153 (4): 273-79, October, 1971.

18. Arnold, L. E.; Strobl, D.; Weisenberg, A. "Hyperkinetic adult: study of the 'paradoxical' amphetamine response." *JAMA* 222 (6): 693–94, November 6, 1972.

19. Wood, D. R.; Reimherr, F. W.; Wender, P. H., et al. "Diagnosis and treatment of minimal brain dysfunction in adults." *Arch Gen Psychiatry* 33 (12): 1453-60, December, 1976.

20. Bellak, L., ed. *Psychiatric aspects of minimal brain dysfunction in adults*. New York, New York: Grune & Stratton, 1979. 208 p.

21. Safer, D. J.; Allen, R.; Barr, E. "Depression of growth in hyperactive children on stimulant drugs." *N Engl J Med* 287: 217-20, August 3, 1972.

22. Oettinger, L.; Majovski, L. V.; Limbeck, G. A. et al. "Bone age in children with minimal brain dysfunction." *Percept Mot Skills* 39 (3): 1127-31, December, 1974.

23. Satterfield, J. H.; Satterfield, B. T.; Cantwell, D. "Multimodality treatment: a two-year evaluation of 61 hyperactive boys." *Arch Gen Psychiatry* 37 (8): 915-19, August, 1980.

24. Cantwell, D. P. "Psychiatric illness in the families of hyperactive children." *Arch Gen Psychiatry* 27 (9): 414-17, September, 1972.

25. Morrison, J. R., and Stewart, M. A. "A family study of the hyperactive child syndrome." *Biol Psychiatry* 3: 189–95, 1971.

26. Morrison, J. R., and Stewart, M. A. "The psychiatric status of the legal families of adopted hyperactive children." *Arch Gen Psychiatry* 28 (6): 888-91, June, 1973.

27. Safer, D. "A familial factor in minimal brain dysfunction." *Behav Genet* 3: 175-86, 1973.

28. Morrison, J. R., and Minkoff, K. "Explosive personality as a sequel to the hyperactive child syndrome." *Compr Psychiatry* 16 (4): 343-48, July-August, 1975.

29. Schuckit, M. A.; Petrich, J.; Chiles, J. "Hyperactivity: diagnostic confusion." *J Nerv Ment Dis* 166 (2): 79-87, February, 1978.

30. Satterfield, J. H.; Cantwell, D. P.; Lesser, L. I., et al. Physiological studies of the hyperkinetic child: I. *Am J. Psychiatry* 128 (11): 1418-24, May, 1972.

31. Shetty, T. "Photic response in hyperkinesis of childhood." *Science* 174: 1356-57, December 24, 1971.

32. Knopp, W.; Arnold, L. E.; Andras, R. L., et al. "Predicting amphetamine response in hyperkinetic children by electronic pupillography." *Pharmakopsychiatry* 6: 158-66, 1973.

33. Coleman, M. "Serotonin concentrations in whole blood of hyperactive children." *J Pediatr* 78 (6): 985-90, June, 1971.

34. Coleman, M.; Steinberg, G.; Tippett, J., et al. "A preliminary study of the effect of pyridoxine administration in a subgroup of hyperkinetic children: a double-blind crossover comparison with methylphenidate." *Biol Psychiatry* 14 (5): 741-51, October, 1979.

35. Harley, J. P.; Matthews, C. G.; Eichman, P. "Synthetic food colors and hyperactivity in children: a double-blind challenge experiment." *Pediatrics* 62 (6): 975-83, December, 1978.

36. Arnold, L. E.; Christopher, J. C.; Huestis, R. D., et al. "Megavitamins for minimal brain dysfunction: a placebo-controlled study." *JAMA* 240 (24): 2642-43, December 8, 1978.

37. Bhatara, V.; Clark, D. L.; Arnold, L. E. "Behavioral and nystagmus response of a hyperkinetic child to vestibular stimulation." *Am J Occup Ther* 32 (5): 311-16, May-June, 1978.

38. Bhatara, V.; Clark, D. L.; Arnold, L. E., et al. "Hyperkinesis treated by vestibular stimulation: an exploratory study." *Biol Psychiatry* 16 (3): 269-79, March, 1981.

39. Silver, A. A., and Hagin, R. A. "Profile of a first grade class." *J Am Acad Child Psychiatry* 11: 645–74, 1972.

40. Arnold, L.E.; Barnebey, N.; McManus, J., et al. "Prevention by specific perceptual remediation for vulnerable first-graders: controlled study and follow-up of lasting effects." *Arch Gen Psychiatry* 34 (11): 1279-94, November, 1977.

41. Gittleman, R. Letter to editor: "Data do not always speak for themselves." *Arch Gen Psychiatry* 35: 1394-95, November, 1978.

42. Arnold, L. E.; Barnebey, N. S.; Smeltzer, D. J. Letter to editor: "Reply to Gittelman." *Arch Gen Psychiatry* 35: 1395, November, 1978.

43. Sprague, R. L., and Sleator, E. K. "Drugs and dosages: implications for learning disabilities." In: Bakker, D. J., ed. *The neuropsychology of learning disorders.* Baltimore, Maryland: University Park Press, 351-66, 1976.

44. Sprague, R. L., and Sleator, E. K. "Methylphenidate in hyperkinetic children:

differences in dose effects on learning and social behavior." *Science* 198: 1274-76, December 23, 1977.

45. Rapoport, J. L.; Buchsbaum, M.S.; Weingartner, H., et al. "Dextraomphetamine: its cognitive and behavioral effects in normal and hyperactive boys and normal men." *Arch Gen Psychiatry* 37 (8): 933-43, August, 1980.

46. Barkley, R. A., and Cunningham, C. E. The effects of methylphenidate or the mother-child interactions of hyperactive children." *Arch Gen Psychiatry* 36 (2) 201-8, February, 1979.

47. Whalen, C. K.; Henker, B.; Dotemoto, S. "Methylphenidate and hyperactivity effects on teacher behaviors." *Science* 208 (4449): 1280–82, June 13, 1980.

48. Shekim, W. O.; Dekirmenjian, H.; Chapel, J. L. "Urinary catecholamin metabolites in hyperkinetic boys treated with d-amphetamine." *Am J Psychiatry* 13 (11): 1276-79, November, 1977.

49. Gittelman-Klein, R.; Klein, Donald F.; Abikoff, H. "Relative efficacy c methylphenidate and behavior modification in hyperkinetic children: an interim report." *J Abnorm Child Psychol* 4 (4): 361-79, 1976.

50. Corson, S. A.; Corson, E. O'L.; Kirilcuk, V., et al. *Experimental control o hyperkinetic and violent behavior in dogs.* Sound 16mm Cinema, Psychologic Cinema Register, Pennsylvania State University, 1974.

51. Conners, C. K., and Taylor E. "Pemoline, methylphenidate, and placebo i children with minimal brain dysfunction." *Arch Gen Psychiatry* 37 (8): 922–30 August, 1980.

SAMPLE BOOK ENTRY

75 Ross, Dorothea M., and Ross, Sheila A. *Hyperactivity: research, theory, and action.* New York, New York: Wiley, 1976. 385 p. (Bibliography.) (Wiley Series on Personality Processes.)

This text provides a general overview of the hyperactive child: clinical description, etiological factors, drug treatment, psychotherapy, educational intervention, prevention, and management. It is concluded that: (1) hyperactivity is one of the most common symptoms of disordered behavior in childhood; (2) hyperactivity may span the major developmental stages, often being apparent from birth to adulthood; (3) progress is being made concerning the etiology of the syndrome (pollutants, environmental factors, and social causes); (4) there is a trend toward a more sophisticated approach to the experimental assessment of drugs; and (5) the on-site management of behavior and learning problems in the school setting is being recognized. An appendix and bibliography are included.

1. Item number
2. Author(s)
3. Title of book
4. Place of publication
5. Publisher
6. Date of publication
7. Number of pages
8. Presence of bibliography
9. Series (if any)
10. Annotation

SAMPLE JOURNAL ENTRY

789 Conners, C. Keith. "The acute effects of caffeine on evoked response, vigilance, and activity level in hyperkinetic children." *J Abnorm Child Psychol* 7 (2): 145-51, June, 1979. (11 References.)

Studies the effects of caffeine on several variables on seventeen hyperkinetic children who had previously responded to sympathomimetic amines. The children were given three different dosages of caffeine in counterbalanced order (placebo, and low and high doses equivalent to one and three cups of coffee). One hour following ingestions they were tested on measures of visual evoked response, alpha time, vigilance, and activity level. There was a significant effect on evoked response. The behavioral measures tended to be affected in a dose-related manner but not to a statistically significant degree. It is concluded that although centrally active, caffeine does not show the congruence between behavioral and central effects that other stimulants useful in behavioral management have shown.

1. Item number
2. Author(s)
3. Title of article
4. Name of journal (abbreviation)
5. Volume and issue number
6. Inclusive pagination
7. Month and year of publication
8. Number of bibliographical references
9. Annotation

ABBREVIATIONS

CNS	Central Nervous System
CSF	Cerebrospinal Fluid
EEG	Electroencephalogram
EKG	Electrocardiogram
EMG	Electromyogram
K-P	Kaiser Permanente
LD	Learning Disabilities, Learning Disabled
MBD	Minimal Brain Dysfunction
MMPI	Minnesota Multiphasic Personality Inventory

THE HYPERKINETIC CHILD

I.
Bibliographies

1 Archuleta, Alyce, J., and Archuleta, Michael J. The hyperactive child: a selected bibliography for parents and educators. San Diego, California: Current Bibliography Series, 1974. 26p.
Consists of a 155-item unannotated bibliography on various aspects of the hyperkinetic syndrome. Entries are arranged by five categories: books, government documents, general periodicals, education journals, and medical and technical journals. "Other sources of information" lists six organizations of interest to parents.

2 Chicorel abstracts to reading and learning disabilities. New York, New York: Chicorel Library Publishing Corporation, 1976. (Chicorel Index Series, Volume 19).
This annual publication abstracts journal literature relating to reading and learning disabilities. Entries are arranged by subject. Cross-references direct the user from one term to another. An author index completes the volume.

3 Chicorel index to learning disorders. New York, New York: Chicorel Library Publishing Corporation, 1975. 2v. (Chicorel Index Series, Volume 18 [A-Hi] and 18A [Hy-Vo]).
Abstracts and indexes approximately 3,000 books that deal with a diverse number of topics in the area of learning disabilities. References are included on hyperactivity.

4 Chicorel index to reading and learning disabilities: an annotated guide. New York, New York: Chicorel Library Publishing Corporation, 1976. 400p. (Chicorel Index Series, Volume 14A).
Lists 1,500 books for professionals and others interested in the field. Subjects covered range from administration to decoding, dyslexia, mental health, hyperactivity, parent education, speech handicapped, vocabulary development, and others.

5 Chicorel index to reading disabilities. New York, New York: Chicorel Library Publishing Corporation, 1974. 500p. (Chicorel Index Series, Volume 14).
More than 600 books dealing with various aspects of reading disabilities are included in this publication. Entries are annotated.

Gluckstein, Fritz P.
see Hyperactivity due to minimal brain dysfunction. (Item No. 13).

Gluckstein, Fritz P.
see Therapy of hyperactivity due to minimal brain dysfunction. (Item No. 14).

6 Harley, J. Preston. "Hyperactivity and food additives: a bibliography." Cat Sel Doc Psychol 8: 42-43, May, 1978. (0 References).
Contains sixty entries (1973-1978, plus one item from 1947) on the topic of hyperactivity and food additives. Many documents pertain to the Feingold hypothesis.

7 Hyperactivity: A selective bibliography. Exceptional child bibliography series no. 643. Reston, Virginia: Council for Exceptional Children, 1975. 20p. (ED 106 995).
This bibliography on hyperactivity contains approximately forty-four general entries and approximately thirty-seven entries dealing specifically with drug treatments for hyperactivity. Each entry includes an abstract, publishing data, and information on the availability of the document from the Educational Resources Information Center (ERIC) Document Reproduction Service. The bibliography has been compiled from holdings at the Information Center of the Council for Exceptional Children.

8 Hyperactivity--drug therapy/food additives/allergies. A selective bibliography. Exceptional child bibliography series no. 602. Reston, Virginia: Council for Exceptional Children, 1976. 19p. (ED 129 029).
Consists of approximately sixty-five abstracts and associated indexing information for documents or journal articles published from 1968 to 1975 and selected from the computer files of the Council for Exceptional Children's Information Services and the Education Resources Information Center (ERIC). Abstracts include bibliographic data (identification or order number, publication date, author, title, source or publisher, and availability); descriptors indicating the subject matter covered; and a summary of the document's contents. Also provided are instructions for using the bibliography, a list of journals from which articles were abstracted, and an order form for ordering microfiche or paper copies of the documents through the ERIC Document Reproduction Service.

9 Hyperactivity--general. A selective bibliography. Exceptional child bibliography series no. 643. Reston, Virginia: Council for Exceptional Children, 1976. 21p. (ED 129 028).
Approximately eighty-four citations for documents or journal articles published from 1967 to 1975 and selected from the computer files of the Council for Exceptional Children's Information Services and the Education Resources Information Center (ERIC), are included in this annotated bibliography. Abstracts include bibliographic data (identification or order number, publication date, author, title, source or publisher, and availability); descriptors indicating the subject matter covered; and a summary of the document's contents.

Kirson, Tamara, et al.
see Bibliography on the hyperkinetic behavior syndrome. (Item No. 12).

10 Reading instruction: remedial and compensatory: abstracts of doctoral dissertations published in Dissertation Abstracts International, July through December, 1977 (Volume 38, Nos. 1-6), pt. 2. 1978. 13p.
Presents a collection of abstracts which provides information on recent doctoral dissertations in the area. Reading acquisition of hyperactive children is one topic considered.

11 Simpson, Richard L. "The hyperactive child: resources." In: Principles and techniques of intervention with hyperactive children. Edited by Marvin J. Fine. Springfield, Illinois: Thomas, 1977. 269-310. (113 References).

This bibliography reviews literature relating not only to hyperactivity but also to various therapeutic intervention techniques that have been used in the educational setting. Entries, categorized under four broad headings, primarily represent the literature of the 1960s and early 1970s. All 113 entries are annotated.

12 U. S. National Institute of Mental Health. Bibliography on the hyperkinetic behavior syndrome. Washington, D.C.: U. S. Government Printing Office, 1978. 40p. (DHEW Publication No. [ADM] 77-449). (ED 152 052).

Cites a group of approximately 800 references of interest to educators, counselors, parents, and researchers who seek information about the behavior of, and appropriate treatment for, the hyperkinetic child. Various dimensions are covered: sociopsychological, physiological, and pharmacological, with emphasis on the last. A list of NIMH research grants is included. Entries are unannotated. The bibliography was prepared by Tamara Kirson, Ronald Lipman, and Natalie Reatig.

13 U. S. National Library of Medicine. Hyperactivity due to minimal brain dysfunction. Prepared by Fritz P. Gluckstein. Bethesda, Maryland: U. S. Department of Health, Education, and Welfare, Public Health Service, National Institutes of Health, 1974. 20p. (Literature Search No. 74-19).

Two hundred fifty-six items comprise this bibliography which is one of a series of computer-generated bibliographies issued by the NLM. Entries are arranged alphabetically by author and include books, articles, and reports. Although unannotated, the liberal use of descriptors provides the reader with a key to the contents of the entries. All aspects except therapy are represented. The period covered is January, 1972 through June, 1974.

14 ———. Therapy of hyperactivity due to minimal brain dysfunction. Prepared by Fritz P. Gluckstein. Bethesda, Maryland: U. S. Department of Health, Education, and Welfare, Public Health Service, National Institutes of Health, 1974. 12p. (Literature Search No. 74-18).

This computer-generated bibliography consists of 167 citations concerning the therapeutic aspects of hyperactivity. Each entry contains a list of descriptors pertinent to the article. The period covered is January, 1972 through June, 1974.

15 Winchell, Carol A. The hyperactive child: a bibliography of medical, educational, and behavioral studies. Westport, Connecticut: Greenwood Press, 1975. 182p.

Over 1,800 medical, educational, and behavioral references (primarily between 1950 and 1974) are cited in this unannotated bibliography on hyperkinesis. Entries have been taken from more than 300 professional journals and from sources such as books, conference reports, government documents, and dissertations. Arrangement is by the following major topics (and typical subtopics in parentheses): introductory research (symptomatology, classification, and epidemiology); etiology (genetic factors, pre- and perinatal complications); diagnosis (neurological, psychological, educational, and behavioral testing); management (clinical, educational, and parental management); and related research (psychological, sociological, and follow-up studies). Appended are lists of research terms applied to hyperkinesis, of drugs used to treat hyperkinesis, and of journal abbreviations. Author and key word subject indexes are provided.

II.
The Hyperactive Child Syndrome

A. COMPREHENSIVE STUDIES

16 Annual progress in child psychiatry and child development, 1974. Edited by Stella Chess and Alexander Thomas. New York, New York: Brunner/Mazel, 1975. 642p. (Bibliography).
Contains thirty-seven papers devoted to twelve topics. The papers are either reports of original work or reviews of knowledge in a particular area of study and deal with one of the following topics: (1) developmental issues; (2) perception and cognition; (3) parent-child interaction; (4) learning issues; (5) brain dysfunction; (6) mental retardation; (7) clinical issues; (8) psychopharmacology; (9) adolescence; (10) drug abuse problems; (11) child abuse; and (12) children and the law. Although the hyperactive syndrome is discussed in many parts throughout the volume, Chapter 15 (Wolff and Hurwitz - Item No. 181) and Chapter 26 (Grinspoon and Singer - Item No. 779) deal specifically with MBD and hyperkinesis.

17 Annual progress in child psychiatry and child development, 1975. Edited by Stella Chess and Alexander Thomas. New York, New York: Brunner/Mazel, 1975. 541p. (Bibliography).
The seventh volume of this series reprints a collection of thirty-three original and review-type articles. Sections of the book focus on the following areas: (1) social issues and public policy; (2) parent-child interaction; (3) developmental issues; (4) adolescence; (5) racial issues; (6) learning disabilities; (7) hyperactivity; (8) child psychosis; (9) clinical issues; (10) family therapy; and (11) mass media. Chapter 20 (Shaffer, et al. - Item No. 1538), and Chapter 21 (Satterfield, et al. - Item No. 1547) are devoted to the hyperactive child syndrome.

18 Annual progress in child psychiatry and child development, 1976. Edited by Stella Chess and Alexander Thomas. New York, New York: Brunner/Mazel, 1977. 744p. (Bibliography).
Forty papers, dealing with research in the fields of child psychiatry and child development, are found in the 1976 edition of this annual publication. Two papers, one by Cunningham, Cadoret, and Loftus (Item No. 297) and the other by Cadoret, Cunningham, and Loftus (Item No. 290), examine the incidence of hyperactivity and other psychiatric conditions in adoptees.

19 Annual progress in child psychiatry and child development, 1977. Edited by Stella Chess and Alexander Thomas. New York, New York: Brunner/Mazel, 1977. 782p. (Bibliography).
A variety of topics is included in this year's contributions: (1) infancy studies; (2) developmental issues; (3) biochemical studies; (4) psychosexual development; (5) sex differences in young children; (6) twin

studies; (7) hyperactive children; (8) clinical issues; (9) psychopathology in adolescence; (10) childhood psychosis; (11) socio-cultural issues; (12) cross-cultural issues; and (13) legal issues. Chapters 20 (Langhorne, et al. - Item No. 109) and 21 (Paternite, et al. - Item No. 473) are concerned with the hyperactive child.

20 Baker, Nancy C. "Why can't Bobby sit still?" Day Care Early Educ 4(5): 12-15, May-June, 1977. (0 References).
According to Dr. James Satterfield of the Gateways Hospital Hyperkinetic Clinic in Los Angeles, hyperactive children may be characterized by excessive motor activity, poor attention span, impulsivity, and irritability. Treatment should involve various approaches--medication, behavior modification techniques, special education, and psychiatry. The success of Gateways Hospital in treating hyperactive children is noted.

21 Barkley, Russell A. "Recent developments in research on hyperactive children." J Pediatr Psychol 3(4): 158-63, 1978. (59 References).
This article introduces a special issue of the journal devoted to hyperactivity and includes an overview of recent research. These topics are addressed: (1) the nature of hyperactivity; (2) the early identification of children at risk for hyperactivity; (3) prognosis; and (4) treatment advances.

22 Bond, Becky, and Rae, Sharon. "Hyperactive children." JAMA 239(10): 968-69, March 6, 1978. (3 References).
Provides brief answers to some of the most frequently asked questions concerning hyperkinesis, such as: (1) What are the symptoms of hyperactivity? (2) What causes hyperkinesis and how is it diagnosed? and (3) Will medication help my hyperactive child perform better in school and improve his behavior?

23 Bryant, N. Dale. "Learning disabilities: a report on the state of the art." Teach Coll Rec 75(3): 395-404, February, 1974. (26 References).
Presents a state-of-the-art report on learning disabilities (LD). The subject is discussed in terms of: (1) problems of definition; (2) incidence rates; (3) types; (4) causes and prediction; and (5) future of LD in the schools. The most serious of the many problems concerning LD is seen to be the lack of a research base for corrective procedures used in the field. The problem of children who cannot learn in spite of normal intelligence is likely to diminish only when this research base is established. Teaching must be upgraded as well.

24 Cantwell, Dennis P. "Hyperkinetic syndrome." In: Child psychiatry: modern approaches. Edited by Michael Rutter and Lionel Hersov. Oxford, England: Blackwell, 1976. 524-55. (197 References).
Presents an overview of the hyperkinetic syndrome. Topics covered include (1) the clinical picture; (2) etiology and classification; (3) epidemiology; (4) physical and neurological findings; (5) laboratory studies; (6) familial-genetic factors; (7) natural history and prognosis; (8) treatment approaches; and (9) directions for future research.

25 ———, ed. The hyperactive child: diagnosis, management, current research. New York, New York: Spectrum Publications, distributed by John Wiley and Sons, 1975. 209p. (Bibliography). (Series on Child Behavior and Development, Volume I).

This text contains twelve chapters focusing on the clinical, research, and management aspects of the hyperactive child syndrome. Part I (three chapters) describes the clinical picture of the hyperactive child and outlines a scheme for evaluation. Part II (three chapters) reviews the etiology of the syndrome (neurophysiological, biochemical, and familial-genetic). Part III (five chapters) deals with several specific types of intervention: stimulant drug treatment, behavioral therapy, videotape training, and educational approaches. The last chapter offers a six-stage model for clinical and research work. A subject index completes the volume.

Contents: Epidemiology, Clinical Picture, and Classification of the Hyperactive Child Syndrome (Cantwell - Item No. 185); Diagnostic Evaluation of the Hyperactive Child (Cantwell - Item No. 481); Natural History and Prognosis in the Hyperactive Child Syndrome (Cantwell - Item No. 1897); Neurophysiologic Studies with Hyperactive Children (Satterfield - Item No. 125); Biochemical Research with Hyperactive Children (Ritvo - Item No. 323); Familial-Genetic Research with Hyperactive Children (Cantwell - Item No. 291); Stimulant Drug Treatment of Hyperactive Children (Fish - Item No. 739); Behavioral Management of the Hyperactive Child (Simmons - Item No. 1097); Videotape Training for Parents as Therapeutic Agents with Hyperactive Children (Feighner - Item No. 1242); Educational Approaches with Hyperactive Children (Forness - Item No. 1010); A Critical Review of Therapeutic Modalities with Hyperactive Children (Cantwell - Item No. 643); A Medical Model for Research and Clinical Use with Hyperactive Children (Cantwell - Item No. 482).

26 Caring about kids: helping the hyperactive child. 1978. 12p. (ED 163 744).
Discusses the hyperactive child in terms of identification, causes, various treatment modalities, prognosis, and resources. The booklet is intended for parents.

27 Carter, Sidney, and Gold, Arnold P. "The syndrome of minimal cerebral dysfunction." In: Carter, Sidney, and Gold, Arnold P. Neurology of infancy and childhood. New York, New York: Appleton-Century-Crofts, 1974. 31-34. (20 References on p. 38).
Briefly considers the clinical manifestations, laboratory findings, diagnosis, and drug treatment of hyperactivity and minimal cerebral dysfunction.

Chess, Stella, ed.
see Annual progress in child psychiatry and child development. (Item Nos. 16, 17, 18, 19).

28 Clarizio, Harvey F., and McCoy, George F. Behavior disorders in children. 2nd ed. New York, New York: Crowell, 1976. 596p. (Bibliography).
Provides an overview of the disturbed child and adolescent. Part I covers basic issues, the incidence of emotional disturbance in youth, and the factors influencing these disturbances. Part II outlines six types of disorders common among deviant youth. Part III deals with intervention and prevention strategies. Learning disabilities, MBD, and hyperactivity are discussed in Chapter 5.

29 Clark, Matt. "Troubled children: the quest for help." Newsweek 83(14): 52-56, 58, April 8, 1974. (0 References).
Generally reviews three childhood emotional disorders: autism, schizophrenia, and hyperkinesis. Within the past few years there has been

increased recognition of the needs of children with these problems. The number of youngsters receiving treatment for emotional problems in institutions and outpatient facilities has risen nearly 60 percent in the last seven years--from 486,000 to 770,000. Hyperkinesis has become the most publicized of the serious childhood behavior disorders. It is emphasized that in order to combat these problems effectively, more private and governmental commitment is necessary. Special training for those children already afflicted is imperative.

30 Codd, J. A. "Hyperactive children: problems, issues, and approaches." NZ Med J 88(622): 333-36, October 25, 1978. (38 References).
This author discusses the hyperkinetic syndrome in regard to: (1) problems of definition and diagnosis; (2) incidence rates; (3) effectiveness of, and justification for, the use of drugs; and (4) alternative approaches to management. The interdisciplinary approach--closer liaison and communication between the educational and medical professions--is urged.

31 "Coming face to face with the impersonal numbers game." J Learn Disabil 11(2): 11-17, February, 1978. (0 References).
Presents a conversation between the editor of the journal and Daniel Ringelheim, director of the Aid to States Division of the U. S. Bureau of Education for the Handicapped (HEW). A few comments concern the hyperactive child.

Denhoff, Eric, ed.
see Minimal brain dysfunction: a developmental approach. (Item No. 64).

32 de Sousa, Alan, and de Sousa, D. A. "Hyperkinesis." Child Psychiatry Q 10(4): 8-13, October, 1977. (21 References).
The hyperkinetic syndrome is discussed according to: (1) etiology; (2) clinical features; and (3) treatment approaches. The syndrome is seen as an aspect of the symptomatology of a number of disorders which are precipitated by stress and tension. Management consists of drugs (methylphenidate, dextroamphetamine, or chlorpromazine), operant conditioning, psychosurgery, and, with less success, psychotherapy.

33 Ellingson, Careth. Speaking of children: their learning abilities/disabilities. New York, New York: Harper & Row, 1975. 285p. (0 References).
Presents an examination of normal and dysfunctional child development and learning processes. Discussed are: (1) patterns and characteristics of learning abilities and disabilities; (2) treatments for these disabilities (e.g., behavior modification and chemotherapy); (3) screening and testing procedures for home and school; (4) various types of cognitive learning styles; and (5) a case study of a clinical school for learning dysfunctions. Hyperactivity is considered in Chapters III and VII. Appendix A contains a list of LD service organizations.

34 Fine, Marvin J. "Hyperactivity: where are we?" In: Principles and techniques of intervention with hyperactive children. Edited by Marvin J. Fine. Springfield, Illinois: Thomas, 1977. 3-46. (90 References).
This first chapter of a collection of seven contributions reviews basic information on the hyperactive child, outlines current beliefs, and describes accepted therapeutic procedures. Also discussed are definitional and conceptual viewpoints and problems, incidence figures, the relation-

ship between hyperactivity and learning problems, and three causal considerations: organic, developmental, and psychological. Various treatment regimens are summarized.

35 Ford, W. "Hyperactive child syndrome: overview." Can Pharm J 111: 410-12, December, 1978. (7 References).
Covers symptoms, possible causes, and drug and alternate treatments of hyperactive children.

36 Fras, Ivan. "The 'real' hyperactive child." Consultant 15(7): 97-103, July, 1975. (0 References).
Outlines typical signs and points out difficulties in diagnosing the syndrome. Treatment includes counseling and pharmacotherapy.

37 Geier, Annette. Hyperactivity: research and treatment alternatives: a review and analysis of recent findings. Highland Park, New Jersey: Essence Publications, 1978. 81p.
Reviews and analyzes recent literature concerning hyperactivity. Emphasis is placed on treatment modalities. The incidence and frequency are discussed, along with diagnosis, symptomatology, definition, etiological theories, and arousal levels. Pros and cons of drug therapy are covered as well as other treatment interventions, e.g., behavior modification and relaxation training.

38 Handbook on learning disabilities: a prognosis for the child, the adolescent, the adult. Edited by the New Jersey Association for Children with Learning Disabilities. Englewood Cliffs, New Jersey: Prentice-Hall, 1974. 257p. (Bibliography).
Comprehensively overviews the subject. References to hyperactivity are scattered throughout the text. No subject index is provided.

39 Harriman, Sarah. "Compulsion." Connecticut 39: 16ff., March, 1976.

40 Havighurst, Robert J. "Choosing a middle path for the use of drugs with hyperactive children." Sch Rev 85(1): 61-77, November, 1976. (16 References).
Describes hyperactivity, children who display it, and drug treatments and their effects. Means of identification are presented, and a survey of teachers' attitudes toward Ritalin and its use is reviewed. Actual biological abnormality exists in some hyperactive children who can be cautiously treated with drugs. The benefits and dangers of classifying children as hyperactive are outlined. It is concluded that: (1) hyperactivity is a real behavior syndrome appearing in a small percentage of children; (2) possibly 1 percent of children five to twelve years old are being treated with Ritalin and approximately half of these benefit from it; and (3) teachers and school nurses are in good positions to assist parents and physician to decide whether to use medication. For a reprint of this study refer to Item No. 744.

41 Hyperactivity. Brooklyn, New York: Parent Press, 1977.

42 Hyperactivity in children: etiology, measurement, and treatment implications. Edited by Ronald L. Trites. Baltimore, Maryland: University Park Press, 1979. 241p. (Bibliography).
This volume represents the proceedings of the Symposium on Hyperactivity in Children held in Ottawa, Canada, February, 1978. The symposium focused on an examination of hyperactivity in terms of prevalence, etiological

factors, problems in measurement, and treatment approaches.

Contents: Models of Hyperactivity: Implications for Diagnosis and Treatment (Kinsbourne and Swanson - Item No. 269); Prevalence of Hyperactivity in Ottawa, Canada (Trites - Item No. 204); Evaluation of Psychophysiological, Neurochemical, and Animal Models of Hyperactivity (Ferguson and Pappas - Item No. 266); Factors Possibly Implicated in Hyperactivity (Tryphonas - Item No. 1376); Can Hyperactives be Identified in Infancy? (Rapoport, et al. - Item No. 512); The Hyperkinetic Syndrome (Kløve and Hole - Item No. 271); Method and Theory for Psychopharmacology with Children (Conners and Wells - Item No. 733); Behavioral Interventions for Hyperactivity (Mash and Dalby - Item No. 1076); Assessment of Intervention (Sprague - Item No. 2016).

Discussion of the articles is also included.

43 Jeffrey, Sophia. "Focus on hyperactivity (report of provincial conference)." Prime Areas 19(2): 22-28, Winter, 1977.

44 Jenkins, R. L. "Behavior disorders of childhood." PA J 5: 13-18, Spring, 1975.

45 Jenkins, Richard L., and Harms, Ernest. Understanding disturbed children: professional insights into their psychiatric and developmental problems. Seattle, Washington: Special Child Publications, 1976. 476p. (Bibliography).

Several chapters briefly refer to the hyperkinetic syndrome.

46 Johnston, Robert B. "Minimal cerebral dysfunction: nature and implications for therapy." In: Medical problems in the classroom: the teacher's role in diagnosis and management. Edited by Robert H. Haslam and Peter J. Valletutti. Baltimore, Maryland: University Park Press, 1975. 281-303. (26 References).

Presents an overview of the minimal cerebral dysfunction (MCD) syndrome. The term "hyperactivity" is briefly discussed as being an inappropriate designation for the syndrome. Comments are made on the role of medication and educational strategies in the management of the MCD child.

47 Juliano, Daniel B., and Gentile, J. Ronald. "Will the real hyperactive child please sit down? Problems of diagnosis and remediation." Child Study J Monogr Nos. 1-6: 1-38, 1974. (188 References).

Reviews the research literature on the symptomatology, etiology, performance, and behavioral management (drug and behavior modification treatments) of hyperactive children with normal intelligence. The major identifying characteristic of hyperactive children is excessive activity or restlessness at inappropriate times. The minimal brain damage hypothesis is concluded to be ambiguous. Most drug treatment studies have been methodologically poor. Behavior modification studies are also reviewed and shown to have some promise in improving the behavior of hyperactive children.

Kalverboer, A. F., ed.
see Minimal brain dysfunction: fact or fiction. (Item No. 65).

48 Kauffman, J. M., and Hallahan, D. P. "Learning disability and hyperactivity (with comments on minimal brain dysfunction)." In: Advances in clinical child psychology. Volume 2. Edited by Benjamin

B. Lahey and Alan E. Kazdin. New York, New York: Plenum, 1978. 71-105. (128 References).

49 Kinsbourne, Marcel. "The hyperactive and impulsive child." Ont Med Rev 42: 657-60, 1975.

50 ———. "Hyperactivity." Paper presented to the Heinz Seminar at the Annual Meeting of the Canadian Paediatric Association, Toronto, Ontario, Canada, 1975. 14p. (ED 112 602).
Discusses hyperactivity in terms of characteristics, precipitating factors, and drug therapy. Emotional stress and food additives are cited as possible causes.

51 Kinsbourne, Marcel, and Caplan, Paula J. Children's learning and attention problems. Boston, Massachusetts: Little, Brown, 1979. 300p. (Bibliography).

52 Knopf, Irwin J. "Abnormalities of middle childhood: language disorders, learning disabilities, and hyperkinesis." In: Knopf, Irwin J. Childhood psychopathology: a developmental approach. Englewood Cliffs, New Jersey: Prentice-Hall, 1979. 267-302. (136 References).
Focuses on clinical features, etiological considerations, and treatment approaches of the hyperactive child as well as several other common problems of the middle childhood period.

53 Kratoville, Betty L., and Schweich, Peter D., eds. Hyperactivity: a meeting of the minds. Brooklyn, New York: Parent Press, 1977. 63p.
Excerpts from a two-day seminar on the daily management of the hyperactive child are reprinted. Comments of nine participants (including psychologists, educators, physicians, and parents) are presented on numerous topics: problems of defining the syndrome; origin of the syndrome; management strategies; methods of dealing with physicians, parents, and siblings; the child's attitude about himself; environmental factors; the child's responsibilities in the home; behavior modification techniques; stimulant drugs; diet; allergies; vitamins; hearing and visual problems; homework; sports activities; and sexuality. The Archway School Professional Advisory Board conducted the symposium.

54 Laufer, Maurice W. "In Osler's day it was syphilis." In: Anthony, E. James, ed. Explorations in child psychiatry. New York, New York: Plenum, 1975. 105-24. (35 References).
Through a physician's personal account, the history and development of the hyperkinetic child syndrome and its treatment methods are set forth. The terminology of the entity is also traced.

55 Laufer, Maurice W., and Shetty, Taranath. "Organic brain syndromes." In: Comprehensive textbook of psychiatry. Volume 2. 2nd ed. Baltimore, Maryland: Williams & Wilkins, 1975. 2200-13. (75 References).
Describes several syndromes, including hyperactivity, which are causally related to cerebral dysfunction. Comments are made on prevalence, mechanism, clinical features, diagnosis, prognosis, and treatment.

56 Lear, Leonard. "Exorcising the demons." Prevention 29: 158ff., July, 1977.

57 Learning disabilities. Part II. Program 114. 1978. 30p. (ED 161 207).
Consists of the second of two transcripts from a radio series on learning disabilities. Discussions concern hyperactivity as well as several other topics. An annotated bibliography accompanies the transcript.

58 Leary, P. M. "Minimal brain dysfunction." S Afr Med J 50(20): 784-86, May 8, 1976. (4 References).
Discusses the minimal brain dysfunction syndrome in terms of etiology, pathology, and management. Hyperactivity is noted as the most prominent characteristic of the syndrome. It is estimated that 5 to 7 percent of the white school children in South Africa show evidence of MBD.

59 Mac Keith, Ronald. "High activity and hyperactivity." Dev Med Child Neurol 16(4): 543-44, August, 1974. (6 References).
Briefly defines the hyperactive syndrome, mentions some of the factors in its diagnosis, and lists the causes of high activity in children. Hyperactivity is viewed as a symptom, although the word is used synonymously with the hyperkinetic syndrome of high activity, distractibility, and learning difficulties. Nine causes are listed, including emotional deprivation, epilepsy, psychiatric disorder, and high drive, which is frequently associated with high intelligence. It is noted that an overlap often exists among these various conditions. Merely arriving at a label should not be the end point of treatment. The use of cerebral stimulants may be necessary with those few children whose high activity is due to the hyperkinetic syndrome.

Mendlewicz, J., ed.
see Minimal brain dysfunction: fact or fiction. (Item No. 65).

60 Millichap, J. Gordon. "Definitions and diagnosis of minimal brain dysfunction." In: Learning disabilities and related disorders: facts and current issues. Edited by J. Gordon Millichap. Chicago, Illinois: Year Book Medical Publishers, 1977. 3-11. (2 References).
The hyperactive syndrome is discussed in terms of definition, incidence, signs and symptoms, neurological abnormalities, the role of the EEG, differential diagnosis, and pathophysiology.

61 ————. "The hyperactive child." Practitioner 217(1297): 61-65, July, 1976. (3 References).
Offers a general review of the MBD syndrome including incidence, causes, symptoms, diagnosis, management, pharmacotherapy, remedial education, psychotherapy, parental counseling, and prognosis.

62 ————. The hyperactive child with minimal brain dysfunction: questions and answers. Chicago, Illinois: Year Book Medical Publishers, 1975. 169p. (Bibliography).
Provides answers to questions most frequently asked regarding hyperactive behavior and related disorders. Included are new and improved treatment measures, informative case studies, and numerous illustrations, charts, and tables. Diagnostic procedures are explained with interpretations of signs and symptoms. The volume is suitable for parents, teachers, and professionals working with the hyperactive child.

Contents: Definitions and Frequency; Causes of Minimal Brain Dysfunction; Symptoms, Signs, and Syndromes; Speech and Language Disorders; Dyslexia and Other Specific Learning Disorders; Diagnostic Evaluation: Pediatric Neurology Examination and the Electroencephalogram; Diagnostic Evaluation: Neuropsychologic Tests, Special Senses--Hearing and Vision Tests; Differential Diagnosis--Related Disorders; Treatment: General and Educational Management; Treatment: Drug Therapy, Diets, and Other Remedies; Prognosis and Prevention; Conclusions and Research Goals; Case Histories.

63 Minde, Klaus K. "Hyperactivity--where do we stand?" In: Topics in child neurology. Edited by Michael E. Blaw, Isabelle Rapin, and Marcel Kinsbourne. Jamaica, New York: Spectrum, 1977. 279-87. (31 References).
Partial proceedings of the conference sponsored by the International Child Neurology Association.

64 Minimal brain dysfunction: a developmental approach. Edited by Eric Denhoff and Leo Stern. New York, New York: Masson Pub. U.S.A., 1979. 198p. (Bibliography).

65 Minimal brain dysfunction: fact or fiction. Edited by A. F. Kalverboer, H. M. van Praag, and J. Mendlewicz. Basel, New York: Karger, 1978. 110p. (Bibliography).
Presents a collection of writings on various problems raised by the MBD syndrome including those of nosology, etiology, and treatment. The latest viewpoints on MBD are expressed from the disciplines of psychology, neurology, psychiatry, pharmacology, and epidemiology.

Contents: Opening Remarks (Mendlewicz); Introduction (van Praag); MBD: Discussion of the Concept (Kalverboer); Longitudinal Research and the Minimal Brain Damage Syndrome (Shaffer - Item No. 1940); Diagnosis: Developmental Psychological Assessment (Yule); Minimal Brain Dysfunction and Minor Neurological Dysfunction (Pyck and Baines - Item No. 2012); Animal Hyperactivity Syndromes: Do They Have Any Relevance to Minimal Brain Dysfunction? (Grahame-Smith - Item No. 1855); Minimal Brain Dysfunction Syndrome and the Plasticity of the Nervous System (Prechtl); Closing Remarks (Mendlewicz).

66 Mordock, John B. The other children: an introduction to exceptionality. New York, New York: Harper, 1975. 734p. (Bibliography).
This introductory text contains one chapter devoted to various aspects of MBD. Hyperactivity is perceived as a learned defensive or avoidance reaction to anxiety-arousing situations. Emphasis is placed on remedial efforts.

67 Neumann, Yvonne. "Minimal brain dysfunction: (MBD)." Phoenix J 7(2): 4-8, June, 1974.
The author discusses minimal brain dysfunction in regard to its definition, etiology, symptoms, diagnosis, and therapy. The lack of a clear definition of the syndrome is noted; two extremely different concepts of MBD are offered. The discussion of etiology centers on cerebral lesions, genetic factors, and environmental influences. A variety of neurological and psychological symptoms accompanies the syndrome. Various diagnostic procedures are examined and evaluated. Comments on drug therapy center on the use of Encephabol.

68 Pasquariello, Patrick S., Jr. "Current thoughts on the hyperkinetic syndrome of childhood." Int J Dermatol 18(5): 383-85, June, 1979. (7 References).

Briefly reviews characteristics, prevalence rates, and diet and drug therapy. It is recommended that caution be used in treating this condition. The importance of the role of the physician in management is stressed. Total involvement with the child and his environment is required in order to afford the maximum results.

69 Peters, John E. "Minimal brain dysfunctions in children." Am Fam Physician 10(1): 115-23, July, 1974. (0 References).
The MBD syndrome is discussed in terms of definition, types, signs, diagnosis, and medical management. The syndrome is comprised of three main groupings: pure hyperkinesis, pure learning disabilities, and mixed. In hyperkinesis, quality of activity is poor, the child is unable to organize his activities, and he cannot remember the sequence of items which must be done. Communication to the child about his disability must be simple, clear, and short. With proper management at home and school the vast majority of MBD children can realize their potential.

70 Piazza, Robert, ed. Readings in hyperactivity. Guilford, Connecticut: Special Learning Corporation, 1979. 117p. (Special Education Series).

71 Renshaw, Domeena C. The hyperactive child. Chicago, Illinois: Nelson Hall, 1974. 197p. (Bibliography).
Provides information derived from clinical and experimental investigation on the nature and management of the hyperactive child. Introductory chapters present an overview of the hyperactive, hyperanxious, and hyperaggressive child. Following chapters cover: (1) definition and diagnosis; (2) epidemiology; (3) pathology; (4) educational management; (5) medical management; (6) prognosis; and (7) prevention. Stressed is the importance of proper diagnosis, the multidisciplinary approach, and special education facilities. A subject index completes the volume.

72 Repetski, N. "The frenzy of the hyperactive child." Read Dig 113: 97-101, December, 1978.

73 ———. "Is he still better?" Canadian 3-9, February 25, 1978.

74 Rie, Herbert E. "Hyperactivity in children." Am J Dis Child 129(7): 783-89, July, 1975. (40 References).
The hyperkinetic syndrome is reviewed according to its definition, causal factors, and drug treatment. The last is seen to be inadequate therapy when used alone since it has a number of poorly studied effects, may mask problems other than hyperactivity itself, and may not improve classroom learning.

75 Ross, Dorothea M., and Ross, Sheila A. Hyperactivity: research, theory, and action. New York, New York: Wiley, 1976. 385p. (Bibliography). (Wiley Series on Personality Processes).
This text provides a general overview of the hyperactive child: clinical description, etiological factors, drug treatment, psychotherapy, educational intervention, prevention, and management. It is concluded that: (1) hyperactivity is one of the most common symptoms of disordered behavior in childhood; (2) hyperactivity may span the major developmental stages, often being apparent from birth to adulthood; (3) progress is being made concerning the etiology of the syndrome (pollutants, environmental factors, and social causes); (4) there is a trend toward a more sophisticated approach to the experimental assessment of drugs; and

(5) the on-site management of behavior and learning problems in the school setting is being recognized. The appendix lists a number of mechanical devices for measuring activity and some of the more standard rating scales commonly used in the direct observation of hyperactive children. A lengthy bibliography and author and subject indexes complete the volume. This book is intended for professionals in the fields of medicine, psychology, and education. The final chapter on management techniques would be appropriate for parents as well.

76 Schain, Richard J. "Hyperactivity in children." In: Schain, Richard J. Neurology of childhood learning disorders. 2nd ed. Baltimore, Maryland: Williams & Wilkins, 1977. 44-51. (20 References).
Several topics are covered in this chapter: (1) the nature of the symptoms; (2) etiologic considerations; (3) developmental hyperactivity; and (4) long-term consequences.

77 Schmitt, Barton D. "The hyperactive child." Paper presented at the University of Kansas Medical Center, Kansas City, Kansas, June, 1974.

78 Solomon, Gail E. "Minimal brain dysfunction." In: Handbook of treatment of mental disorders in childhood and adolescence. Edited by Benjamin B. Wolman. Englewood Cliffs, New Jersey: Prentice-Hall, 1978. 128-43. (61 References).
Discusses the MBD syndrome in regard to its incidence, diagnostic procedures, therapeutic modalities, and prognosis.

79 Stamm, J. S., and Kreder, S. V. "Minimal brain dysfunction: psychological and neurophysiological disorders in hyperkinetic children: a review." In: Neuropsychology: handbook of behavioral neurobiology. Volume 2. Edited by M. S. Gazzaniga. New York, New York: Plenum, 1978. 119-50. (109 References).

Stern, Leo, ed.
see Minimal brain dysfunction: a developmental approach. (Item No. 64).

80 Suran, Bernard G., and Rizzo, Joseph V. "Children with learning disabilities." In: Suran, Bernard G., and Rizzo, Joseph V. Special children: an integrative approach. Glenview, Illinois: Scott, Foresman, 1979. 244-77. (Bibliography).
Focuses on learning disabilities in terms of: (1) definition and classification; (2) incidence and etiology; (3) diagnosis and identification; (4) developmental consequences; and (5) intervention. Hyperactivity is briefly mentioned in the chapter.

Thomas, Alexander, ed.
see Annual progress in child psychiatry and child development. (Item Nos. 16, 17, 18, 19).

Trites, Ronald L., ed.
see Hyperactivity in children: etiology, measurement, and treatment implications. (Item No. 42).

81 Van Osdol, Bob M., and Carlson, Larry. "A study of developmental hyperactivity." In: Frazier, James R., and Frazier, Dianne M. Exceptional children: biological and psychological perspectives.

New York, New York: MSS Information Corporation, 1974. 220-34. (64 References).
Reprints an article from Mental Retardation 10(3): 18-24, June, 1972.

van Praag, H. M., ed.
see Minimal brain dysfunction: fact or fiction. (Item No. 65).

82 Weiss, Gabrielle, and Hechtman, Lily. "Hyperactive child syndrome." Science 205(4413): 1348-54, September 28, 1979. (74 References).
The hyperkinetic syndrome is reviewed according to: (1) problems of definition and terminology; (2) diagnosis; (3) the value of multidisciplinary assessment; (4) prevalence; (5) etiologies; (6) stimulant drug therapy; and (7) other forms of therapy.

83 Wender, Paul H. "Diagnosis and management of minimal brain dysfunction." In: Manual of psychiatric therapeutics: practical psychopharmacology and psychiatry. Edited by Richard I. Shader. Boston, Massachusetts: Little, Brown, 1975. 163-69. (0 References). (Basic Medical Sciences Series).
Explores the relationship between hyperactivity and MBD. Brief references are made to characteristics, incidence, prognosis, etiology, diagnosis, and management. Some of the most frequently used drugs are summarized and comments made on problems of terminology.

84 ————. "Minimal brain dysfunction in children." In: Frazier, James R., and Frazier, Dianne M. Exceptional children: biological and psychological perspectives. New York, New York: MSS Information Corporation, 1974. 235-50. (24 References).
Reprints an article from Pediatric Clinics of North America 20(1): 187-202, February, 1973.

85 ————. "The minimal brain dysfunction syndrome." Annu Rev Med 26: 45-62, 1975. (58 References).
Reviews characteristics, prevalence, diagnosis, prognosis, and management aspects of minimal brain dysfunction. This syndrome occurs frequently on a genetic basis, possibly due to an abnormality in monoamine metabolism. The administration of medication as an efficacious treatment regimen is upheld.

86 ————. "Peck's bad boys--a growing concern." US News World Rep 76(21): 72-75, May 27, 1974. (0 References).
Uses an interview format with Dr. Paul Wender, Professor of Psychiatry, University of Utah College of Medicine, to discuss many of the issues relating to the hyperactive child. Dr. Wender comments on the frequency of the problem, its symptoms and characteristics, drug therapy, and the roles of teachers, physicians, and parents in managing the behavior disorder.

87 Wender, Paul H., and Eisenberg, Leon. "Minimal brain dysfunction in children." In: American handbook of psychiatry. Volume II. New York, New York: Basic Books, 1974. 130-46. (54 References).
Focuses on various aspects of the MBD syndrome: (1) characteristics; (2) diagnosis; (3) prevalence; (4) etiology; (5) mechanism; (6) prognosis; and (7) management.

88 Werry, John S. "Minimal brain dysfunction (neurological impairment) in children." NZ Med J 80(521): 94-100, August 14, 1974. (36 References).

This review article discusses the MBD syndrome in terms of: (1) history of the concept; (2) psychotropic drugs and children; (3) diagnosing in psychiatry; (4) safety of psychotropic drugs in children; and (5) ethical issues. Also reviewed are the main themes presented at the Minimal Brain Dysfunction Conference held in New York in 1972.

89 Whalen, Carol K., and Henker, Barbara, eds. Hyperactive children: the social ecology of identification and treatment. New York, New York: Academic Press, 1980. 407p. (Bibliography).

B. CHARACTERISTICS/SYMPTOMATOLOGY

90 Ando, Haruhiko, and Yoshimura, Ikuko. "Speech skill levels and prevalence of maladaptive behaviors in autistic and mentally retarded children: a statistical study." Child Psychiatry Hum Dev 10(2): 85-90, Winter, 1979. (13 References).
Assesses speech skill levels and maladaptive behaviors in a group of forty-seven autistic and 128 mentally retarded children (ages six to fourteen years) attending a special school. Nine maladaptive behaviors (self-injury, attacks on others, destruction of property, hyperactivity, withdrawal, lack of eye contact, stereotyped behavior, tantrums, and fear) were studied. Results indicate that the mentally retarded children with withdrawal had significantly lower speech skill levels than those without withdrawal; the autistic children with self-injury had significantly lower speech skill levels than those without self-injury.

91 Bryan, Tanis H., and Bryan, James H. "Behavior of the learning disabled." In: Bryan, Tanis H., and Bryan, James H. Understanding learning disabilities. Port Washington, New York: Alfred Publishing Company, 1975. 113-42. (Bibliography).
Hyperactivity is reviewed according to: (1) definition; (2) types; and (3) characteristics. The relationships among hyperactivity, brain damage, and learning disabilities are explored. A subject index is included in the volume which is directed primarily toward parent and teacher.

92 Chapel, James L., and Bradshaw, Jennifer. "The natural history of hyperactivity in children." Res Relat Child 41: 114, March, 1978-August, 1978. (0 References).
Abstracts a report of research in progress or recently completed research. Data are provided on: name of investigator(s), purpose of the study, number and kind of subjects used, methodology, principal findings, duration of research, cooperating group(s), and availability of publication(s). Research Relating to Children is compiled by the ERIC Clearinghouse on Early Childhood Education.

93 Cohen, Arnold R. "Hyperkinetic syndrome." In: Clinican's handbook of childhood psychopathology. Edited by Martin M. Josephson and Robert T. Porter. New York, New York: Aronson, 1979. 307-22. (9 References).
Describes the characteristics of hyperkinesis and notes the primary deficit as the inability to maintain purposeful attention. Comments are also made on incidence, etiology, diagnosis, and treatment.

94 Edwards, Eileen M. "The hyperactive young child with normal intelligence." Aust Fam Physician 5(9): 1281-82, 1285-88, October, 1976. (9 References).

Defines the hyperactive syndrome as total daily motor activity which is significantly greater than the norm for age level. Behavior is characterized by: (1) early sensitivity to sensory stimuli; (2) excessive crying in the first year; (3) poor sleeping and eating patterns; (4) impulsive behavior; and (5) emotional lability. Management consists of reducing sensory stimulation, setting up routines at home, channeling random activity, and properly administering medication and diet.

95 Evans, James R., and Smith, Linda J. "Common behavioral SLD characteristics." Acad Ther 12(4): 425-27, Summer, 1977. (0 References).
Discusses hyperactivity in relation to a larger entity, the minimal brain dysfunction syndrome. Sixty cases of specific learning disabilities (SLD), which were being treated by private practice, were used to determine the frequency of overactivity. Forms completed by parents showed that overactivity was infrequently reported; sensitivity to criticism, short attention span, and discouragement at home and at school were reported in approximately half the cases. No symptoms were reported in more than 57 percent of the cases.

96 Firestone, Philip; Lewy, Fran; Douglas, Virginia I. "Hyperactivity and physical anomalies." Can Psychiatr Assoc J 21(1): 23-26. February, 1976. (14 References).
Investigates the relationship between hyperactivity and the incidence of physical anomalies. Twenty-four nine-year-old boys, previously judged hyperactive, were matched for age and IQ with twenty-four normal boys. The subjects were examined individually for physical anomalies and were given a weighted anomaly score, the weighing depending on the degree to which each anomaly deviated from the normal. A difference between weighted anomaly scores of the two groups supports the hypothesis that a relationship exists between the two concepts.

97 Firestone, Philip, and Peters, Susan. "Minor physical anomalies in hyperactive, mentally retarded, and normal children." Res Relat Child 40: 30, September, 1977-February, 1978. (0 References).
Abstracts a report of research in progress or recently completed research. Data are provided on: name of investigator(s), purpose of the study, number and kind of subjects used, methodology, principal findings, duration of research, cooperating group(s), and availability of publication(s). Research Relating to Children is compiled by the ERIC Clearinghouse on Early Childhood Education.

98 Firestone, Philip; Peters, Susan; Rivier, Marlene; et al. "Minor physical anomalies in hyperactive, retarded and normal children and their families." J Child Psychol Psychiatry 19(2): 155-60, April, 1978. (25 References).
Studies rates of incidence of minor physical anomalies (MPA) in three groups of children, their siblings, and their parents. Hyperactive, retarded, and normal children and their siblings and parents were examined for the frequency of MPA. The results indicate that the hyperactive, retardates, their siblings and parents had equal numbers of MPA that were significantly higher than in the normal control children and their families who did not differ from each other. In addition, there were more fathers absent due to divorce or separation in the two patient groups than in the normal group.

99 Foreman, B. D., and McKinney, J. P. "A comparison of classroom behavior ratings of learning disabled and nonlearning disabled children." Paper presented at the Annual Meeting of the Southeastern Psychological Association, Hollywood, Florida, May, 1974.

100 Friend, J. C. M. "Syndrome of childhood hyperactivity: I." Med J Aust 1(21): 782-84, May 21, 1977. (0 References).
The characteristics of the syndrome are set forth. Brief information is also provided on the etiology, epidemiology, and natural history of hyperactivity. This paper is part one of a two-part series published in this journal. For part two of this study refer to Item No. 612.

101 Halverson, Charles F., and Victor, James B. "Minor physical anomalies and problem behavior in elementary school children." Child Dev 47(1): 281-85, March, 1976. (19 References).
Updates an earlier study which examined the relationship between minor physical anomalies (MPA) and problem behaviors of 100 elementary schoolchildren. Teachers and peers were the judges of problem behavior. A problem checklist and a teacher ranking of hyperactivity were related to the incidence of MPA for boys. A negative peer factor was also consistently related to the incidence of minor physical anomalies for both boys and girls. The behavior of high-anomaly girls was not easily characterized in terms of any one type of problem behavior. Sex differences and their implications are explored.

102 Hart, Donna R. "Minor physical anomalies and language and behavior variables in selected two-year-old children." For a summary see: Diss Abstr Int 39A(4): 2180, October, 1978. (0 References).

103 Hook, Ernest B. "Methodology questioned." Pediatrics 57(2): 292, February, 1976. (1 Reference).
Letter to editor.

104 "Hyperkinesis." People 4: 64-68, December 8, 1975.
Interview.

105 Johnson, Charles F. "Hyperactivity and abnormal palmar creases." Clin Pediatr 16(7): 647, July, 1977. (5 References).
Comments on a study by Robert J. Lerer (Item No. 110).

106 Lambert, Nadine M., and Windmiller, Myra. "An exploratory study of temperament traits in a population of children at risk." J Spec Educ 11(1): 37-47, Spring, 1977. (6 References).
Uses a factor analysis to examine temperament traits in a group of hyperkinetic children. Parents of 327 hyperactive elementary schoolchildren and controls were interviewed on questions pertaining to their children's early history. Six traits were examined: (1) attention span; (2) threshold level; (3) activity level; (4) distractibility; (5) adaptability; and (6) rhythmicity. Temperament patterns of the subject groups were compared by ANOVA and Scheffe contrasts which indicated that the hyperactive group showed the most extreme scores on all dimensions except for distractibility. Effects of these traits on parents, teachers, and the child are detailed.

107 Langhorne, John E., Jr., and Loney, Jan. "A four-fold model for subgrouping the hyperkinetic/MBD syndrome." Child Psychiatry Hum Dev 9(3): 153-59, Spring, 1979. (15 References).

Assesses the direct and interactive effects of aggression and hyperactivity on sixteen measures obtained during three periods: (1) at referral; (2) during treatment with methylphenidate; and (3) at five-year follow-up. Eighty-six hyperactive/MBD boys (ages six to twelve years) were surveyed. The major finding of the study was that the presence or absence of aggressive symptomatology differentiated the boys. Further, there were no significant interactions between aggression and hyperactivity. Results demonstrate the value of differentiating between the two symptoms.

108 Langhorne, John E., Jr.; Loney, Jan; Paternite, Carl E.; et al. "Childhood hyperkinesis: a return to the source." J Abnorm Psychol 85(2): 201-9, April, 1976. (50 References).
Reports the use of a factor analysis procedure to examine core symptoms of hyperkinesis in a group of children. Ninety-four boys seen at a child psychiatry clinic between 1967 and 1972 served as subjects. A factor analysis was performed on measures of the most widely agreed upon symptoms. Results of this multivariate research are given in detail. For a commentary on this study refer to Item No. 215.

109 ————. "Childhood hyperkinesis: a return to the source." In: Annual progress in child psychiatry and child development, 1977. Edited by Stella Chess and Alexander Thomas. New York, New York: Brunner/Mazel, 1977. 327-41. (50 References).
Reprints an article from the Journal of Abnormal Psychology 85(2): 201-9, April, 1976. (Item No. 108).

110 Lerer, Robert J. "Do hyperactive children tend to have abnormal palmar creases? -- report of a suggestive association." Clin Pediatr 16(7): 645-47, July, 1977. (6 References).
Investigates the incidence of simian and Sydney palmar creases in two groups of children. The palms of 307 hyperactive children and 452 control children were examined and compared. Results of the research show the incidence of simian and Sydney creases was two to three times higher in the hyperactive population than in the controls. The presence of this anomaly may point to other abnormalities which may manifest themselves subsequently as behavioral and/or learning problems. An editorial commentary points out that: (1) the term "simian line" should be replaced by the term "single palmar crease"; (2) control groups should be evaluated as thoroughly as hyperactive groups; and (3) crease abnormalities are not of specific diagnostic value. For a commentary on the study refer to Item No. 105.

111 Moore, Mildred J. "Formulation of hyperactive profiles in children." For a summary see: Diss Abstr Int 37A(8): 5041, February, 1977. (0 References).

112 O'Donnell, James P., and Van Tuinan, Mark. "Behavior problems of preschool children: dimensions and congenital correlates." J Abnorm Child Psychol 7(1): 61-75, March, 1979. (33 References).
Attempts to compile, categorize, and correlate several behavior problems, including hyperactivity. Factor analysis of a revised Behavior Problem Checklist for a sample of preschool children yielded six oblique primary factors and two orthogonal second-order factors. Scores on these factors were correlated with activity level, gross- and fine-motor incoordination, minor physical anomalies, and sociability. Results show that: (1) there are sex differences and factor differences in the resulting patterns of

correlations; and (2) the patterns of correlations indicate that the six primary factors could be collapsed into two broad (Conduct and Personality) and two narrow (Distractibility and Attention Seeking) factors.

113 Ottenbacher, Kenneth. "Hyperactivity and related behavioral characteristics in a sample of learning disabled children." Percept Mot Skills 48(1): 105-6, February, 1979. (5 References).
Identifies the behavioral characteristics of a sample of learning-disabled children and determines the prevalence of hyperactive behaviors in that sample. Sixty-four LD and twelve MBD children were evaluated by their teachers on eleven categories of behavior. Analysis showed that behavioral characteristics associated with hyperactivity did not differentiate among subjects. Teachers rated poor motor coordination as the outstanding trait of this sample.

114 "Physical anomalies predict hyperactivity." Sci News 113(6): 86, February, 1978. (0 References).
Announces recent research by the National Institute of Mental Health (NIMH) which identified a constellation of physical anomalies that could be indicative of the later development of hyperactivity.

115 Prinz, Robert, and Loney, Jan. "Teacher-rated hyperactive elementary school girls: an exploratory developmental study." Child Psychiatry Hum Dev 4(4): 246-57, Summer, 1974. (12 References).
Reports the evaluation by an art teacher of sixteen elementary schoolgirls (previously diagnosed as hyperactive) and sixteen normal control classmates. Interpretation of the data indicates that: (1) no significant differences existed between hyperactive girls and controls as to general adjustment; (2) hyperactive girls were significantly lower than controls in measures of art proficiency; (3) hyperactive girls were lower on impulse control; and (4) both groups had similar ratings in self-esteem. When these data are compared with a study on hyperactive boys, important differences occur.

116 Quinn, Patricia O., and Rapoport, Judith L. "Minor physical anomalies and neurologic status in hyperactive boys." Pediatrics 53(5): 742-47, May, 1974. (29 References).
Attempts to show a relationship between the presence of minor physical anomalies (MPA) and neurological status in hyperactive boys. Previous studies are cited which indicate that high ratings of MPA were associated with school failure. As part of an outpatient study which compared imipramine and methylphenidate, stigmata were measured in the present study for the total evaluation of behavioral, neurologic, and cognitive status. Eighty-one middle-class hyperactive boys (ages six to twelve years) served as subjects. After a medical examination, a battery of psychological tests, and an EEG, the children were examined for stigmata and assigned to imipramine or methylphenidate treatment groups. MPA charted included head circumference, presence of whorls, hypertelorism, low-set ears, high palate, furrowed tongue, curved fifth finger, palmar creases, gaps between toes, etc. "Soft" neurological signs charted included gait, skipping, broad jump, etc. Results showed that the evaluation of these eighty-one boys replicated previous studies which have found increased minor physical anomalies in hyperactive children. Thus, further evidence is provided for congenital contributors to behavior disorders.

117 ————. "Minor physical anomalies and plasma dopamine-beta-hydroxylase activity in hyperactive boys." Pediatr Res 8(4): 464, April, 1974. (0 References).
Abstract of a conference paper presented at the annual meeting of the American Pediatric Association and the Society for Pediatric Research.

118 Quinn, Patricia O.; Renfield, Marilyn; Burg, Cheryl; et al. "Minor physical anomalies: a newborn screening and one-year follow-up." J Am Acad Child Psychiatry 16(4): 662-69, Autumn, 1977. (18 References).
Reports on a study which screened normal newborns for minor physical anomalies. The infants were then evaluated one year later in order to compare high and low anomaly groups with respect to later behavior and development. Nine hundred thirty-three infants were screened at birth according to the Waldrop scoring method. The infants were grouped into high, middle, and low anomaly categories. One hundred twenty-three of these infants were evaluated at one year of age using the Bayley Scales of Infant Development. The anomaly scores were found to be reliable and stable over time and to correlate with infant irritability at one year. In the high-anomaly group there was a positive correlation of irritability and hyperactivity with family history of hyperactivity and/or behavioral disorders or obstetrical complications. These findings may indicate a congenital contribution to behavior disorders for nonretarded preschool children.

119 Rapoport, Judith L., and Quinn, P. O. "Minor physical anomalies and hyperactivity." Pediatrics 55(4): 573, April, 1975. (5 References).
Letter to editor.

120 ————. "Minor physical anomalies (stigmata) and early developmental deviation: a major biologic subgroup of 'hyperactive children'." Int J Ment Health 4(1-2): 29-44, Spring-Summer, 1975. (29 References).
Summarizes a series of ongoing studies on the relation between anomalies (stigmata) and hyperactivity in children. The present study surveyed eighty-two hyperactive boys and their siblings for the presence of stigmata. The authors conclude that: (1) the boys' stigmata scores had a significant positive relationship to reports of paternal hyperactivity; (2) stigmata are significant measures of minor developmental defects of the CNS; (3) the presence of stigmata may aid in diagnostic evaluation; and (4) stigmata scores may aid in the identification of a specific drug-responsive subgroup. For a reprint of this study refer to Item No. 688.

121 ————. "Minor physical anomalies (stigmata) and early developmental deviation--a major biologic subgroup of hyperactive children." In: Mental health in children. Volume 3. Edited by D. V. Siva Sankar. Westbury, New York: PJD Publications, 1977. 271-90. (20 References).

122 Rapoport, Judith L.; Quinn, Patricia O.; Lamprecht, Friedhelm. "Minor physical anomalies and plasma dopamine-beta-hydroxylase activity in hyperactive boys." Am J Psychiatry 131(4): 386-90, April, 1974. (25 References).
Compares the presence of plasma dopamine-beta-hydroxylase (DβH) and minor physical anomalies (stigmata) to activity level and behavior in hyper-

active boys. Seventy-six boys (ages six to twelve years) were selected for the longitudinal study and were examined and scored for the presence of anomalies. Behavior ratings were obtained from teachers and parents, medical histories and blood samples collected, and DβH activity measured. Findings indicate that the presence of multiple minor physical anomalies was associated with severity of hyperactivity. In addition, children with high stigmata scores had higher than normal DβH activity. DβH was not related to behavioral activity ratings but specifically to stigmata score. Both imipramine and methylphenidate significantly increased plasma DβH activity; however, clinical improvement did not parallel change. It is noted that these children are an important subgroup within the hyperactive population.

123 Rapoport, Judith L., and Steg, J. "Minor physical anomalies and early developmental deviation." Paper presented at the American Academy of Child Psychiatry, St. Louis, Missouri, 1975.

124 Santostefano, Sebastiano. "MBD: time to take a new look." Med Times 103(9): 82-87, 91-94, 99, September, 1975. (0 References).
Discusses minimal brain dysfunction in terms of definition and characteristics of the syndrome. The stages in the intellectual and emotional development of children are traced. One case study and treatment suggestions are offered.

125 Satterfield, James H. "Neurophysiologic studies with hyperactive children." In: Cantwell, Dennis P., ed. The hyperactive child: diagnosis, management, current research. New York, New York: Spectrum Publications, distributed by John Wiley and Sons, 1975. 67-82. (45 References). (Series on Child Behavior and Development, Volume I).
Reviews four studies supporting the view that hyperactive children differ from nonhyperactive children on measures which are indicators of central nervous system function. Due to conflicting earlier studies, this report presents findings from the same laboratory in which the groups were more homogeneous and in which the experimental methodology was identical in three of the four studies. The principal findings are: (1) there is an identifiable subgroup of "good responder" hyperactive children who have low CNS arousal levels; (2) the pretreatment CNS arousal level is negatively correlated with the severity of the child's behavioral disturbance; (3) stimulant medication in these low arousal hyperactive children functions like a stimulant in that it increases CNS arousal level; and (4) those children with the greatest increases in CNS arousal level resulting from stimulant medication obtained the best clinical response as measured by teacher rating scales. It is recommended that two forms of treatment (medical and psychological) be used together to obtain maximal benefits for the hyperactive child.

126 Schain, Richard J. "Minor physical anomalies and hyperactivity." Pediatrics 54(4): 522, October, 1974. (3 References).
Letter to editor.

127 Spezzano, Charles J. "The intellectual, neuropsychological, social, and emotional characteristics of children referred because of hyperactivity." For a summary see: Diss Abstr Int 37B(3): 1451, September, 1976. (0 References).

128 Steg, John P., and Rapoport, Judith L. "Minor physical anomalies in normal,neurotic, learning disabled, and severely disturbed children." J Autism Child Schizophr 5(4): 299-307, December, 1975. (18 References).
Compares the incidence of anomalies in children to various learning/behavior impairments and examines the relationship between incidence of anomaly and background factors of prenatal trauma and/or family pathology. One hundred eight boys from four different clinical populations were examined and anomaly scores obtained. Children with academic/behavior problems were found to have a higher incidence of anomalies and common backgrounds of family pathology and/or prenatal trauma.

129 Stewart, Mark A.; Palkes, Helen S.; Young, Carol; et al. "Intellectual ability and school achievement of hyperactive children, their classmates, and their siblings." In: Life history research in psychopathology. Volume III. Edited by David F. Ricks, Alexander Thomas, and Merrill Roff. Minneapolis, Minnesota: University of Minnesota Press, 1974. 68-86. (23 References).
Reprints three papers presented during a two-day conference held at Columbia University.

130 Tignor, Beverly S. "The relationship between minor physical anomalies and measures of attention and school achievement in primary school children." For a summary see: Diss Abstr Int 35B(8): 4200, February, 1975. (0 References).

131 Waldrop, Mary F.; Bell, Richard Q.; McLaughlin, Brian; et al. "Newborn minor physical anomalies predict short attention span, peer aggression, and impulsivity at age three." Science 199(4328): 563-65, February 3, 1978. (14 References).
Studies the association between minor physical anomalies (MPA) and later hyperactivity. Thirty male newborn children, as part of a newborn examination, were checked for the presence of sixteen MPA (abnormal head circumference, low-set ears, high steepled palate, curved fifth finger, single palmar crease, etc.). An additional thirty-six nursery schoolboys were included in the sample. The newborns were again assessed at age three. The number of MPA was significantly related to a cluster of behaviors which included hyperactivity, short attention span, peer aggression, and impulsivity. The predictive value of minor physical anomalies is assessed.

132 Walsh, Thomas H. "Anhedonia as a symptom of minimal brain dysfunction in children." For a summary see: Diss Abstr Int 36B(9): 4714, March, 1976. (0 References).

133 Williams, B. J.; Vincent, J.; Elrod, J. T. "Preliminary draft of the behavioral components of hyperactivity." Paper presented at the Annual Meeting of the American Psychological Association, San Francisco, California, August, 1977.

C. CLASSIFICATION/NOMENCLATURE

134 Arieff, Alex J. "Neurology--epilepsy and learning disorders." Ill Med J 146(5): 467-70, November, 1974. (2 References).
Offers eight possible causes of learning disorders. Six specific kinds are delineated: (1) developmental dyslexia; (2) developmental spelling disability; (3) developmental writing disability; (4) developmental

dyscalculia; (5) drawing disability; and (6) developmental dyspraxia. Two other conditions, hyperkinesis and epilepsy, are also discussed. Proper diagnostic testing is imperative to the welfare of the child.

135 Baumann, Robert J. "Minimal brain dysfunction." JAMA 236(14): 1577, October 4, 1976. (1 Reference).
Letter to editor.

136 Bax, Martin. "Who is hyperactive?" Dev Med Child Neurol 20(3): 277-78, June, 1978. (2 References).
This editorial comments on current labeling practices. Emphasized is the need for proper clinical service in the child's own environment--the playground and the school.

137 Block, Walter M. "Cerebral dysfunctions: an attempt at clarification." Behav Neuropsychiatry 6(1-12): 3-5, April-December, 1974-January-March, 1975. (6 References).
Attempts to separate and define some of the conditions included in the term "minimal brain dysfunction." In studying data of 465 children examined in a multidisciplinary diagnostic clinic, four behavior groups were delineated: (1) organic brain damage (encephalopathy); (2) hyperkinetic behavior syndrome; (3) specific learning disability (subgroup: dyslexia); and (4) vague cerebral dysfunction. Each classification, based on primary symptomatology, was designed to narrow the concept of cerebral dysfunction for better communication among professionals.

138 ————. "Cerebral dysfunctions--clarification, delineation, classification." PDM 5-6(9-12; 1-8): 21-25, January-December, 1974. (7 References).
Because of the continuing controversy surrounding the terminology applied to the concept of cerebral dysfunctions, the author proposes that these disorders be separated into five distinct groups: (1) organic brain damage (encephalopathy); (2) hyperkinetic brain syndrome; (3) specific learning disabilities (e.g., dyslexia); (4) maturational lag; and (5) vague cerebral dysfunction. These distinctions were made on the basis of a multidisciplinary study of 365 children in a diagnostic clinic. It is further recommended that no child be called "brain damaged" unless there is evidence of anatomical damage, and that the term "minimal" brain damaged be permanently abolished. Four case histories illustrate the applicability of the proposed classification.

139 ————. "Cerebral dysfunction--clarification, delineation, classification." Behav Neuropsychiatry 5(7-12): 13-17, October, 1973-March, 1974. (7 References).

140 Campbell, M., and Shapiro, T. "Therapy of psychiatric disorders of childhood." In: Manual of psychiatric therapies: practical psychopharmacology and psychiatry. Edited by Richard I. Shader. Boston, Massachusetts: Little, Brown, 1975. 137-62. (6 References). (Basic Medical Sciences Series).
Discusses hyperactivity as one of a number of personality disorders based on the Group for the Advancement of Psychiatry (GAP) system of classification. Therapy includes treatment of the child, the parents, and the family. A guide to drug therapy accompanies the article.

141 Campbell, Susan B. "Hyperactivity: course and treatment." In: Child personality and psychopathology: current topics. Volume 3.

Edited by Anthony Davids. New York, New York: Wiley, 1976. 201-36. (110 References).
Deals with definitional problems and reviews, from a developmental perspective, a series of studies on a clearly defined subgroup of hyperactive children. The syndrome is traced through infancy, preschool, school age, adolescence, and adulthood. Studies are included which examine the effects of stimulant medication. Alternative treatment methods are briefly covered.

142 Cantwell, Dennis P. "The hyperactive child." Hosp Pract 14(1): 65-73, January, 1979. (4 References).
Points out common myths surrounding the hyperkinetic syndrome and advocates the use of a new designation, "attentional deficit disorder" (ADD). ADD children may suffer from some form of brain damage or dysfunction which is possibly genetic in origin. The role of the physician and the value of early diagnosis and educational remediation are emphasized.

143 Carey, William B.; McDevitt, Sean C.; Baker, David. "Differentiating minimal brain dysfunction and temperament." Dev Med Child Neurol 21(6): 765-72, December, 1979. (20 References).
Studies the relationship between children's negative behavior traits and MBD in a group of sixty-one schoolchildren presenting with learning/behavior problems. The children were assigned to one of four diagnostic groups: (1) MBD; (2) hyperactivity; (3) learning disability; and (4) other criteria. Their temperament profiles were then determined by the Behavioral Style Questionnaire. The disproportionately large number of children with more difficult temperament diagnoses in the referred population indicates that teachers and physicians may have misinterpreted bad behavior as evidence of neurological dysfunction. Those diagnosed clinically as having MBD were less adaptable, less persistent, more active, and more negative than the control population, suggesting that MBD overlaps with difficult temperament. Children in the other three groups were temperamentally similar to the MBD group, which raises doubt about the advisability of diagnosing MBD on the basis of behavior alone. A comprehensive neurobehavioral profile is recommended to separate clearly the various factors contributing to problems in school performance.

144 Clements, Sam D., and Hicks, Tom J. "Physically and neurologically impaired." In: Wisland, Milton V., ed. Psychoeducational diagnosis of exceptional children. Springfield, Illinois: Thomas, 1974. 213-32. (35 References).
Differentiates hyperactivity as one of twelve subgroups of the minimal brain dysfunction syndrome. The activity levels and patterns of behavior are similar to those of children who have a known history of brain damage. The syndrome is not seen as a major characteristic of children with LD or MBD; rather, it should be associated with children of superior intelligence.

145 Cohen, Donald J.; Granger, Richard H.; Provence, Sally A.; et al. "Mental health services." In: Issues in the classification of children: a sourcebook on categories, labels, and their consequences. Volume II. Edited by Nicholas Hobbs. San Francisco, California: Jossey-Bass, 1975. 88-122. (61 References). (Jossey-Bass Behavioral Science Series).
Investigates the relationship between diagnostic classification and children's mental health services. Discussion centers on four questions: (1) Does labeling help or hinder such services? (2) Do labels facilitate

or interfere with early recognition? (3) Do labels facilitate or interfere with organizing useful services for a community? and (4) Do labels place the child at a disadvantage by the meanings they have for the schools and other parts of the community? The hyperkinetic behavioral disturbance is one of several labels discussed in the chapter.

146 Conners, C. Keith. "Minimal brain dysfunction and psychopathology in children." In: Child personality and psychopathology: current topics. Volume 2. Edited by Anthony Davids. New York, New York: Wiley, 1975. 137-68. (24 References).
Argues that the idea of minimal brain dysfunction is a useful heuristic concept--one that has stimulated research in other meaningful ways of conceptualizing certain childhood disorders whose bases lie in the development and function of the central and peripheral nervous system. In addition to exploring biological causes, the concept of an underlying brain dysfunction encourages investigation into somatic therapies.

147 de Hirsch, Katrina. "Learning disabilities: an overview." Bull NY Acad Med 50(4): 459-79, April, 1974. (40 References).
Delineates, defines, and discusses four categories of learning disorders: (1) psychogenic; (2) neurogenic; (3) disorders related to developmental language disabilities; and (4) disorders that stem primarily from environmental conditions. Although these diagnostic categories are likely to overlap and interact, they can be valuable in planning appropriate remedial measures for the learning-disabled child.

148 Denckla, Martha B. "MBD." In: Education and the brain. The 77th Yearbook of the National Society for the Study of Education, Part II. Edited by Jeanne S. Chall and Allan F. Miraky. Chicago, Illinois: The National Society for the Study of Education, 1978. 223-68. (48 References).
Reviews the hyperkinetic syndrome in terms of history of terminology, phenomenology, and therapy. Arguments are given both in favor of the use of the word "hyperkinesis" and against the use of the term. Appropriate therapies include medical treatment, educational remediation, and counseling.

149 Donaldson, John Y. "Some considerations in the treatment of hyperactive children." Nebr Med J 60(6): 194-96, June, 1975. (3 References).
Differentiates three categories of childhood hyperkinesis: (1) that which is due to MBD; (2) that which is caused by intensive levels of anxiety; and (3) that which can be attributed to poor socialization and lack of internalized control. Each type of hyperkinesis necessitates a different treatment method. Group I responds to drugs which increase brain norepinephrine levels. Group II responds best with psychotherapy and environmental changes, and, as a last resort, tranquilizers. Group III's response to medication is minimal; therefore, a program of social intervention must be undertaken in the management of this type of hyperkinesis.

150 Fleischmann, David J. "Etiological subgrouping of hyperkinetic boys." For a summary see: Diss Abstr Int 38B(7): 3391, January, 1978. (0 References).

151 Freeman, Roger D. "Minimal brain dysfunction, hyperactivity, and learning disorders: epidemic or episode?" Sch Rev 85(1): 5-30, November, 1976. (148 References).

Delves into the confusing terminology and ill-defined parameters of minimal brain dysfunction, hyperactivity, and learning disorders. Research into current practices from a social and ideological view is lacking and must be pursued in the interest of developing a coherent picture of the conditions, their management, and the social side effects of present treatment approaches. It is concluded that "There is no epidemic but, rather, an unfortunate episode in the history of progressive medicalization of deviant or troublesome behavior." For a reprint of this study refer to Item No. 744.

152 Gellis, Sydney S. "MBD." Am J Dis Child 129(11): 1324, November, 1975. (0 References).
Comments on studies by Barton D. Schmitt (Item No. 173), and Jerome S. Haller, et al. (Item No. 1470).

153 Gittelman-Klein, Rachel; Spitzer, Robert L.; Cantwell, Dennis. "Diagnostic classifications and psychopharmacological indications." In: Pediatric psychopharmacology: the use of behavior modifying drugs in children. Edited by John S. Werry. New York, New York: Brunner/Mazel, 1978. 136-67. (Bibliography).
Describes all phases of the concept of diagnostic classification and emphasizes two classification systems, the American Psychiatric Association's Diagnostic and Statistical Manual (DSM-III) and the Ninth Edition of the International Classification of Diseases (ICD-9). Hyperkinesis is included in the DSM-III under "Attention Deficit Disorder with Hyperactivity" and "Attention Deficit Disorder without Hyperactivity." The latter disorder is not present in ICD-9. "Attention Deficit Disorder with Hyperactivity" of DSM-III is equivalent to the ICD-9 "Simple Disturbance of Activity and Attention." Other differences in the classification systems are noted.

154 Glazzard, Peggy. "Special touches." Early Years 9(6): 48, 75, February, 1979.
Points out several variables involved in labeling a child hyperactive. Among factors discussed are hunger, level of difficulty of the work assignment, prerequisite skills, fatigue, illness, sensory difficulties, family environment, and tight underwear. Remedial approaches are briefly considered.

155 Glenn, Hugh W. "The myth of the label 'learning disabled child'." Elem Sch J 75(6): 357-61, March, 1975. (15 References).
Calls attention to the fallacies involved in applying the label "learning disabled" to children who are not performing effectively in school. The term is said to have no clear definition, is not potentially useful to educators, and does not pinpoint the skills which the child must acquire. Attention should be devoted to language-centered programs which focus on developing language behaviors.

156 Gordon, N. S. "Minimal brain dysfunction--reply." Dev Med Child Neurol 20(4): 532, August, 1978. (1 Reference).
Letter to editor.

157 Hussey, Hugh H. "Minimal brain dysfunction." JAMA 235(2): 183, January 12, 1976. (0 References).
Concerns diagnostic terminology. Three previous studies are referred to in the editorial.

158 "Hyperactivity." Lancet 2(8089): 561, September 9, 1978. (3 References).
Briefly considers terminology problems surrounding the use of the word "hyperactive."

159 "Is there a hyperkinetic syndrome?" Br Med J 1(6162): 506-7, February 24, 1979. (6 References).
Traces the history of the term "hyperkinesis" and concludes that, appropriate or not, this rubric is likely to remain.

160 Joost, Michael G. "Quantifying hyperactivity in children." For a summary see: Diss Abstr Int 38B(2): 837, August, 1977. (0 References).

161 Lahey, Benjamin B.; Stempniak, Michael; Robinson, Earl J.; et al. "Hyperactivity and learning disabilities as independent dimensions of child behavior problems." J Abnorm Psychol 87(3): 333-40, June, 1978. (25 References).
Points out definitional problems surrounding the terms "hyperactivity" and "learning disabilities" and argues for the existence of dimensions of behavior (intercorrelated core characteristics). In an experiment a broad item pool containing many items putatively related to the syndromes was utilized and independent factors extracted. Nineteen teachers generated 404 ratings of fourth to eighth graders from two schools which had both regular and special education classes. It is concluded that independent dimensions of problem behavior that correspond to "learning disabilities" and "hyperactivity" may be identifiable. Implications are discussed.

162 ————. "Hyperactivity and learning disabilities as independent dimensions of child behavior problems." In: Behavior therapy with hyperactive and learning disabled children. Edited by Benjamin B. Lahey. New York, New York: Oxford University Press, 1979. 92-99. (25 References).
Reprints an article from the Journal of Abnormal Psychology 87(3): 333-40, June, 1978. (Item No. 161).

163 Loney, Jan; Langhorne, John E.; Paternite, Carl E. "An empirical basis for subgrouping the hyperkinetic/minimal brain dysfunction syndrome." J Abnorm Psychol 87(4): 431-41, August, 1978. (38 References).
Reports the results of a factor analysis of medical chart ratings using primary and secondary symptoms in a group of hyperactive/MBD boys. One hundred thirty-five boys (ages four to twelve years) served as subjects. Six primary symptoms (including hyperactivity, inattention, and fidgetiness) and four secondary symptoms (including compulsivity and aggression) were rated. Results of the tally show that: (1) aggression accounted for 44.6 percent of the factor variance and hyperactivity for 23.4 percent; and (2) correlations between scores on these variables and descriptors from parent and teacher rating scales provide evidence for concurrent validity.

164 Neisworth, John T.; Kurtz, P. David; Jones, Russell T.; et al. "Biasing of hyperkinetic behavior ratings by diagnostic reports." J Abnorm Child Psychol 2(4): 323-29, 1974. (11 References).
Sets forth some of the problems of assigning diagnostic labels to "deviant" children and examines the impact of labeling on observer judgments

of child behavior. Two preschool children, one "hyperkinetic" and one "normal" were observed by four pairs of raters over a ten-day interval using the Davids scale. Raters who had been given diagnostic reports suggesting hyperactivity in the child they observed produced significantly higher ratings of hyperkinesis than raters who had not been given diagnostic reports. Thus, prior knowledge increased the chances that a child would be perceived to be hyperkinetic. The impact of labeling on the child is assessed.

165 Neisworth, John T., and Smith, Robert M. "An analysis and redefinition of 'developmental disabilities'." Except Child 40(5): 345-47, February, 1974. (2 References).
Comments on the legal definition of the term "developmental disabilities" as set forth in Public Law 91-517. Major objections include: (1) imprecision of terminology; (2) lack of clarity concerning the character of developmental disabilities; (3) failure to recognize the fallacies involved in establishing a cause-and-effect relationship; and (4) difficulty in establishing age limits. A redefinition of "developmental disabilities" is proposed which specifies domains of functional competence and allows for objective measurement of various conditions.

166 Newton, Jerry. "Minimal brain dysfunction." JAMA 236(14): 1577-78, October 4, 1976. (1 Reference).
Letter to editor.

167 Ney, Philip G. "Four types of hyperkinesis." Can Psychiatr Assoc J 19(6): 543-50, December, 1974. (27 References).
Predicts the characteristics of four types of hyperkinesis: constitutional, conditioned, chemical, and chaotic. Each type is discussed in detail; each is thought to be sufficiently distinct to warrant specific diagnosis and treatment. Although hyperactivity was the feature common to all four types, the four types were different with respect to sex ratio, family history, type of parenting, learning disability, and type of treatment.

168 Oettinger, Leon, Jr. "Minimal brain dysfunction." Dev Med Child Neurol 20(4): 531-32, August, 1978. (4 References).
Letter to editor.

169 Ross, Alan O. "Is something wrong with their brains?" In: Ross, Alan O. Learning disability: the unrealized potential. New York, New York: McGraw-Hill, 1977. 44-60. (7 References).
Discusses problems of terminology. The author concludes that emphasis should be shifted to the use of remedial intervention--both educational and medical--since many currently used labels are not in the best interests of the child.

170 Rutter, Michael. "Emotional disorder and educational underachievement." Arch Dis Child 49(4): 249-56, April, 1974. (48 References).
Reviews data on the association between emotional or behavioral disorders and educational underachievement. Educational underachievement is defined by the degree of deviation from normal achievement as well as by the prognosis for improvement. Underachievement can be classified in three ways: (1) according to the scholastic skill involved; (2) general backwardness versus specific retardation; and (3) failure to acquire educational skills versus loss of these skills. Studies are cited which

indicate that underachievement in all subjects is associated with behavioral disturbance. There is some association with emotional difficulties, but the stronger association is with disorders of conduct. The relationship between other learning disabilities and emotional disorder is analyzed in terms of the following six mechanisms: temperamental influences, anxiety, stress at a critical period, lack of motivation, avoidance of learning, and generally impaired psychological functioning.

171 Sandberg, S. T.; Rutter, M.; Taylor, E. "Hyperkinetic disorder in psychiatric clinic attenders." Dev Med Child Neurol 20(3): 279-99, June, 1978. (97 References).
Tests the validity of the concept of the hyperkinetic syndrome in children. Sixty-eight boys (ages five to eleven years) referred to a child psychiatric clinic participated in the survey. Their rates of hyperactivity were measured by the Conners' Teacher Questionnaire, the Conners' Parent Questionnaire, and observations during testing. When compared with psychiatrically abnormal children without hyperkinesis, few differences were found on cognitive functioning, perinatal history, neurological examination, congenital anomalies, and psychosocial circumstances. The researchers conclude that no evidence exists for the validity of a broad concept of hyperkinetic syndrome.

172 Saravia-Campos, J. "Minimal brain dysfunction: an oversimplification?" Dev Med Child Neurol 18(2): 246-48, April, 1976. (9 References).
Expresses concern about the chaotic classification and terminology of the MBD syndrome. "Post-encephalitic behavior disorder" (aetiological) or "minimal cerebral palsy" (descriptive) are suggested as alternatives for the over-inclusive "minimal brain dysfunction."

173 Schmitt, Barton D. "The minimal brain dysfunction myth." Am J Dis Child 129(11): 1313-18, November, 1975. (44 References).
Focuses on some of the fallacies surrounding the MBD syndrome. Highlighted are problems of terminology ("MBD has become an all-embracing wastebasket diagnosis for any child who does not quite conform to society's stereotype of normal children"), the fallibility of diagnostic tests, and the potential harmful effects of labeling to the child, his family, his school, his physician, the therapeutic process, and research. Practical approaches to treating general symptoms (such as hyperactivity and problems in learning) without using the MBD label are offered. For a commentary on this study refer to Item No. 152.

174 Schuckit, Marc A.; Petrich, John; Chiles, John. "Hyperactivity: diagnostic confusion." J Nerv Ment Dis 166(2): 79-87, February, 1978. (37 References).
Describes the primary symptoms of hyperactivity and attempts to clarify some of the diagnostic difficulties surrounding the syndrome. In an experiment two samples of adolescents were surveyed, one from a psychiatric clinic and the other from a drug abuse treatment program. Histories were gathered and evaluated for all patients; each individual was also evaluated for evidence of the hyperkinetic syndrome. Findings indicate that more than one in five adolescents had shown hyperactivity, but almost all of these developed symptoms of other psychiatric problems (especially antisocial personality) by late adolescence. This picture is felt to reflect the inaccurate use of hyperactive labels in difficult-to-manage children.

175 Sella, Jeanne G. "Differential performance on perceptual discrimination and sensory motor tasks by normal and learning disabled children." For a summary see: Diss Abstr Int 39B(12, pt. 1): 6142, June, 1979. (0 References).

176 Shaffer, D., and Greenhill, L. "A critical note on the predictive validity of 'the hyperkinetic syndrome'." J Child Psychol Psychiatry 20(1): 61-72, January, 1979. (63 References).
Argues that the diagnosis of "hyperactivity syndrome" tells little about etiology and does not permit generalizations to be made about clinical state. Its usefulness in predicting response to drug or other forms of treatment has yet to be demonstrated. A series of follow-up studies has been reviewed in order to determine whether a diagnosis of hyperactivity syndrome will allow predictions to be made about natural history. The literature reveals widely differing outcome in different samples. It may be that this inconsistency simply reflects methodological variation between the studies. However, it can also be taken that the lack of consistency further weakens the validity or clinical usefulness of this diagnostic concept.

177 Shaywitz, B. A.; Cohen, Donald J.; Shaywitz, Sally E. "New diagnostic terminology for minimal brain dysfunction." J Pediatr 95(5, pt. 1): 734-36, November, 1979. (0 References).
Discusses DSM III (Diagnostic and Statistical Manual of the American Psychiatric Association) nomenclature for minimal brain dysfunction. ADD (Attention Deficit Disorder) is the new label replacing the term MBD in this categorization system.

178 Stephenson, P. Susan. "The hyperactive child: some misleading assumptions." Can Med Assoc J 113(8): 764-69, October 18, 1975. (62 References).
Points out the controversies and ambiguities surrounding the hyperkinetic syndrome, especially problems of terminology. It is contended that the term "hyperkinesis" should be restricted to the definition used in British studies. Hyperkinesis, which has a large number of underlying causes, should be considered only a symptom. Thus, management plans must be individualized to fit individual needs.

179 ————. "What is a hyperactive child?" Can Ment Health 23(4): 5-6, 1975. (10 References).
Attributes the confusion surrounding the "hyperactive" label to disagreement among experts as to causal factors, treatment approaches, and definition of the problem. Hyperactivity should not be perceived as a single entity which responds to a single treatment modality. Complaints about a child's hyperactivity must therefore be examined carefully in light of all factors in his development and environment, including home, school, and community. Eleven underlying causes of hyperactivity are listed.

180 Williams, Noel H. "Hyperkinesis: the need for both a physiological and behavioural assessment." Paper presented at the First World Congress on Future Special Education, Stirling, Scotland, June 25-July 1, 1978. 12p. (ED 157 360).
The hyperkinetic child is discussed in terms of assessment and management. An evaluation procedure which identifies the subgroups of hyperkinetic children is included.

181 Wolff, Peter H., and Hurwitz, Irving. "Functional implications of the minimal brain damage syndrome." In: Annual progress in child psychiatry and child development, 1974. Edited by Stella Chess and Alexander Thomas. New York, New York: Brunner/Mazel, 1975. 249-76. (32 References).
Examines and compares the definitions and functional implications of minimal brain damage and synonymous diagnostic terms and reports a study exploring the relation of choreiform movements to behavior disturbances in a classroom of presumably normal children. The results suggest that more extensive systematic studies will be necessary before it can be determined whether the confused, but nevertheless extensive, domain of mixed behavioral and neurologic disabilities in school-age children belong to one global syndrome, or should be classified separately according to differences in etiology, functional significance, and response to therapeutic intervention.

182 Wolkind, S. N., and Everitt, B. "A cluster analysis of the behavioural items in the pre-school child." Psychol Med 4(4): 422-27, November, 1974. (13 References).
Outlines the difficulties of developing a system of classification of non-psychotic disorders of early childhood and describes the usefulness of a cluster analysis technique in developing a diagnostic system based on symptom groups. One hundred three-year-old children, who attended three nursery schools in a London borough, and thirty-one "high-risk" children served as subjects. Mothers and mother substitutes were interviewed, and three different methods of cluster analysis were used--Ward, Wolfe, and McRae. Among the clusters found were two suggesting conduct and neurotic disorders. Evidence is presented which suggests that the clusters produced are clinically meaningful and have prognostic significance.

183 Wright, William H. "MBD." JAMA 235(18): 1967, May 3, 1976. (2 References).
Letter to editor.

D. EPIDEMIOLOGY

184 Akhurst, Bertram A. "The prevalence of behaviour problems among children in care." Educ Res (U.K.) 17(2): 137-42, February, 1975. (11 References).
Surveys the incidence of behavior problems among 182 children undergoing long-term residential care in sixty-two children's homes run by local authorities and voluntary bodies. The Rutter Scales were used as a measuring device to assess the level of behavior problems as reported by houseparents and teachers. Results, as in numerous previously cited studies, show the child care population to exhibit physical, social, and educational maladjustments considerably higher than that of the general population. The possible implications of diagnostic groupings, patterns of reporting, and child-care variables are addressed.

185 Cantwell, Dennis P. "Epidemiology, clinical picture, and classification of the hyperactive child syndrome." In: Cantwell, Dennis P., ed. The hyperactive child: diagnosis, management, current research. New York, New York: Spectrum Publications, distributed by John Wiley & Sons, 1975. 3-16. (68 References). (Series on Child Behavior and Development, Volume I).
Reviews terminology, epidemiology, and clinical picture (hyperactivity, distractibility, impulsivity, excitability, antisocial behavior, cognitive

and learning disabilities, and other emotional symptoms) of the hyperactive child. It is concluded that: (1) the term "hyperactive child syndrome" should be used to denote a behavioral syndrome only, with no implications as to etiology; (2) the syndrome is more common in boys, begins early in life, and is characterized by four cardinal symptoms: hyperactivity, impulsivity, distractibility, and excitability; (3) antisocial behavior, specific learning disabilities, and depressive symptoms occur in many but not all children with the syndrome; (4) children with this syndrome form a heterogeneous group; and (5) epidemiological studies indicate that the syndrome is relatively common in the general population and is a leading cause of referral to child guidance clinics.

186 ————. "Prevalence of psychiatric disorder in a pediatric clinic for military dependent children." J Pediatr 85(5): 711-14, November, 1974. (20 References).
Investigates the prevalence of psychiatric disorder among a group of children attending a pediatric clinic in a military unit in the Southern California area. One hundred children (fifty boys and fifty girls, ages eight to eleven years) served as subjects. Data were acquired by parent interview, a behavior questionnaire administered to the child's teacher, and a one-half hour diagnostic play interview with the child. A judgment was then made as to the presence or absence of psychiatric disorder. Tabulation reveals that clinically significant psychiatric disorder was present in thirty-five of the 100 children (twenty-three boys and twelve girls). Conduct disorders were more common in boys; neurotic disorders in girls. Only three of the thirty-five children were currently receiving treatment from a psychiatrist, and four hyperactive children were receiving medicine. In general, mothers of psychiatrically disturbed children were about the same as mothers of normal children in regard to their assessments of their children's behavior.

187 Conners, C. Keith. Discussion of "Prevalence of hyperactivity in Ottawa." In: Hyperactivity in children: etiology, measurement, and treatment implications. Edited by Ronald L. Trites. Baltimore, Maryland: University Park Press, 1979. 57-59. (4 References).
Comments on a study by Ronald L. Trites (Item No. 204).

188 Gill, David H. "The young and the restless. Critique of a combined medical-nursing audit of hyperkinetic reaction of childhood." QRB 3(7): 14-23, July, 1977.
Reports on a medical-nursing audit of hyperkinetic reaction of childhood. The site of the audit was a 500-bed general hospital with a 100-bed private psychiatric unit with a children's ward. The audit was completed by a committee over a period of twenty-two months. During this time 264 children were admitted to the unit; 116 (44 percent) were discharged with the diagnosis of hyperkinesis. Numerous tables detail all phases of the project.

189 How many children in District 4J are receiving medication for "hyperactivity"? 1976. 12p. (ED 135 175).
Examines incidence of hyperactivity, the process of identifying such children, and the extent and type of medication used to control the hyperactivity of elementary schoolchildren in the Eugene, Oregon school district. The percentage of children identified as hyperkinetic was comparable to other empirically demonstrated percentages.

190 Howell, D. C., and Huessy, H. R. "Long-term follow-up of hyperkinetic and non-hyperkinetic children." Am J Epidemiol 110(3): 360, 1979. (0 References).
Abstract of a meeting.

191 Huessy, Hans R. "Epidemiology of behavior disorders and learning disabilities." Res Relat Child 40: 129, September, 1977-February, 1978. (0 References).
Abstracts a report of research in progress or recently completed research. Data are provided on: name of investigator(s), purpose of the study, number and kind of subjects used, methodology, principal findings, duration of research, cooperating group(s), and availability of publication(s). Research Relating to Children is compiled by the ERIC Clearinghouse on Early Childhood Education.

192 "Hyperactivity in children." Br Med J 4(5989): 123-24, October 18, 1975. (38 References).
Compares epidemiology statistics of the United States with those of the United Kingdom. The diagnosis of hyperactivity is made at a much higher rate in the United States than it is in the United Kingdom. In one survey 40 percent of the children seen by child psychiatrists in Washington were labeled hyperkinetic, while a survey of psychiatrically disordered children (ages nine to eleven years) in the Isle of Wight found only 1.6 percent of them labeled hyperkinetic. Factors accounting for such differences are suggested.

193 Kahn, David A., and Gardner, George E. "Hyperactivity: predominant diagnosis in child referrals." Front Psychiatry 5(9): 3, May 1, 1975. (0 References).
Briefly summarizes a study by these two physicians who examined 240 rural and urban children referred to child psychiatrists by pediatricians. Hyperactivity was diagnosed in 30 percent of all urban children and 26 percent of the rural referrals. The importance of early referrals is emphasized.

194 Lambert, Nadine M.; Sandoval, Jonathan H.; Sassone, Dana M. "Multiple prevalence estimates of hyperactivity in school children." In: R. Halliday (chair). The hyperactive child: fact, fiction and fantasy. Symposium presented at the Meeting of the American Psychological Association, San Francisco, California, 1977.

195 ———. "Prevalence estimates of hyperactivity in schoolchildren." Pediatr Ann 7(5): 330-38, May, 1978. (14 References).
Offers a number of definitions of hyperactivity based on information from several sources: home, school, and physician. Thus, several prevalence rates are produced, based on different defining systems. The data presented do not indicate an increase in the number of hyperactive children from the past decade.

196 ———. "Prevalence of hyperactivity in elementary school children as a function of social system definers." Am J Orthopsychiatry 48(3): 446-63, July, 1978. (32 References).
Reviews epidemiological studies and details a new study which seeks to reconcile the widely varying estimates of prevalence of hyperactivity in children. The sample of the new study involved over 5,000 children from the population of California public and private school children. Parents, teachers, and physicians were then asked to identify hyperactive children.

The data indicate: (1) the overall prevalence rate of children identified as hyperactive by the home, the school, and the physician was only 1.19 percent of an elementary school population; (2) approximately 5 percent were considered hyperactive by at least one rating group; and (3) prevalence rates were relatively constant from kindergarten through fifth grade. The data presented do not support the belief that there are currently more hyperactive children than there were in the past.

197 Lewis, Margaret A. "Hyperactivity and variations in prevalence rates for assignment to special classes among Black, White and Spanish surnamed students in twenty-five urban and suburban school districts in New Jersey." For a summary see: Diss Abstr Int 34A(7): 4040, January, 1974. (0 References).

198 Minde, Klaus K., and Cohen, Nancy J. "Hyperactive children in Canada and Uganda." J Am Acad Child Psychiatry 17(3): 476-87, June, 1978. (19 References).

Reports on a cross-cultural study of the incidence of hyperactivity among primary schoolchildren in Uganda and Canada. The Peterson-Quay questionnaire was found to correctly identify hyperactives and controls in both cultures. Ugandan children showed more antisocial behavior as well as evidence of the existence of the hyperkinetic syndrome. Problems of methodology are noted.

199 Richman, N.; Stevenson, J. E.; Graham, P. J. "Prevalence of behaviour problems in 3-year-old children: an epidemiological study in a London borough." J Child Psychol Psychiatry 16(4): 277-87, October, 1975. (13 References).

Studies the prevalence, classification, and factors associated with the appearance and prognosis of behavior problems in a sample of three-year-old children living in a section of London. Data on the children of 705 families were gathered through questionnaires and social interviews. Using this data, a final rating of the child's behavioral status was made. Interpretation of the statistics shows that: (1) 7 percent of the children had behavior problems in the moderate to severe range; (2) 15 percent exhibited mild behavior problems; (3) there were no significant class differences; (4) boys were more hyperactive while girls were more fearful; and (5) the rate of behavior and emotional disorder in the preschool period is similar to that in later childhood and early adolescence.

200 Rutter, Michael; Yule, William; Berger, Michael; et al. "Children of West Indian immigrants. I. Rate of behavioral deviance and of psychiatric disorder." J Child Psychol Psychiatry 15(4): 241-62, October, 1974. (30 References).

This epidemiological study examines hyperactivity as one of many deviant traits found in a sample of children. A total population survey was made of all ten-year-old children in an inner London borough. Comparisons were then made between children born to West Indian migrants and children from nonimmigrant families, and within the West Indian group, between children born abroad and those born in Great Britain. Results indicate that West Indian children showed more behavioral difficulties at school, but not at home. Details on prevalence, type of disorder, and pattern of disorder are given.

201 Schultz, Edward W.; Salvia, John A.; Feinn, Jonathan. "Prevalence of behavioral symptoms in rural elementary school children." J Abnorm Child Psychol 2(1): 17-24, 1974. (6 References).

Discusses hyperactivity as one of fifty-five problem behaviors surveyed in a group of elementary school children. One thousand five hundred seventy-five third- and fourth-grade students attending school in two rural counties in east central Illinois participated in the study. The Behavior Problem Checklist (Quay and Peterson) was used to gather data from each child's classroom teacher. Results show: (1) the prevalence of symptoms was fairly high for the population; (2) boys exhibited a significantly greater mean number of problem behaviors than girls, although girls exhibited the more neurotic forms of behavior; (3) fewer mean symptoms were found in general as compared with other studies; and (4) fourth-grade girls, as opposed to third-grade girls, demonstrated an increased frequency in behavior common to the conduct disorder cluster. Two tables are included.

202 Sprague, Robert L. Discussion of "Prevalence of hyperactivity in Ottawa." In: Hyperactivity in children: etiology, measurement, and treatment implications. Edited by Ronald L. Trites. Baltimore, Maryland: University Park Press, 1979. 53-56. (12 References).
Comments on a study by Ronald L. Trites (Item No. 204).

203 Sprague, R. L.; Cohen, M. N.; Eichlseder, W. "Are there hyperactive children in Europe and the South Pacific?" In: R. Halliday (chair). The hyperactive child: fact, fiction and fantasy. Symposium presented at the Meeting of the American Psychological Association, San Francisco, California, 1977.

204 Trites, Ronald L. "Prevalence of hyperactivity in Ottawa, Canada." In: Hyperactivity in children: etiology, measurement, and treatment implications. Edited by Ronald L. Trites. Baltimore, Maryland: University Park Press, 1979. 29-52. (27 References).
Presents a demographic study of a large population (14,083) of Canadian children. The Conners' Teacher Rating Scale was used to gather data. Attention is called to the methodology problems caused by existing imprecise definitions of the syndrome. For commentaries on this study refer to Item Nos. 187 and 202.

205 Trites, Ronald L.; Dugas, Erika; Lynch, George; et al. "Prevalence of hyperactivity." J Pediatr Psychol 4(2): 179-88, June, 1979. (17 References).
Reports results of the Conners Teacher Rating Scale completed for a random sample of 14,083 elementary schoolchildren (kindergarten to Grade 6) in Ontario, Canada. Prevalence estimates of hyperactivity and other problems showed marked consistency across age and teachers. Boys tended to be identified as problems more frequently than girls. Prevalence rates obtained in this study are compared with others obtained using the same instrument in other countries. The problems of using arbitrary cutoff scores with such instruments are discussed.

206 Waechter, Donna; Anderson, Robert P.; Juarez, Leo J.; et al. "Ethnic group, hyperkinesis, and modes of behavior." Psychol Sch 16(3): 435-39, July, 1979. (19 References).
Examines modes of behavior across different ethnic groups of children. One hundred thirty-two black, white, and Mexican-American children were rated as hyperactive through the use of the Abbreviated Conners Teacher Rating Scale. Score patterns were studied through analysis of variance. The research indicates that: (1) there are behavioral differences across ethnic groups; (2) black children scored significantly higher than white

or Mexican-American children on three scale items; and (3) the mean total score of black children was higher than the other two groups. Sociological implications are interpreted.

207 Walzer, Stanley; Richmond, Julius B.; De Buno, Theodore. "Epidemiology and disordered learning." In: Advocacy for child mental health. Edited by Irving N. Berlin. New York, New York: Brunner/Mazel, 1975. 46-67. (59 References).
Focuses on the problems of surveying the incidence of learning disorders in children. The primary aim of epidemiological investigation should be to provide a framework for introducing meaningful intervention and prevention programs.

E. ATTITUDES, MISCONCEPTIONS, AND CONTROVERSIES

208 Adelman, Howard S. "The myth of the hyperactive child." J Learn Disabil 11(8): 10-11, October, 1978. (0 References).
Letter to editor.

209 Akins, Keith. "The hyperkinetic child." Can Med Assoc J 114(9): 767-68, May 8, 1976. (11 References).
Letter to editor.

210 Becker, R. D. "Minimal cerebral (brain) dysfunction--clinical fact or neurological fiction? The syndrome critically re-examined in the light of some hard neurological evidence." Isr Ann Psychiatry 12(2): 87-106, June, 1974. (49 References).
Critically appraises some of the current theoretical, empirical, and clinical controversies in the field. The use of the term "minimal brain dysfunction" is advocated. The author attempts to redefine the etiological, symptomatic, neuropsychological, and behavioral correlates of the MBD syndrome. Also discussed are: (1) the diagnostic value of "hard" and "soft" neurological signs; (2) equivocal and/or nonspecific outcomes of neurological examinations; (3) secondary emotional consequences of the syndrome; (4) other corollaries of MBD; and (5) guidelines for early recognition and diagnosis.

211 Bosco, J. J., and Robin, S. S. "Symposium: Stimulant drugs and the schools: Dimensions in remediation of social toxicity. III. Three perspectives on the use of Ritalin: Teachers, prospective teachers, and professors. II. An examination of problems of attitude formation and professional practice." Paper presented at the Annual Meeting of the Council for Exceptional Children, New York, New York, April, 1974.

212 Bryan, Tanis H. "Learning disabilities: a new stereotype." J Learn Disabil 7(5): 304-9, May, 1974. (18 References).
Refutes some of the most popular stereotypes associated with learning disabilities, claiming that these stereotypes have not been borne out in the literature by empirical support. There is no systematically gathered evidence demonstrating that LD children actually have the variety of characteristics frequently attributed to them--perceptual problems, hyperactivity, difficulty with cross-modal integrations, MBD, or normal intelligence. They do seem to have difficulty paying attention, using language, and coping with complex auditory and visual presentations. Professionals in the field are urged to be aware of inappropriate stereotypes and be sensitive to, and supportive of, research efforts in behalf of the LD child.

213 Campbell, Elizabeth S., and Redfering, David L. "Relationship among environmental and demographic variables and teacher-rated hyperactivity." J Abnorm Child Psychol 7(1): 77-81, March, 1979. (9 References).
Studies the influence of environmental and demographic factors on the occurrence of teacher-rated hyperactivity. In an experiment seventy-nine hyperactive and eighty-one nonhyperactive children (ages five to twelve years) were studied. Parents of the subjects were interviewed to obtain information regarding the environmental and demographic factors of sex, race, birth order, number of siblings, frequency of change of residence, income level, mother's age, father's age, educational level of mother, educational level of father, parents' marital status, and the method of child discipline used in the home. Comparison between the hyperactive and nonhyperactive groups suggested nonsignificant differences with the exception of sex in which the ratio of hyperactive males to hyperactive females was 5:1.

214 Campbell, Susan B.; Schleifer, Michael; Weiss, Gabrielle. "Continuities in maternal reports and child behaviors over time in hyperactive and comparison groups." J Abnorm Child Psychol 6(1): 33-45, March, 1978. (15 References).
This article examines: (1) consistencies in maternal reports and child behaviors over time; and (2) the relationship of maternal reports to teacher ratings in elementary school. Data were available for a group of hyperactive and control children who had participated in a longitudinal study. The two-year follow-up sample consisted of twenty hyperactive children (fifteen boys and five girls) and twenty-one controls; the three-year follow-up involved twelve hyperactive boys and three hyperactive girls and sixteen controls. Data, given in detail, provide some evidence of consistency in maternal ratings of behavior problems across time periods for both groups. These findings suggest that data from several sources should be considered when evaluating both degree of pathology and changes in behavior over time.

215 DeFilippis, Nick A. "Source of data as a factor in assessing symptoms of hyperkinesis." J Consult Clin Psychol 47(6): 1115-16, December, 1979. (3 References).
Comments on studies by John E. Langhorne, et al. (Item No. 108) and Patricia G. Zukow, et al. (Item No. 609). The present study corroborates the conclusions of Langhorne which found a lack of agreement between teachers and parents in assessing the symptoms of hyperactivity in children.

216 Divoky, Diane, and Schrag, Peter. "The invention of a disease." Edcentric 35: 4-8, 22-26, July-August, 1975. (0 References).
Reprints excerpts from a book by Peter Schrag and Diane Divoky, The myth of the hyperactive child and other means of child control (Item No. 238).

217 "Do guilt-ridden mothers conceal hyperactivity of their children?" Can Fam Physician 21(7): 25, July, 1975. (0 References).
Many mothers of hyperactive children possess guilt feelings concerning their own performance as parents, and for this reason, often fail to seek clinical attention for their children. According to Dr. Marcel Kinsbourne, a favorable prognosis for hyperkinesis can be hampered if the proper diagnostic and treatment steps are not taken.

218 "Drugs--specific cure or social change?" Except Parent 6(2): 11-17, April, 1976. (0 References).

The case of a hyperactive eleven-year-old boy is described from the viewpoint of the child's mother, father, teacher, and pediatrician. Reasons for continuing medication and designing a structured educational program are discussed by the psychological consultant.

219 Early, Kathleen. "The hyperactive child: is he a myth or society's victim?" Town Ctry 130: 150-51ff., November, 1976. (0 References).
Uses a case study of a five-year-old girl to point out some of the major controversies surrounding the hyperkinetic syndrome. Success is reported with the Feingold diet.

220 Eisenberg, Leon. "Hyperkinesis revisited." Pediatrics 61(2): 319-21, February, 1978. (10 References).
Comments on studies by James S. Miller (Item No. 1920) and Susan G. O'Leary and William E. Pelham (Item No. 1084).

221 Hampe, Edward. "Parents' and teachers' perceptions of personality characteristics of children selected for classes for the learning disabled." Psychol Rep 37(1): 183-89, August, 1975. (9 References).
Assesses the influence of parents' and teachers' perceptions of behavior problems on special class placement of children. Forty-five learning-disabled children (ages five to thirteen years) served as subjects. Evidence from the study suggests that children are selected for special classes not only because of poor academic performance, but also on factors such as activity level, impulse control, attention span, and distractibility. Data were obtained from the Louisville Behavior Checklist (parents) and the School Behavior Checklist (teachers).

222 Hegeman, Gail A. "Parental perceptions of the hyperactive child: a hyperactivity scale for the Personality Inventory for Children." For a summary see: Diss Abstr Int 38B(6): 2862, December, 1977. (0 References).

223 Howells, J. G. "Is there a hyperkinetic syndrome?" Br Med J 1 (6164): 685, March 10, 1979. (0 References).
Letter to editor.

224 "Hyperkinetic behavior syndrome [is] no myth." AORN J 23(6): 1140, May, 1976. (0 References).
Reprints comments by J. Gordon Millichap. The statements were made at a two-day symposium on MBD.

225 Kalechstein, Melvin; Hansen, Phillip; Kalechstein, Pearl B. "Hyperactivity: pediatricians' and teachers' perspectives." J Sch Health 49(1): 20-23, January, 1979. (22 References).
Documents the results of a questionnaire developed to compare the responses of a group of eighty pediatricians and a group of 302 master's degree candidates in special education (79.18 percent of whom were teachers with an average of 4.72 years of teaching experience). The groups were queried on four variables relating to the hyperkinetic syndrome in children: etiology, diagnosis, treatment, and labels. Tables show group and intragroup similarities and differences. Most disagreement between the two groups was in the preferred method of treatment. The necessity for a multidisciplinary approach is stressed.

226 Loney, Jan; Whaley-Klahn, Mary A.; Weissenburger, Fred E. "Responses of hyperactive boys to a behaviorally focused school attitude questionnaire." Child Psychiatry Hum Dev 6(3): 123-33, Spring, 1976. (21 References).
Examines the responses to a questionnaire administered to three groups of elementary schoolboys. The boys were divided into: (1) those considered by a teacher as hyperactive and referrable; (2) those considered as among the most active but not referrable; and (3) normoactive classmates. All groups were given the Teacher Approval-Disapproval Scale. The scale consisted of various items which queried the child about the amount of approval or disapproval directed toward himself personally or toward the rest of the class, or about the frequency of his own happiness and unhappiness in the classroom or that of the rest of the class. Generally, hyperactive boys said they received significantly less approval and significantly more disapproval from teachers than did the other groups.

227 McMahon, Robert C.; Kunce, Joseph T.; Salamak, Martin. "Diagnostic implications of parental ratings of children." J Clin Psychol 35(4): 757-62, October, 1979. (4 References).
Investigates the association between clinical judgment and parental ratings using a refinement of the Missouri Children's Behavior Checklist. The study sought to compare parents' descriptions of their children with the collective diagnostic impressions of a professional interdisciplinary university medical center team. One hundred twenty children and a cross-validation sample of sixty-seven children were used for the data base. In general, the results indicate that: (1) parental ratings show consistent relationships to selected interdisciplinary staff diagnoses; (2) hyperkinesis may be related more strongly to aggressiveness than to the lack of socially responsible behavior; and (3) parental ratings are potentially valuable in the diagnostic process.

228 Nader, Philip R. "Minimal brain dysfunction myth." Am J Dis Child 130(7): 779, July, 1976. (1 Reference).
Letter to editor.

229 O'Malley, John E. "The hyperkinetic syndrome revisited: myths and mayhem." In: Mental health in children. Volume II. Edited by D. V. Siva Sankar. Westbury, New York: PJD Publications, 1976. 303-17. (27 References).
The author discusses the hyperkinetic syndrome in regard to its: (1) clinical description; (2) prevalence; (3) natural history; (4) etiology; and (5) treatment approaches. Myths and mayhem surrounding the syndrome are outlined.

230 Pollack, Stephen L. "Reactivity in the classroom observation of hyperactive children." For a summary see: Diss Abstr Int 39B(11): 5578-79, May, 1979. (0 References).

231 Rapoport, Judith L., and Benoit, Marilyn. "The relation of direct home observations to the clinic evaluation of hyperactive school age boys." J Child Psychol Psychiatry 16(2): 141-47, April, 1975. (12 References).
Compares data from clinic behavioral measures to direct home observations of twenty hyperactive elementary schoolboys. During one-hour home visits, frequency counts of shifts in activity, negative interpersonal interaction, and global estimates of hyperactivity were made. The home observation figures were then compared with parent and teacher rating

scales, mothers' reports, and psychologists' behavior ratings. Statistics reveal a significant correlation between home observations and teachers' and psychologists' ratings. Hyperactivity was a pervasive characteristic in both structured and unstructured settings.

232 Rich, H. Lyndall. "The syndrome of hyperactivity among elementary resource students." Educ Treat Child 2(2): 91-100, Spring, 1979.
Investigates the accuracy of teachers' identification of hyperactive behavior based on perceptions of student motor activity and the extent to which these perceptions influenced the quantity and quality of teacher talk and behavior problem assessment. Activity levels were computed for twenty-eight elementary students, fourteen ranked active and fourteen inactive. Data were collected using activity level counters, a behavior checklist, and observation. Analysis of results did not support the accuracy of teachers' perceptions of motor activity. Perceived student motor activity, conduct problems, and teacher talk formed a cluster of significant variables, while actual student motor activity alone was not a significant variable.

233 Robin, S. S., and Bosco, J. J. "Symposium: Stimulant drugs and the schools: Dimensions in remediation of social toxicity. II. Three perspectives on the use of Ritalin: Teachers, prospective teachers and professors. I. Description of attitude, knowledge and role." Paper presented at the meeting of the Council for Exceptional Children, New York, New York, April, 1974.

234 Ross, Irwin. "Exclusion and discrepancy as criteria for identifying children with learning disabilities." For a summary see: Diss Abstr Int 35A(1): 289, July, 1974. (0 References).

235 Russman, Barry S. "Minimal brain dysfunction myth." Am J Dis Child 130(4): 445, April, 1976. (3 References).
Letter to editor.

236 Schmitt, Barton. "The minimal brain dysfunction myth." Am J Dis Child 130(8): 901-2, August, 1976. (0 References).
Letter to editor.

237 ———. "The minimal brain dysfunction myth: reply." Am J Dis Child 130(7): 779, July, 1976. (0 References).
Letter to editor.

238 Schrag, Peter, and Divoky, Diane. The myth of the hyperactive child and other means of child control. New York, New York: Pantheon, 1975. 285p. (Bibliography).
Protests methods currently being used to treat the hyperactive child. The authors state that although only a small percentage of the population actually suffers from brain damage, schools, doctors, and juvenile authorities have begun to attribute similar or related symptoms to millions of children in the United States. Simultaneously, traditional treatment methods of management and control have been replaced by psychosocial and psychochemical techniques which view almost every form of bad behavior as a medical ailment. Also included in the volume are personal examples as illustrations, an appendix on the elements of self-defense, bibliographical notes on each chapter, and a subject and name index.

239 Simeon, Jovan; Coffin, Charles; Marasa, John. "Videotape techniques in pediatric psychopharmacology research." In: Psychopharmacology of childhood. Edited by D. V. Siva Sankar. Westbury, New York: PJD Publications, 1976. 7-27. (14 References).
Advocates the use of videotape techniques to improve the validity of pediatric psychopharmacology programs and to determine the degree of agreement among parents and professionals in their assessments of children's behavior during treatment. In the experiment, children were taped during free behavior, task behavior, and social interaction. The tapes were then blindly viewed and rated. Significant differences between parental ratings and professional ratings were found. Advantages of the method are listed.

240 Sprague, Robert L. "Counting jars of raspberry jam." In: Learning disability/minimal brain dysfunction syndrome: research perspectives and applications. Edited by Robert P. Anderson and Charles G. Halcomb. Springfield, Illinois: Thomas, 1976. 94-125. (27 References).
Critically reviews some of the misconceptions and fallacies in the area of LD and MBD. The main points of the presentation are: (1) established organizations or bureaucracies often serve their own ends, rather than the populations which they are supposed to serve; (2) too much emphasis is placed on theory and speculation about the causes of MBD, rather than working to improve the child's behavior; (3) LD and MBD children are capable of performing at a much higher level than is expected of them; and (4) behavioral management may be more effective than drugs in the modification of hyperactivity.

241 Spring, Carl; Greenberg, Lawrence M.; Yellin, Absalom M. "Agreement of mothers' and teachers' hyperactivity ratings with scores on drug-sensitive psychological tests." J Abnorm Child Psychol 5(2): 199-204, June, 1977. (6 References).
Studies differences between parents' and teachers' ratings in order to test the hypothesis that certain correlations would be expected with psychological tests that require sustained attention. Forty-five children (thirty-eight boys and seven girls) previously diagnosed as hyperactive participated in the study. The Hyperactivity Rating Scale (HRS) was used to obtain parent and teacher reports. Teachers' ratings, but not parents' ratings, were negatively correlated with performance on the psychological tests that require sustained attention and on which performance is improved by stimulant drugs. Reasons for this pattern of correlation are offered.

242 Stephenson, P. S. "The hyperkinetic child." Can Med Assoc J 114 (9): 768, May 8, 1976. (2 References).
Letter to editor.

243 Stevens, Theodore. "Activity level: a comparison between objective and subjective measures and a classroom management approach." For a summary see: Diss Abstr Int 39B(8): 4055-56, February, 1979. (0 References).

244 Stevens, Theodore M.; Kupst, Mary Jo; Suran, Bernard G.; et al. "Activity level: a comparison between actometer scores and observer ratings." J Abnorm Child Psychol 6(2): 163-73, June, 1978. (25 References).

Explores the relationships between observer ratings gathered from a variety of sources with actometer-measured activity level in several different settings with particular reference to the prediction of the mechanically defined criterion of activity level. Thirteen boys (ages nine to thirteen years) from a day hospital program participated in the study. The actometer, a modified wristwatch which measures muscle movement, was used to measure activity. Ratings were obtained from mothers and six clinical staff members. Comparisons between measures showed that staff ratings correlated significantly with actometer activity in the classroom. Mothers' ratings correlated significantly with actometer activity in some situations and with overall activity. Cautious optimism should be used with assessment tools.

245 Swazey, J. P. "Myths, muckraking, and hyperactive children." Hastings Cent Rep 6(2): 16-18, 1976. (2 References).

246 Treegoob, Mark R. "A contrast of the knowledge and attitudes of special education teachers and elementary teachers about Ritalin in its use with hyperkinetic children." For a summary see: Diss Abstr Int 37A(6): 3555-56, December, 1976. (0 References).

247 Ullmann, Rina, and Sprague, Robert L. "Convergence of teacher ratings of classroom behaviors with direct systematic observation of the same behavior." Res Relat Child 40: 128-29, September, 1977-February, 1978. (0 References).
Abstracts a report of research in progress or recently completed research. Data are provided on: name of investigator(s), purpose of the study, number and kind of subjects used, methodology, principal findings, duration of research, cooperating group(s), and availability of publication(s). Research Relating to Children is compiled by the ERIC Clearinghouse on Early Childhood Education.

248 Wender, Paul H., and Wender, Esther H. "The minimal brain dysfunction myth." Am J Dis Child 130(8): 900-901, August, 1976. (0 References).
Letter to editor.

249 Wickman, E. K. "Teachers' list of undesirable forms of behaviour." In: Behaviour problems in school: a source book of readings. Edited by Phillip Williams. London, England: University of London Press, 1974. 6-15. (References).
Hyperactivity is included as one item on a classified list of problem behaviors as reported by a group of twenty-seven British teachers. Comparisons are made to other such lists and to parental ratings. The majority of the items represent an undesirable action, rather than an action which a child would fail to do. Most behavior problems surveyed represent disturbances of classroom order of some kind.

250 Zinna, Ros. "Is there a hyperkinetic syndrome?" Br Med J 1(6164): 685, March 10, 1979. (0 References).
Letter to editor.

251 Ziv, A. "Children's behaviour problems as viewed by teachers, psychologists and children." In: Williams, Philip, comp. Behaviour problems in school: a source book of readings. London, England: University of London Press, 1974. 39-45. (References).

Compares points of view of two groups of professionals (teachers and psychologists) and children on what constitutes bad behavior. By means of a checklist, thirty problem behaviors were rated and correlated. Results show similarities between teachers' and psychologists' rankings and similarities between children's and teachers' rankings. Hyperactivity was rated higher on the psychologists' list. The study took place in Israel.

252 Zuckerman, Robert. "Minimal brain dysfunction myth." Am J Dis Child 130(8): 900, August, 1976. (0 References).
Letter to editor.

III.
Etiology

A. CAUSAL STUDIES

253 Arnold, L. Eugene. "Causes of hyperactivity and implications for prevention." Sch Psychol Dig 5(4): 10-22, Fall, 1976. (23 References).
Hyperactivity is reviewed in relation to its: (1) definition; (2) multiple causation of symptoms; (3) specific causes; and (4) possibilities for prevention. Specific causes are attributed to MBD, genetic factors, neurophysiological factors, the peripheral nervous dysfunction hypothesis, nutrition, hypersensitivity, radiation, and psychosocial stress. Possibilities for prevention include natural childbirth, prenatal care, breast feeding, nontoxic environment, and prompt remediation of deficient perceptual skills in kindergarten or first grade.

254 Frazier, Shervert. "Two differing opinions. Minimal brain dysfunction." Med Times 103(9): 68, September, 1975. (0 References).
Presents contrasting statements by two physicians, Dr. Salvatore V. Ambrosino and Dr. Sebastiano Santostefano, concerning MBD. Although both physicians stress that MBD children represent an increasingly large clinical population which has been neglected by physicians, they differ as to the etiology and approach to the problem. Dr. Ambrosino attributes the cause of MBD to neurological dysfunction and advocates the use of stimulant drugs in its management. Dr. Santostefano believes that these children represent a developmental lag in the areas of cognitive and emotional growth. He cautions against the use of medication in favor of other treatment modalities.

255 Goggin, James E. "Sex differences in the activity level of preschool children as a possible precursor of hyperactivity." J Genet Psychol 127(1st half): 75-81, September, 1975. (11 References).
Attempts to determine whether or not preschool age boys have a higher activity level than girls. The activity levels of preschool children from a normal sample were measured randomly by an observation technique as the children took part in a nursery school program. The results show that boys were more active than girls and that the boys' behavioral activity was manifested in patterns similar in nature to those often included as part of the various definitions of hyperactivity. The implications of the results are discussed and future research needs delineated.

256 Griffiths, Allen D., and Griffiths, Patricia W. "Learning disabilities: etiology." Optom Wkly 65(34): 928-32, October, 1974. (28 References).
Discusses learning disabilities in terms of: (1) definitions of the syndrome; (2) characteristic symptoms; and (3) categories of etiology. A

list of identifying behaviors is included as well as a list of nine symptoms and manifestations which an LD child might exhibit. Three categorical designations of organic etiology are discussed: minimal brain damage syndrome, minimal brain dysfunction, and minimal cerebral dysfunction. The effects of neurological dysfunction on visual perception are outlined, along with emotional and developmental types of functional etiology.

257 "Hyperkinesis: opinions vary on cause and treatment." Mod Med 46(7): 82-92, April 15, 1978. (0 References).
Four clinicians (Patricia O. Quinn, Alan C. Levin, Esther H. Wender, and Dennis P. Cantwell) discuss the observed relationships between hyperactivity in children and other factors--social, environmental, biochemical, and nutritional.

258 Levine, Edward M., et al. "Hyperactivity among white middle-class children: psychogenic and other causes." Child Psychiatry Hum Dev 7(3): 156-68, Spring, 1977. (16 References).
Investigates the problem of hyperactivity through a literature review, examinations of thirty-seven hyperactive grade-school children, and field interviews with Chicago area school nurses, social workers, psychologists, teachers, and principals. Research indicates that although constitutional factors are sometimes responsible for this problem, hyperactivity is often due to psychogenic factors. School teachers seem overly inclined to identify hyperactivity in their students and to recommend that it be counteracted with drugs. It is recommended that any child thought to be hyperactive undergo a comprehensive examination before drugs are prescribed.

259 Marcea, Anita. "The problem of hyperactivity." Acad Ther 13(3): 277-84, January, 1978. (20 References).
Causal factors of hyperkinesis include neurological disorders, biological disorders, developmental disorders, and the allergic process. Each of these causes is defined and delineated. It is urged that: (1) children presenting with symptoms of hyperactivity be examined by a physician; (2) parents, teachers, and physicians be aware of the multiple factors involved in this syndrome; and (3) careful diagnosis be made so that faulty classifications do not take place.

260 Neeman, Renate L. "Minimal brain dysfunction and specific learning disabilities." J Rehabil Asia 16(4): 23-25, October, 1975.
Briefly describes the salient characteristics of the MBD syndrome and outlines various theories concerned with its etiology. The paper is an outgrowth of the March, 1972 Conference on Minimal Brain Dysfunction sponsored by the New York Academy of Sciences, the National Institute of Child Health and Human Development, and the National Institute of Neurological Diseases and Stroke.

261 Renshaw, Domeena C. "Understanding the hyperactive child." Ill Med J 149(4): 351-54, April, 1976. (8 References).
Hyperactivity is defined as a collection of behavioral manifestations which forms a clinical entity. The hyperkinetic child syndrome, traditionally oversimplified and overgeneralized, has been attributed to many causal factors--induced labor, prematurity, birth trauma, immaturity of the central nervous system, enzyme deficiency, neurohormone imbalance, and broken homes. A changing society, with its emphasis on competitiveness, expanding knowledge, and accelerated living may be a possible cause as well.

262 Stewart, Mark A. "Is hyperactivity abnormal? and other unanswered questions." Sch Rev 85(1): 31-42, November, 1976. (37 References).
A review of research on the etiology of hyperactivity indicates that there is much disagreement on many aspects of the syndrome. Little is known of the extent to which the behaviors that comprise hyperactivity cluster together; what constitutes an abnormal level of activity; and whether the syndrome is physiological or behavioral in origin. Although diagnosis rests on parents' and teachers' reports, clinical observations have not distinguished such children. Likewise, little is known about the developmental history of hyperactive children. Comments are made on stimulant drug therapy versus behavioral approaches. For a reprint of this study refer to Item No. 744.

B. THEORETICAL MODELS

263 Arnold, L. Eugene. "Minimal brain dysfunction: a hydraulic parfait model." Dis Nerv Syst 37(4): 171-73, April, 1976. (4 References).
Uses a Venn diagram to show the overlap of MBD, behavior disorders, and learning disorders. Figure 2 shows a hydraulic parfait model of MBD. Figure 3 illustrates the relationship between MBD symptoms and diagnosis. Implications of the three models are briefly discussed.

264 Conners, C. Keith. Discussion of "Models of hyperactivity." In: Hyperactivity in children: etiology, measurement, and treatment implications. Edited By Ronald L. Trites. Baltimore, Maryland: University Park Press, 1979. 21-23. (0 References).
Comments on a study by Marcel Kinsbourne and James M. Swanson (Item No. 269).

265 Douglas, Virginia L. Discussion of "The hyperkinetic syndrome." In: Hyperactivity in children: eitology, measurement, and treatment implications. Edited by Ronald L. Trites. Baltimore, Maryland: University Park Press, 1979. 137. (0 References).
Comments on a study by Hallgrim Kløve and Kjell Hole (Item No. 271).

266 Ferguson, H. Bruce, and Pappas, Bruce A. "Evaluation of psychophysiological, neurochemical, and animal models of hyperactivity." In: Hyperactivity in children: etiology, measurement, and treatment implications. Edited by Ronald L. Trites. Baltimore, Maryland: University Park Press, 1979. 61-92. (131 References).
Reviews the literature of some of the proposed models of hyperactivity--psychophysiological, neurochemical, and animal.

267 Hebb, D. O. "Physiological learning theory." J Abnorm Child Psychol 4(4): 309-14, 1976. (9 References).
This theoretical article speculates on the importance of inhibitory neurons and the role of neural connections in attention. The hyperactive child is inattentive; the cause could be a primary disorder of attention or an earlier failure of perceptual learning. Attention is seen as an aspect or consequence of perception and the concurrent cognitive activity. The problem of attention is more likely to come from internal, rather than external, noise. Inhibition is briefly discussed, and it is suggested that the child with MBD may have suffered a selective loss of inhibitory neurons.

268 Kinsbourne, Marcel. Response to discussion of "Models of hyperactivity." In: Hyperactivity in children: etiology, measurement, and treatment implications. Edited by Ronald L. Trites. Baltimore, Maryland: University Park Press, 1979. 24-27. (0 References).
Comments on his study (Item No. 269) and C. Keith Conners' criticism of it (Item No. 264).

269 Kinsbourne, Marcel, and Swanson, James M. "Models of hyperactivity: implications for diagnosis and treatment." In: Hyperactivity in children: etiology, measurement, and treatment implications. Edited by Ronald L. Trites. Baltimore, Maryland: University Park Press, 1979. 1-20. (49 References).
Describes three models (deficit, delay, and difference) of hyperactivity and reviews the literature in those areas. The question of etiology is seen as only indirectly relevant to the management of hyperactivity and does not as yet have implications for diagnosis and treatment. For commentaries on this study refer to Item Nos. 264 and 268.

270 Kløve, Hallgrim. Response to discussion of "The hyperkinetic syndrome." In: Hyperactivity in children: etiology, measurement, and treatment implications. Edited by Ronald L. Trites. Baltimore, Maryland: University Park Press, 1979. 138-39. (0 References).
Comments on his study (Item No. 271) and Virginia Douglas' discussion of it (Item No. 265).

271 Kløve, Hallgrim, and Hole, Kjell. "The hyperkinetic syndrome: criteria for diagnosis." In: Hyperactivity in children: etiology, measurement, and treatment implications. Edited by Ronald L. Trites. Baltimore, Maryland: University Park Press, 1979. 121-36. (17 References).
Presents evidence in support of two hypotheses: (1) stimulant drugs, rather than having a "paradoxical" effect, are most likely acting on a hypoactive central nervous system; and (2) if stimulant drugs are acting on a hypofunctional nervous system, there should be independent evidence supporting the hypothesis of a dysfunctional nervous system. Early development histories of the sixty-two patients in the study have been analyzed in detail in support of the second hypothesis. A high incidence of "risk factors" in pregnancy and delivery was associated with hypoaroused hyperactive children. For commentaries on this study refer to Item Nos. 265 and 270.

272 Knopf, Irwin J. "Conceptual models of psychopathology." In: Knopf, Irwin J. Childhood psychopathology: a developmental approach. Englewood Cliffs, New Jersey: Prentice-Hall, 1979. 90-123. (74 References).
Defines and analyzes various conceptual models in order to explain abnormal childhood behaviors. Models considered are: (1) genetic; (2) biochemical; (3) neurophysiological; (4) psychoanalytic; (5) sociocultural; (6) learning; and (7) humanistic.

273 Leonard, B. E. "Pharmacological and biochemical aspects of the hyperkinetic disorder." Neuropharmacology 18(12): 923-29, December, 1979. (78 References).
Reviews some of the pharmacological, neurological, and biochemical theories aimed at explaining the etiology of the hyperkinetic syndrome.

274 Porges, Stephen W. "Peripheral and neurochemical parallels of psychopathology: a psychophysiological model relating autonomic imbalance to hyperactivity, psychopathy, and autism." In: Advances in child development and behavior. Volume 11. Edited by Hayne W. Reese. New York, New York: Academic Press, 1976. 35-65. (75 References).

275 Rourke, Byron P. "Brain-behavior relationships in children with learning disabilities: a research program." Am Psychol 30(9): 911-20, September, 1975. (37 References).
Offers a neuropsychological approach to the explanation of learning disabilities and studies the factors associated with such disabilities. Also discussed are EEG abnormalities, laterality, attentional deficits, and differential score approaches.

276 Schierberl, James P. "Physiological models of hyperactivity: an integrative review of the literature." J Clin Child Psychol 8(3): 163-72, Fall, 1979. (173 References).
Reviews existing literature on the physiological concommitants of hyperactivity and organizes the findings around several basic theoretical models--biophysical, arousal, and attentional. Emphasis is placed on theoretical implications of the studies reviewed.

277 Shaywitz, Sally E.; Cohen, Donald J.; Shaywitz, Bennett A. "The biochemical basis of minimal brain dysfunction." J Pediatr 92(2): 179-87, February, 1978. (62 References).
Reviews studies that support the belief that MBD fits a medical model and suggests a biochemical basis for MBD. Central monoaminergic mechanisms may be fundamental in the pathogenesis of the clinical syndrome of MBD. Hyperactivity is discussed as a prominant symptom in MBD. Further investigation is deemed necessary.

278 Stern, W. C. A physiological model of childhood hyperkinesis. Shrewsburg, Massachusetts: Worcester Foundation for Experimental Biology, 1975.
Research in progress.

279 Williams, N. "Hyperkinesis: a behavioral and physiological comparison." Ment Retard Bull 4(1): 48-61, Spring, 1976.
Attempts to verify the hypothesis that physiological arousal is positively related to behavioral arousal and, therefore, the hyperkinetic child is physiologically overaroused. Fifty-one learning-disabled boys were used as subjects and were administered the Child Rating Scale and the Galvanic Skin Response (GSR) to measure their level (high, normal, low) of arousal. The author concludes that hyperkinesis does not reflect a state of physiological arousal, and that the child in the classroom is likely to be underaroused, rather than overaroused, in terms of GSR. Success of treatment (medication or behavior modification) is a function of the origin of the hyperactivity.

280 Zentall, Sydney S. "Effects of stimulation on activity and task performance in hyperactive children with learning and behavior disorders." For a summary see: Diss Abstr Int 35A(9): 5977, March, 1975. (0 References).

281 ———. "Environmental stimulation model." Except Child 43(8): 502-10, May, 1977. (83 References).

Suggests an alternative theoretical model of hyperactivity based on the proposition that environmental stimulation serves to decrease, rather than to increase, hyperactive behavior in the child. This understimulation model is supported by a large number of studies. Classroom treatment techniques, designed to increase stimulation and based on the above model, can include: (1) large, bright classrooms; (2) forms of movement in the classroom (pets, mobiles, moving children); (3) shortened and easier self-paced tasks; (4) frequent changes of tasks; and (5) active tasks. The roles of isolation and reinforcement are outlined.

282 ————. "Optimal stimulation as theoretical basis of hyperactivity." Am J Orthopsychiatry 45(4): 549-63, July, 1975. (81 References).
Describes the stimulus reduction theory and suggests an alternate hypothesis. Current theory and practice in the clinical and educational management of hyperactive children recommend a reduction in the amount of environmental stimulus a hyperactive child receives--assuming that the hyperactive behavior is due to overstimulation. However, through a review of existing research, evidence is presented which suggests that hyperactive behavior may result from a homeostatic mechanism that functions to increase stimulation for a child experiencing insufficient sensory stimulation.

283 Zentall, Sydney, and Zentall, Thomas R. "Activity and task performance of hyperactive children as a function of environmental stimulation." J Consult Clin Psychol 44(5): 693-97, October, 1976. (29 References).
Studies the role of environmental stimulation on activity level and task performance of a group of hyperactive children. Eleven hyperactive children (ages seven to eleven years) in a high-stimulation environment were significantly less active and performed an academically related task no poorer than when placed in a low-stimulation environment. Understimulation, rather than overstimulation, apparently precipitates hyperactive behavior; thus, the traditional theory is not upheld by this research.

C. GENETIC FACTORS

284 Abe, K. "Parent-child similarity in hyperkinesis (marked restlessness) and fear of strangers in early childhood." Jpn J Hum Genet 20(4): 288-89, 1976. (0 References).
Abstract of a conference paper.

285 Adams, Richard M. "Medication and hyperkinesis: a new concept." J Sch Health 49(4): 226, April, 1979. (2 References).
Comments on the theory that certain types of hyperkinesis associated with MBD may represent inborn errors of metabolism in which selected brain catecholamines are deficient. A more precise method of quantifying hyperkinesis is necessary before medications can be more appropriately prescribed.

286 Bannatyne, Alexander. The spatially competent child with learning disabilities (SCLD): the evidence from research. 1975. 47p. (ED 111 133).
Reviews research on hyperactive children as well as children with learning disabilities. The author supports the hypothesis that the majority (60 to 80 percent) of LD children are not brain damaged. They do, however, have above-average spatial ability and major deficits in auditory-vocal memory processing. The latter are likely to be genetic in origin.

287 ———. "The spatially competent LD child." Acad Ther 14(2): 133-35, November, 1978. (43 References).
Presents characteristics of the spatially competent learning-disabled (SCLD) child. Hyperactivity is discussed as one characteristic of the Spatial Competency with Poor Auditory Vocal Memory Functioning (SCLD) list. Emphasis is placed on inherited and situation-specific types of hyperactivity. The list is based on an earlier classification by the author. Such children are seen to be normal in spite of a right hemisphere spatial ability which dominates. The author contends that SCLD children comprise 60 to 80 percent of the LD population in schools.

288 Bernstein, Joel E.; Page, John G.; Janicki, Robert S. "Some characteristics of children with minimal brain dysfunction." In: Clinical use of stimulant drugs in children. Edited by C. Keith Conners. Amsterdam: Excerpta Medica, 1974. 24-35. (26 References). (International Congress Series, No. 313).
Focuses on some characteristics of a large group of children referred for evaluation and treatment of hyperactivity. Four hundred thirteen children (aged six to thirteen years) referred to twenty-one medical centers participated in the study. Their parents were questioned about the gestational and developmental histories of their children and about familial relationships. The parents' replies to more than 100 descriptive items were recorded on a standardized case report form. Among the most significant characteristics were: (1) a high incidence of birth complications; (2) a significant incidence of left-handedness and ordinal position; (3) frequent retardation in developmental milestones; and (4) increased incidence in hyperactivity and learning problems among the parents. General discussion follows.

289 Cadoret, Remi J.; Cunningham, Lynn; Loftus, Rosemary; et al. "Studies of adoptees from psychiatrically disturbed biologic parents. II. Temperament, hyperactive, antisocial, and developmental variables." J Pediatr 87(2): 301-6, August, 1975. (9 References).
Continues an earlier report which studied psychiatric disability in two groups of adoptees (Item No. 296). The present study analyzes other important childhood behaviors in the adoptees and relates these behaviors to the psychiatric diagnosis of the biologic parents. Two groups, experimental and control, were used to assess temperamental, hyperactive, antisocial, and developmental variables. Results of the study show: (1) male experimental adoptees had an excess number of temperament traits and antisocial behaviors; (2) no differences for females in the two groups were evident; and (3) hyperactive behavior in the adoptees of each sex was associated more with antisocial parentage than in those of "normal" parentage.

290 ———. "Studies of adoptees from psychiatrically disturbed biologic parents. II. Temperament, hyperactive, antisocial and developmental variables." In: Annual progress in child psychiatry and child development, 1976. Edited by Stella Chess and Alexander Thomas. New York, New York: Brunner/Mazel, 1977. 258-68. (9 References).
Reprints an article from the Journal of Pediatrics 87(2): 301-6, August, 1975. (Item No. 289).

291 Cantwell, Dennis P. "Familial-genetic research with hyperactive children." In: Cantwell, Dennis P., ed. The hyperactive child: diagnosis, management, current research. New York, New York:

Spectrum Publications, distributed by John Wiley and Sons, 1975. 93-105. (36 References). (Series on Child Behavior and Development, Volume 1).

Reviews currently available research evidence relating to families of hyperactive children. Discussed are psychiatric illness in the family, environmental aspects, and genetic transmission. Principal findings include: (1) a significant number of the parents of hyperactive children were themselves hyperactive as children and have increased rates of alcoholism and sociopathy; (2) there is support for the hypothesis that genetic factors play an important role (twin and adoption studies); (3) support exists for the hypothesis that there is a genetic relationship between the hyperactive child syndrome and alcoholism, sociopathy, and hysteria; and (4) little evidence is available on the effect of family environment on the hyperactive child.

292 ———. "Genetic factors in the hyperkinetic syndrome." J Am Acad Child Psychiatry 15(2): 214-23, Spring, 1976. (48 References).

Examines the role of genetic factors in the hyperkinetic syndrome. Two family studies suggest that the hyperkinetic syndrome is a familial disorder which passes from generation to generation. Adoption studies suggest that the mechanism of transmission is genetic rather than environmental. The limited evidence available from twin studies is also consistent with the notion that genetic factors play an important role in the hyperkinetic syndrome. The possible genetic mechanisms of transmission are considered: chromosome anomaly, simple autosomal dominant and simple autosomal recessive transmission, sex linkage, and polygenic inheritance. The available data best fit a polygenic model. Suggestions for future research are made.

293 ———. "Genetic studies of hyperactive children: psychiatric illness in biologic and adopting parents." In: American Psychopathological Association. Genetic Research in Psychiatry: Proceedings of the 63rd Annual Meeting of the American Psychopathological Association. Edited by Ronald R. Fieve, David Rosenthal, and Henry Brill. Baltimore, Maryland: Johns Hopkins University Press, 1975. 273-80. (28 References).

Reports the results of a study to test the hypothesis that the association between the hyperactive child syndrome and three adult psychiatric disorders (alcoholism, sociopathy, and hysteria) is genetic and that the syndrome is genetically transmitted. The data reveal that: (1) a significant percentage of the biologic parents of hyperactive children are psychiatrically ill; and (2) high rates of alcoholism, sociopahty, and hysteria are present. Further research is warranted.

294 ———. "Genetics of hyperactivity." J Child Psychol Psychiatry 16(3): 261-64, July, 1975. (18 References).

Provides evidence of a genetic component in the hyperactive child syndrome. Studies are cited which examine the biologic parents of hyperactive children, hyperactivity in twins, polygenic inheritance, and adoption. It is concluded that, according to the existing body of literature on the subject, the syndrome is a familial disorder, rather than an environmental one. Additional research is needed to support this hypothesis.

295 ———. "Minimal brain dysfunction in adults: evidence from studies of psychiatric illness in the families of hyperactive

children." In: Adult MBD Conference, Scottsdale, Arizona, 1978. Psychiatric aspects of minimal brain dysfunction in adults. Edited by Leopold Bellak. New York, New York: Grune & Stratton, 1979. 37-44. (12 References).
Reviews data on the prevalence and types of psychiatric illness in the families of hyperactive children. These conclusions are reached: (1) there seems to be an increased prevalence of the hyperactive child syndrome in the close relatives of hyperactive probands; (2) there is an increased prevalence of other psychiatric disorders in close relatives; (3) the syndrome is a familial disorder that is transmitted from generation to generation; (4) a strong genetic component operates in the genesis of the syndrome; and (5) the hyperactive syndrome may manifest itself in adults in the form of alcoholism, sociopathy, and hysteria.

296 Cunningham, Lynn; Cadoret, Remi J.; Loftus, Rosemary; et al. "Studies of adoptees from psychiatrically disturbed biological parents: psychiatric conditions in childhood and adolescence." Br J Psychiatry 126: 534-49, June, 1975. (26 References).
Assesses psychiatric problems in two groups of adoptees: group I of fifty-nine adoptees were born of psychiatrically disturbed biological parents; group II consisting of fifty-four adoptees had psychiatrically "normal" biological parents. All children had been separated from their biological parents at birth. Data were obtained through interviews with the adopting parents. The results of the research find that: (1) the incidence of psychiatric conditions was significantly higher in group I; (2) more boys than girls showed disturbance, with hyperactivity being common among the boys; and (3) there was some evidence of correlation of the type of psychiatric diagnosis of the biological parent with that of the adoptee. For a continuation study refer to Item No. 289.

297 ————. "Studies of adoptees from psychiatrically disturbed biological parents: psychiatric conditions in childhood and adolescence." In: Annual progress in child psychiatry and child development, 1976. Edited by Stella Chess and Alexander Thomas. New York, New York: Brunner/Mazel, 1977. 233-57. (26 References).
Reprints an article from the British Journal of Psychiatry 126: 534-49, June, 1975. (Item No. 296).

298 Denson, R.; Nanson, J. L.; McWatters, M. A. "Hyperkinesis and maternal smoking." Can Psychiatr Assoc J 20(3): 183-87, April, 1975. (25 References).
Investigates the role of tobacco addiction in the etiology of the hyperkinetic syndrome. The syndrome is portrayed as the result of several causes with a single causal agent being difficult to discern. Mothers of methylphenidate-sensitive hyperactive children reported smoking two to three times as many cigarettes as the mothers of dyslexic and normal controls; the reported cigarette consumption of the fathers showed no significant difference. These findings support the hypothesis that smoking during pregnancy is a factor in childhood hyperkinesis.

299 Glow, Peter H., and Glow, Roslyn A. "Hyperkinetic impulse disorder: a developmental defect of motivation." Genet Psychol Monogr 100(2): 159-231, November, 1979. (251 References).
This literature review presents and examines a theory which proposes that the hyperkinetic impulse disorder is determined interactively by polygenically inherited and environmental factors. The theory holds that the hyperkinetic impulse disorder is a developmental disorder of intrinsic

motivation, characterized by poor appreciation of the contingencies between behavior and environmental events. Characteristics of hyperkinetic impulse disorder (overactivity, impulsivity, impersistence, inattention, and underachievement in academic and social skills) are accounted for, and implications for treatment and management are explored.

300 Hersher, Leonard. "Cacography in mothers of children with LD." Pediatr Res 11(4): 562, April, 1977. (0 References).
Abstract of a conference paper presented at the Annual Meeting of the American Pediatric Society and the Society for Pediatric Research.

301 Hersher, Leonard, and Presser, Stephen E. "Cacography in the mothers of hyperactive children with learning disorders." Percept Mot Skills 46(3, pt. 2): 1041-42, June, 1978. (2 References).
Establishes a relationship between mothers' spelling errors and children with behavior and learning problems. Mothers of twenty such children completed questionnaires concerning the histories and current problems of their children. In comparison with a group of twenty control mothers, the mothers of children with learning disorders made significantly more spelling errors per 100 words. Possible reasons for this frequency are offered.

302 Miller, Lawrence G. "Genetic disease and social pathology." Ethics Sci Med 4(1-2): 29-50, 1977. (113 References).
Discusses the formulation and implications of the category of genetic disease while questioning the utility of genetic disease as a medical category. The hyperkinetic syndrome in children and the XYY abnormality are cited and examined as two types of genetic disease. The author believes that the category of genetic disease serves to place excessive emphasis on innate as opposed to environmental factors and tends to seek medical solutions to social problems.

303 Morrison, James R. "Hereditary factors in hyperkinesis." Am J Psychiatry 131(4): 472, April, 1974. (6 References).
Letter to editor.

304 Morrison, James R., and Stewart, Mark A. "Bilateral inheritance as evidence for polygenicity in the hyperactive child syndrome." J Nerv Ment Dis 158(3): 226-28, March, 1974. (15 References).
Cites recent evidence indicating that the hyperactive child syndrome can be inherited. Two modes of transmission are compatible with currently known family data: dominance with reduced penetrance and polygenetic inheritance. The present study analyzes, by methods of Slater, the family histories of twelve hyperactive children. Data analyzation shows that relatives with this syndrome or with related psychiatric conditions were found on both sides of the families more often than would be expected if the genetic component were the result of a dominant gene. Polygenic inheritance is the likely mode of transmission. These conclusions are viewed as tentative; other family studies need to be undertaken.

305 Nichols, Paul L. "Minimal brain dysfunction--genetic studies." Behav Genet 7(1): 80-81, January, 1977. (0 References).
Abstract of a paper presented at the 6th annual meeting of the Behavior Genetics Association.

306 Plomin, Robert, and Foch, Terryl. "Hyperactivity-related behaviors in a normal population of young twins." Behav Genet 8(6): 561-62, November, 1978. (0 References).

Abstract of a paper presented at the 8th annual meeting of the Behavior Genetics Association.

307 Rieder, Ronald O., and Nichols, Paul L. "Offspring of schizophrenics. III: Hyperactivity and neurological soft signs." Arch Gen Psychiatry 36(6): 665-74, June, 1979. (49 References).
Seeks to determine if the offspring of schizophrenics have an increased frequency of behavorial or neurological abnormalities by age seven. Twenty-nine male offspring of schizophrenics, plus controls, were given neurological and psychological examinations at age seven. Eight of the twenty-nine were found to have high ratings on a factor score that was termed "hyperactive" (increased activity, impulsivity, distractibility, and emotional lability); three of these boys had high ratings for neurological signs as well. These frequencies were significantly greater than in the control group. Fifteen female offspring of schizophrenics were not found to differ from their controls on these measures. Previous studies of the childhoods of male schizophrenics have found behavior patterns similar to the behavior of the boys who scored high on the hyperactive factor. It is thus likely that the "hyperactive" cases in this sample are even more at risk for developing schizophrenia in later life than the other offspring of schizophrenic parents.

308 Ruff, Carol F.; Ayers, Joyce L.; Templer, Donald I. "Hyperactivity of alcoholics and their children." Cat Sel Doc Psychol 5: 333, Fall, 1975.

309 Siggers, D. C. "Human behavioural genetics." Dev Med Child Neurol 19(6): 818-20, December, 1977. (12 References).
Hyperactivity is cited as one of several behavioral abnormalities which has genetic involvement in its etiology.

310 Welner, Zila; Welner, Amos; Stewart, Mark A.; et al. "A controlled study of siblings of hyperactive children." J Nerv Ment Dis 165(2): 110-17, August, 1977. (30 References).
Reports on a study of eighty-nine siblings of forty-three eleven-year-old hyperactive boys and 104 siblings of thirty-eight nonhyperactive boys. Among the findings it is revealed that: (1) more brothers of the hyperactive boys showed signs of hyperactivity than did the brothers of the control group; (2) both hyperactive boys and their brothers showed more depression-anxiety symptoms than did the controls; (3) the hyperactive boys, but not their siblings, presented with more antisocial symptoms than controls; and (4) WISC and Jastak Achievement Test scores were within normal limits for all groups involved in the study.

311 Wender, Paul H. "A possible monoaminergic basis for minimal brain dysfunction." Psychopharmacol Bull 11(3): 36-37, July, 1975. (0 References).
Briefly outlines the etiology, characteristics, and drug treatment for the MBD syndrome. The hypothesis is offered that MBD has a possible genetic basis and that some forms of the genetic disorder may occur as a manifestation of monoamine metabolism abnormalities. The relevance of animal models is discussed.

312 ————. "Some speculations concerning a possible biochemical basis of minimal brain dysfunction." Life Sci 14(9): 1605-21, May 1, 1974. (0 References).

Comprehensively reviews characteristic features, prevalence rates, and prognosis of the minimal brain dysfunction (MBD) syndrome. It is hypothesized that MBD is a genetic disorder of monoamine metabolism; evidence is presented in support of this hypothesis.

313 ———. "Some speculations concerning a possible biochemical basis of minimal brain dysfunction." Psychopharmacol Bull 10(4): 35-36, October, 1974. (0 References).
Delineates three genetically related groups of MBD children: (1) those with behavioral difficulties alone (often referred to as hyperactive or hyperkinetic children); (2) those with behavioral and cognitive difficulties; and (3) those with cognitive difficulties alone (usually referred to as "learning-disabled" children). Reference is made to possible biochemical etiologies.

314 ———. "Speculations concerning a possible biochemical basis of minimal brain dysfunction." Int J Ment Health 4(1-2): 11-28, Spring-Summer, 1975. (40 References).
Defines minimal brain dysfunction (MBD) and offers two hypotheses regarding this designation: (1) MBD is a broad family of disorders whose boundaries are unclear; and (2) MBD is a genetic disorder of monoamine metabolism. The conclusions of two naturalistic studies (Holman and Wender) suggest the possibility of biochemical enzyme deficit. Several methods for the assessment of monoamine metabolism are offered. For a reprint of this study refer to Item No. 688.

315 ———. "Speculations concerning a possible biochemical basis of minimal brain dysfunction." In: Learning disabilities and related disorders: facts and current issues. Edited by J. Gordon Millichap. Chicago, Illinois: Year Book Medical Publishers, 1977. 13-24. (38 References).
Reprints an article from the International Journal of Mental Health 4(1-2): 11-28, Spring-Summer, 1975. (Item No. 314).

316 Yonge, Olive, et al. "Behavioral antecedents of hyperactivity." Ment Retard Bull 6(1): 14-25, Summer, 1978. (19 References).
Reports on a questionnaire administered to fifty mothers, twenty-five of whom had hyperactive sons and twenty-five of whom had nonhyperactive sons. The questionnaire focused on the behavioral antecedents of the hyperactive syndrome. Results of the questionnaire indicate that: (1) many hyperactive boys had relatives with similar symptoms to hyperactivity; (2) hyperactive boys were more prone to come from single-parent homes; (3) fathers of such children had a greater incidence of learning problems; and (4) hyperactive boys had more difficulty with discipline and sociality.

D. NEUROLOGICAL DYSFUNCTION

317 de Quirós, Julio B., and Schrager, Orlando L. Neuropsychological fundamentals in learning disabilities. San Rafael, California: Academic Therapy, 1978. 268p. (Bibliography).
Supports a neurological basis for overt learning disorders. Neuropsychology is the study of the pathways between objective disturbances (in behavior, movement, or perception) and the cerebral or central nervous system disorders from which such disturbances originate. Discussion centers on terminology, normal developmental stages of learning, dysfunctions, current neurological examination techniques, and methods of therapy. The book is intended for teachers, psychologists, therapists, and doctors who work with LD children.

318 Dubey, Dennis R. "Organic factors in hyperkinesis: a critical evaluation." Am J Orthopsychiatry 46(2): 353-66, April, 1976. (51 References).
Evaluates data derived from studying the role of organic factors in hyperkinesis. Focus is placed on electroencephalographic, neurological, biochemical, pregnancy and birth, and genetic research. The investigation shows that the majority of hyperkinetic children do not suffer from biological dysfunction; hence, assessment should be multimodal and take educational and sociological factors into account.

319 ————. "Organic factors in hyperkinesis: a critical evaluation." In: Behavior therapy with hyperactive and learning disabled children. Edited by Benjamin B. Lahey. New York, New York: Oxford University Press, 1979. 39-48. (51 References).
Reprints an article from the American Journal of Orthopsychiatry 46(2): 353-66, April, 1976 (Item No. 318).

320 Dykman, Roscoe A., and Peters, John E. "Children with minimal brain dysfunction, frontal and temporal lobe types." Res Relat Child 37: 48, March, 1976-August, 1976. (0 References).
Abstracts a report of research in progress or recently completed research. Data are provided on: name of investigator(s), purpose of the study, number and kind of subjects used, methodology, principal findings, duration of research, cooperating group(s), and availability of publication(s). Research Relating to Children is compiled by the ERIC Clearinghouse on Early Childhood Education.

321 Flores, Eduardo G. "Hyperkinetic behaviour and absence attacks with left cerebral atrophy in children." Can J Neurol Sci 4(3): 238, August, 1977. (0 References).
Abstract of a paper.

322 Kinsbourne, M. "Mechanism of hyperactivity." In: Topics in child neurology. Edited by Michael E. Blaw, Isabelle Rapin, and Marcel Kinsbourne. Jamaica, New York: Spectrum, 1977. 289-306. (15 References).
Partial proceedings of the conference sponsored by the International Child Neurology Association.

323 Ritvo, Edward R. "Biochemical research with hyperactive children." In: Cantwell, Dennis P., ed. The hyperactive child: diagnosis, management, current research. New York, New York: Spectrum Publications, distributed by John Wiley and Sons, 1975. 83-91. (5 References). (Series on Child Behavior and Development, Volume I).
Reviews two principles of neurobiochemistry and neuropharmacology: (1) there are chemicals within the central nervous system (CNS) that transmit messages from one nerve cell to another; and (2) the CNS contains systems which work in opposition to each other to modulate or regulate functioning. Also discussed are the hypotheses set forth in a book by Paul Wender, Minimal Brain Dysfunction in Children (1971), in which Wender offers an explanation of the reaction of drugs on children with MBD. The experimental studies of Rapoport, Coleman, and Arnold are cited; findings are reviewed. Evidence to date indicates that there may be specific neurobiochemical dysfunctions within the CNS which cause hyperactivity in certain children.

324 Werry, John. "Organic factors in childhood psychopathology." In: Quay, Herbert C., and Werry, John S., eds. Psychopathological disorders of childhood. 2nd ed. New York, New York: Wiley, 1979. 542p. (Bibliography).

E. PRE- AND PERINATAL COMPLICATIONS

325 Brown, J. K.; Purvis, R. J.; Forfar, J. O.; et al. "Neurological aspects of perinatal asphyxia." Dev Med Child Neurol 16(5): 567-80, October, 1974. (10 References).
Investigates the occurrence of perinatal asphyxia and possible long-term sequelae, especially those of a neurological and intellectual nature. This study presents neurological findings for ninety-four infants who were selected from 760 asphyxiated infants born in Scotland. Abnormal behavior after an asphyxial birth and neurological examination can be used in the neonatal period to detect potentially brain-damaged infants and to make an accurate prognosis of long-term mental and neurological handicaps.

326 Colligan, Robert C. "Psychometric deficits related to perinatal stress." J Learn Disabil 7(3): 154-60, March, 1974. (14 References).
Based on the postulate that there is a continuum of reproductive casualty, it was hypothesized that potentially stressful perinatal experience could subsequently produce measurable effects on certain psychologic tests. Data were reviewed from 386 seven-year-old children whose histories confirmed that they were neurologically normal. A perinatal stress score was obtained for each child by counting the deviant symptoms during pregnancy, delivery, and puerperium. Although results marginally support the hypothesis of the study, they are not clear or systematic. Because of this, the results were not an important factor in affecting or predicting results of later psychologic tests. Difficulties in methodology are pointed out.

327 Gorman, R. F. "Minimal brain dysfunction." Med J Aust 1(8): 284, February 23, 1974. (2 References).
Letter to editor.

328 Handford, H. Allen. "Brain hypoxia, minimal brain dysfunction, and schizophrenia." Am J Psychiatry 132(2): 192-94, February, 1975. (5 References).
Seeks to establish a relationship among brain hypoxia, MBD, and schizophrenia. It is hypothesized that individuals who have survived prenatal, perinatal, or immediate postnatal hypoxia are at risk for the development of MBD, and, subsequently, schizophrenia in adulthood. Severity depends on numerous factors such as the stage of brain development when hypoxia occurred, the degree of hypoxia and resulting damage, the extent of the effects, and the patient's interaction with his family and social environment. The hypothesis and its implications for the child with MBD are discussed. Emphasis is placed on early intervention and multidisciplinary management during childhood and adolescence.

329 Husain, Arshad, and Kasham, Javad. "Maternal medication and minimal brain dysfunction." Mo Med 75(10): 508-11, October, 1978. (17 References).
Reviews the literature on the effect of drugs and chemical agents during the developmental years and reports the results of a study designed to determine if maternal medication has a causal relationship to MBD in children. From a larger population of patients referred to a pediatric devel-

opmental evaluation clinic, charts were reviewed when it was indicated that the mother had taken medication during pregnancy. The children were also evaluated for symptoms of MBD, LD, and hyperactivity. These symptoms were found for thirty-one of the sixty-two children (50 percent) in the sample; only one of the children (8.3 percent) in the control group exhibited MBD symptoms. The need for extreme caution in prescribing medication for pregnant women is emphasized.

330 Lewis, Richard S. "The brain-injury syndrome: the search for cause." In: Lewis, Richard S. <u>The other child grows up</u>. New York, New York: Times Books, 1977. 59-82. (24 References).
Identifies hyperactivity as one of several conspicuous behavior problems of the brain-injured child as well as other children who have not suffered head trauma. Several case studies of hyperactive children are documented throughout the volume. A subject index is included.

331 Lievens, Paul. "The organic psychosyndrome of early childhood and its effects on learning." <u>J Learn Disabil</u> 7(10): 626-31, December, 1974. (1 Reference).
Investigates the effect of the organic psychosyndrome--a group of psychic symptoms generally attributed to mild diffuse brain damage--on the intellectual and emotional development of a group of elementary schoolchildren. Twenty-two Belgian children (ages seven to twelve years) served as participants. The case histories of these children showed only one abnormal feature: neonatal cerebral trauma. Effects were manifested in inadequate attention and motor, emotional, and thymic control. A discussion of these effects is included.

332 Lubchenco, Lula O.; Bard, Harry; Goldman, Alan L.; <u>et al</u>. "Newborn intensive care and long-term prognosis." <u>Dev Med Child Neurol</u> 16(4): 421-31, August, 1974. (24 References).
Reports on a retrospective follow-up study to determine if low birth weight infants show a higher incidence of CNS handicaps than do other children. One hundered and fifty-one children were evaluated on incidence, type, and severity of handicaps at four years of age. Preterm children who had birth weights appropriate-for-dates had approximately the same incidence of handicap as children born at term but small-for-dates. Preterm infants cared for in the intensive care nursery and provided with intravenous fluid therapy had fewer handicaps than children cared for in the regular nursery or children in the intensive care nursery who had received only oral feedings. A high incidence of CNS disturbances, including cerebral palsy, mental retardation, and hyperactivity, was found for children who weighed more than 2500 grams at birth but were of less than thirty-eight weeks gestational age.

333 Nichols, Paul L. "Minimal brain dysfunction: associations with perinatal complications." Paper presented at the Society for Research in Child Development, New Orleans, Louisiana, March 17-20, 1977. 13p. (ED 142 017).
The relationships among perinatal complications and hyperactivity and MBD are examined. Over 28,000 seven-year-old children were surveyed. Ten perinatal antecedents were studied for possible associations. Results are reported.

334 Nichols, P. L.; Chen, T. C.; Pomeroy, J. D. "Minimal brain dysfunction: association among symptoms." Paper presented at the 84th Annual Meeting of the American Psychological Association, Washington, D. C., 1976.

335 Rubin, Rosalyn A., and Balow, Bruce. "Perinatal influences on the behavior and learning problems of children." In: Advances in clinical child psychology. Volume 1. Edited by Benjamin B. Lahey and Alan E. Kazdin. New York, New York: Plenum, 1977. 119-60. (123 References).
Briefly discusses hyperactivity as one of several problem behaviors which shows a causal relationship between perinatal influences and insults and later behavior disorders.

336 Towbin, Abraham. "Cerebral dysfunctions related to perinatal organic damage: clinical-neuropathologic correlations." J Abnorm Psychol 87(6): 617-35, December, 1978. (100 References).
Neuropathology studies in recent years have defined basic mechanisms involved in the pathogenesis of fetal-neonatal brain damage contributing to sequelant, syndromic cerebral dysfunctions. These investigations identify hypoxic processes as the main cause of perinatal cerebral damage. The acute cerebral lesions present at birth, with transition to chronic scar lesions, are correlated organically with chronic functional sequels, with elements of the syndromic tetralogy of mental retardation, cerebral palsy, epilepsy, and related psychopathy, and patterns of minimal brain dysfunction. The gestational age at the time of the hypoxic exposure and the severity of the hypoxia essentially determine the location and the extent of the damage in the cerebrum and, correspondingly, influence the pattern and severity of the sequelant cerebral dysfunctions.

F. DISEASE SEQUELAE

337 Alon, Uri; Naveh, Yehezkel; Gardos, Michael; et al. "Neurological sequelae of septic meningitis." Isr J Med Sci 15(6): 512-17, June, 1979. (32 References).
Traces the neurological sequelae of septic meningitis in a long-term follow-up study. Seventy-two children who survived septic meningitis were reevaluated after three to eleven years. Thirty-four (52 percent) of sixty-five children were found to have neurological sequelae. Of the thirty-four, fifteen had major sequelae and nineteen showed evidence of only minimal brain dysfunction--namely, hyperkinetic behavior, organic learning disturbances and minor motor disabilities. Acute-phase findings that were significantly associated with the rate of neurological sequelae were age, time between onset and admission, seizures, spinal fluid glucose level, and the number of polymorphonuclear cells. Because of the high frequency of late neurological sequelae, children who survive septic meningitis should be monitored closely in order to detect evidence of minimal brain dysfunction. An early diagnosis will help in proper management.

338 Friedman, Nathan. "Part II: Is reading disability a fusional-eye movement disability." J Am Optom Assoc 45(6): 727-82, June, 1974. (14 References).
Attributes children's learning and reading problems to fusional stresses and eye movement restrictions. Unfortunately, routine eye examinations do not usually reveal these abnormalities. Poor readers are dismissed as visually "normal." Because children with serious reading problems have fusional pain and other annoyances, they avoid reading and become hyperactive as a result of tension. A training procedure to correct these restrictions using the author's Visual Training Reading Aid (illustration included) is described. Part I of this study considers the reading disability, dyslexia, which is also attributed to fusional dysfunction.

339 Gubbay, Sasson S. The clumsy child: a study of developmental apraxia and agnostic ataxia. London, England: Saunders, 1975. 194p. (Bibliography). (Major Problems in Neurology, Volume 5).
This book is devoted to a discussion of the many neurological disorders which may cause abnormalities of motor development. Special attention is paid to the child whose clumsiness arises from a failure of the development of normal praxis--a clumsiness often observed within the symptomatology of minimal cerebral dysfunction. Hyperactivity is briefly discussed as one of the disorders allied to developmental apraxia within the spectrum of minimal cerebral dysfunction. Included are case studies, tables, and a subject index. The volume is directed toward the professional.

340 Klein, Pnina S.; Forbes, Gilbert B.; Nader, Philip R. "Effects of starvation in infancy (pyloric stenosis) on subsequent learning abilities." J Pediatr 87(1): 8-15, July, 1975. (32 References).
Traces the effects of early starvation and malnutrition on later intellectual functioning. Previous studies have shown the nutritional deficits suffered during critical periods of early life were associated with reductions in the number of brain cells, the brain being most vulnerable at this time. But because of the presence of socioeconomic and cultural variables, the effects of malnutrition on intellectual functioning have been difficult to isolate. The present study uses a naturally occurring type of malnutrition, congenital hypertrophic pyloric stenosis, to investigate the effect of malnutrition on cognitive development. Pyloric stenosis, which is disassociated with poverty or social deprivation, involves a malfunctioning of an intestinal valve. The severity ranges from minimal dehydration to gross starvation and requires surgical correction. Fifty subjects (ages five to fourteen years) who had pyloric stenosis in infancy were compared with forty-four siblings and fifty matched controls for number of specific learning disabilities and general adjustment. Learning ability was negatively correlated with the degree of severity of the starvation. Starvation resulting in a reduction of more than 10 percent of the expected body weight in infancy was associated with poorer learning abilities, especially those involving short-term memory, attention, and overactivity.

341 Nagaraja, Jaya. "The hyperactive child." Child Psychiatry Q 9(2): 1-4, 1976. (5 References).
Details a study of fifty children referred to a psychiatric facility in Hyderabad because of hyperkinetic behavior. The children (ages two to ten years) represented both urban and rural areas and exhibited overactivity, distractibility, aggressiveness, destructiveness, and excitability. Twenty-eight of the fifty were retarded. The hypothesis that the hyperkinetic syndrome can be ascribed to brain damage as a result of sequelae to disease, rather than to environment causes, is supported.

342 Thompson, Robert J., Jr., and Schindler, Francis H. "Embryonic mania." Child Psychiatry Hum Dev 6(3): 149-54, Spring, 1976. (8 References).
Documents a case study of a five-year-old boy who was originally thought to be hyperactive. The case is cited as evidence for the existence of an embryonic stage of mania--a condition not to be confused with childhood hyperkinesis. Hyperactivity is seen as an unlikely form of manic-depressive disorder, although some hyperactive youngsters can exhibit an embryonic form of mania. Caution is to be used in differentiating between hyperactivity and embryonic mania.

343 Weinberg, Warren A., and Brumback, Roger A. "Mania in childhood: case studies and literature review." Am J Dis Child 130(4): 380-85, April, 1976. (42 References).
Hyperactivity is designated as one criterion for the diagnosis of mania, an episodic disorder characterized by marked irritability and agitation, push of speech, sleep disturbance, distractibility, and noticeable mood instability for longer than one month. Five case studies are documented. The criteria for mania in children, rather than those used for adults, are discussed.

344 Wender, Esther H.; Palmer, Frederick B.; Herbst, John J.; et al. "Behavioral characteristics of children with chronic nonspecific diarrhea." Am J Psychiatry 133(1): 20-25, January, 1976. (16 References).
Discusses hyperactivity as one of numerous problems associated with chronic nonspecific diarrhea. This common syndrome of early childhood is characterized by sleep problems, crying and irritability, resistance to discipline, digestive problems, and overactivity. Possible etiologies are suggested.

G. CONCOMITANT DISORDERS

345 Authier, Jerry; Donaldson, John; Prica, George; et al. "Hyperactivity: a symptom--not a disease entity." J Fam Pract 4(5): 965-70, May, 1977. (5 References).
Uses a discussion format to explore some of the facets of the hyperkinetic syndrome. Emphasis is placed on hyperactivity as a presenting symptom of such problems as mental retardation, childhood schizophrenia, minimal brain dysfunction, neurotic conditions, or lack of discipline and internal controls. A table of symptoms is included.

346 Brumback, Roger A., and Weinberg, Warren A. "Relationship of hyperactivity and depression in children." Percept Mot Skills 45(1): 247-51, August, 1977. (23 References).
Assesses the relationship between hyperactivity and depression in a group of children manifesting school problems. Two hundred and twenty-three white middle- or upper-class children (ages six to twelve years) served as subjects and were evaluated for the presence or absence of depression and/or hyperactivity. Data show that although hyperactivity and depression can occur independently, they are frequently associated.

347 Conners, C. Keith. "Pediatric psychopharmacology and childhood depression." In: Depression in childhood: diagnosis, treatment, and conceptual models. Edited by Joy G. Schulterbrandt and Allen Raskin. New York, New York: Raven Press, 1975. 101-4. (10 References).
Comments on a study by Judith L. Rapoport (Item No. 354).

348 Hersher, Leonard. "Minimal brain dysfunction and otitis media." Percept Mot Skills 47(3, pt. 1): 723-26, December, 1978. (8 References).
Compares the frequency of otitis media among twenty-two hyperactive LD children with a sample of 772 normal children. A significantly higher percentage of hyperactive children (54 percent) had more than six episodes of otitis media; the normal group had only 15 percent. Thirty-six percent of the hyperactive group had more than ten episodes compared to 5 percent in the normal group.

349 ————. "Otitis media in hyperactive children with learning disorders." Pediatr Res 11(4): 562, April, 1977. (0 References).
Abstract of a conference paper presented at the annual meeting of the American Pediatric Society and the Society for Pediatric Research.

350 Kissel, S., and Freeling, N. W. "A brief note on the relationship between hyperkinesis and depression." New York, New York: Rochester Mental Health Center, 1974.

351 Kron, Leo; Katz, Jack L.; Gorzynski, G.; et al. "Hyperactivity in anorexia nervosa: a fundamental clinical feature." Compr Psychiatry 19(5): 433-40, September-October, 1978. (27 References).
Explores the association between heightened physical activity and anorexia nervosa. In reviewing the charts of thirty-three patients hospitalized with this illness during the past ten years, the researchers noted the presence of hyperactivity in twenty-five patients. Hyperactivity is viewed as an early and enduring clinical feature of anorexia nervosa.

352 Miller, Freeman, and Wenger, Dennis R. "Femoral neck stress fracture in a hyperactive child: a case report." J Bone Joint Surg 61(3): 435-37, 1979. (16 References).
Presents a case study of a fourteen-year-old hyperactive girl with both a stress fracture of the femoral neck and bilateral ischial epiphysis avulsion. The extreme activity of the girl produced excessive forces on the pelvis and was the probable cause of this rare combination of stress-related pelvic injuries.

353 Philips, Irving, and Williams, Nancy. "Psychopathology and mental retardation: a statistical study of 100 mentally retarded children treated at a psychiatric clinic: II. Hyperactivity." Am J Psychiatry 134(4): 418-19, April, 1977. (9 References).
In a study surveying 100 mentally retarded children referred to a University of California psychiatric clinic, thirty-nine children were diagnosed as hyperactive. No important relationship between hyperactivity and mental retardation (with or without psychosis) or brain damage was found. Further, when compared with a group of seventy-nine nonretarded children, no significant differences were noted. It is concluded that hyperkinesis is not an inevitable concomitant of mental retardation.

354 Rapoport, Judith L. "Pediatric psychopharmacology and childhood depression." In: Depression in childhood: diagnosis, treatment, and conceptual models. Edited by Joy G. Schulterbrandt and Allen Raskin. New York, New York: Raven Press, 1975. 87-100. (55 References).
Examines the relationship among hyperactivity (and other symptoms) and depression and psychopharmacology. For a commentary on this study refer to Item No. 347.

355 Snow, P. G. "Hyperkinesis and chronic constipation." NZ Med J 81(541): 515-17, June 11, 1975. (3 References).
Briefly discusses the problems of the hyperactive child who, because of soiling, has become emotionally disturbed. Frequently, the child's colon has been chronically distended due to febrile illness, but there also exists a relationship between colon stasis and hyperactivity. The condition may be exaggerated due to the smaller role of the family doctor and a diet high in carbohydrates. Eleven case reports are documented.

356 Thomas, Ellidee D. "Hyperactivity not associated with MBD." J Pediatr Psychol 1(3): 42-44, 1976. (11 References).
Reviews selected literature concerning conditions other than MBD which may have hyperactivity as a symptom. An example of this is shown by case studies of two five-year-old children whose hyperactivity was associated with sensory impairment. Other causes could be encephalitis and emotional and behavior problems. Suggestions for management of hyperactivity associated with varying underlying etiologies are offered.

357 White, James H., and O'Shanick, Greg. "Juvenile manic-depressive illness." Am J Psychiatry 134(9): 1035-36, September, 1977. (8 References).
Investigates a possible link between the hyperkinetic syndrome and manic-depressive illness. Studies are reviewed which show a positive correlation between the two syndromes; some previous reports cite cases in which manic-depressive children were often misdiagnosed as hyperactive. A case report of one fifteen-year-old boy is documented.

H. ENVIRONMENTAL INFLUENCES

1. ALLERGY

358 Cook, W. G. "Allergy, nutrition, and hyperactivity." J Learn Disabil 7(8): 524, October, 1974. (0 References).
Letter to editor.

359 Havard, Janice G. "The relationship between allergic conditions and language and/or learning disabilities." For a summary see: Diss Abstr Int 35A(11): 6940, May, 1975. (0 References).

360 Hoffer, A. "Hyperactivity, allergy, and megavitamins." Can Med Assoc J 111(9): 905, 907, November 2, 1974. (1 Reference).
Letter to editor.

361 Mayron, Lewis W. "Allergy, learning, and behavior problems." J Learn Disabil 12(1): 32-42, January, 1979. (83 References).
Examines the relationships among allergy (food, chemical, or inhalant), academic performance, and behavior problems, including hyperactivity. The allergic-tension-fatigue syndrome is discussed as well as the procedures for the diagnosis of immunologic sensitivity disease.

362 Philpott, W. H.; Mandell, M.; von Hilsheimer, G. "Allergic, toxic and chemically defective states as causes and/or facilitating facets of emotional reactions, dyslexia, hyperkinesis, and learning problems." In: Selected papers on learning disabilities. Our challenge: the right to know. Edited by A. Ansara. Pittsburgh, Pennsylvania: Association for Children with Learning Disabilities, 1975.

363 Rapp, Doris T. Allergies and the hyperactive child. New York, New York: Sovereign Books, 1979. 212p.

364 Von Hilsheimer, George. Allergy, toxins, and the learning disabled child. San Rafael, California: Academic Therapy Publications, 1974. 61p. (Bibliography).
Studies the relationship of metabolic efficiency and systemic disease to learning disabilities, behavior disorders, and emotional disturbances.

Conditions thought to be related to allergies and toxins include: (1) hyperactivity; (2) unusual fat metabolism; (3) hypothyroidism; (4) insufficient absorption of vitamins; (5) high values of lead, toxic metals, and chemicals; and (6) inability to process gluten, corn, colors, and flavorings. Methods of screening children and treatment regimens are included.

2. DIET

365 "Artificial additives and hyperactivity." Compr Ther 5(4): 7, April, 1979.

366 Banville, Thomas G. "Hyperactivity or chocolate milk?" Educ Dig 42(9): 48-49, May, 1977. (0 References).
Presents a case study of a third-grade boy who, through psychological evaluation, was found to have an allergy to chocolate milk (chocolate and milk). When these two items were eliminated from his diet, the boy's behavior improved. It is estimated that one in five children under age fifteen have some allergy, but only about one-third of these children receive treatment. The tension-fatigue syndrome is briefly discussed.

367 Boykin, Lorraine. "Nutrition and hyperkinesis: is there an association?" J Psychiatr Nurs 16(12): 45-46, December, 1978. (3 References).
Briefly discusses the role of nutrition in hyperkinesis. Evidence is presented which relates food and overactivity.

368 Brown, George W. "Food additives and hyperactivity." J Learn Disabil 7(10): 652-53, December, 1974. (0 References).
Letter to editor.

369 Burns, A. "Another approach to learning disabilities: the role of food colorings and flavors in producing hyperkinesis with learning disabled children." NYSSNTA 7(3): 29-30, Spring, 1976.

370 Crook, William G. "Adverse reactions to food can cause hyperkinesis." Am J Dis Child 132(8): 819-20, August, 1978. (9 References).
Letter to editor.

371 ———. "Food allergy--the great masquerader." Pediatr Clin North Am 22(1): 227-38, February, 1975. (55 References).
Describes the systemic and nervous system symptoms which can often be attributed to food allergies. Although these allergens are different from those causing respiratory or skin problems, they can produce symptoms of abdominal pain, headache, limb pain, fatigue, irritability, hyperactivity, cough, and secondary school and behavior problems. The "allergic tension-fatigue syndrome" is defined, and suggestions are given for diagnosing the child who might have a food allergy. The elimination diet is advocated.

372 ———. "More on food additives and hyperkinesis." Am J Dis Child 133(10): 1080-81, October, 1979. (3 References).
Letter to editor.

373 "Diet [is] not [the] cause of hyperactivity." Sci News 111(26): 406-7, June 25, 1977. (0 References).
Reports on research by a Wisconsin team of psychologists and neurologists who studied the effects of food additives on hyperactivity. No evidence

was found to support the theory that additives cause excessive motor activity. Dr. Feingold disputes these findings.

374 Divoky, Diane. "Can diet cure the LD child? You are what you eat is not necessarily so." Learning 6(7): 56-57, March, 1978. (0 References).
Critically appraises Dr. Benjamin Feingold's theory that synthetic food additives are etiological in hyperactivity and learning disorders, and that modification of the diet is the best means of treating children suffering from these disorders. Among the objections raised by the author to the Feingold K-P diet is that the treatment may mask underlying emotional and/or learning deficiencies. Educational and psychological remediation should play a part in the total treatment regimen. These therapies may be neglected when treatment is based on a purely medical model.

375 Feingold, Ben F. "Adverse reactions to food additives with special reference to hyperkinesis and learning difficulty (H-LD)." In: Man/Food Equation Symposium, London, 1973. Man/Food equation: proceedings of a symposium held at the Royal Institution, London, September, 1973. Edited by F. Steele and A. Bourne. London, New York: Academic Press, 1975. 215-34. (21 References).
Defines and classifies various kinds of food chemicals and lists the clinical patterns of disease attributed to food additives. The pharmacological interrelationships are examined, and a hypothesis is evolved which implicates food additives as etiologic agents of disease, especially childhood hyperkinesis. Also discussed are the features of the chemical patterns encountered and management aspects of children on a salicylate-free diet. Three case studies are documented.

376 ———. "Hyperkinesis and learning disabilities linked to artificial food flavors and colors." Am J Nurs 75(5): 797-803, May, 1975. (17 References).
Investigates the link between hyperkinesis and learning disabilities and artificial food flavors and colors. Feingold reports a rapid improvement in behavior and learning abilities in hyperkinetic and learning-disabled children following dietary management eliminating artificial food colors and flavors and naturally occurring salicylates. Approximately 50 percent of such children respond to strict elimination diets. Losses of hyperactivity, aggression, and impulsiveness are the initial changes observed, followed by improvement in muscular coordination, writing and drawing abilities, speech, and loss of clumsiness. Cognition and perception are usually the last symptoms to respond to the diet. All behavior-modifying drugs should be stopped while the diet is being implemented. An elimination diet is described.

377 ———. "Hyperkinesis and learning disabilities linked to the ingestion of artificial food colors and flavors." J Learn Disabil 9(9): 551-59, November, 1976. (21 References).
Reviews the background of hyperkinesis and learning disabilities, food additives, and the Kaiser-Permanente (K-P) diet, which eliminates all synthetic colors and flavors and foods containing salicylates from the diet of hyperkinetic children. Age was found to be inversely related to the speed and degree of responsiveness to dietary management. The role of artificial food colors and flavors as etiologic agents is explained and supported by the favorable response of 30 to 50 percent of various samples of hyperkinetic and learning-disabled children managed with the K-P diet.

378 ————. "The role of the school luncheon program in behavior and learning disabilities." In: U.S. Congress. House. Committee on Education and Labor. Subcommittee on Elementary, Secondary, and Vocational Education. Oversight hearings on the school lunch program: hearing. 94th Congress, Second Session. Washington, D.C.: U.S. Government Printing Office, 1976. 518-27. (0 References).
Consists of a prepared statement presented to the committee by Dr. Feingold. The statement briefly discusses characteristics, terminology, etiologic factors, classification of international additives, adverse reactions induced by flavors and colors, and the K-P diet. Three supplements accompany the statement.

379 Fitzsimon, M.; Holborow, P.; Berry, P.; et al. "Salicylate sensitivity in children reported to respond to salicylate exclusion." Med J Aust 2(12): 570-72, December 2, 1978. (21 References).
Reports on a trial designed to assess whether a reaction to salicylates could be induced in children who were thought to be sensitive to these substances, and for that reason had been maintained on the K-P diet. Twelve children (ages six to thirteen years) were selected for the study on the basis of their apparent response to the K-P diet. The children were challenged-tested with 40 mg of acetylsalicylic acid in a double-blind, crossover trial with ascorbic acid as a placebo. All children were rated according to a battery of psychological and neurological tests. Results indicate that general cognitive capacity, line-walking, and the finger-to-nose test may be impaired after the ingestion of acetylsalicylic acid. Some sleep disturbances are noted.

380 "Food additives and hyperactive kids." Sci Dig 80: 13, November, 1976.

381 Gale, Allen E. "Food additives and hyperactivity." Med J Aust 2(14): 546-47, October 2, 1976. (4 References).
Letter to editor.

382 Gaylin, Jody. "Research disputes link between hyperactivity and food additives." Psychol Today 11(5): 46, 152, October, 1977. (0 References).
Briefly reports on contradictory studies by Dr. J. Preston Harley and Dr. Ben Feingold concerning the effects of diet on hyperactive behavior in children.

383 Glaisher, I. L. "Hyperkinesis and sensitivity to aniline food dyes." J Orthomol Psychiatry 5(4): 270, 1976. (1 Reference).
Letter to editor.

384 Goyette, Charles H., and Conners, C. Keith. "Reply to Miller." Pediatrics 61(2): 327-28, February, 1978. (1 Reference).
Letter to editor.

385 Goyette, Charles H.; Conners, C. Keith; Petti, Theodore; et al. "Effects of artificial colors on hyperkinetic children: a double-blind challenge study." Psychopharmacol Bull 14(2): 39-40, April, 1978. (5 References).
Two experiments were used to evaluate the effects of artificial colors on a group of hyperkinetic children. A total of twenty-four children participated in the double-blind trials and were given challenge cookies containing artificial dyes and also placebo. Artificial food dyes are thought to

be particularly disruptive to younger children. It will be important to delineate characteristics of those who are sensitive to the dyes and to examine the possible mechanisms whereby these chemicals act on the CNS.

386 Graham, D. M. "Food additives and hyperactivity." Cereal Foods World 21(6): 248, 1976. (0 References).

387 Hawley, Clyde D. "Hyperkinesis and sensitivity to aniline food dyes." J Orthomol Psychiatry 5(4): 271, 1976. (1 Reference).
Letter to editor.

388 Hawley, Clyde, and Buckley, Robert E. "Hyperkinesis and sensitivity to aniline food dyes." J Orthomol Psychiatry 5(2): 129-37, 1976. (15 References).
Outlines the identifying characteristics of the hyperkinetic syndrome and relates those characteristics to food allergies and sensitivities. A simple method for performing the sublingual food dye sensitivity test, used to determine food allergy, is given. Two case reports are cited.

389 ————. "Sensitivity to food dyes in hyperkinetic children." J Appl Nutr 26(4): 57-61, 1974.

390 Hughes, Everett C.; Oettinger, Leon, Jr.; Johnson, Fordyce; et al. "Chemically defined diet in diagnosis and management of food sensitivity in MBD: a case report." Ann Allergy 42(3): 174-76, March, 1979. (12 References).
Describes a case illustrating both a definite etiology of food sensitivity in minimal brain dysfunction and the procedure which evolved while using diet modification on an eleven-year-old boy.

391 Institute of Food Technologists' Panel on Food Safety and Nutrition and the Committee on Public Information. "Diet and hyperactivity: any connection?" Nutr Rev 34(5): 151-58, May, 1976. (22 References).
Presents a summary statement by the Institute of Food Technologists' Expert Panel on Food Safety and Nutrition and the Committee on Public Information. The Feingold hypothesis is discussed. Further study into the relationship between diet and hyperkinesis is recommended.

392 Jani, Subhash N., and Jani, Linda A. "Nutrition deprivation and learning disabilities--an appraisal." Acad Ther 10(2): 151-58, Winter, 1974-75. (14 References).
Offers an appraisal of nutritional deprivation and learning disabilities. Internal and external aspects of deprivation are outlined. Ignorance of, or lack of concern for good nutritional habits, ingestion of interfering substances, or lack of adequate foods are cited as external causes. Internal causes include genetic defects or dependencies, stress, and malabsorption as a result of disease. More research is necessary to study fully the significance of malnutrition to the classroom teacher, and to offer practical suggestions for improved nutrition education.

393 Larkin, T. "Food additives and hyperactive children." Cereal Foods World 22(11): 582ff, 1977.

394 ————. "Food additives and hyperactive children." FDA Consum 11: 18-21, March, 1977.

Discusses the possibility of a link between hyperactive children and synthetic colors and flavors used in food. The FDA's response to this recent theory has been to require all manufacturers of foods and beverages to state on the label when artificial colors or flavors have been added, and to set up a study group, the Interagency Collaborative Group on Hyperkinesis, to further explore this area and determine the validity of this theory.

395 McDonald, K. D. "Diet and hyperactivity." Psychol Today 12(11): 7, November, 1979. (1 Reference).
Letter to editor.

396 Miller, James S. "The diet wasn't controlled." Pediatrics 61(2): 326-28, February, 1978. (0 References).
Letter to editor.

397 Norwood, Christopher. "Diet for a small madman: food chemicals and behavior." New York 10: 46-52, August 8, 1977.

398 O'Banion, Dan; Armstrong, Betty; Cummings, Ruth A.; et al. "Disruptive behavior: a dietary approach." J Autism Child Schizophr 8(3): 325-37, September, 1978. (19 References).
Investigates the effect of several foods on levels of hyperactivity, uncontrolled laughter, and disruptive behaviors of an eight-year-old autistic boy. The setting for the experiment was the boy's own room. Data were gathered during four phases: (1) while the child was fed a normal American diet; (2) while a six-day fasting period was in effect; (3) while individual foods were then presented; and (4) while foods were presented which had not provoked a reaction in phase 3. Certain foods (wheat, corn, tomatoes, sugar, mushrooms, and dairy products) were found to be instrumental in producing behavioral disorders with this child.

399 Piepho, Robert W. "Diet and MBD." J Am Pharm Assoc 17(12): 726, December, 1977. (2 References).
Letter to editor.

400 Powers, Hugh, and Presley, James. Food power: nutrition and your child's behavior. New York, New York: St. Martin's Press, 1978. 230p. (Bibliography).
Studies the relationship between diet and behavioral problems in children from infancy to adolescence. Chapter 1 includes sections on orthomolecular psychiatry and evaluation of medical care. Chapter 2 deals with glucose and the brain, the four food groups, and diet deficiencies. The malnutrition of affluence is explained in Chapter 3. The fourth chapter covers resistance to illness in terms of nutritional needs considered from prenatal through adolescent development, chronic illness, hospitalization, allergies, drugs, alcohol, and stress. In Chapter 5 these subjects are discussed: serotonin, hyperactivity, hyperkinetics, and blood sugar. Clues to future learning problems, effects of caffeine, and ways nutrition relates to behavior are explored in Chapter 6. In the final chapter tips are given that incorporate nutritional principles advocated by the authors. Numerous case studies are cited. A lengthy source list is included and appended are a homeostasis test description, and two food lists that contain the high nutrients, and the hidden sugar foods. The book is directed toward parents in particular.

401 "Pure food for healthier children." Prevention 29: 85, June, 1977.

402 Rapp, Doris J. "Does diet affect hyperactivity?" Ann Allergy 40(4): 293-94, April, 1978. (0 References).
Abstract of a conference paper.

403 ———. "Does diet affect hyperactivity?" J Learn Disabil 11(6): 56-62, June-July, 1978. (22 References).
Reports on a study in which the basic aims were: (1) to determine if dyes, foods, or allergies relate to increased activity in some children; (2) to determine if sublingual foods or food colorings are of diagnostic value; and (3) to evaluate the benefit of a diet that omits suspect foods and food colorings. Twenty-four hyperactive nonasthmatic children were referred for study. The children were tested with sublingual foods and dyes, followed by a seven-day special diet, and then by individual ingestion challenges with the same food items. Parental evaluation noted that twelve children had a moderate-to-marked improvement after the one-week diet, indicating that even a simple one-week experimental diet can be used to detect a subgroup of children whose hyperactivity can be traced to specific food dyes or foods.

404 ———. "Hyperactivity and food allergy: are they related?" Ann Allergy 40(4): 297-98, April, 1978. (0 References).
Abstract of a conference paper.

405 Relationships of hunger and malnutrition to learning ability and behavior. 1978. 24p. (ED 164 122).
Surveys the literature relative to learning and behavior and hunger, undernutrition, and malnutrition. The causal implications of nutritional problems on the hyperkinetic syndrome of childhood are evaluated.

406 Rose, Terry L. "The functional relationship between artificial food colors and hyperactivity." J Appl Behav Anal 11(4): 439-46, Winter, 1978. (28 References).
Examines the causal relationship between the ingestion of artificial food colors and an increase in selected hyperactive behaviors of two children in the regular classroom setting. Two hyperactive girls (ages eight years) were measured on out-of-seat, on-task, and physically aggressive behaviors. Research results indicate the existence of a functional relationship between the ingestion of artificial food colors and an increase in the frequency and duration of hyperactive behaviors.

407 ———. "An investigation of the functional relationship between food additives and hyperactivity." For a summary see: Diss Abstr Int 38A(11): 6653, May, 1978. (0 References).

408 Rowe, K. S., et al. "Artificial food colorings and hyperkinesis." Aust Paediatr J 15(3): 202, 1979. (0 References).
Abstract of a paper.

409 Sheridan, M. J. "Diet and hyperactivity: is there a relationship?" Am Baby 41: 26ff, August, 1979.

410 Smith, Lendon H., and Leavitt, Jerome E. Nutrition, pressures, and discipline: their impact on learning. 1979. 20p. (ED 164 144).

411 Sobotka, T. J. "Hyperkinesis and food additives: a review of experimental work." FDA By-Lines 4: 493, 1978.

412 Sprague, R. L. "Critical review of food additive studies." Paper presented at a Meeting of the American Psychological Association, Washington, D.C., September, 1976.

413 Swanson, J. "Behavioral responses to artificial color." Paper presented at the American College of Allergists Second International Food Allergy Symposium, Mexico City, Mexico, October 16-20, 1978.

414 Taub, Samuel J. "Allergies may lead to minimal brain dysfunction in children." Eye Ear Nose Throat Mon 54(4): 168-69, April, 1975. (1 Reference).
Attempts to show a connection between food allergies and subsequent learning and behavior problems in children. Cited is a pilot study conducted by Dr. Fred Kittler with twenty children (fifteen boys and five girls, ages six to seven years) who were diagnosed as having MBD. All children had abnormal EEGs and positive skin tests to inhalants; nine had apparent milk allergy; fifteen had positive skin tests to food, with milk being the most common offender. After six months of diet restriction, the children with normal intelligence showed a marked improvement in behavior and learning performance.

415 Taylor, Eric. "Food additives, allergy, and hyperkinesis." J Child Psychol Psychiatry 20(4): 357-63, October, 1979. (30 References).
Finds no persuasive evidence that intolerance to food additives is a major cause of hyperactivity. Alteration of diet should not be recommended as a routine clinical procedure. However, the controversy concerning diet does seem to indicate that more experimental work is needed.

416 Tryphonas, Helen, and Trites, Ronald. "Food allergy in children with hyperactivity, learning disabilities and/or minimal brain dysfunction." Ann Allergy 42(1): 22-27, January, 1979. (21 References).
Investigates the presence, incidence, and significance of food allergies in hyperactive, learning-disabled, and MBD children. Ninety hyperactive children, twenty-two children with learning disabilities, and eight emotional-inattentive children were selected from a larger pool and received a battery of various tests. All were tested for allergy to forty-three food extracts using the in vitro Radioallergosorbent test (RAST). Blood samples were collected and RAST scores obtained. Fifty-two percent of all children tested exhibited allergy to one or more of the food extracts. A statistically significant association was found between the number of allergies and teachers' scores of hyperactivity with the LD group. A weak association was found between a small number of children clinically diagnoseable as hyperactive and the number of allergies.

417 U. S. Congress. Senate. Committee on Labor and Public Welfare. Subcommittee on Health. Hyperactive children: examination into the causes of hyperactive children and the methods used for treating these young children: Joint hearing. 94th Congress, 1st Session, September 11, 1975. Washington, D.C.: U. S. Government Printing Office, 1976. 428p. (Bibliography). (ED 138 021).
Reprints the text of a Congressional hearing held September 11, 1975, Senator Edward Kennedy presiding. The purpose of the hearing was to investigate hyperactivity--its etiology and treatment. The thrust of the report is on the role of food additives and diet on the syndrome. Sections cover witnesses' testimony, statements, and additional information consisting of articles and reports from individuals and groups. Some reports are reprinted in full. Witnesses include Dr. Ben Feingold, Sen. J. Glenn Beall, Jr., and FDA representatives.

418 von Hoffman, N. "Chemical additives, crime and hyperkinesis." NYSSNTA 6(2): 31-32, Winter, 1975.

3. LEAD

419 Barocas, Ralph, and Weiss, Bernard. "Behavioral assessment of lead intoxication in children." Environ Health Perspect 7: 47-52, May, 1974. (15 References).
Considers two problems related to lead exposure: (1) definition of the behavioral consequences of asymptomatic lead absorption; and (2) identification of better behavioral assessment procedures. A brief review of the literature suggests ways to detect a child who, without showing blatant symptoms, might be suffering from lead intoxication. It is suggested that various techniques, e.g., psychometric testing and psychopharmacology, be used to supplement traditional assessment procedures. Emphasis is placed on examining a specific target behavior in a specified natural setting, rather than in the laboratory setting. Time sampling as a means of aiding the assessment is explored.

420 Bloom, H.; Lewis, I. C.; Noller, B. N. "A study of lead concentrations in blood of children (and some adults) of Southern Tasmania." Med J Aust 2(22): 823-24, November 30, 1974. (4 References).
Letter to editor.

421 Bryce-Smith, D., and Waldron, H. A. "Blood-lead levels, behaviour, and intelligence." Lancet 1: 1166-67, June 8, 1974. (9 References).
Letter to editor.

422 ————. "Blood levels, behaviour, and intelligence." Lancet 2: 44-45, July 6, 1974. (0 References).
Letter to editor.

423 ————. "Hyperactivity in children." Br Med J 4(5995): 521, November 29, 1975. (7 References).
Letter to editor.

424 Chaiklin, Harris, and Mosher, Barbara. "Maternal anxiety and lead levels in children." Paper presented at the Annual Meeting of the National Council on Family Relations, Philadelphia, Pennsylvania, October 19-22, 1978. 19p. (ED 169 451).
Examines the relationship between maternal anxiety and lead levels in children as evidenced in a study of the mothers of fifteen children with normal lead levels and fifteen children with elevated levels.

425 David, Oliver J. "Association between lower level lead concentrations and hyperactivity in children." Environ Health Perspect 7: 17-25, May, 1974. (17 References).
Briefly reviews the literature relating to lead levels and the hyperkinetic syndrome in children and reports on a study designed to test the hypothesis that hyperactive children have higher blood-lead levels than normal children. The subjects, all outpatients of a New York clinic, were classed as hyperactive or nonhyperactive on the basis of a doctor's diagnosis, a teachers' rating scale, and a parent questionnaire. These measures were scored: (1) blood-lead levels; (2) post penicillamine urine lead levels; and (3) scores on a lead exposure questionnaire. Data analyzation reveals that: (1) the hyperactive group had significantly

higher scores on all measures than controls; (2) there is an association between hyperactivity and raised lead levels; and (3) physicians should be aware that raised lead levels can be a causal factor in children with hyperactivity.

426 ————. "Blood-lead levels, behaviour, and intelligence." Lancet 1: 866, May 4, 1974. (1 Reference).
Letter to editor.

427 ————. "CNS effects of lower lead levels." Res Relat Child 42: 76, September, 1978-February, 1979. (0 References).
Abstracts a report of research in progress or recently completed research. Data are provided on: name of investigator(s), purpose of the study, number and kind of subjects used, methodology, principal findings, duration of research, cooperating group(s), and availability of publication(s). Research Relating to Children is compiled by the ERIC Clearinghouse on Early Childhood Education.

428 ————. "The food additive hypothesis, lead, and hyperactivity." Pediatrics 57(4): 576, April, 1976. (1 Reference).
Letter to editor.

429 ————. "Lead and hyperactivity." Res Relat Child 37: 90-91, March, 1976-August, 1976. (0 References).
Abstracts a report of research in progress or recently completed research. Data are provided on: name of investigator(s), purpose of the study, number and kind of subjects used, methodology, principal findings, duration of research, cooperating group(s), and availability of publication(s). Research Relating to Children is compiled by the ERIC Clearinghouse on Early Childhood Education.

430 David, Oliver J.; Hoffman, Stanley P.; Sverd, Jeffrey; et al. "Lead and hyperactivity." Res Relat Child 33: 75, March, 1974-August, 1974. (0 References).
Abstracts a report of research in progress or recently completed research. Data are provided on: name of investigator(s), purpose of the study, number and kind of subjects used, methodology, principal findings, duration of research, cooperating group(s), and availability of publication(s). Research Relating to Children is compiled by the ERIC Clearinghouse on Early Childhood Education.

431 ————. "Lead and hyperactivity. Behavioral response to chelation: a pilot study." Am J Psychiatry 133(10): 1155-58, October, 1976. (10 References).
Tests the hypothesis that chronically elevated lead levels in the blood may be directly etiological in some cases of childhood hyperactivity. Thirteen hyperactive children presenting with elevated blood and urine lead levels were administered a lead-chelating medication. The effects of deleading were compared for two groups: (1) six children in whom a probable etiology for hyperactivity could be determined; and (2) seven children in whom no other known cause for hyperactivity could be determined. Research results indicate that group one showed little improvement; marked improvement in behavior occurred in group two. It is concluded that the hypothesis tested could be supported by this research. Lead level measurements should be a part of the diagnostic evaluation of children with hyperactive behavior.

432 ————. "Lead and hyperactivity: lead levels among hyperactive children." J Abnorm Child Psychol 5(4): 405-16, December, 1977. (17 References).

Cites previous studies which have demonstrated an association between increased body lead burdens and hyperactive behavior in children. The present study shows that within a group of hyperactive children those for whom an organic etiology is present have lead burdens lower than in those for whom no definite etiology could be found. Eighty-four children (seventy-four boys and ten girls, mean age 8.3 years) were selected for study. All children went through an etiologic categorization procedure. The authors conclude that hyperactivity per se is not responsible for the acquisition of elevated lead levels. Implications of the findings are discussed.

433 ————. "The role of lead in hyperactivity." Psychopharmacol Bull 12(2): 11-13, April, 1976. (4 References).

Evidence is presented to test the hypothesis that minimally elevated lead levels can be etiologic in some cases of hyperkinesis, and that deleading these cases should ameliorate their hyperactive condition. Thirteen leaded hyperactive children (mean age 8.2 years), seven of whom had no known cause of their hyperactivity except increased lead levels, and six other children who had a probable other cause for their hyperactivity, were treated with a chelating agent (penicillamine [PCA]). Treatment covered a twelve-week period. Assessments were then made by various behavioral scales and questionnaires. Results show that although all but one child had significantly lower levels of lead, the behavioral effects of chelation were different for the two groups. From the data it is concluded that if an increased body lead burden can be determined as the only possible cause for the hyperactivity, more promising will be the treatment with a deleading regimen. Difficulties with methodology are pointed out as well as a need for more controlled replication.

434 Duva, Nicholas A. "Effects of asymptomatic lead poisoning of psychoneurological functioning school-age urban children: a follow-up study." For a summary see: Diss Abstr Int 38A(1): 168, July, 1977. (0 References).

435 Hole, K.; Dahle, H.; Kløve, H. "Lead intoxication as an etiologic factor in hyperkinetic behavior in children: a negative report." Acta Psychiatr Scand 68(5): 759-60, September, 1979. (15 References).

Reports on a study done in Scandinavia (Bergen) which measured lead concentration in the hair of a group of hyperkinetic children. Nineteen hyperactive boys and twenty-two controls served as subjects. Samples of 100 mg of hair were obtained and analyzed by means of atomic absorption spectrophotometry. Findings indicate that lead intoxication was not an important etiologic factor in hyperkinetic behavior in children in Bergen.

436 Landrigan, Philip J.; Whitworth, Randolph H.; Baloh, Robert W. "Blood-lead levels, behaviour, and intelligence." Lancet 1: 1167, June 8, 1974. (0 References).

Letter to editor.

437 Lansdown, R. G.; Clayton, B. E.; Graham, P. J.; et al. "Blood-lead levels, behaviour, and intelligence: a population study." Lancet 1: 538-41, March 30, 1974. (16 References).

Investigates relationships among place of residence (past and present), blood-lead levels, intelligence, reading attainments, and behavior. Four hundred and seventy-six children, under the age of sixteen (the total population of children in the East End of London), who had lived within 500 miles of a factory, were identified. Blood samples were collected from these children--all of whom had been exposed to undue amounts of lead. Various intelligence tests and behavior questionnaires were administered. Data analyzation shows that distance from the factory producing the lead pollution was related to blood-lead level, but there was no relationship between blood-lead level and mental intelligence. Lower levels of intelligence and higher rates of disturbance were seen to result from social factors. Overactivity was frequently found in those children exhibiting high lead levels.

438 ————. "Blood-lead levels, behaviour, and intelligence." Lancet 1: 1167-68, June 8, 1974. (6 References).
Letter to editor.

439 McCabe, Edward B. "Blood-lead levels, behaviour, and intelligence." Lancet 2(7885): 896, October 12, 1974. (0 References).
Letter to editor.

440 MacIsaac, David S. "Learning and behavioral functioning of low income, Black preschoolers with asymptomatic lead poisoning." For a summary see: Diss Abstr Int 37A(5): 2747, November, 1976. (0 References).

441 Millichap, J. Gordon. "Neuropsychological manifestations of lead poisoning." Ill Med J 147(2): 170-71, February, 1975. (4 References).
Outlines eight neuropsychological manifestations of lead poisoning in children: (1) acute lead encephalitis; (2) chronic lead encephalitis; (3) cerebellar ataxia; (4) convulsive disorder; (5) behavior disorder; (6) learning and perceptual disorders; (7) mental retardation; and (8) peripheral neuropathy. Early recognition of signs and symptoms and prompt therapy can reduce the number of fatalities and permanent neurologic sequelae for children suffering from lead poisoning.

442 Rummo, Judith H. "Intellectual and behavioral effects of lead poisoning in children." For a summary see: Diss Abstr Int 35B(6): 3035-36, December, 1974. (0 References).

4. LIGHTING

443 Arehart-Treichel, Joan. "School lights and problem pupils." Sci News 105(16): 258-59, April, 1974. (0 References).
Summarizes research conducted by John Ott of the Environmental Health and Light Research Institute in Sarasota, Florida. Ott maintains that inadequate and harmful fluorescent lights in school rooms can cause or aggravate hyperactivity. Through numerous classroom, plant, and animal experiments it was found that people are healthier when exposed to the total light spectrum available in nature. If deprived of specific wavelengths, particularly long ultraviolet ones, disease states--such as hyperactivity --can occur. Additional research in the area is called for.

444 Mayron, Lewis W. "Hyperactivity from fluorescent lighting--fact or fancy: a commentary on the report by O'Leary, Rosenbaum, and

Hughes." J Abnorm Child Psychol 6(3): 291-94, September, 1978. (5 References).
Comments on a study by K. Daniel O'Leary, et al. (Item No. 448) which produced negative results in a study comparing two types of fluorescent lighting, and Lewis Mayron, et al. study (Item No. 446) which produced positive results. Experimental differences in the general categories of subjects, lights, measurements, and design, are commented on.

445 Mayron, Lewis W., and Kaplan, Ervin. "Bioeffects of fluorescent lighting." Acad Ther 12(1): 75-90, Fall, 1976. (22 References).
Studies the effect of fluorescent lighting on bean seeds. The research corroborates and extends an earlier experiment (Item No. 446) in which the use of full-spectrum fluorescent lighting and radiation shielding decreased the hyperactive behavior of first-grade students in classrooms lighted previously by cool-white fluorescent lighting. Academic achievement of this group of children also improved.

446 Mayron, Lewis W.; Ott, John; Nations, Rick; et al. "Light, radiation, and academic behavior: initial studies on the effects of full-spectrum lighting and radiation shielding on behavior and academic performance of school children." Acad Ther 10(1): 33-47, Fall, 1974. (6 References).
Provides the details of a pilot experiment designed to establish and document the value of full-spectrum lighting and radiation shielding on the behavior of a group of elementary schoolchildren. Four first-grade classrooms were used, two experimental and two control. The lighting in the experimental rooms was adapted from white fluorescent bulbs. A 16mm camera, hidden from view, was used to record the motor activity of the students. Each student's behavior was rated by use of the SCORE student performance objectives. Findings indicate that the hyperactive behavior of children in the two experimental rooms decreased. Academic achievement also was shown to be significantly different among the four classrooms, but in such a way that it was unclear whether the differences resulted from the experimental conditions or from teacher differences. There appeared to be no relationship between academic achievement and decrease in hyperactive behavior. For a commentary on this study refer to Item No. 444.

447 O'Leary, K. Daniel; Rosenbaum, Alan; Hughes, Philip C. "Direct and systematic replication: a rejoiner." J Abnorm Child Psychol 6(3): 295-97, September, 1978. (11 References).
Comments on the procedural and methodological differences between a prior study by these authors (Item No. 448) and one by Mayron, et al. (Item No. 446). The two studies reached different conclusions regarding the effects of fluorescent lighting on hyperactive children's behavior.

448 ———. "Fluorescent lighting: a purported source of hyperactive behavior." J Abnorm Child Psychol 6(3): 285-89, September, 1978. (8 References).
Compares the effects of standard cool-white fluorescent lighting with a broad-spectrum fluorescent system on the hyperactive behavior of a group of schoolchildren. Seven first-grade children attended full-day sessions at a laboratory school classroom during an eight-week period. The classroom lighting conditions were alternated each week between the two types of fluorescent lighting systems. Results, assessed by independent observations of task orientation and ratings of activity level, showed no effects of lighting conditions on hyperactive behavior. For a commentary on this study refer to Item No. 444.

449 Ott, John N. "Influence of fluorescent lights on hyperactivity and learning disabilities." J Learn Disabil 9(7): 417-22, August-September, 1976. (7 References).
A pilot project was conducted by the Environmental Health and Light Research Institute in four first-grade windowless classrooms of a school in Sarasota, Florida. In two of the rooms standard fluorescent lights were used; in the experimental rooms fluorescent lights more closely duplicating natural daylight were installed. The research shows that the behavior of hyperactive children dramatically improved in the experimental room. Time-lapse pictures are included.

450 Painter, Marylyn. "Fluorescent lights and hyperactivity in children: an experiment." Acad Ther 12(2): 181-84, Winter, 1976-1977. (0 References).
Compares the effects of fluorescent and incandescent classroom lighting on the behavior of nine elementary schoolchildren. A Santa Cruz, California teacher substituted incandescent for fluorescent lights in her classroom. The hyperactive behavior of her autistic and emotionally disturbed pupils decreased by 32.3 percent. Cited are cases of other school districts' positive results obtained by replacing fluorescent lights.

5. SOCIETY/FAMILY

451 Ackerman, Peggy T.; Elardo, Phyllis T.; Dykman, Roscoe A. "A psychosocial study of hyperactive and learning-disabled boys." J Abnorm Child Psychol 7(1): 91-99, March, 1979. (17 References).
Compares three groups of boys (hyperactive, normally behaved learning-disabled (LD), and normal controls) on tests measuring personality traits, cognitive role-taking, and moral reasoning. The boys were rated by parents and teachers on a number of behaviors; parents were interviewed to assess home stimulation potential. Hyperactive boys were rated more aggressive and anxious than LD boys and controls and had not been encouraged as much by parents to achieve. Hyperactives had been born to younger parents, on the average, and 25 percent lived with their mothers and stepfathers. None of the LD or control boys had stepfathers. The groups did not differ significantly in moral reasoning ability, cognitive role-taking, or locus of control; on the Junior Personality Inventory hyperactives tended to have elevated scores on the neuroticism scale while LD boys had higher scores on the lie scale.

452 Alley, Gordon R.; Forsyth, Robert A.; Snider, Bill; et al. "Comparative parental MMPI protocols of children evaluated at a child development clinic." Psychol Rep 35(3): 1147-54, December, 1974. (10 References).
Reports on a study which examined the relationship between parental psychopathology and childhood behavior disorders. All parents at a clinic completed the Minnesota Multiphasic Personality Inventory (MMPI) upon evaluation of their child; 144 pairs of parents were selected for the study. This sample was divided according to the diagnostic categories of the child: (1) MBD; (2) behavior disorder; and (3) normal. Analysis of the data acquired by comparing MMPI scores and clinical scores showed significant differences when both mothers' and fathers' scores were combined. Although parents could not be differentiated on the basis of MMPI scales, they could be identified by the test-taking attitude of the mothers of the behaviorally disturbed children.

453 Anderson, Daniel R.; Levin, Stephen R.; Lorch, Elizabeth P. "The effects of TV program pacing on the behavior of preschool children." AV Commun Rev 25(2): 159-66, Summer, 1977. (15 References).
Examines the short-term effects of TV program pacing on the subsequent behavior of young children. Also tested was the hypothesis that TV in general, and Sesame Street in particular, produces hyperactivity, impulsivity, disorganized behavior, and shortened attention spans in preschool children. Seventy-two children (age four years) were given a forty-minute medium experience followed by a twenty-minute testing and observation session. No support was found for any immediate effects of TV program pacing on the behavior of preschool children.

454 Blair, Carole. "Hyperactivity in children: viewed within the framework of synergistic man." Nurs Forum 18(3): 293-303, 1979. (19 References).
Discusses the synergistic school of thought which suggests that the range of behaviors displayed by the hyperactive child reflects a changing pattern of interaction with the environment. Man is viewed as a whole and cannot be perceived or predicted from viewing the parts. Diversity and variability within and between individuals must be respected. Implications for the hyperactive child are discussed.

455 Block, Gerald H. "Hyperactivity: a cultural perspective." J Learn Disabil 10(4): 236-40, April, 1977. (30 References).
Contrary to existing studies which attribute the etiology of hyperactivity to organic or emotional factors originating within the child or his immediate home environment, this study suggests that cultural factors can also be a source of such behavior. These cultural changes include: (1) family factors; (2) diet; (3) accelerated pace of life; (4) crowding; and (5) exposure to lead, noise, etc. A new direction for research is called for which requires the involvement of an interdisciplinary team.

456 Conrad, Peter. "Situational hyperactivity: a social system approach." J Sch Health 47(5): 280-85, May, 1977. (26 References).
Offers a sociological approach to explain the hyperactive syndrome in children. This approach is often termed "labeling" or "interactionist perspective" and focuses on social reaction to behavior. Deviance is defined by a social audience and is viewed as a status attributed by others as a response to behavior. The hyperactive child is seen as an actor in a social system. The social system approach is offered as a contrasting model to the medical-clinical model. Two case studies of situational hyperactivity are cited.

457 Cunningham, Charles E., and Barkley, Russell A. "The role of academic failure in hyperactive behavior." J Learn Disabil 11(5): 274-80, May, 1978. (47 References).
Explores the possibility of academic failure as a cause of the behavioral patterns observed in many hyperactive children. These negative behavioral patterns may persist due to inadvertent social responses of both teachers and peers. Treatment predictions, confirmed by outcome research, indicate that interventions directed only toward behavior will not result in improvements in academic achievement. It was found, however, that if remedial measures are taken to improve academic performance, behavior will improve as well.

458 Fouts, Gregory T. Effect of social reinforcement on infant activity: a pilot study. 1974. 10p. (ED 103 103).

This pilot study was designed to suggest an experimental interpretation of the development of extreme activity levels in infants and to demonstrate maternal influence on that level. It is suggested that early infancy be established as the target age for prevention/elimination of hyperactivity.

459 Friedman, Ronald J. "MMPI characteristics of mothers of preschool children who are emotionally disturbed or have behavior problems." Psychol Rep 34(3, pt. 2): 1159-62, June, 1974. (5 References).
Reports the use of the Minnesota Multiphasic Personality Inventory (MMPI) in identifying psychological deviancy patterns in parents of children showing emotional or behavioral problems. MMPI profiles were obtained for mothers of a group of preschool children. Mothers of children with emotional problems scored higher than controls in the areas of depression, psychopathic deviate, psychasthenia, schizophrenia, and hypomania; mothers of children with behavior problems differed from controls only on the hypomania scale. A discussion of the causes or effects of maternal maladjustment on deviant behavior in children follows.

460 Halpern, Werner I. "Turned-on toddlers: the effects of television on children and adolescents." J Commun 25(4): 66-70, Autumn, 1975. (13 References).
Assesses the role of television as a contributing factor to childhood behavior disorders. Since parents depend more and more on television as a baby-sitter and teacher of their children, many children are the recipients of a daily stimulus--a rich, one-way, jived-up, and repetitious auditory and visual experience. The result is a sensory overkill for many children, especially the immature child whose neurological equipment is underdeveloped. The sensory overload may precipitate more than transient behavior problems. The situation becomes educationally counterproductive "because it violates a necessary synthesis between developmental readiness and responsible adult responsiveness to the receptive child."

461 Henderson, Arvin; Dahlin, Irmeli; Partridge, Cloyd; et al. "Reply to Dr. Oettinger." Pediatrics 54(4): 514, October, 1974. (0 References).
Letter to editor.

462 Horner, Peter L. "Effects of physical-environmental stimulation on hyperactive child behaviors." For a summary see: Diss Abstr Int 39B(5): 2502-3, November, 1978. (0 References).

463 Langmeier, J., and Matějček, Z. Psychological deprivation in childhood. Edited by G. L. Mangan. New York, New York: Wiley, 1975. 496p. (Bibliography).
Chapter 10, "A theory of psychological deprivation," compares and contrasts hyperactive and hypoactive children and the effect of deprivation upon them. Institutionalized children were used to identify these two basic types.

464 Langsdorf, Richard; Anderson, Robert P.; Waechter, Donna; et al. "Ethnicity, social class, and perception of hyperactivity." Psychol Sch 16(2): 293-98, April, 1979. (11 References).

Examines the relationship between ethnicity and hyperactivity and challenges the assumption that hyperactivity is uniformly distributed across ethnic groups. One thousand seven hundred nineteen black, white, and Mexican-American elementary schoolchildren were surveyed. The Abbreviated Conners Teacher Rating Scale was used to identify the hyperactive groups. Two findings emerged: (1) the 15 percent overall incidence rate is substantially higher than previously reported in the literature for large samples; and (2) in those schools with nonwhite majorities, teachers rated black children as significantly more often hyperactive and Mexican-American children as significantly less often hyperactive than would be expected, based on their representation in the general student body. These findings are interpreted from a sociological perspective.

465 Lewis, Barbara J. "Sensory deprivation in young children." Child Care Health Dev 4(4): 229-38, July-August, 1978.
Discusses sensory deprivation in young children. Focus is placed on the implications of sensoristasis for those children whose environments do not provide sufficient stimulation (often resulting in hyperactivity or withdrawal), or for those prevented from exploring their environments because of motor deficits. Experimental work and research in the area are reviewed.

466 Lowitt, Michael F., et al. "Family psychopathology in parent-child relationships." Paper presented at the 52nd Annual Meeting of the American Orthopsychiatric Association, Washington, D.C., March 22-24, 1975. 18p. (ED 113 636).
Comments on how parents' personalities and child-raising techniques influence the development and pathology of their offspring.

467 Mayron, Lewis. "Ecological factors in learning disabilities." J Learn Disabil 11(8): 40-50, October, 1978. (103 References).
The link between environmental causes and learning and behavior disorders is investigated. Five classifications, considered etiological, that involve factors in the environment of the child are discussed: anxiety, malnutrition, toxicity, allergy, and technical pollution. Hyperactivity is perceived as the result of anxiety or chronic arousal due to constant internal or external pressure.

468 Morrison, James R. "Parental divorce as a factor in childhood psychiatric illness." Compr Psychiatry 15(2): 95-102, March-April, 1974. (16 References).
Examines the relationship between divorce of parents and psychiatric disturbance in children. Also considered are the antecedents of the divorce or the possibility that parental divorce and childhood psychiatric illness may both be related secondarily to a common background factor. Personal interviews to determine psychiatric status were conducted with the parents of 127 children in 1971/1972. The interviewer was unaware of the status and history of the child. Detailed tables display these findings and correlations. Research indicates that the question of etiology of psychopathology cannot be conclusively answered at this time. More studies involving a larger population are needed before determining what is cause and what is effect.

469 Oettinger, Leon, Jr. "Hyperactivity: the Henderson-Dahlin-Partridge-Engelsing hypothesis." Pediatrics 54(4): 514, October, 1974. (1 Reference).
Letter to editor.

470 Panton, W. D. "The hyperactive child." Can Med Assoc J 112(9): 1042, May 3, 1975. (0 References).
Letter to editor.

471 Paternite, Carl E. "Childhood hyperkinesis: a cross-sectional and longitudinal examination of the relationships and symptomatology and the home or family subenvironment." For a summary see: Diss Abstr Int 38B(7): 3411, January, 1978. (0 References).

472 Paternite, Carl E.; Loney, Jan; Langhorne, John E., Jr. "Relationships between symptomatology and SES-related factors in hyperkinetic/MBD boys." Am J Orthopsychiatry 46(2): 291-301, April, 1976. (30 References).

Studies the relationship among symptomatology, socioeconomic status (SES), and parenting styles in a group of children. One hundred and thirteen hyperkinetic/MBD boys (mean age 8.2 years), outpatients at a child psychiatric clinic, and living with their families, served as subjects. Five pieces of information gathered from the boys' case histories were used to classify the sample into SES groups. Primary symptoms (e.g., hyperactivity) did not vary as a function of SES, but SES-related differences emerged for secondary symptoms (e.g., aggressive behavior, self-esteem deficits, etc.) and for parenting variables. Parenting variables were found to be better predictors of secondary symptoms than was SES. The need for replication and extension of these findings is stressed.

473 ————. "Relationships between symptomatology and SES-related factors in hyperkinetic/MBD boys." In: Annual progress in child psychiatry and child development, 1977. Edited by Stella Chess and Alexander Thomas. New York, New York: Brunner/Mazel, 1977. 342-55. (30 References).

Reprints an article from the American Journal of Orthopsychiatry 46(2): 291-301, April, 1976 (Item No. 472).

474 ————. "Relationships between symptomatology and SES-related factors in hyperkinetic/MBD boys." In: Behavior therapy with hyperactive and learning disabled children. Edited by Benjamin B. Lahey. New York, New York: Oxford University Press, 1979. (30 References).

Reprints an article from the American Journal of Orthopsychiatry 46(2): 291-301, April, 1976 (Item No. 472).

475 Whaley-Klahn, Mary Anne, and Loney, Jan. "A multivariate study of the relationship of parental management to self-esteem and initial drug response in hyperkinetic/MBD boys." Psychol Sch 14(4): 485-92, October, 1977. (14 References).

Studies the parenting characteristics of the mothers and fathers of a group of hyperkinetic boys, the self-esteem of these boys at referral, and their response to CNS medication. Eighty-three boys (ages four to twelve years), predominantly white, and all students at an outpatient child psychiatry clinic, served as subjects. Results of the research show: (1) mothers of children with more severe self-esteem deficits did not describe themselves as too strict, were rated higher in the direction of hostility, listed fewer self-reported shortcomings, and described their husbands as too demanding; and (2) fathers of these lower self-esteem boys tended not to describe themselves as too demanding. Also identified were four predictors of response to CNS stimulant medication and mother and father variables contributing to their child's response. Implications of the findings are discussed.

476 Zassler, Philip H. "Neurological disorganization and socioeconomic status." For a summary see: Diss Abstr Int 34A(12, pt. 1): 7616-17, June, 1974. (2 References).

IV. Diagnosis

A. DIAGNOSTIC EVALUATION

477 Adler, Sidney, and Steinberg, Russell M. "The pediatric examination and MBD." In: Learning disabilities and related disorders: facts and current issues. Edited by J. Gordon Millichap. Chicago, Illinois: Year Book Medical Publishers, 1977. 39-43. (15 References).
Offers suggestions to the physician for differential diagnosis. Nineteen major entities are given and eleven "hallmarks" of learning disabilities are listed.

478 Ament, Aaron. "The learning-disabled or hyperactive child." JAMA 235(15): 1552-53, April 12, 1976. (1 Reference).
Letter to editor.

479 Anderson, Robert P., et al. "The assessment and modification of hyperkinesis: a review of programmatic research at Texas Tech University." Paper presented at the 3rd International Scientific Conference of IFLD, Montreal, Canada, August 9-13, 1976. 15p. (ED 135 127).
Reviews studies on hyperkinesis in learning-disabled children conducted at Texas Tech University over the past ten years.

480 Boyle, J. P. "Psychophysiological support for differentiated diagnosis in the hyperactivity syndrome." Greeley, Colorado: University of Northern Colorado, 1974.
Unpublished manuscript.

481 Cantwell, Dennis P. "Diagnostic evaluation of the hyperactive child." In: Cantwell, Dennis P., ed. The hyperactive child: diagnosis, management, current research. New York, New York: Spectrum Publications, distributed by John Wiley and Sons, 1975. 17-50. (45 References). (Series on Child Behavior and Development, Volume I).
Outlines evaluation procedures which should ideally be carried out with every child referred for hyperactivity. Covered are: (1) interview with the parents; (2) interview with the child; (3) behavior rating scales; (4) physical examination; (5) neurologic examination; and (6) laboratory studies. A twenty-seven point sample interview with the child is reprinted.

482 ———. "A medical model for research and clinical use with hyperactive children." In: Cantwell, Dennis P., ed. The hyperactive child: diagnosis, management, current research. New York, New

York: Spectrum Publications, distributed by John Wiley and Sons, 1975. 193-205. (20 References). (Series on Child Behavior and Development, Volume I).
Sets forth a six-stage model for clinical and research work with hyperactive children. The model integrates data from the previous chapters of the book into the following stages of investigation: (1) clinical description of the behavior problem; (2) systematic physical and pediatric neurologic examination; (3) investigation of laboratory results; (4) study of psychiatric disorder in, and the relationship between, family members; (5) use of prospective and retrospective follow-up studies; and (6) subdivision of the index population of patients according to response to treatment.

483 ————. "A model for the investigation of psychiatric disorders of childhood: its application in genetic studies of the hyperkinetic syndrome." In Anthony, E. James, ed. Explorations in child psychiatry. New York, New York: Plenum, 1975. 57-79. (46 References).
Presents a six-stage model for investigating the hyperkinetic syndrome: (1) clinical description; (2) physical and neurologic factors; (3) laboratory studies; (4) family studies; (5) natural history studies; and (6) treatment studies. Applications for the model are provided. The author outlines some common misconceptions surrounding the syndrome.

484 Clements, Sam D. "The clinical psychological assessment of minimal brain dysfunctions." In: Clinical use of stimulant drugs in children. Edited by C. Keith Conners. Amsterdam: Excerpta Medica, 1974. 36-43. (1 Reference). (International Congress Series, No. 313).
Examines the relationship between an evaluating psychologist or team and the school system with reference to the detection and treatment of MBD. Also discussed are: (1) the importance of preassessment data; (2) diagnostic labels; (3) the role of special education; and (4) the value of the multidisciplinary team.

485 Cole, Sherwood O., and Moore, Samuel F. "The hyperkinetic child syndrome: the need for reassessment." Child Psychiatry Hum Dev 7(2): 103-12, Winter, 1976. (31 References).
Some of the relevant issues pertaining to the hyperactive child are discussed in terms of: (1) diagnostic practices; (2) treatment practices; and (3) changing views about the nature of the disorder itself. Rather than focusing on the child as a source of the problem (as had typically been the case), future research and practices need to demonstrate a broad-based perspective on the adjustment problems of these children that examines "situational" determinants and institutional policies.

486 Duncan, Melba H. "Attention deficit disorder (ADD) 1980: unnecessary mistakes in diagnosis and treatment of learning and behavior problems of the MBD/hyperactive syndrome." J Clin Child Psychol 8(3): 180-82, Fall, 1979. (8 References).
Calls attention to errors which can occur in the diagnosis and management of hyperactivity. Such mistakes include: (1) inflexible family-centered diagnostic orientation; (2) deficient habits in obtaining histories, report-writing, and postdiagnostic follow-up; and (3) special education semantic errors that lead in wrong directions.

487 Fremont, Theodore S.; Seifert, David M.; Wilson, John H. Informal diagnostic assessment of children. Springfield, Illinois: Thomas, 1977. (Bibliography).
Divided into four major chapters, this book covers classroom evaluation, developmental history, brain dysfunctions, and emotional evaluation. Chapter III on brain dysfunctions explores indicators which suggest neurological and perceptual malfunctioning. Hyperactivity is considered as one of nine diagnostic components of MBD.

488 Gardner, Richard A. The objective diagnosis of minimal brain dysfunction. New Jersey: Creative Therapeutics, 1979. 452p.
Presents a comprehensive overview for the practicing psychologist, pediatrician, and educator. Topics covered include: hyperactivity, attentional deficit and distractibility, impulsivity, motor coordination, soft neurological signs, auditory and visual processing, aphasias, agnosias and apraxias, intelligence, and socialization problems.

489 Keele, Marjorie S., and Huizinga, Raleigh J. "Role of special pediatric evaluation in the evaluation of a child with learning disabilities." J Learn Disabil 8(1): 40-45, January, 1975. (15 References).
Investigates three aspects of the special pediatric examination of the child with LD: (1) the reliability of the examination in correctly identifying the child with LD; (2) the proportion of LD children who show signs; and (3) the identification of LD children who are benefited by a special pediatric evaluation. Two pediatric specialists, utilizing nine pediatric factors, diagnosed LD correctly in 91 percent of the 629 cases evaluated, but overdiagnosed it in 30 percent of nonlearning-disabled children. Thus, it is recommended that the special pediatric evaluation by a specialist is indicated for a LD child with motor hyperactivity and in certain other instances.

490 Kinsbourne, Marcel. "Hyperactivity: diagnosis." Except Parent 8(4): 9-12, August, 1978.
Describes characteristics and identification techniques in the infant, preschool child, kindergarten, and elementary school student.

491 Klein, Donald F., and Gittelman-Klein, Rachel. "Diagnosis of minimal brain dysfunction and hyperkinetic syndrome." In: Clinical use of stimulant drugs in children. Edited by C. Keith Conners. Amsterdam: Excerpta Medica, 1974. 1-11. (3 References). (International Congress Series, No. 313).
Calls attention to the difficulties involved in diagnosing hyperkinesis and MBD. The question of predicting good and poor drug responders is also addressed. General discussion follows.

492 ————. "Problems in the diagnosis of minimal brain dysfunction and the hyperkinetic syndrome." Int J Ment Health 4(1-2): 45-60, Spring-Summer, 1975. (8 References).
Reports on a study conducted with 155 children in an attempt to identify those who were "pervasively hyperactive." Since school was the usual source of complaint of hyperactivity, only children who showed hyperactivity in at least one other setting besides the school were selected. A scale was used to measure activity at home. On eleven items, scored on a five-point scale, the child had to obtain a minimum score of twenty-eight (of a possible forty-four) to be considered hyperactive at home. Among the children who were evaluated as hyperactive, some of them had

such severe family pathology as to give the impression that the child had an adjustment reaction. It is pointed out that when diagnosing hyperactivity, cultural factors cannot be ruled out since there may be subcultural standards for activity level at variance with general standards. For a reprint of this study refer to Item No. 688.

493 Lambert, C. Timothy; O'Donell, Alice A.; Caldwell, Bill S., Jr. "Evaluation of the hyperactive child." J Fam Pract 2(6): 465-70, December, 1975. (4 References).
Uses a discussion format to comment on some of the important issues in evaluating the hyperactive child. Topics covered include: history-taking, psychological testing, and neurological examination.

494 Lambert, Nadine; Yandell, Wilson; Sandoval, Jonathan. "Factors associated with identification and treatment of hyperactive children." Res Relat Child 34: 142, March, 1974-August, 1974. (0 References).
Abstracts a report of research in progress or recently completed research. Data are provided on: name of investigator(s), purpose of the study, number and kind of subjects used, methodology, principal findings, duration of research, cooperating group(s), and availability of publication(s). Research Relating to Children is compiled by the ERIC Clearinghouse on Early Childhood Education.

495 Morgan, L. Y.; Juberg, R. C.; Hardman, R. P. "Digital, palmar, and hallucal dermatoglyphics of hyperactive subjects." Clin Res 26(6): A813, December, 1978. (0 References).
Abstract of a conference paper presented at a meeting of the Southern Society for Pediatric Research.

496 Sambrooks, J., and Robards, M. "The hyperactive child: objective assessment." Arch Dis Child 51(9): 732, September, 1976. (2 References).
Abstract of a conference paper presented at the Paediatric Research Society of London.

497 Schain, Richard J. "Etiology and early manifestations of MBD." In: Learning disabilities and related disorders: facts and current issues. Edited by J. Gordon Millichap. Chicago, Illinois: Year Book Medical Publishers, 1977. 25-31. (2 References).
Discusses numerous factors, e.g., tests, EEG, conversation with the child, and seizure history, which can aid the physician in the diagnosis of hyperactivity. Characteristic symptomatology is given.

498 Stevens, Gwendolyn R. "Socio-cultural variables and assessment: a test of the interactionist position on the assessment of the hyperkinetic syndrome." For a summary see: Diss Abstr Int 39A(5): 2846, November, 1978. (0 References).

499 Sulzbacher, Stephen I. "The learning-disabled or hyperactive child." JAMA 235(15): 1553, April 12, 1976. (0 References).
Letter to editor.

500 ———. "The learning-disabled or hyperactive child: diagnosis and treatment." JAMA 234(9): 938-41, December 1, 1975. (9 References).
Proposes a diagnostic procedure which emphasizes the acquisition of differential diagnostic information. Properly performed, the procedure is

useful in choosing the most valuable mode of treatment for a given child. Basically, the technique calls for: (1) conducting a complete clinical examination; (2) investigating the referral complaint; (3) pinpointing the problem behavior by recording the frequency of specific behavior deviations in the classroom and at home; and (4) determining the correct dosage of medication. Several new ideas in the treatment of MBD that are reviewed are: (1) encouraging the child and teaching him how to express anger constructively; (2) using encounter techniques; and (3) encouraging biofeedback or autosuggestion to help the child develop self-control.

501 Svoboda, William B. "Specific learning disabilities in children." W Va Med J 70(1): 1-4, January, 1974. (0 References).
The concepts of specific learning disabilities and the manifestations related to these problems are presented with the concept of diagnostic approaches for the specific disabilities to derive specific remediative approaches. Specific learning disability is defined as a cluster of learning problems which results from a disorder of one or more of the basic psychologic processes involved in the understanding or usage of spoken or written language. Although the syndrome is shrouded by numerous diagnostic terms of nonspecific nature, certain manifestations point to its existence: (1) a child who performs beneath his ability; (2) a child who learns through hearing and is unable to learn by sight; (3) a child who experiences difficulties in recognizing and processing stimuli; (4) a child who exhibits spatial confusion; and (5) a child who is uncoordinated or hyperkinetic. The importance of the medical history is emphasized. The diagnostic approaches as utilized by the West Virginia Medical Center Learning Disabilities Clinic are outlined and the aims of remedial approaches briefly presented.

502 Willoughby, Robert H. "Behavioral assessment of childhood hyperactivity." Res Relat Child 41: 111-12, March, 1978-August, 1978. (0 References).
Abstracts a report of research in progress or recently completed research. Data are provided on: name of investigator(s), purpose of the study, number and kind of subjects used, methodology, principal findings, duration of research, cooperating group(s), and availability of publication(s). Research Relating to Children is compiled by the ERIC Clearinghouse on Early Childhood Education.

503 Walker, Sydney. "Drugging the American child: we're too cavalier about hyperactivity." Psychol Today 8(7): 43-48, December, 1974. (0 References).
Presents medical case histories from the files of a neuropsychiatrist. The cases illustrate the need for a multidimensional approach to the diagnosis of hyperactivity, rather than the prescription of drugs. Cited are examples of hyperactivity due to poor oxygenation, low glucose level, ingestion of inedible substances, brain lesions, and mixed dominance. Care must be used that psychoactive stimulants do not merely mask, without curing, the symptoms of hyperactivity.

504 ———. "Drugging the American child: we're too cavalier about hyperactivity." J Learn Disabil 8(6): 354-58, June, 1975. (0 References).
Reprints an article from Psychology Today 8(7): 43-48, December, 1974. (Item No. 503).

B. EARLY IDENTIFICATION

505 Appelbaum, Alan S. "Diagnostic considerations in the evaluation of hyperkinetic children." J Pediatr Psychol 3(3): 24-26, Summer, 1975.
Stresses the importance of early identification of the hyperactive child and the value of obtaining a detailed medical and behavioral history for proper diagnosis. Neurological examination, psychological testing, and psychiatric interviews may also be helpful. It is important to survey the total functioning of the family as an aid in the management of the child.

506 Bailey, Edward N.; Kiehl, Phyllis S.; Akram, Dure S.; et al. "Screening in pediatric practice." Pediatr Clin North Am 21(1): 123-65, February, 1974. (273 References).
This lenghty review article is devoted to several components of pediatric care: screening, preventive care, and health maintenance. Emphasis is placed on the importance of early diagnosis and the screening tests used for evaluation. Behavioral disorders and MBD are discussed as well as growth, vision, hearing and speech disorder, heart disease, hypertension, anemia, lead poisoning, congenital hip disease, developmental disorders, metabolic disease, etc. Recommendations for early screening are outlined for each syndrome, providing measures are available. An accompanying table summarizes the recommendations made in the text.

507 Burg, Cheryl; Quinn, Patricia O.; Rapoport, Judith L. "Clinical evaluation of one-year-old infants: possible predictors of risk for the 'hyperactivity syndrome'." J Pediatr Psychol 3(4): 164-67, 1978. (16 References).
Evaluates the usefulness of temperament and anomaly measures in predicting later behavior problems, including the hyperkinetic syndrome. One hundred and twenty-three infants were selected from a normal newborn screening of 933 infants on the basis of minor physical anomalies. At one year of age the infants were rated by parents and a psychologist. Significant associations indicate the usefulness of a temperament scale for infant behavior studies. Some association was found between anomaly score and fussy irritable behavior.

508 Cantwell, Dennis. "Early interventions with hyperactive children." J Oper Psychiatry 5: 56-67, 1974.

509 Fidone, George S. "Recognizing the precursors of failure in school." Clin Pediatr 14(8): 768-70, 75-78, August, 1975. (21 References).
Emphasizes the need to identify educationally high-risk children in the preschool years. Early identification can aid in proper planning and management of the child's needs. The physician must be aware of the relationship between high-risk categories and future educational failure and accept responsibility for the child's well-being. Also discussed are the characteristics of certain educationally vulnerable children. Some practical suggestions regarding their early management are offered.

510 Kinsbourne, Marcel. Discussion of "Can hyperactives be identified in infancy?" In: Hyperactivity in children: etiology, measurement, and treatment implications. Edited by Ronald L. Trites. Baltimore, Maryland: University Park Press, 1979. 116-19. (1 Reference).
Comments on a study by J. L. Rapoport, et al. (Item No. 512).

511 Lodge, Ann. "Determination and prevention of infant brain dysfunction: sensory and nonsensory aspects." In: Winter Conference on Brain Research: Environments as therapy for brain dysfunction. Edited by Roger N. Walsh and William T. Greenough. New York, New York: Plenum Press, 1976. 310-42. (135 References). (Advances in Behavior Biology, Volume 17).
Discusses available assessment procedures and some therapeutic approaches relating to infant brain dysfunction. Emphasized is the need for more precise identification of both the sensory and nonsensory factors which affect infant neurodevelopmental processes and the nature of their susceptibility to environmental influences. This paper is part of the proceedings of a workshop series at the Winter Conference on Brain Research held in Steamboat Springs, Colorado, January, 1975.

512 Rapoport, J. L.; Quinn, P. O.; Burg, C.; et al. "Can hyperactives be identified in infancy?" In: Hyperactivity in children: etiology, measurement, and treatment implications. Edited by Ronald L. Trites. Baltimore, Maryland: University Park Press, 1979. 103-15. (25 References).
Studies the prediction of hyperactivity in infancy. The authors conclude that the combination of temperament, background factors, and anomalies may prove helpful in predicting later problems. Research is cited which supports the idea of congenital contributors to behavior. Table 1 lists the anomalies and scoring weights for obtaining the Minor Physical Anomaly Score. For a commentary on this study refer to Item No. 510.

513 Wilson, Richard G. "The clumsy child." Midwife Health Visit 10: 53-55, February-March, 1974. (5 References).
Briefly alludes to the hyperkinetic syndrome which may be one of a multiplicity of symptoms and signs found in the clumsy child. Emphasis must be placed on early recognition so that emotional complications can be avoided.

514 Wolinsky, Gloria F. "Some factors to be considered in early pinpointing of a learning disabled child." Rehabil Lit 38(1): 2-4, 15, January, 1977. (12 References).
Discusses early diagnosis: who should make it; how early; and its advantages. Activity level is one of several factors of observed behavior that may aid in early diagnosis.

C. NEUROLOGICAL MANIFESTATIONS

515 Adams, Richard M. "Neurological examination of the child." Am J Dis Child 129(6): 748, June, 1975. (0 References).
Letter to editor.

516 Adams, Richard M., and Estes, Robert E. "Soft neurological signs in learning-disabled children and controls." Am J Dis Child 129(6): 748-49, June, 1975. (0 References).
Letter to editor.

517 Adams, Richard M.; Kocsis, Jenci J.; Estes, Robert E. "Soft neurological signs in learning-disabled children and controls." Am J Dis Child 128(5): 614-18, November, 1974. (24 References).
Compares learning-disabled children and controls for incidence of selected neurological signs. Neurological signs are broadly defined as those neurological variations that are equivocal or intermittent and consequent-

ly may be overlooked during neurological examination. Three hundred and sixty-eight fourth-grade boys and girls (ages nine to eleven years) served as subjects and were grouped as normal, borderline, or LD. A variety of motor and sensory factors were evaluated as possible correlates of LD: eye-hand preference, balance, stereognosis, graphesthesia, hand-finger immobility, finger localization, diadochokinesia, color vision, and head circumference. Research results indicate that two of the functions tested, graphesthesia and diadochokinesia, were significantly depressed in the LD group, although the magnitude of difference was not great enough for clinical usefulness. Classroom observation and psychoeducational testing are apt to be more accurate indications of LD than the soft neurological signs outlined in this study.

518 Aron, Alan M. "Neurologic conditions." In: Clinican's handbook of childhood psychopathology. Edited by Martin M. Josephson and Robert T. Porter. New York, New York: Aronson, 1979. 263-78. (12 References).
Comments briefly on organically driven hyperactivity. The syndrome is perceived to be associated with many different disease states. The first step in management is to establish its genesis by medical history, detailed physical and neurological examination, and psychiatric evaluation.

519 Barlow, Charles F. "Neurological examination of the child." Am J Dis Child 129(6): 747-48, June, 1975. (0 References).
Letter to editor.

520 ————. "'Soft signs' in children with learning disorders." Am J Dis Child 128(5): 605-6, November, 1974. (6 References).
Refutes the hypothesis that soft neurological signs are relevant in children with learning disorders. A more refined neuropsychological study of the child may be the most expeditious way to proceed; solutions will probably come from the fields of psychology and special education. Some problems involved in using signs in the diagnostic procedure are given.

521 Bergström, Kjell, and Bille, Bo. "Computed tomography of the brain in children with minimal brain damage: a preliminary study of 46 children." Neuropaediatrie 9(4): 378-84, November, 1978. (12 References).
Investigates the occurrence of morphological changes in a series of cases of minimal brain damage (MBD) by means of computed cranial tomography (CT). Forty-six MBD children (ages four to fifteen years) underwent CT. The criteria used for a diagnosis of MBD was the presence of clinical features of a developmental disturbance of the central nervous system causing incoordination. CT revealed abnormalities in fifteen cases (32.6 percent), consisting in cerebral atrophy, asymmetry or an anomaly.

522 Brase, David A., and Loh, Horace H. "Possible role of 5-hydroxytryptamine in minimal brain dysfunction." Life Sci 16(7): 1005-15, April, 1975. (81 References).
Reviews studies investigating the role of 5-hydroxytryptamine-containing neurons in some cases of hyperkinetic behavior and its involvement in the mechanisms by which amphetamine-like drugs are beneficial in the treatment of MBD. However, it is emphasized that a balance between various neurotransmitter mechanisms may be involved and that the possibility of the presence of a metabolic dysfunction should not be overlooked.

523 Camp, Janet A.; Phil, M.; Bialer, Irv; et al. "Clinical usefulness of the NIMH physical and neurological examination for soft signs." Am J Psychiatry 135(3): 362-64, March, 1978. (7 References).
Reports on a pilot study designed to examine the clinical validity of the Physical and Neurological Examination for Soft Signs (PANESS), an examination used for diagnostic purposes. Thirty-two hyperactive boys and 111 controls participated in the test. PANESS was administered by child psychiatrists or medical students. Forty-three items were scored. Data from the study indicate that the PANESS does not appear to be clinically valid because of its inability to discriminate effectively between the hyperactive and normal samples at any of the age levels studied. Further refinements are necessary before the test can be a useful diagnostic tool. PANESS was developed by the Pharmacology and Research Branch of the Early Clinical Drug Evaluation Unit in the National Institute of Mental Health. For another study on PANESS refer to Item No. 543.

524 Burnett, Loring L., and Struve, Frederick A. "The value of EEG study in minimal brain dysfunction." J Clin Psychol 30(4): 489-95, October, 1974. (91 References).
Assesses conflicting views concerning the role of the electroencephalogram in the diagnosis of MBD. The general value and limitations of this test in diagnosis, prognosis, and follow-up are described. A major difficulty in considering the potential usefulness of the EEG in the area of MBD revolves around the multiplicity of terms that refer to the concept. Because of false-negative findings and perhaps because some authorities do not recognize standards of normality, EEGs can have reduced importance. It is suggested that the EEG be used in conjunction with medical history, intellectual-perceptual tests, and neurological examination for optimal clinical usefulness.

525 Dayton, Delbert H., and Blanco, Richardo A. "Timing of neurological development in rural Guatemalan children." Pediatrics 53(5): 726-36, May, 1974. (53 References).
Supplies data concerning the relationship between stigmata score and genetic and perinatal factors in a group of elementary schoolchildren. Eighty-one Guatemalan boys (ages six to twelve years) participated in an outpatient study at a hyperactive clinic. Minor physical anomalies were scored with the neurological examination. Findings show that: (1) data on the relation of stigmata score to genetic and perinatal factors showed a significant relationship between the presence of pregnancy complications and the number of stigmata in the offspring of that pregnancy; (2) eighteen fathers (25 percent) reported childhood hyperactivity; (3) positive paternal history was associated with a higher stigmata score; and (4) the unsocialized aggressive children had the highest and the anxious-neurotic group the lowest mean stigmata scores.

526 Denckla, Martha B., and Rudel, Rita G. "Anomalies of motor development in hyperactive boys." Ann Neurol 3(3): 231-33, March, 1978. (15 References).
Reports on a study to determine whether hyperactive children who have neither learning disabilities nor subtle traditional neurological soft signs have measurable anomalies for their age observable on a five-minute examination of coordination. Forty-eight hyperactive boys and fifty control boys were selected from a larger population and were given a variety of tests and examinations. Discriminant function scores for speed, rhythm, and overflow correctly classified 89 percent of the boys as those with hyperactive versus normal behavioral histories. The value of the neurological examination in this area is upheld.

527 DeSouza, S. W., and Milner, R. D. G. "Clinical and CSF studies in newborn infants with neurological abnormalities." Arch Dis Child 49(5): 351-58, May, 1974. (28 References).
Compares seventy-three newborn infants for abnormal behavior and cerebrospinal fluid (CSF) abnormalities. Thirty-four infants with abnormal neurological signs of no specific etiology and forty-nine normal infants served as subjects for the experiment. Following detailed neurological examination, the hyperexcitability syndrome was diagnosed in eighteen abnormal infants and the apathy syndrome in sixteen of the abnormal infants. The majority of the abnormal infants had either blood-stained or xanthochromic CSF. The study points out the diagnostic importance of the apathy or hyperexcitability syndrome.

528 Everett, Guy M. "Dopamine and the hyperkinetic child." Adv Biochem Psychopharmacol 16: 681-82, 1977. (4 References).
Four studies which support the hypothesis of norepinephrine and dopamine involvement in MBD are reviewed. The role of drugs on these brain systems is briefly discussed since drugs clinically activate the inadequate existing dopamine systems or act as specific inhibitors of overactive dopamine systems. Further pharmacological research is necessary.

529 Gross, Mortimer D., and Wilson, William C. Minimal brain dysfunction. New York, New York: Brunner/Mazel, 1974. 206p. (Bibliography).
Presents data based on the neuropsychiatric, psychological, and electroencephalographic (EEG) examination of a large group of children who were consecutive patients at an Illinois mental health center. Of 1056 subjects (ages two to eighteen years), 77 percent were diagnosed as having MBD. This diagnosis was determined on the basis of classical MBD history, abnormal EEG, test results, and abnormal neuropsychiatric findings. It is concluded from the data that MBD represents a very common, real entity requiring a specific treatment program. Major factors distinguishing MBD from normal children are restlessness and distractibility. In children with MBD, the EEG is abnormal in more than one-half of the cases. Psychological tests frequently demonstrate significant defects in perception. The most convincing approach to MBD is through a therapeutic trial of medication, with norepinephrine enhancers or anticonvulsants producing dramatic improvement. A glossary of approximately 150 terms is provided. Appended are outlines of symptomatology and diagnostic evaluation; EEG data; findings when more than one sibling was examined; EEG data of monozygotic twins; a list of exercises to develop psychomotor skills; the questionnaire used to elicit MBD symptoms; and a chart illustrating types of EEG waves.

530 Houghton, Robert R., and Tabachnick, Barbara G. "Muller-Lyer illusion in hyperactive boys." J Learn Disabil 12(2): 77-81, February, 1979. (7 References).
Examines changes in magnitude of Muller-Lyer illusion (lines between forks and arrows) as a function of age. Forty-eight hyperactive and forty-eight nonhyperactive boys (ages six to nine years) were studied. As expected, a decreasing linear trend in magnitude of illusion was found with increasing age from six to nine years for nonhyperactive boys. For hyperactive boys, illusion increased from six to seven years and then decreased. Differences in illusion with age for hyperactives resembled J. Piaget's hypothesized developmental curve for primary illusion moved forward in years, supporting the notion of a lag rather than an aberrancy in perceptual development. Peak illusion was found for six-year-old non-

hyperactive and seven-year-old hyperactives. By ages eight and nine, no significant differences were found between the two groups.

531 Kinsbourne, Marcel. "MBD--a fuzzy concept misdirects therapeutic effort." Postgrad Med 58(3): 211-12, September, 1975. (0 References).
Differences between hard and soft neurological signs are distinguished. Diagnosis should not emphasize the lumping together of trivial findings; rather, attention should be directed to the child's learning problems.

532 Laxton, Georgia A. "40Hz. activity in MBI, LLD and normal children: a comparative EEG study." For a summary see: Diss Abstr Int 38B(1): 408, July, 1977. (0 References).

533 Koupernik, Cyrille; Mac Keith, Ronald; Francis-Williams, Jessie. "Neurological correlates of motor and perceptual development." In: Cruickshank, William M., and Hallahan, Daniel P., eds. Perceptual and learning disabilities in children: II. Research and theory. Syracuse, New York: Syracuse University Press, 1975. 105-35. (59 References).
This chapter generally focuses on the neurological aspects of the psychological areas of perceptual and motor development in infancy through childhood. A discussion of the concept of MBD and hyperkinesis outlines the characteristics, problems, and drug treatment. The use of the label "MBD" is questioned.

534 Lerer, Robert J., and Lerer, Pamela B. "Soft neurological signs in learning-disabled children and controls." Am J Dis Child 129(6): 748, June, 1975. (0 References).
Letter to editor.

535 McMahon, Shirley A., and Greenberg, Lawrence M. "Serial neurologic examination of hyperactive children." Pediatrics 59(4): 584-87, April, 1977. (18 References).
Reports the results of several neurological examinations given to hyperactive children and analyzes the value of soft neurological signs in the diagnosis and assessment of hyperkinesis. Forty-two of 102 boys (ages 6.5 to eleven years), undergoing drug treatment for hyperactivity, served as subjects and were given serial neurological examinations on five different occasions. The responses to three of these signs were studied: heel gait, toe gait, and diadochokinesis. A high degree of variability of response within individuals was documented. There was no evidence of interaction between treatment and the subjects' responses. The degree of variability was such that to have used these data as measures of "improvement" would have been misleading. Thus, the report concludes that caution is to be used in assessing the value of soft neurological signs for diagnostic purposes.

536 Newton, Jerry. "Neurological examination of the child." Am J Dis Child 129(6): 747, June, 1975. (0 References).
Letter to editor.

537 Peters, John E.; Dykman, Roscoe A.; Ackerman, Peggy T.; et al. "The special neurological examination." In: Clinical use of stimulant drugs in children. Edited by C. Keith Conners. Amsterdam: Excerpta Medica, 1974. 53-66. (8 References). (International Congress Series, No. 313).

A special neurological examination developed by the authors is described. Eighty-two MBD boys and thirty-four controls participated in the study. Hyperactivity is viewed as an unessential and often overemphasized component of the MBD/LD child.

538 Peters, J. E.; Romine, J. S.; Dykman, R. A. "A special neurological examination of children with learning disabilities." Dev Med Child Neurol 17(1): 63-78, February, 1975. (32 References).
Describes in detail a special neurological examination designed to study the incidence of MBD signs, subtypes of disabilities, and the decrease in signs with increasing age. Eighty-two boys with learning and/or behavior problems and forty-five controls served as subjects. An analysis of the results of the examination shows that the boys with learning disabilities had significantly more minor neurological signs than control children. It is noted that many of these signs become less obvious or disappear by age eleven, pointing to the similarity between older cases and controls. Younger children show deficits in CNS functioning in the areas of language, fine motor coordination, and cross-modality integrations.

539 Satterfield, James H.; Cantwell, Dennis P.; Saul, Ronald E.; et al. "Intelligence, academic achievement, and EEG abnormalities in hyperactive children." Am J Psychiatry 131(4): 391-95, April, 1974. (19 References).
Investigates EEG, neurological, psychological, and behavioral measures in a group of school-age children. One hundred and twenty hyperactive boys (ages five to ten years) served as subjects. The boys were administered numerous tests: WISC, WRAT, ITPA, Goodenough-Harris Drawing Test, Bender-Gestalt, and others. Results reveal that EEGs were normal for sixty-three children, borderline for thirty-five children, and abnormal for twenty-two children. The abnormal group scored significantly higher on intelligence tests and other measures of cognitive performance than hyperactive children with normal EEGs. The authors caution that an abnormal EEG finding should not necessarily indicate the need for special education.

540 Small, Joyce G.; Milstein, Victor; Jay, Sara. "Clinical EEG studies of short and long term stimulant drug therapy of hyperkinetic children." Clin Electroencephalogr 9(4): 186-94, October, 1978. (24 References).
Assesses the value of the EEG in diagnosis and treatment of hyperkinetic children and examines the effect of pemoline on the EEG and MBD-related behaviors. The goals of the study were to obtain extensive EEG studies on twenty-one hyperkinetic children and sixteen sex- and age-matched normal controls. In the experimental group, the EEG was evaluated after nine weeks of either drug or placebo treatment. Those children remaining on active drugs were to receive complete EEG studies after six months or more of continuous drug treatment. Magnesium pemoline is shown to be effective in improving the behavior of hyperactive children as rated by parents, teachers, and professional staff. However, the results of the study basically do not demonstrate any EEG correlates of changes in the behavioral state.

541 Stine, Oscar C.; Saratsiotis, John B.; Mosser, Robert S. "Relationships between neurological findings and classroom behavior." Am J Dis Child 129(9): 1036-40, September, 1975. (5 References).
Attempts to establish a relationship between the presence of certain neurological signs and classroom behaviors of a sample of children. Five hundred and seventy-five children (ages ten to twelve years) from low-income

urban neighborhoods were examined by pediatricians for certain neurological signs, while classroom teachers ranked each child according to types of behavior. Data were studied on neurological signs found in more than fifteen children and on types of classroom behavior clinically expected to be related to central nervous system defects. Analyzation shows: (1) significant positive associations were found among nystagmus and hyperactivity, mixed dominance and hyperactivity, as well as between mixed dominance and variable day-to-day performance; (2) errors in moving parts of the body on verbal command were associated with distractibility and underachievement; and (3) head circumference greater than the 90th percentile for age was associated with unvarying behavior and clumsiness, tactile agnosia with unvarying behavior, asymmetry of the eyes with hyperactivity, and asymmetrical position of the child's head with underachievement.

542 Touwen, B. C. L., and Sporrel, T. "Soft signs and MBD." Dev Med Child Neurol 21(4): 528-30, August, 1979. (24 References).
Calls attention to the pitfalls in the use of the term "neurological soft signs" in the diagnosis of MBD.

543 Werry, John S., and Aman, Michael G. "The reliability and diagnostic validity of the physical and neurological examination for soft signs (PANESS)." J Autism Child Schizophr 6(3): 253-62, September, 1976. (17 References).
Reports on a study to investigate the value and reliability of the neurological examination in the diagnosis of hyperkinesis. PANESS, a neurological examination recommended by the National Institute of Mental Health for psychotropic drug studies in children, was used. Twenty-one children (mean age eight years) served as subjects and were examined on two separate occasions by two pediatric residents. Results show: (1) one-half of the children were hyperactive; (2) one-fourth had histories pointing to brain damage; and (3) one-fourth were normal. Since many of the signs, though reliable, did not occur in the majority of the children, the PANESS should be regarded as experimental rather than definitive. For another study on PANESS refer to Item No. 523.

544 White, Leonard. "Diagnostic classification and equivocal neurological signs in childhood schizophrenia and minimal brain dysfunction: a factorial study of GSR conditioning." For a summary see: Diss Abstr Int 34B(7): 3512-13, January, 1974. (0 References).

D. TESTS, SCALES, AND OTHER SCREENING DEVICES

545 Abikoff, Howard; Gittelman-Klein, Rachel; Klein, Donald. "Validation of a classroom observation code for hyperactive children." J Consult Clin Psychol 45(5): 772-83, October, 1977. (40 References).
The development and use of a classroom observation code that would correctly identify hyperactive children are reported. Sixty children (ages six to twelve years), who had been referred to an outpatient clinic for hyperactivity, and sixty normal children served as subjects. A fourteen-category observation code was used to record the classroom behavior of all subjects. Among other results, the research indicated that the subjects referred for hyperactivity had significantly higher scores than controls on twelve of the categories. Thus, the code is considered to be a reliable and valid instrument for the objective quantification of classroom behavior in hyperactive children. For a commentary on this study refer to Item No. 568.

546 Adams, Jerry; Hayden, Benjamin S.; Canter, Arthur. "The relationship between the Canter Background Interference Procedure and the hyperkinetic behavior syndrome." J Learn Disabil 7(2): 110-15, February, 1974. (17 References).

This study tests the hypothesis that children with hyperkinesis have a significantly greater deficit in performance on the Canter Background Interference Procedure (Canter BIP) than do normal children. One group of forty hyperkinetic boys and one group of thirty-eight control boys served as subjects. The standard Bender-Gestalt designs were administered in the usual manner and then readministered a short time later using special Canter BIP paper. Findings show that while the groups did not differ on the Bender-Gestalt Test (with IQ partialed out), the hyperkinetic group showed a greater deterioration of performance on the Canter BIP. It is emphasized that the magnitude of the difference was too small to yield reliable classification of the individual child. Caution is required in the clinical use of this technique. The Canter BIP is briefly described.

547 Adams, Jerry; Kenny, Thomas J.; Peterson, Rolf A.; et al. "Age effects and revised scoring of the Canter BIP for identifying children with cerebral dysfunction." J Consult Clin Psychol 43(1): 117-18, February, 1975. (3 References).

Reports on a study which undertook an item analysis of the Canter Background Interference Procedure (BIP) in order to select and weigh items which would more accurately distinguish between children with cerebral dysfunction and normal children. One hundred and sixty-eight children (ages eight to twelve years) were scored by the Canter system, which included eighty-three possible errors. Attempts to improve discrimination between normal and cerebral dysfunction children were successful only after age differences were considered.

548 Anderson, Robert P., et al. "Relationship between performance based and observer based measures of hyperactivity. Trends in research with hyperactive children." Paper presented at the 24th Annual Meeting of the Southwestern Psychological Association, Fort Worth, Texas, April 21-23, 1977. 19p. (ED 144 965).

Discusses the WARD model, an assessing system for measuring hyperactivity. The WARD model uses a mobile, portable, digital logic system which controls a basic vigilance task. Measures produced are compared to teacher observation of hyperactivity. Teachers appear to be making fairly accurate judgments about hyperactive children.

549 Arnold, L. Eugene, and Smeltzer, Donald J. "Behavior checklist factor analysis for children and adolescents." Arch Gen Psychiatry 30(6): 799-804, June, 1974. (9 References).

Presents a factor analysis of two behavior checklists used at a child psychiatry clinic to help parents evaluate and objectify their feelings about their child's behavior and symptoms. Parents were asked to fill out this form during the initial consultation. Three hundred and fifty-one checklists (216 for boys, 135 for girls) were available for the factor analysis. One checklist was for children age twelve and under; one concerned the group ages thirteen to eighteen. Comparison of the factors by age group revealed several trends: (1) teenagers experience much the same problems as younger children do; (2) teenagers' problems are complicated by additional symptoms; and (3) hyperactivity is still present in the teenage group. Detailed tables are included.

550 Barkley, Russell A., and Ullman, Douglas G. "A comparison of objective measures of activity and distractibility in hyperactive and non-hyperactive children." J Abnorm Child Psychol 3(3): 231-44, 1975. (13 References).
Compares measures of activity and distractibility in three groups of boys (ages four to twelve years). Subjects consisted of sixteen boys referred to a clinic for possible hyperactivity, sixteen boys referred to the same center for problems other than hyperactivity, and twenty normal controls. In a fifteen-minute free-play and a five-minute test session, thirteen measures of activity, distractibility, and parental ratings of activity were obtained. Results show that the multiple measures had significant but relatively low order correlations among themselves and varied as a function of the subject group. There was no consistent relationship between the measures of activity and distractibility. These findings are discussed in detail.

551 Beatty, James R. "The analysis of an instrument for screening learning disabilities." J Learn Disabil 8(3): 180-86, March, 1975. (26 References).
Reports on the use of a screening device, the Classroom Screening Instrument (CSI), as an aid in the early diagnosis of children with learning disabilities. The CSI was used to collect data for 400 children. The data were then factor analyzed to locate the common factor space and to determine the number of original items contributing to the factor space. Of the original eighty items, forty-eight were found to be loading on ten factors. Forty of those items were of complexity one, seven were of complexity two, and one item was of complexity three. The factor solution based upon forty-eight items was of different structure than the original instrument. It is indicated that the CSI consists of factors relevant to the screening and diagnosis of LD.

552 Behar, Lenore, and Stringfield, Sam. Manual for the Preschool Behavior Questionnaire. 1974. 17p. (ED 167 576).
Describes the development, norming, and validation of the Preschool Behavior Questionnaire (PBQ), a screening instrument used for the detection of children's behavior problems.

553 Blunden, Dale; Spring, Carl; Greenberg, Lawrence M. "Validation of the Classroom Behavior Inventory." J Consult Clin Psychol 42(1): 84-88, February, 1974. (7 References).
Uses factor analytic methods to assess construct validity of the Classroom Behavior Inventory (CBI), a scale developed by L. M. Greenberg for rating hyperactive behavior. Three hundred and twenty kindergarten boys from twenty classes in nine public schools served as subjects. The boys were then rated by their teachers on the forty-item inventory. The CBI was found to measure three dimensions of behavior: hyperactivity, hostility, and sociability. Correlations of CBI ratings and classroom observations were used to measure concurrent validity. Significant concurrent validity was obtained only for the CBI impulsiveness category. Applications of the CBI and clinical relevancy are discussed.

554 Bowers, A. J. "Can we effectively assess hyperactivity in schools?" Child Care Health Dev 4(6): 411-20, November-December, 1978. (34 References).
Critically appraises some of the measures commonly used to assess activity levels within the classroom setting. Measures covered are behavioral rating scales, direct observation, and mechanical assessment (pedometer,

actometer, and ballistograph). Although rating scales are thought to be the most practical means of assessment, improvements need to be made.

555 Burns, Edward, and Jenkins, Ellen. "Stability of Q-sorts in assessing descriptions of hyperactivity." Percept Mot Skills 40(3): 694, June, 1975. (0 References).
Documents the use of Q-sorts to assess the meaning of the term "hyperactivity." A seventy-five item Q-sort, composed of adjectives which could describe hyperactive children, was given to ten professionals familiar with behavioral disorders. The test was administered on two occasions. The Q-sort method is considered a valid method for the assessment of the term "hyperactivity."

556 Burns, Edward, and Lehman, Lyle C. "An evaluation of summated rating and pair comparison measures of hyperkinesis." J Learn Disabil 7(8): 504-7, October, 1974. (5 References).
Uses two methods, summated ratings and pair comparisons, to determine hyperkinetic behavior in a group of school-age children. Twenty children (mean age 9.5 years), who had been referred because of behavioral and/or academic problems, were subjects for the five-week program. Each child was rated by the RSH (Davids, 1971, Rating Scale of Hyperkinesis). Results reveal that the ratings method was internally consistent and reliable for measuring hyperkinesis and that pair comparisons were valuable for specifying the importance of each subcategory on an individual basis.

557 Chamberlin, Robert W. "The use of teacher checklists to identify children at risk for later behavioral and emotional problems." Am J Dis Child 130(2): 141-45, February, 1976. (26 References).
Examines the role and validity of teacher checklists in evaluating children with emotional/behavioral problems. The report concludes that: (1) such measures are not very accurate predictors of behavior in settings other than the classroom; (2) checklists do not predict the development of later behavioral/emotional problems; and (3) much observable behavior is transient and situational and best managed by passage of time or behavior modification.

558 Conners, C. Keith. "Psychological evaluations and visual perception." In: Learning disabilities and related disorders: facts and current issues. Edited by J. Gordon Millichap. Chicago, Illinois: Year Book Medical Publishers, 1977. 93-98. (0 References).
Reviews some of the well-known psychological and visual perception tests which can aid the clinical psychologist in his diagnosis of children with learning and behavioral problems.

559 ————. "Rating scales for use in drug studies with children." In: Assessment manual. Rockville, Maryland: Early Clinical Drug Evaluation Unit, National Institute of Mental Health, 1976.

560 Copeland, Anne P., and Weissbrod, Carol S. "Behavioral correlates of the hyperactivity factor of the Conners Teacher Questionnaire." J Abnorm Child Psychol 6(3): 339-43, September, 1978. (4 References).
Assesses the usefulness of the Conners Teacher Questionnaire, Hyperactivity Factor, in discriminating hyperactive children. Sixteen hyperactive boys and sixteen controls participated in the study. The boys were videotaped alone in a playroom and then shown a videotaped model. The boys'

activity levels, judgments about their behavior, and other interview questions were compared with the boys' scores on the Teacher Questionnaire. Several of the measures had a significant correlation with the Teacher Questionnaire scores, suggesting that this rating scale is a useful assessment tool.

561 Cratty, Bryant J. "Evaluative instruments." In: Cratty, Bryant J. Remedial motor activity for children. Philadelphia, Pennsylvania: Lea and Febiger, 1975. 69-92. (Health Education, Physical Education, and Recreation Series). (53 References).
Briefly reviews some of the most frequently used tests available for inclusion in batteries intended to survey the motor abilities of children and youth. One section, Tests of Impulse Control, Attention, and Hyperactivity, discusses: (1) the Hewett's Assessment of Attention; and (2) the Impulse Control (or Line Drawing) test.

562 Das, J. P. "Diagnosis and measurement of hyperactivity." Ment Retard Bull 3(2-3): 182-88, 1975-76.
A three-part program for the detection and measurement of hyperactivity is presented. Part I consists of the Child Rating Scale which teachers can use to help them determine the extent of a child's classroom misbehavior. Part II of the program discusses physiological measures of arousal--heart rate, respiration, and skin conductance. Part III consists of a battery of tests to measure dimensions of information processing. It is stressed that adequate and accurate diagnosis of the hyperactive child can be beneficial in planning appropriate treatment.

563 Dykman, Roscoe A.; Ackerman, Peggy T.; Peters, John E.; et al. "Psychological tests." In: Clinical use of stimulant drugs in children. Edited by C. Keith Conners. Amsterdam: Excerpta Medica, 1974. 44-52. (16 References). (International Congress Series, No. 313).
Summarizes standard psychological tests and laboratory procedures which have been found to differentiate MBD and LD children from normal children. Table I lists twelve tests reviewed in the text: WISC Full Scale IQ; WISC Verbal IQ; WISC Subtest (5); Bender-Gestalt Development Errors; Wide Range Achievement Test; Gray Oral Reading Test; Tone Discrimination; Physiological Reactivity to Meaningful Stimuli, Tapping Speed, DeRenzi-Vignolo Token Test; Reaction Time; and Impulsive Errors. The researchers believe that the more basic deficits of LD children can be uncovered with laboratory tests, rather than existing psychological and educational tests. General discussion is included.

564 Forbes, Gordon B. "Comparison of hyperactive and emotionally-behaviorally disturbed children on the Devereux Child Behavior Rating Scale: a potential aid in diagnosis." J Clin Psychol 34(1): 68-71, January, 1978. (8 References).
Compares two groups of children on the Devereux Child Behavior Rating Scale (DCB). Twenty hyperactive and twenty emotionally-behaviorally disturbed children (ages five to eleven years) were rated according to the scale. Ratings of the two groups exceeded the normative population on all DCB factors, although there were differences between the two groups. Generally, the hyperactive children received the most extreme scores. It is concluded that the DCB can differentiate between hyperactive children and children with symptoms similar to those of hyperactivity.

565 Forness, Steven R., and Esveldt, Karen C. "Classroom observation of children with learning and behavior problems." J Learn Disabil 8(6): 382-85, June-July, 1975. (8 References).

Uses direct observation to determine whether children in the process of being referred for academic and behavior problems exhibit certain behaviors that are observably different from their peers and whether such behaviors relate to subsequent special education needs. Twenty-four boys were observed. The technique is advocated and, although not mentioning hyperactivity specifically, might be applied to such cases.

566 Gardner, Richard A.; Gardner, Andrew K.; Caemmerer Alexander; et al. "An instrument for measuring hyperactivity and other signs of MBD." J Clin Child Psychol 8(3): 173-79, Fall, 1979. (33 References).
Describes the development of the steadiness tester, an instrument designed to detect the presence of several signs of MBD and hyperactivity. Data are provided for 500 normal children and 356 children with MBD. Results demonstrate a statistically significant difference between the performance of normal and MBD children over the whole range of ages studied (five to 15.5 years). The steadiness tester is not viewed as a screening test for MBD; but it should be used as one criterion for determining whether a child exhibits hyperactivity.

567 Golinko, Barry E. "Hyperactivity: operationalization of traits using a structured behavioral interview: a pilot study." J Pediatr Psychol 3(1): 35-44, 1978. (26 References).
Focuses on the development of a behavioral interview to be used in the assessment of hyperactivity. The interview was tested with the mothers of eighteen hyperactive children (ages five to twelve years). The means, standard deviations, and interrater reliabilities for individual items and for the interview as a whole are reported; the predictive validity and possible uses of this structured interview are discussed.

568 Haynes, Stephen N., and Kerns, Robert D. "Validation of a behavioral observation system." J Consult Clin Psychol 47(2): 397-400, April, 1979. (11 References).
Comments on a study by Howard Abikoff, et al. (Item No. 545). The authors' methodology is reviewed and suggestions offered for future validation studies of observation systems.

569 Hull, Grafton H., Jr. "Utilization of the Conners Abbreviated Symptom Questionnaire for diagnosing hyperactivity." For a summary see: Diss Abstr Int 40A(3): 1281-82, September, 1979. (0 References).

570 Humphreys, Lewis E., and Ciminero, Anthony R. "Parent report measures of child behavior: a review." J Clin Child Psychol 8(1): 56-63, Spring, 1979. (47 References).
Reviews several methods used to collect parent report data on children. The specific methods are categorized and discussed in three general categories: (1) checklists; (2) rating scales; and (3) structured interviews. Each specific device is described in terms of its content, scoring, reliability, validity, factor structure, normative samples, and other findings regarding its application in clinical and research settings. Since very few scales came close to meeting all of the psychometric standards that are important in evaluating self-report instruments, more work is needed to improve the quality of this method of assessment.

571 Joost, Michael G., and Salvendy, Gavriel. "The development and validation of an objective method for quantifying hyperactivity in children." Jpn Psychol Res 21(1): 18-28, May, 1979. (29 References).

Expresses concern about the lack of objective, reliable, and quantitative methods to assess hyperactivity. This study discusses how objective measures, using sinus arrhythmia and force platform scores, were developed and validated on thirty boys (fifteen hyperactive and fifteen controls). The hypothesis that discrimination between the two groups could be obtained using objective measures is supported.

572 Kaufman, Nadeen L., and Kaufman, Alan S. "Comparison of normal and minimally brain dysfunctioned children on the McCarthy Scales of Children's Abilities." J Clin Psychol 30(1): 69-72, January, 1974. (7 References).

Evaluates the McCarthy Scales of Children's Abilities (MSCA), an assessment tool for children with learning disabilities and MBD. The MSCA contains eighteen tests grouped into six scales: Verbal, Perceptual-Performance, Quantitative, General Cognitive, Memory, and Motor. Twenty-two minimally brain-dysfunctioned children (ages five to nine years), drawn from several New York public elementary schools, were administered the MSCA. Their scores were compared to scores obtained by twenty-two matched controls. Data analyzation shows: (1) MBDs scored lower than controls on most of the tests; (2) the groups did not differ significantly on the establishment of hand dominance; and (3) the MBDs' low mean General Cognitive Index score was more consistent with their low level of school achievement than with their mean IQ. It is indicated that the MSCA can be a useful tool for assessing LD children.

573 Kupfer, David J.; Detre, Thomas; Koral, Jacqueline. "Deviant behavior patterns in school children, application of KDS™-14." Psychol Rep 35(1, pt. 1): 183-91, August, 1974. (10 References).

Recommends the use of a rating scale, the KDS™-14, to help teachers identify deviant behavior patterns in schoolchildren, and to study incidence rates of such children. By means of a preliminary survey, three types of problem students were identified: aggressive children, children with learning difficulties, and shy-withdrawn children. Further identification was made by using the KDS™-14 to determine the overall incidence of certain behaviors in the population of a school system. Seventeen thousand students in five small Connecticut towns constituted this population.

574 Kupietz, Samuel S., and Botti, Elaine. "Behavior measurement in pediatric psychopharmacology." Am J Psychiatry 131(1): 106, January, 1974. (4 References).

Letter to editor.

575 Leonard, Dwight J. "WISC pattern analysis: a comparison of techniques for the diagnosis of MBD in school age children." For a summary see: Diss Abstr Int 36A(2): 708, July, 1975. (0 References).

576 Manni, John L., et al. "Hyperactivity: a strategy for evaluating intervention strategies." Devereux Forum 14(1): 38-44, Summer, 1979.

Suggests a strategy which can be used to evaluate referrals made on the basis of hyperactive behavior as well as measure the effectiveness of intervention programs. Following initial sections on stimulant drugs and the role of school personnel, a six-step intervention procedure is outlined: (1) operationalize the behavior(s); (2) collect baseline data; (3) perform situation validation; (4) select an intervention strategy; (5) assess treatment effects; and (6) modify intervention if necessary.

577 Menkes, John H. "The clinical evaluation of school difficulties." Neuropaediatrie 5(3): 217-23, August, 1974. (16 References).
Evaluates numerous tests useful in the proper diagnosis of the learning-disabled child. Included are: (1) intelligence tests; (2) Auditory-Visual Integration Test; (3) Right-Left Discrimination Test; (4) the Bender-Gestalt Test; (5) Auditory Comprehension and Discrimination Test; and (6) the Finger Recognition Test. Once a child has been evaluated, a complex program designed to adjust family and school environment, and less importantly, supportive drug therapy, must be undertaken.

578 Murley, Harris D.; Milam, Donald R.; Gorman, Warren. "Objective psychiatric and psychologic signs of brain disorders." Ariz Med 33(11): 891-95, November, 1976. (25 References).
Describes two simple screening devices which the physician and others can use to detect MBD. The neurologic examination requires brief observations of cranial nerves, motor and sensory status, an estimate of IQ, plus ten simple observations for stance, coordination, and verbal skills. The psychologic test monitors impairment of the right and left cerebral hemispheres by a drawing of Greek Cross, Bender Visual-Motor Test, and the Wechsler Memory Scale.

579 Owen, Joan E. "The identification of characteristics of the hyperactive child through objective evaluation." For a summary see: Diss Abstr Int 37B(11): 5840-41, May, 1977. (0 References).

580 Paulsen, Karen, and O'Donnell, James P. "Construct validation of children's behavior problem dimensions: relationship to activity level, impulsivity, and soft neurological signs." J Psychol 101 (2nd half): 273-78, March, 1979. (16 References).
A construct validation study of dimensions of children's behavior problems was carried out using multiple linear regression. Seventy-six latency-aged boys in residential treatment served as subjects. The dimensions involved were Conduct Disorder and Inadequacy-Immaturity. The predictor variables were activity level, impulsivity, and soft signs of neurological damage. Results indicate that Conduct Disorder was significantly predicted by activity level, in combination with impulsivity. Inadequacy-Immaturity was significantly predicted by activity level and soft signs. A third dimension, Personality Disorder, was found to be uncorrelated with the three predictor variables.

581 Poggio, John P., and Salkind, Neil J. "A review and appraisal of instruments assessing hyperactivity in children." Learn Disabil Q 2(1): 9-22, Winter, 1979.
Critically appraises and reviews a selected group of nine observational instruments commonly used to assess activity level (and in particular, hyperactivity) in young children. Information is provided on reliability, validity, norms, recommendations, and references for each of the nine instruments reviewed, which include the Child Rating Scale, the Classroom Behavior Inventory, the Classroom Observation Code, the Hyperactivity Rating Scale, the Rating Scales for Hyperactive and Withdrawn Children, the Schenectady Kindergarten Rating Scales, the Teachers Rating Scale, the Parent Rating Scale, and the Werry-Weiss-Peters Activity Scale. Most instruments were seen to have serious flaws that limit their effectiveness in the assessment of hyperactivity in children. An annotated bibliography is included of thirteen newer or less popular instruments.

582 Proger, Barton B., et al. Discriminators of clinically defined emotional maladjustment: the predictive validities of the Quay and

Devereux Scales. Blue Bell, Pennsylvania: Montgomery City Intermediate Unit 23, 1974. 20p. (ED 090 721).
Tests the predictive validity of the Quay Behavior Problem Checklist and the Devereux Elementary School Behavior Rating Scale. The tests were administered to ninety-five boys (ages seven to fourteen years) who had been clinically diagnosed as aggressive, hyperactive, or withdrawn.

583 Proger, Barton B.; Mann, Lester; Green, Paul A.; et al. "Discriminators of clinically defined emotional maladjustment: predictive validity of the Behavior Problem Checklist and Devereux Scales." J Abnorm Child Psychol 3(1): 71-82, 1975. (33 References).
Compares the accuracy of two rating scales with psychiatrists' diagnoses for screening emotional maladjustment in a group of schoolchildren. Ninety-six boys (ages eight to fourteen years), who were enrolled in special classes for emotionally disturbed children in the suburban Greater Philadelphia area, served as subjects. Thirty-two of the boys were aggressive, thirty-two hyperactive, and thirty-two withdrawn; all were administered the Behavior Problem Checklist (BPC) and the Devereux Elementary School Behavior rating scales (DESB). A descriptive intercorrelation matrix was generated for the four BPC scales only and the fourteen DESB scales. Three stepwise discriminant analyses were run: (1) BPC scales only; (2) DESB scales only; and (3) BPC and DESB scales combined. Results of the research show that the four BPC subscales used alone attained the optimal predictive accuracy of 65 percent (or sixty-two of ninety-five) of the children correctly identified.

584 Quay, Lorene C.; Popkin, Michael; Weld, Gary; et al. "Responses of normal and learning disabled children as a function of the stopwatch in the Matching Familiar Figures Testing situation." J Exp Child Psychol 26(2): 383-88, October, 1978. (8 References).
Reports on an experiment designed to ascertain whether normal and hyperactive learning-disabled children differ in their responses to the Matching Familiar Figures Test (MFFT) as a function of a temporal cue. Sixteen learning-disabled and fifteen normal boys (ages eight to nine years) served as subjects. A counterbalanced design, in which each boy was administered one-half of the test with a stopwatch and the other one-half of the test without a stopwatch, was used. Among other results research indicates that normal and LD boys respond in a different manner to the temporal cue.

585 Rie, Ellen D.; Rie, Herbert E.; Henderson, Douglas B. "A parent-teacher behavior rating scale for underachieving children." J Learn Disabil 11(10): 59-61, December, 1978. (3 References).
Reports on the development of a behavior rating scale designed to measure overt behavioral characteristics of LD children and to measure change in these characteristics with drug administration. The scale, usable by parents and teachers, includes activity level as one item of seven categories.

586 Routh, Donald K., and Schroeder, Carolyn S. "Standardized playroom measures as indices of hyperactivity." J Abnorm Child Psychol 4(2): 199-207, 1976. (16 References).
Examines some standardized types of observation of children's behavior in a playroom situation, developed in research with normal children, as measures of certain aspects of hyperactivity. Three groups of children served as subjects: two groups of normal and mentally retarded hyperactive children and one group of normal children. All children were ob-

served in a standardized playroom, under varying conditions, for two fifteen-minute sessions. Hyperactive children were found to be more active under all conditions than controls, a fact upheld by parental ratings.

587 Routh, Donald K.; Schroeder, Carolyn S.; O'Tuama, Lorcan A. "Development of activity level in children." Dev Psychol 10(2): 163-68, March, 1974. (15 References).
Studies the relationship of age to an open-field measure of activity and to a parental rating scale commonly used in the assessment of hyperactivity. One hundred and forty children (ages three to nine years) served as participants. Open-field activity was observed for two fifteen-minute sessions under varying conditions. Parents filled out an activity scale (Werry-Weiss-Peters). Among other results it was confirmed that open-field activity decreased with age--a fact which was upheld by parents' ratings. There were no significant sex differences on either open-field measures or parental ratings. A discussion of these findings is included.

588 Sandoval, Jonathan. "The measurement of the hyperactive syndrome in children." Rev Educ Res 47(2): 293-318, Spring, 1977. (88 References).
Critically appraises various instruments that have been used to measure different aspects of the hyperactive syndrome in children. Measures are classified into five types: (1) behavioral ratings; (2) observation schedules; (3) direct physical measurements; (4) simple performance tests; and (5) higher-order cognitive tests. Each type is reviewed in detail in terms of reliability and validity. Evidence is presented which indicates that the most commonly used measures are still in a developmental phase and, therefore, merit additional study.

589 Sandoval, Jonathan, and Lambert, Nadine M. "Reliability and validity of teacher rating procedures in the assessment of hyperactivity as a function of rating scale format." Paper presented at the 62nd Annual Meeting of the American Educational Research Association, Toronto, Canada, March 27-31, 1978. 30 p. (ED 160 614).
Investigates the effects of varying the formats of behavior rating scale items on teacher ratings of student hyperactivity. Two hundred and forty-two teachers and four scales were studied. The items on the scales were varied in format and were positively or negatively worded. The experiment showed that precision of rating scales can effect reliability and validity of teacher ratings.

590 Saxon, Samuel A.; Dorman, Layton B.; Starnes, K. Diane. "Construct validity of three rating scales for hyperactivity." J Clin Child Psychol 5(2): 56-58, Fall, 1976. (14 References).
Assesses the construct validity of three previously published rating scales used to screen hyperactive children. Scales under study were the BRS by C. Keith Conners (1969), Davids (1971), and Bell's (1970). Fifty children (mean age 5.8 years), who had been referred to a center because of learning/behavior disorders, served as subjects. The children were rated by their parents and three objective measures of activity. The rating scale scores of the children did not predict their activity level; further, no support for the scales having construct validity was found. More objective measures should therefore be used in evaluating the hyperactive child.

591 Schain, Richard J. "Tests of attention and achievement." In: Learning disabilities and related disorders: facts and current issues.

Edited by J. Gordon Millichap. Chicago, Illinois: Year Book Medical Publishers, 1977. 73-75. (6 References).
Briefly surveys some of the most commonly used tests and scales for diagnosing learning and behavioral disorders.

592 Schwartz, Sheila C. "An inventory and analysis of psychometric predictor variables used in the diagnosis of hyperkinesis." For a summary see: Diss Abstr Int 37B(10): 5375-76, April, 1977. (0 References).

593 Simensen, R. J., and Sutherland, J. "Psychological assessment of brain damage: the Wechsler Scales." Acad Ther 10(1): 69-81, Fall, 1974. (51 References).
The value of the WISC as a psychological means of diagnosing children with neurologically based learning disorders is assessed. The hypothesis that the WISC might provide an index to cerebral damage is not supported by research. Further, subtest patterns are not reliable predictors of CNS involvement. The authors find that no satisfactory method of distinguishing learning-disabled populations is currently available. A review of the literature is included.

594 Simonds, John F. "Relationship between children's learning disorders and emotional disorders at a mental health clinic." J Clin Psychol 30(4): 450-58, October, 1974. (14 References).
Reports on a study which attempted to ascertain the usefulness of tests as screening tools for LD children and to identify the variables that would determine whether patients screened for LD could be grouped clinically according to the prominence of learning or emotional symptoms. One hundred and fourteen children (ages ten to thirteen years), who were patients at a mental health center, served as subjects and were classified according to the prominence of emotional or learning symptoms. Age, sex, test scores, diagnostic testing, and historical data were used to delineate three clinical groups: (1) prominent learning symptom; (2) prominent emotional symptom; and (3) equally prominent learning and emotional symptoms. It is concluded from the data that tests do enable the professional to screen for learning disabilities and help in the analysis of the effects of emotional problems on the learning process.

595 Sines, Jacob O. "Assessment of children's environments." Res Relat Child 39: 99, March, 1977-August, 1977. (0 References).
Abstracts a report of research in progress or recently completed research. Data are provided on: name of investigator(s), purpose of the study, number and kind of subjects used, methodology, principal findings, duration of research, cooperating group(s), and availability of publication(s). Research Relating to Children is compiled by the ERIC Clearinghouse on Early Childhood Education.

596 Smith, Sara F. "The construction and validation of the screening test of educational prerequisite skills." For a summary see: Diss Abstr Int 37A(6): 3504-5, December, 1976. (0 References).

597 Sprague, R. L.; Cohen, M. N.; Werry, J. S. Normative data on the Conners' Teacher Rating Scale and Abbreviated Scale. Urbana, Illinois: Children's Research Center, University of Illinois, 1974.
Technical report.

598 Spring, Carl; Blunden, Dale; Greenberg, Lawrence; et al. "Validity and norms of a hyperactivity rating scale." J Spec Educ 11(3): 313-21, Fall, 1977. (10 References).
Reports on a study in which 1,337 elementary schoolchildren were rated by their teachers to determine norms for the Hyperactivity Rating Scale. Forty-five hyperactive children referred by physicians were also rated. Norm data were factor analyzed, and a hyperactivity factor was identified. Behaviors with the highest loading on the hyperactivity factor yielded the largest differences between hyperactive and norm groups. Black children had the highest hyperactive ratings within the norm group, and boys had higher ratings than girls in the hyperactive group.

599 Stone, F. Beth. "Assessment of children's activity level." Am J Orthopsychiatry 44(2): 250, March, 1974. (0 References).
Abstract of a paper which reviews various methods of assessing hyperactivity, including rating scales, questionnaires, and other traditional methods. Emphasis is placed on the author's recent use of a stabilimetric chair as an innovative means of objectively measuring activity level.

600 Vincent, J. P.; Williams, B. J.; Elrod, T. "Ratings and observations of hyperactivity by the multitrait-multimethod analyses." In: The hyperactive child: fact, fiction, and fantasy. Symposium presented at the meeting of the American Psychological Association, San Francisco, California, August, 1977.

601 Werry, John S., and Hawthorne, Daniel. "Conners Teacher Questionnaire: norms and validity." Aust NZ J Psychiatry 10(3): 257-62, September, 1976. (10 References).
Tests the validity of a commonly used rating scale, the Conners Teacher Questionnaire. The questionnaire has four factors: Conduct Problem, Hyperactivity, Inattentive-Passive, and Tension. (A fifth factor, Sociability, appeared in an original version of the scale.) Various samples were used to compare norms and validity. These revealed that Conners' original factor structure appeared stable across studies. The tendencies for males to be rated higher on acting out behaviors and females on neurotic symptoms are consistent with clinical experience as well as previous studies.

602 Werry, John S.; Sprague, Robert L.; Cohen, Miye N. "Conners' Teacher Rating Scale for use in drug studies with children--an empirical study." J Abnorm Child Psychol 3(3): 217-29, 1975. (17 References).
Evaluates the Conners' Teacher Rating Scale, a widely used scoring system for hyperactive children on medication. Two hundred and ninety-one elementary schoolchildren were rated by their teachers using this scale. Scores were significantly lower than those for a similar group of ninety-two New York children and considerably less than those scores of a group of sixty-four children. Boys tended to act out while girls scored higher on neuroticism. A detailed factor study comparing the present scale to the original model is given.

603 Whaley, M. A., and Loney, J. "The Teacher Approval-Disapproval Scale (TADS): from the mouths of babes." Paper presented at the American Psychological Association, 1974.

604 Williams, B., and Vincent, J. HABOS: Code system for hyperactivity. Houston, Texas: Baylor School of Medicine and University of Houston, 1977. Unpublished manuscript.

605 Williams, Ben J.; Vincent, John R.; Elrod, Tom. "A naturalistic study of hyperactive children." Res Relat Child 36: 41, September, 1975-February, 1976. (0 References).
Abstracts a report of research in progress or recently completed research. Data are provided on: name of investigator(s), purpose of the study, number and kind of subjects used, methodology, principal findings, duration of research, cooperating group(s), and availability of publication(s). Research Relating to Children is compiled by the ERIC Clearinghouse on Early Childhood Education.

606 Wright, William H. "The development and validation of a scale for school observation of characteristics associated with minimal brain dysfunction and learning disabilities in elementary school boys." For a summary see: Diss Abstr Int 38A(8): 4707, February, 1978. (0 References).

607 Wright, William H., and Michael, William B. "The development and validation of a scale for school observation of characteristics associated with learning disabilities and minimal brain dysfunction in elementary school boys." Educ Psychol Meas 37(4): 917-28, Winter, 1977. (6 References).
Traces the development and validation of a new instrument, the School Observation Scale (SOS). The SOS was designed for elementary schoolteachers as an aid in recording and assessing behavior patterns characteristic of children with LD and MBD. The SOS contains sixty-three variables organized into five sections: (1) motor coordination and activity; (2) lack of attention and distraction; (3) learning and cognition difficulties; (4) emotionality; and (5) personal social response. The reliability of the SOS in differentiating behavior in groups of normal and educationally handicapped children is documented. The scales provide adequate reliability and validity in this area.

608 Zentall, Sydney S., and Barack, Robin S. "Rating scales for hyperactivity: concurrent validity, reliability, and decisions to label for the Conners and Davids Abbreviated Scales." J Abnorm Child Psychol 7(2): 179-90, June, 1979. (22 References).
Examines the concurrent validity and inter- and intrarater reliability for the Abbreviated Teacher Questionnaire (ATQ, Conners, 1973) and the Rating Scales for Hyperkinesis (Davids, 1971). Sixteen teachers from two special and two regular schools (grades one to four) rated 211 normal and forty-nine special children using both scales. High correlations were found suggesting excellent predictability between scales and considerable stability across time and rater. Lower scores on a subsequent rating relative to an initial rating were demonstrated, dependent on time between ratings but independent of teacher expectation of treatment gains, bias produced by rating selected children, and whether children were hyperactive or normal. Use of initial and infrequent rating scores versus subsequent, closely spaced ratings was related to the rater's objective (e.g., diagnosis, treatment, or assessment).

609 Zukow, Patricia G.; Zukow, Arnold H.; Bentler, P. M. "Rating scales for the identification and treatment of hyperkinesis." J Consult Clin Psychol 46(2): 213-22, April, 1978. (32 References).
Reports the development of parent and teacher rating scales in response to the need for a simple instrument to aid in the diagnosis and treatment of hyperkinesis. Seventy-eight hyperactive children and eighty-two controls (ages two to eleven years) were rated by parents. Multivariate

analysis produced three factors: Excitability, Motor Coordination, and Directed Attention. An analysis of the teacher form on thirty-six hyperactive and seventy-eight controls yielded two similar factors: Attention/ Excitability, and Motor Coordination. Success of the scales in identifying hyperactive and normal children is discussed. For a commentary on this study refer to Item No. 215.

V. Management

A. OVERVIEW

610 Cohen, Donald J. "Minimal brain dysfunction: diagnosis and therapy." In: Current psychiatric therapies. Volume 17. Edited by Jules H. Masserman. New York, New York: Grune & Stratton, 1977. 57-70. (11 References).
Reviews characteristics, diagnostic methods, and five therapeutic interventions for the MBD child. Interventions include parental guidance, special education, psychotherapy, physical education, and medication.

611 Erickson, C. K. "Therapy of childhood hyperkinesis." US Pharm 2: 29-34, August, 1977. (17 References).
Hyperkinesis, also called minimal brain damage or minimal brain dysfunction, is presented with regard to diagnosis, etiology, significance, consequences, stimulant and nonstimulant drug therapy, and behavioral and psychotherapeutic measures.

612 Friend, J. C. M. "Syndrome of childhood hyperactivity: II." Med J Aust 1(22): 819-23, May 28, 1977. (10 References).
Outlines steps in diagnosis and offers suggestions for successful management of the hyperkinetic syndrome. Comments on the Feingold diet are included. For Part I of this study refer to Item No. 100.

613 Greenberg, Jerrold S. "The use of drugs to calm kids." Paper presented at the New York State Federation of Chapters of the Council for Exceptional Children, Buffalo, New York, November, 1974. 19p. (ED 101 268).
Reviews the literature and describes the present state of knowledge regarding the hyperkinetic syndrome. Problems of hyperkinesis persist after the hyperkinesis ceases. A team approach is necessary to respond to these problems.

614 Greene, Charles A., and Rao, V. S. "Management of the hyperactive child: an overview." Paediatrician 8(3): 140-44, 1979.
Describes the identifying characteristics of the hyperkinetic syndrome and reviews four modalities of therapy: behavioral modification, environmental modification, nutritional therapy, and drug therapy.

615 Halpern, Werner I., and Kissel, Stanley. Human resources for troubled children. New York, New York: Wiley, 1976. 263p. (Bibliography). (Wiley Series on Personality Processes).
Summarizes intervention strategies for the practicing clinician. Strategies discussed include: (1) environmental resources; (2) programs for learning problems; (3) parent education and counseling; (4) family ther-

apies; (5) group and individual treatment methods; (6) behavior modification; and (7) pharmacotherapy. Hyperactivity is discussed in Chapter 11 on the medical treatment of behavior disorders. Author and subject indexes are included.

616 Harshbarger, Mary E. "The role of drugs, diet, and food additives in hyperactivity." Paper presented at the 3rd Annual Meeting of the International Reading Association, Great Lakes Regional Conference, Cincinnati, Ohio, October 12-14, 1978. 17p. (ED 163 439).
The hyperkinetic syndrome is covered in terms of causes and treatments--the latter including drugs, diet, megavitamins, behavior therapy, and manipulation of the educational environment. A multidisciplinary approach is advocated.

617 Hill, Charles H., and Gattis, Linda J. "Teaching the restless ones." Read World 16(1): 28-34, October, 1976. (24 References).
Examines attending behavior and its effect on reading achievement in hyperactive children. Studies are cited which show that the child with rapidly shifting attention who cannot focus an adequate amount of attention for a reasonable duration of time on a specific stimulus can be labeled incorrectly. Remedial procedures include: (1) chemical therapy; (2) operant conditioning; (3) use of cubicles to discourage distractibility; (4) short assignments; (5) familiarity with the task; (6) "re-audorizing", i.e., teaching children to rehear by talking to themselves; and (7) lowering educational expectations to accommodate this type of student.

618 Kinsbourne, Marcel. "Hyperactivity: treatment." Except Parent 8(5): 7-11, October, 1978.

619 Knopf, Irwin J. "Treatment approaches." In: Knopf, Irwin. Childhood psychopathology: a developmental approach. Englewood Cliffs, New Jersey: Prentice-Hall, 1979. 161-98. (161 References).
Surveys a representative sample of treatment approaches used to remove or alleviate abnormal behaviors in children. Treatment methods discussed include: (1) psychological approaches (play, individual, group and family, behavior therapy); (2) somatic approaches (shock therapy, psychosurgery, and psychoactive drugs); and (3) milieu approaches (residential treatment centers, special education, summer camps). Hyperkinesis is considered under drug therapy.

620 Landsberg, M. "Loving prescription for hyperactive kids." Chatelaine 51: 24, March, 1978.

621 Renshaw, Domeena. "The hyperkinetic child." Compr Ther 2(2): 36-40, February, 1976. (1 Reference).
Discusses the management of the syndrome of MBD in terms of: (1) diagnosis and evaluation; (2) education of adults, especially in areas of guilt feelings and the importance of the parental role; (3) the importance of psychopharmacotherapy in the treatment; (4) educational ramifications of the child both in school and at home; and (5) follow-up. Emphasis is placed on behavior modification, the contract system, and psychotherapy as necessary components for the successful management of the syndrome.

622 Safer, Daniel J., and Allen, Richard P. Hyperactive children: diagnosis and management. Baltimore, Maryland: University Park Press, 1976. 239p. (Bibliography).

The ten chapters of this book survey many topics related to the hyperactive child, but emphasis is placed on the practical aspects of daily clinical management. Chapters cover the historical background of the disorder, issues in the pharmacological management of hyperactivity, clinical forms and evaluative tests, home management and parental counseling, behavior management in the classroom, educational considerations, and coordination in management. The authors provide evidence for the following conclusions: (1) the school is a vital area for management intervention; (2) multiple modes of intervention are generally more valuable than unidimensional efforts; and (3) some professional approaches (stimulant medication and behavior therapy) are more efficacious than others. The volume is directed toward the professional.

623 Saxon, Samuel A. "Hyperactivity in children." In: Finch, A. J., and Kendall, Philip C. Clinical treatment and research in child psychopathology. New York, New York: SP Medical & Scientific Books, a division of Spectrum Publications, 1979. 103-36. (60 References). (Child Behavior and Development Series, Volume 3).
Proposes a model for conceptualizing the causes, characteristic behaviors, and treatments of hyperactivity. Topics include: (1) definitions of hyperactivity; (2) review of relevant research on causes and therapies; and (3) summary of treatment efforts of the Center for Developmental and Learning Disorders at Birmingham, Alabama.

624 Schechter, Marshall D. "Psychiatric aspects of learning disabilities." Child Psychiatry Hum Dev 5(2): 67-77, Winter, 1974. (0 References).
Details the differential diagnostic and treatment processes required for working with learning-disabled children. Special consideration is given to the psychiatric implications of symptoms which accompany minimal cerebral dysfunction--anxiety, depression, disturbance in primary attachment to adults, and negative self-image. Included are three case vignettes of three seven-year-old boys who, although intellectually within the normal range, were not performing up to their potential. A variety of treatment approaches, including psychotherapy and medication, is recommended.

625 Schnackenberg, Bob C. "Minimal brain dysfunction syndrome in children." Psychiatr Forum 7(1): 26-32, Fall, 1977.
Generally reviews the MBD syndrome--the most commonly diagnosed syndrome in child psychiatry. Treatment approaches include chemotherapy, major tranquilizers, psychotherapy, group therapy, special education, perceptual-motor training, and behavior therapy. A multidisciplinary approach to the syndrome is most effective. One subsyndrome, the dopamine-beta-hydroxylase deficiency, is briefly discussed.

626 Svoboda, William B. "The hyperkinetic syndrome." W Va Med J 71(12): 347-51, December, 1975. (20 References).
Briefly reviews the definition and clinical manifestations of the hyperkinetic syndrome. Five principle cause-types are differentiated and explained: (1) environmental (emotional); (2) sensory reception problems; (3) neural arousal; (4) receptive language processing; and (5) too low or too high intelligence level. Diagnostic approaches include complete history-taking, interviews with parent and child, neurophysical examination, and physical examination. Therapeutic approaches should be directed toward: (1) correcting any identified handicaps of learning; (2) altering the child's environment as necessary; (3) counseling the parents in techniques of child management; and (4) prescribing drugs only as a

temporary initiation to counseling. Successful prognosis depends on the ability of the child to develop self-control.

627 Varga, James R. "The hyperactive child: should we be paying more attention?" Am J Dis Child 133(4): 413-18, April, 1979. (40 References).
Calls attention to some of the current trends in the diagnosis and treatment of hyperkinesis. Comments are made concerning: (1) the value of a more comprehensive, multidisciplinary approach to the problem; (2) professional awareness of the role of the family; (3) the importance of appropriate educational placement; and (4) the controversial aspects of pharmacologic manipulation.

628 Walker, Sydney. Help for the hyperactive child. Boston, Massachusetts: Houghton Mifflin, 1977. 211p. (Bibliography).
Covers etiology, identification, and treatment of hyperactivity. Case histories are used to discuss sources of the syndrome. Sections focus on medication abuse, the myth of "outgrowing" hyperactivity, and the promotional merchandising of pharmaceutical companies regarding medication. Alternative treatment methods, such as diet therapy, patterning, megavitamins, and brain surgery are assessed. The multidimensional approach is stressed. The book is intended for parents, teachers, and professionals who diagnose hyperactive children.

629 Watras, Joseph. "Constructive criticism?" J Thought 11(4): 313-36, November, 1976.
Focuses on issues and attitudes concerning methods of dealing with hyperactive students. Comments are made on drug therapy, educational management, and public opinion.

B. PHARMACOLOGY

1. GENERAL DRUG TREATMENT

630 Adler, Sol. "Pediatric psychopharmacology and the language-learning impaired child." ASHA 16(6): 299-304, June, 1974. (22 References).
This review article is divided into nine sections: (1) behavior modification strategies versus psychopharmacotherapy; (2) drug therapy: an historical overview; (3) social and political issues; (4) stimulants versus tranquilizers and sedative-type drugs; (5) the clinician's role; (6) changes in language-learning behavior; (7) drug use; (8) side effects; and (9) drug use in treatment of communication problems. An appendix lists psychopharmacological agents by type.

631 Allen, R. P. "Drug treatment of hyperactivity." Paper presented at the Meeting of the Association for the Advancement of Behavior Therapy, Atlanta, Georgia, December, 1977.

632 Anders, Thomas F., and Ciaranello, Roland D. "Pharmacological treatment of minimal brain dysfunction syndrome." In: Psychopharmacology: from theory to practice. Edited by Jack D. Barchas, Philip A. Berger, and Roland D. Ciaranello, et al. eds. New York, New York: Oxford University Press, 1977. 425-35. (14 References).
Considers the MBD and hyperactive child in terms of: (1) history of the syndrome; (2) incidence and symptomatology; (3) biochemical and neurophysiological correlates; (4) family and genetic studies; (5) clinical

evaluations; and (6) psychopharmacological and nonpharmacology management. Hyperactivity per se does not represent a syndrome; rather, it is a symptom within a spectrum of diagnostic entities.

633 ———. "Psychopharmacology of childhood disorders." In: Psychopharmacology: from theory to practice. Edited by Jack D. Barchas, Philip A. Berger, and Roland D. Ciaranello, et al. eds. New York, New York: Oxford University Press, 1977. 407-24. (11 References).
Sets forth general principles of psychopharmacology in childhood disorders and cites their use as adjuncts to other therapies. Hyperactivity is covered briefly as a symptom of depression.

634 Baxley, Gladys B.; Turner, Paul F.; Greenwold, Warren E. "Hyperactive children's knowledge and attitudes concerning drug treatment." J Pediatr Psychol 3(4): 172-76, 1978. (10 References).
Surveys a group of hyperactive children's knowledge, attitudes, and perceptions of drug treatment. Twenty-six hyperactive boys (mean age 11.7 years) were interviewed and their responses audiotaped, content-analyzed, and categorized. The boys' responses showed that they were generally knowledgeable about the purpose of their medication, presented mixed attitudes about having to take medication, and associated not taking the medication with certain negative consequences. The clinical relevance of the findings is discussed.

635 Berwick, Donald M. "Prevalence and management of hyperactive children." N Engl J Med 292(10): 536-37, March 6, 1975. (0 References).
Letter to editor.

636 Blau, Stephen. "A guide to the use of psychotropic medication in children and adolescents." J Clin Psychiatry 39(10): 766-72, October, 1978. (70 References).
Cites several clinical entities, including hyperactivity, in which medication can be a useful adjunct to the total therapeutic regimen.

637 Box, Steven. "Hyperactivity." New Soc 42(793): 590, December 15, 1977. (0 References).
Letter to editor.

638 Bryce-Smith, D. "Hyperactivity." New Soc 42(793): 590, December 15, 1977. (0 References).
Letter to editor.

639 Campbell, Barbara A. "Monitoring the child on drug therapy in the public schools of Connecticut." For a summary see: Diss Abstr Int 38A(8): 4469-70, February, 1978. (0 References).

640 Campbell, Magda. "Psychopharmacology in childhood psychosis." Int J Ment Health 4(1-2): 238-54, Spring-Summer, 1975. (74 References).
Reviews the literature on psychopharmacology. The author provides evidence for the following conclusions: (1) diphenhydramine is effective in very disturbed schizophrenic children, particularly those with high IQs; (2) benzedrine and dextroamphetamine, even in very low doses, often worsen psychosis; (3) both chlorpromazine and thioridazine, though widely used, have negative effects on cognitive behavior and learning in general in childhood; (4) trifluperidol has proved more effective than other

drugs; (5) thioxanthene, molindone hydrochloride, hallucinogens, and megavitamins are also used with different effects; (6) lithium decreases such symptoms as hyperactivity and aggressiveness; and (7) the therapeutic effects of levodopa in schizophrenic children have been investigated. Since the purpose of drug treatment is to make the child more amenable to other forms of therapy, it is suggested that a particular drug therapy should be discontinued if it interferes in any way with maturation, development, and learning. For a reprint of this study refer to Item No. 688.

641 Campbell, Magda, and Small, Arthur M. "Chemotherapy." In: Handbook of treatment of mental disorders in childhood and adolescence. Edited by Benjamin B. Wolman. Englewood Cliffs, New Jersey: Prentice-Hall, 1978. 9-27. (141 References).
Presents an overview of pharmacology for children and adolescents. Topics covered include: methodology, choice of drug, drug administration, and classification of drugs.

642 ————. "The use of psychotherapeutic drugs in pediatrics." In: Drug treatment of mental disorders. Edited by Lance L. Simpson. New York, New York: Raven Press, 1976. 209-36. (178 References).
Reviews the major classes of drugs used to treat a variety of disturbances of childhood. The researchers provide evidence for the following conclusions: (1) psychomotor stimulants have been demonstrated to be superior to placebos in treating hyperactive children; (2) neuroleptics comprise an important treatment modality; (3) the superiority of one neuroleptic over another has not been documented with controlled studies; (4) polypharmacy, frequent change of drugs, or unnecessary dose escalation are bad practices; (5) possible hazards of drug use must be weighed against the hazards of the untreated illness; (6) pharmacotherapy versus other treatment modalities has not yet been critically assessed; (7) drug treatment is not indicated for all childhood illnesses; and (8) children's psychopharmacology will remain on an empirical basis until diagnostic entities are more precisely defined.

643 Cantwell, Dennis P. "A critical review of therapeutic modalities with hyperactive children." In: Cantwell, Dennis P., ed. The hyperactive child: diagnosis, management, current research. New York, New York: Spectrum Publications, distributed by John Wiley and Sons, 1975. 173-89. (83 References). (Series on Child Behavior and Development, Volume I).
By means of a literature review, several treatment modalities are summarized. The author concludes that: (1) most of the existing literature consists of drug studies; (2) these drug studies indicate that CNS stimulants are effective for some symptoms with some children, but little is known about how to predict a child's response or what the long-term effects might be; (3) studies of the other treatment approaches are few in number; and (4) involvement of the family is critical to the success of any management program, a fact rarely stressed in the literature.

644 ————. "Drug treatment of the hyperactive syndrome in children." In: Psychopharmacology in the practice of medicine. Edited by Murray E. Jarvik. New York, New York: Appleton-Century-Crofts, 1977. 291-306. (52 References).
Reviews eight general principles of drug therapy and includes remarks concerning safety and efficacy of specific drugs used to treat hyperactive children. Among the types of drugs commented on are: CNS stimu-

lants, antidepressants, sedatives, antipsychotic agents, antihistamines, anticonvulsants, and lithium carbonate. The following conclusions are reached: (1) CNS stimulants are effective for some symptoms with some children, with methylphenidate being the preferred drug; (2) other drugs have not proven to be as effective as the stimulant group; (3) response to drugs is difficult to predict; (4) more information is needed about the long-term efficacy and safety of the medication currently used; (5) there are fewer studies of other treatment modalities; (6) present studies do not reflect the importance of the family in the management program; and (7) a multiple treatment approach can best aid the hyperactive child.

645 ————. "Psychopharmacologic treatment of the minimal brain dysfunction syndrome." In: Psychopharmacology in childhood and adolescence. Edited by Jerry M. Wiener. New York, New York: Basic Books, 1977. 119-48. (141 References).
Considers terminology, classification, definition, diagnostic evaluation, and general problems in evaluating drug treatment of childhood disorders. Emphasis is placed on the use of psychopharmacologic means to treat the MBD syndrome. Findings show that: (1) CNS stimulants are effective for some symptoms of some children for short-term; (2) other drugs have not been as promising as the CNS stimulants; (3) certain factors can be used to predict drug response; (4) more information is needed about the long-term efficacy and safety of the currently used drugs; (5) few studies exist of other treatment modalities, particularly those which combine the other treatment modality with drug treatment; (6) involvement of the family is critical to the success of any management program; and (7) successful management will involve the use of multiple treatment approaches.

Cohen, Michael J., ed.
see Drugs and the special child. (Item No. 650).

646 Conway, Allan. "An evaluation of drugs in the elementary schools: some geographic considerations." Psychol Sch 13(4): 442-44, October, 1976. (5 References).
Examines the relationship between type of school and the frequency of the prescription of medication in a group of hyperactive elementary schoolchildren. Questionnaires were given to school psychologists, administrators, faculty, and mental health professionals in forty-three public schools in rural mid-state New York. The hypothesis that there would be a positive correlation between geographic location and frequency of resorting to psychoactive drugs was supported by comparing the findings of this study with those which surveyed urban-based primary grade facilities. Factors influencing prescription frequency include population density, expanding school districts, lack of professional staff for dealing with the student's problems, and family mobility.

647 Covi, Lino, and Alessi, Larry. "Pharmacological treatment of personality disorders." In: Lion, John R., ed. Personality disorders: diagnosis and management. Baltimore, Maryland: Williams & Wilkins, 1974. 406-18. (63 References).
Briefly describes several studies which have used various drugs to treat the hyperkinetic syndrome. The rest of the chapter concerns drug treatment of other personality disorders such as alcoholism, drug addiction, sexual deviance, and behavior disorders of old age.

648 Critchley, Macdonald. "Biochemistry on the horizon?" J Learn Disabil 8(1): 56-57, January, 1975. (0 References).

Reprints a portion of an opening address by Macdonald Critchley, eminent English physician and president of the World Federation of Neurology. Dr. Critchley spoke at the 25th Annual Meeting of the Orton Society, the World Congress on Dyslexia, which centered on the problems of the learning-disabled child.

649 DeLong, Arthur R. "Drug research: a foundation for decision making." In: Drugs and the special child. Edited by Michael J. Cohen. New York, New York: Gardner Press, 1979. 1-31. (90 References).
Summarizes the state of the art of drug research on hyperactive children. The author arrives at the following conclusions: (1) although drug research has become more sophisticated, it has not yet advanced to the point where answers can be considered final; (2) the more research that is available, the more focus will center on individual differences; and (3) among the crucial aspects of individual situations are various physical and environmental factors affecting the child, the quality of research, the goals to be achieved by treatment, alternative treatments, and the awareness of possible side effects.

650 Drugs and the special child. Edited by Michael J. Cohen. New York, New York: Gardner Press, 1979. 258p. (Bibliography).
Presents a collection of nine original articles addressing the major issues relating to drug therapy for hyperactive children. Contents: Drug Research: a Foundation for Decision Making (DeLong - Item No. 649); Drug Therapy with Children and Adolescents (Silver - Item No. 697); Drugs: Classroom Learning Facilitators? (Murray - Item No. 1499); Perspectives on Drug Treatment for Hyperactivity (Weithorn - Item No. 987); Drug Therapy for Hyperactivity: Existing Practices in Physician-School Communication (Ross - Item No. 1526); Drugs and the Family (Eisenpreis - Item No. 1240); Hyperactive Children at Risk (Preis and Huessy - Item No. 1932); Long-Term Effects of Stimulant Therapy for HA Children: Risk Benefit Analysis (Allen and Safer - Item No. 943); Drug Therapy--Children's Rights (Weithorn - Item No. 1992).

651 "Drugs help, but won't cure, most hyperactive children." JAMA 232 (12): 1205, 1208, 1215-16, June 23, 1975. (0 References).
Summary of a seminar devoted to pharmacologic treatment of hyperkinetic children.

652 Ellis, Teresa, and Justen, Joseph E. "Drug therapy for the hyperkinetic child: some commonly asked questions and answers." Spec Child 2(1): 5-11, 23, Summer-Fall, 1975.
Responses to common questions concerning drug therapy for the hyperkinetic child are given. Topics addressed include most frequently prescribed drugs, possible side effects, and length of treatment.

653 Forman, Phillip M. "Pharmacological intervention." In: Progress in learning disabilities. Edited by Helmer R. Myklebust. New York, New York: Grune & Stratton, 1975. 151-60. (13 References).
Provides brief answers to these questions: What are we treating? Who should we treat? Why does the drug work? What drug should we use? How do we use the drug? How do we know if the drug is helpful? How do we know if the drug is harmful?

654 Gadow, Kenneth D. Children on medication: a primer for school personnel. 1979. 116p. (ED 170 978).

This book discusses children whose various disorders (hyperkinesis, epilepsy, enuresis, school phobia, cerebral palsy, and childhood psychosis) require them to be on medication. The behavioral effects of various drugs, along with their major side effects, are described. Included in the appendixes are a psychotropic drug chart, a classification of epilepsies, and the Conners' Abbreviated Teacher Rating Scale. A glossary completes the report.

655 ———. "Pills and preschool: medication usage with young children in special education." Paper presented at the Illinois Council for Exceptional Children, Chicago, Illinois, October, 1975.

656 ———. "Psychotropic and anticonvulsant drug usage in early childhood special education programs. III. A preliminary report: parent interviews about drug treatment." Paper presented at the 55th Annual International Convention, the Council for Exceptional Children, Atlanta, Georgia, April 11-15, 1977. 105p. (ED 139 182).

Reports on interviews with parents of 115 children receiving medication for hyperactivity, convulsive disorders, or other reasons. The Children's Medication Chart and telephone interviews were used to collect data on such aspects as frequency of administration, therapeutic response, side effects, physician referral, drug-free periods, and dosage.

657 Gadow, K. D., and Sprague, R. L. Children's medication chart. Champaign, Illinois: Institute for Child Behavior and Development, University of Illinois, 1975.

658 Gellis, Sydney S. "MBD." JAMA 235(18): 1967, May 3, 1976. (0 References).

Letter to editor.

659 Gittelman-Klein, Rachel. "Psychopharmacological treatment of anxiety disorders, mood disorders, and tic disorders of childhood." In: Psychopharmacology: a generation of progress. Edited by Morris A. Lipton, Alberto DiMascio, and Keith F. Killam. New York, New York: Raven, 1978. 1471-80.

Gittelman-Klein, Rachel, ed.
see Recent advances in child psychopharmacology. (Item No. 688).

660 Gossel, Thomas A. "Drug therapy and hyperkinetic children." Ohio Pharm 24(6): 22-27, June, 1975. (26 References).

Briefly reviews characteristics, incidence, and pathological causes of the hyperkinetic syndrome. Three stimulant drugs, methylphenidate, dextroamphetamine, and deanol, are of primary interest to the pharmacist. Thirteen other drugs which have limited to moderate effectiveness are listed in Table II. Table III lists four agents believed to be "possibly effective" in the management of behavior problems. Several generalities are drawn: (1) all children displaying general symptoms of the hyperkinetic syndrome are not candidates for drugs; (2) children displaying symptoms should never be given the drugs on a test basis in an attempt to diagnose the disorder; (3) other tests must always be performed before drugs are routinely prescribed; and (4) nonmedical methods should be tried before drugs are administered.

661 Graham, Philip. "Hyperactivity." New Soc 42(793): 589, December 15, 1977. (0 References).

Letter to editor.

662 "Hyperkinesis can have many causes, symptoms." JAMA 232(12): 1204, 1208, June 23, 1975. (0 References).
Summary of a seminar devoted to pharmacologic treatment of hyperkinetic children.

663 "I got my Rit-lin you got your dex...more on the drugging of children." This Mag 10(4): 10-11, August-September, 1976.

664 Johnstone, David G. R. "Hyperactivity." New Soc 42(793): 590, December 15, 1977. (0 References).
Letter to editor.

665 Kehne, Christine W. "Control of the hyperactive child via medication--at what cost to personality development; some psychological implications and clinical interventions." Am J Orthopsychiatry 44(2): 237-38, March, 1974. (0 References).
Digest of a paper which discusses some of the psychological issues involved for both parent and child when the child is receiving medication for hyperkinesis. Professionals are urged to be in touch with the child's and the parents' feelings about medication and the role it will play in treatment.

666 Kenny, Thomas J., and Clemmens, Raymond L. Behavioral pediatrics and child development: a clinical handbook. Baltimore, Maryland: Williams & Wilkins, 1975. 209p. (Bibliography).
This primer is devoted to the key issues in the area of the psychologic aspects of pediatrics. Part I is a summary of child development; Part II concerns itself with some of the common disorders of child development: mental retardation, learning disorders, and problems of speech and hearing. The diagnostic procedures usually involved when dealing with exceptional children are discussed in Part III; Part IV covers various phases of management: psychotherapy, behavior modification, medication, etc. The hyperkinetic syndrome is defined early in the volume and is again briefly discussed in Chapter 12, Psychotropic Drug Therapy. One case study of a five-year-old girl is cited. The book is aimed at all professionals who deal with children: nurses, psychologists, psychiatrists, educators, language pathologists, and social workers.

667 King, Alan R. "Hyperactivity." New Soc 42(793): 590, December 15, 1977. (0 References).
Letter to editor.

668 Kline, Carl L. "Prevalence and management of hyperactive children." N Engl J Med 292(10): 536, March 6, 1975. (0 References).
Letter to editor.

669 Kornetsky, Conan. "Minimal brain dysfunction and drugs." In: Cruickshank, W. M., and Hallahan, D. P., eds. Perceptual and learning disabilities in children: II. Research and theory. Syracuse, New York: Syracuse University Press, 1975. 447-81. (86 References).
Reviews research on the use of drugs in the treatment of learning problems in children. The pharmacological, behavioral, neurological, etiological, and long-term treatment aspects of drugs used with minimal brain dysfunction (e.g., methylphenidate hydrochloride) are discussed, and the social and political implications of drug treatment for this population are examined.

670 Krager, John M., and Safer, Daniel J. "Type and prevalence of medication used in the treatment of hyperactive children." N Engl J Med 291(21): 1118-20, November 21, 1974. (9 References).
Presents the results of a 1971 and 1973 survey on the use of medication for hyperactivity in 1,894 elementary schoolchildren in Baltimore County, Maryland. School nurses were asked to list the names of children receiving such medication, the name(s) of the drug(s), the reason for its administration, and the person who administered it. In 1971 in Baltimore County public schools, nurses reported that 1.07 percent of the children were on such medication; in 1973, this had increased to 1.73 percent. Results also show that in 1971, 76.2 percent of the children given medication for hyperactivity received stimulants (methylphenidate or dextroamphetamine), whereas by 1973 this had increased to 88.2 percent. A consistent finding was that children in wealthier areas received medication more often than those in lower socioeconomic areas of the county.

671 Lambert, Nadine M.; Sandoval, Jonathan; Sassone, Dana. "Prevalence of treatment regimes for children considered to be hyperactive." Am J Orthopsychiatry 49(3): 482-90, July, 1979. (13 References).
Explores the prevalence of the use of medication for the treatment of hyperactivity in a school population. In a representative sample of San Francisco Bay Area schoolchildren, 1.2 percent were identified as hyperactive by parents, teachers, and physicians. Estimates of the prevalence of various treatment regimens indicate that 58 percent of those so identified received medication in one year, but a much larger number (86 percent) will be given medication at some time. Multiple treatment approaches generally employed in the area are surveyed.

672 Leopold, N. "Medical management of movement disorders." Hosp Formul 12: 519-21, August, 1977.
Discusses the treatment of hypokinesis and hyperkinesis using drugs to maintain the dopamine-acetylcholine neurotransmitter balance.

673 Levitis, Karen A. "Need for medication in minimal brain dysfunction." Pediatrics 54(3): 388, September, 1974. (2 References).
Letter to editor.

674 May, Elsie. "Drugs in use in schools for severely subnormal children." Child Care Health Dev 2(5): 261-66, October, 1976.
Surveys the use of drug administration in two special schools in Birmingham, England. Forty-two severely subnormal children were given haloperidol, procyclidine HCl, phenobaritone, and phenytoin. Problems encountered in such a program are discussed in terms of: (1) the responsibilities of the teaching and nonteaching staff who must monitor side effects of medication; (2) parents who do not wish their children to have medication and thus will not administer weekend doses, causing their children to come to school disorderly, and disrupting long-term therapy; and (3) the need for trained nurses in schools having such drug therapy programs.

675 "MBD, drug research and the schools." Hastings Cent Rep 1-23, June, 1976.

676 McNeil, H. Graham, Jr.; Rogers, Michael V.; Matthews, Hewitt W. "Drug therapy in the hyperkinetic syndrome." Urban Health 5(4): 12-14, August, 1976. (17 References).
Briefly discusses the use of drug therapy as a treatment modality for the hyperkinetic syndrome. The nature and effects of selected drugs are

described. Proper diagnostic procedures and therapeutic measures are deemed necessary for effective and efficient control of this disorder.

677 Millichap, J. Gordon. "Drugs in the management of learning and behavior disorders in school children." Ill Med J 145(4): 322-23, April, 1974. (5 References).
Agents used in treating children with MBD and hyperkinesis are listed in order of choice according to effectiveness and toxicity: stimulants, antianxiety and antipsychotic agents, and anticonvulsants. Stimulant medications should be used as adjuncts to other types of treatments, especially remedial education. Studies have failed to reveal an association between the medical use of stimulants in children and later drug abuse.

678 ————. "Medications as aids to education in children with minimal brain dysfunction." In: Learning disabilities and related disorders: facts and current issues. Edited by J. Gordon Millichap. Chicago, Illinois: Year Book Medical Publishers, 1977. 111-17. (2 References).
Reviews various classes of drugs: CNS stimulants, antianxiety and antipsychotic agents, antidepressants, antihistaminics, and anticonvulsants. Names, suggested dosages, and principal side effects are shown. The following conclusions are reached: (1) certain medications have proven value for the LD child; (2) drugs should be an adjunct treatment to remedial education; (3) careful monitoring is essential; and (4) dosage should be kept to a minimum.

679 Minimal brain dysfunction. Compendium, Volume 2, No. 15. Summit, New Jersey: CIBA-Geigy Pharmaceutical Company, 1974.

680 Mitchell, Donald P. "Drugs: a limited view?" Educ Leadership 31(5): 451-52, February, 1974. (0 References).
Letter to editor.

681 Moxley, Richard T. "Pharmacopeia: drugs to control hyperactivity." In: Principles of pediatrics: health care of the young. Editor-in-Chief, Robert A. Hoekelman. New York, New York: McGraw-Hill, 1978. 969-71. (1 Reference).
Briefly reviews the use of dextroamphetamine, methylphenidate, and pemoline in hyperkinesis.

682 Muiva, P. M. "Hyperactive child." East Afr Med J 56(5): 237-40, May, 1979. (7 References).

683 Nestadt, Allan. "A review of medication for children with specific learning disabilities." Phoenix J 9(4): 3, 5, 7-8, December, 1976.
Five types of drugs most frequently administered to children with learning disabilities or behavior problems are examined. The names and properties are given for stimulant, anticonvulsant, metabolic, antidepressant, and tranquilizer drugs. Among the most popular of the commonly used drugs is the central nervous stimulant, methylphenidate (Ritalin). Guidelines for its proper use are offered.

684 Nissen, G. "Behavioural disorders in children and the possibilities offered by drugs in their treatment." In: Epileptic seizures, behaviour, pain. Edited by Walther Birkmayer. Bern, Switzerland: Hans Huber, 1976. 230-42. (30 References).

Discusses various types of behavioral disorders in children relating to: (1) nosology; (2) prevalence; and (3) drug therapy, primarily stimulant drug therapy. The papers are an outgrowth of an international symposium held in St. Moritz, January 6-7, 1975.

685 Oettinger, Leon, Jr. "Comment on medication for hyperkinetic children." Pediatrics 58(2): 303, August, 1976. (2 References).
Letter to editor.

686 Piepho. Robert W.; Gourley, Dick R.; Hill, John W. "Minimal brain dysfunction." Am Pharm 17(8): 500-504, August, 1977. (29 References).
MBD is discussed in terms of: (1) pathogenesis; (2) diagnostic and clinical findings; (3) treatment; (4) pharmacotherapy; and (5) therapeutic considerations. MBD is seen as a cognitive/behavioral disorder of unknown etiology. Drug therapy, especially that which uses methylphenidate and dextroamphetamine, is the single most effective treatment, although remedial education, psychotherapy, and family counseling are valuable adjunct therapies. Methylphenidate and dextroamphetamine work primarily on the behavioral symptoms of MBD; cognitive problems may still persist. Other drugs such as pemoline, chlorpromazine, or thioridazine may be useful, but tricyclic antidepressants, antianxiety agents, and anticonvulsants have little or no effect. Information is provided on actions, interactions, dosage, and side effects.

687 Psychopharmacology in childhood and adolescence. Edited by Jerry M. Wiener. New York, New York: Basic Books, 1977. 226p. (Bibliography).
Assesses the current clinical usage of psychopharmacologic agents in childhood and adolescence. Part I covers history, classification, methodological considerations, and the interaction of drugs and development. Part II is devoted to the clinical applications of psychopharmacologic treatment. Conclusions and summary are presented in Part III. An index is provided. The book is intended primarily for clinicians: child psychiatrists, pediatricians, and family practitioners.

Contents: History of Drug Therapy in Childhood and Adolescent Psychiatric Disorders (Wiener - Item No. 714); The Classification and Pharmacology of Psychoactive Drugs in Childhood and Adolescence (Yaffe and Danish - Item No. 717); Methodological Considerations in Drug Research with Children (Conners - Item No. 1997); Developmental Considerations in Psychopharmacology: the Interaction of Drugs and Development (Shapiro); Treatment of Childhood and Adolescent Schizophrenia (Campbell); Psychopharmacologic Treatment of the Minimal Brain Dysfunction Syndrome (Cantwell - Item No. 645); Treatment of Depressive States (Lucas); Treatment of Mild Symptomatic Anxiety States (Patterson and Pruitt); Use of Drugs in Special Syndromes: Enuresis, Tics, School Refusal, and Anorexia Nervosa (Greenberg and Stephans); Summary (Wiener).

688 Recent advances in child psychopharmacology. Edited by Rachel Gittelman-Klein. New York, New York: Human Sciences Press, 1975. 272p. (Bibliography). (Child Psychiatry and Psychology Series).
Presents sixteen papers on current investigations in child psychopharmacology with emphasis on the use of medications in disturbed children.

Contents: Speculations Concerning a Possible Biochemical Basis of Minimal Brain Dysfunction (Wender - Item No. 314); Minor Physical Anomalies (Stigmata) and Early Developmental Deviation--a Major Biologic Subgroup of

Hyperactive Children (Rapoport and Quinn - Item No. 120); Problems in the Diagnosis of Minimal Brain Dysfunction and the Hyperkinetic Syndrome (Klein and Gittelman-Klein - Item No. 492); Controlled Trial of Methylphenidate in Preschool Children with Minimal Brain Dysfunction (Conners - Item No. 812); What is the Proper Dose of Stimulant Drugs in Children? (Sprague and Sleator - Item No. 761); Side Effects from Long-Term Use of Stimulants in Children (Safer and Allen - Item No. 1722); Methylphenidate in Children--Effects Upon Cardiorespiratory Function on Exertion (Aman and Werry - Item No. 1649); A Placebo-Crossover Study of Caffeine Treatment of Hyperactive Children (Conners, et al. - Item No. 790); Clinical Pharmacological Management of Hyperkinetic Children (Katz, et al. - Item No. 1472); Are Behavioral and Psychometric Changes Related in Methylphenidate-Treated, Hyperactive Children? (Gittelman-Klein and Klein - Item No. 889); Are Drugs Enough?--To Treat or to Train the Hyperactive Child (Douglas - Item No. 1054); The Natural History of Hyperactivity in Childhood and Treatment with Stimulant Medication at Different Ages--a Summary of Research Findings (Weiss - Item No. 834); Psychopharmacology in the Prevention of Antisocial and Delinquent Behavior (Satterfield and Cantwell - Item No. 1939); Psychopharmacology in Childhood Psychosis (Campbell - Item No. 640); Pharmacotherapy and Management of Pathological Separation Anxiety (Gittelman-Klein).

These papers are reprints from articles appearing in the Spring-Summer issue of the International Journal of Mental Health.

689 Renshaw, M. C. "Psychopharmacotherapy in children." In: F. J. Ayd, Jr., ed. Rational psychopharmacotherapy and the right to treatment. Baltimore, Maryland: Ayd Medical Communications, 1975.

690 Ross, Alan O. Psychological aspects of learning disabilities and reading disorders. New York, New York: McGraw-Hill, 1976. (Bibliography). (McGraw-Hill Series in Special Education).

Examines the psychological aspects of learning and behavior in the context of educational methodology. Chapter 5 is devoted to hyperactivity and the effect of medication on the syndrome. Topics discussed are: (1) the relationship between hyperactivity and learning disorders; (2) the relationship between hyperactivity and cerebral damage; (3) characteristics; (4) the influence of the environment on the syndrome; and (5) the use of drugs. Drugs should be used after much circumspection, with drug-free alternative interventions given priority. Author and title indexes complete the volume.

691 Saccar, Connie L. "Drug therapy in the treatment of minimal brain dysfunction." Am J Hosp Pharm 35(5): 544-52, May, 1978. (99 References).

Reviews the use of psychotherapeutic agents in the treatment of minimal brain dysfunction. These include: anticonvulsants, antidepressants, central nervous system stimulants, antianxiety agents, antipsychotic agents, and miscellaneous agents. It is concluded that when drugs are indicated for treatment of this syndrome: (1) CNS stimulants are the preferred choice of treatment; (2) tricyclic antidepressants are still in the investigational stage; (3) anticonvulsants are ineffective in controlling behavior problems; and (4) antianxiety and antipsychotic agents are not as desirable as the CNS stimulants.

692 Safer, Daniel J., and Krager, John J. "Prevalence and management of hyperactive children." N Engl J Med 292(10): 537, March 6,

1975. (19 References).
Letter to editor.

693 Schnackenberg, Bob C. "A plea for comprehensive treatment for the hyperkinetic child." Child Welfare 56(4): 231-37, April, 1977. (18 References).
Recommends the use of a combination of treatment modalities in treating the hyperkinetic child. Suggested approaches involve the use of psychostimulants, positive reinforcement, special education, group therapy, psychotherapy, and diet adjustments. Prevention includes the entire spectrum, from preventing birth defects to preschool screening for hyperactivity.

694 Sedgwick, Peter. "Hyperactivity." New Soc 43(796): 31, January 5, 1978. (0 References).
Letter to editor.

695 Shopsin, Baron, and Greenhill, Laurence. "The psychopharmacology of childhood: a profile." In: Psychopharmacology of childhood. Edited by D. V. Siva Sankar. Westbury, New York: PJD Publications, 1976. 179-207. (112 References).
Reviews the major drugs used to treat hyperkinesis and MBD. Comments are also made on other treatments: diet, orthomolecular, and hypnotics. The authors conclude that: (1) more well-designed controlled studies are needed; (2) many drugs have proved ineffectual; and (3) other treatments (diet, vitamins) have not been proven to be successful in treating the hyperkinetic child.

696 Silbergeld, Ellen K. "Neuropharmacology of hyperkinesis." Curr Dev Psychopharmacol 4: 179-214, 1977. (118 References).

697 Silver, Larry B. "Drug therapy with children and adolescents." In: Drugs and the special child. Edited by Michael J. Cohen. New York, New York: Gardner Press, 1979. 33-62. (23 References).
This chapter comprehensively covers the major drugs used to treat hyperkinesis and MBD.

698 Silverstone, Trevor, and Turner, Paul. "Child psychiatry." In: Silverstone, Trevor, and Turner, Paul. Drug treatment in child psychiatry. London, England: Routledge & Kegan Paul. 201-6. (5 References). (Social and Psychological Aspects of Medical Practice Series).
Hyperkinesis is perceived as one of several syndromes which benefit from psychotropic drug treatment.

699 Simeon, Jovan. "Pediatric psychopharmacology--a review of our findings and experience." In: Psychopharmacology of childhood. Edited by D. V. Siva Sankar. Westbury, New York: PJD Publications, 1976. 139-78. (49 References).
Studies drug-induced associations between behavior, brain function, and learning. Hyperkinesis and MBD are included in the discussion.

700 Simeon, J.; Utech, C.; Simeon, S.; et al. "Pediatric psychopharmacology outside the U.S.A." Dis Nerv Syst 35(7, pt. 2): 37-47, July, 1974. (2 References).
Describes research designed to obtain data on the use of psychotropic drugs in children outside the United States. Questionnaires were sent to 251 institutions in fifty-three countries. Of these, seventy-three from

thirty-four countries were returned and analyzed. The percentage of children receiving drugs ranged from 0 to 100 percent (mean 39 percent). Data analyzation reveals that: (1) fifty-six different drugs were administered for eleven psychiatric disorders; (2) the most popular drugs in use were diazepam, thioridazine, chlorpromazine, chlordiazepoxide, imipramine, amitriptyline, haloperidol, and methylphenidate; and (3) the most frequently used drug for hyperkinesis was thioridazine. The problems in interpreting cross-cultural data are discussed.

701 Simon, G. B. "A teachers' guide to 'drugs'." Spec Educ Forward Trends 1(1): 25-28, March, 1974. (0 References).
Briefly reviews various drugs currently used to treat conditions commonly encountered by teachers in the classroom. Covered are anticonvulsants, tranquilizers, antidepressants, and stimulants. Teachers are urged to become familiar with these drugs and their effects. A Table of Names and Substances is included.

702 Sprague, Robert L. "Pediatric psychopharmacology." Psychopharmacol Bull 10(2): 64, April, 1974. (0 References).
Abstract.

703 ————. "Psychopharmacotherapy in children." In: Child psychiatry: treatment and research. Proceedings of the 10th Annual Symposium, September 29-October 1, 1976, Texas Research Institute of Mental Sciences, Houston, Texas. Edited by M. F. McMillan and Sergio Henao. New York, New York: Brunner/Mazel, 1977. 315p. (Bibliography).

704 Sprague, R. L., and Sleator, E. K. "Drugs and dosages: implications for learning disabilities." Paper presented at NATO Conference on the Neuropsychology of Learning Disorders: Theoretical Approaches, Korsør, Denmark, June, 1975.

705 Sprague, Robert L., and Werry, John S. "Psychotropic drugs and handicapped children." In: Second review of special education. Edited by Lester Mann and David A. Sabatino. Philadelphia, Pennsylvania: JSE Press, 1974. 1-50. (Bibliography). (JSE Press Series in Special Education).
Comprehensively reviews studies which pertain to the educational endeavor and the use of psychotropic drugs. The main topics discussed are: (1) the history of psychotropic drug usage; (2) various pharmacological issues; (3) the role of the educator in pediatric psychopharmacology; (4) hyperactivity and MBD; (5) studies of attention, learning performance, arousal theories, activity level, and state-dependent learning; (6) mental retardation; and (7) emotionally disturbed children. The authors provide evidence for the following conclusions: (1) in spite of the vastness of the literature, few studies deal specifically with the MR and ED child; (2) new studies are needed which examine how best to combine special education programs and psychotropic drug treatment; (3) multidisciplinary cooperation is much needed; and (4) existing evidence clearly demonstrates the efficacy of drugs on certain childhood behavior problems.

706 Sroufe, L. Alan. "Drug treatment of children with behavior problems." In: Review of child development research. Volume 4. Edited by Frances D. Horowitz. Chicago, Illinois: University of Chicago Press, 1975. 347-407. (191 References).

This chapter is divided into several sections: (1) Overview of Studies on Drug Effects with Children; (2) The Science of Child Psychopharmacology: Current Status; (3) Problems in Evaluating Drug Treatment of Children; and (4) The Practice of Drug Treatment. Each section is summarized. It is concluded that: (1) existing literature lacks critical analysis; (2) existing information concerning the effects of stimulant drugs on cognitive development, the persistence of behavioral effects, and the long-term physical and psychological consequences is too limited to justify the current level of drug treatment; (3) medication is not appropriate for a great many children currently being treated in this manner; and (4) treating hundreds of thousands of children with stimulant medication in the absence of clear medical need would have serious negative consequences.

707 Stewart, Mark A., and Haller, Ida P. "Hyperactive children." JAMA 231(2): 134-35, January 13, 1975. (3 References).
Letter to editor.

708 Tingergen, N. "Hyperactivity." New Soc 43(796): 31, January 5, 1978. (0 References).
Letter to editor.

709 Varga, James R. "Hyperactivity and medication: reply." Am J Dis Child 133(12): 1288, December, 1979. (1 Reference).
Letter to editor.

710 Wender, Paul H. "Diagnosis and management of minimal brain dysfunction." In: Manual of psychiatric therapies: practical psychopharmacology and psychiatry. Edited by Richard I. Shader. Boston, Massachusetts: Little, Brown, 1975. 137-62. (6 References). (Basic Medical Sciences Series).
Hyperactivity is reviewed as one of several personality disorders based on the Child Psychiatry of the Group for the Advancement of Psychiatry (GAP) system of classification. Therapy must involve the child, the parent, and the family. A complete guide to drug therapy is included.

711 Werry, John S. "The use of psychotropic drugs in children." J Am Acad Child Psychiatry 16(3): 446-68, Summer, 1977. (118 References).
Comprehensively surveys the use of psychotropic drugs in children in terms of clinical use, methods of evaluation, safety, and efficacy. Most cases of hyperkinesis warrant an empirical trial of medication, and, although the literature on pharmacotherapy is abundant, there is a need for a more medical and scientific approach to the use of psychotropic drugs in the treatment of hyperkinesis.

712 Wessel, Morris A. "Prevalence and management of hyperactive children." N Engl J Med 292(10): 536-37, March 6, 1975. (0 References).
Letter to editor.

713 White, James H. "Pharmacologic treatment by target symptoms." In: White, James H. Pediatric psychopharmacology: a practical guide to clinical application. Baltimore, Maryland: Williams & Wilkins, 1977. 88-157. (Bibliography).
Hyperactivity is one of thirteen target symptoms considered in this chapter. Seven case studies are utilized to show ways in which the different drugs prescribed for hyperactivity can be prescribed for different types of patients.

714 Wiener, Jerry M., and Jaffe, Steven. "History of drug therapy in childhood and adolescent psychiatric disorders." In: Psychopharmacology in childhood and adolescence. Edited by Jerry M. Wiener. New York, New York: Basic Books, 1977. 9-40. (164 References).
This historical overview of childhood psychopharmacology covers the 1930s to the present. The major drugs and drug studies are reviewed. Table 1 illustrates the years of introduction and/or use for the major pharmacologic agents in child and adolescent psychiatry.

Wiener, Jerry M.
see Psychopharmacology in childhood and adolescence. (Item No. 687).

715 Winsberg, Bertrand G.; Yepes, Luis E.; Bialer, Irv. "Pharmacologic management of children with hyperactive/aggressive/inattentive behavior disorders: suggestions for the pediatrician." Clin Pediatr 15(5): 471-77, May, 1976. (21 References).
Focuses on some of the pharmacological choices open to the physician in treating hyperactive children. The most effective drugs are psychostimulants, tricyclic compounds, neuroleptics, phenothiazines, and butyrophenones. Although most of these agents have a relatively low rate of side effects, long-term effects are unknown and should be carefully monitored.

716 Woffinder, Margaret, and Purvis, Richard. "Hyperactivity." New Soc 42(793): 590, December 15, 1977. (0 References).
Letter to editor.

717 Yaffe, Sumner J., and Danish, Michele. "The classification and pharmacology of psychoactive drugs in childhood and adolescence." In: Psychopharmacology in childhood and adolescence. Edited by Jerry M. Wiener. New York, New York: Basic Books, 1977. 41-57. (55 References).
This chapter reviews drugs commonly used to treat behavior disturbances in children. Included are: antipsychotic agents, stimulants, antidepressants, and tranquilizers. Classification is made according to accepted chemical use and, within each chemical situation, by chemical structure. However, other considerations, such as data regarding mechanism and site of action, pharmacodynamics, and disposition should be studied for a more accurate classification.

2. SPECIFIC DRUGS

a. Stimulants

i. General

718 Adelman, Howard S., and Compas, Bruce E. "Stimulant drugs and learning problems." J Spec Educ 11(4): 377-416, Winter, 1977. (144 References).
Reviews the current status of stimulant drug research as it relates to children with learning/behavior problems. In addition to summarizing and organizing work in the area, the paper criticizes some of the research and most current applications and attempts to help counteract the premature, widespread application of stimulants as a treatment for learning problems. Areas covered are: "Status of Stimulant Drug Research," "Key Methodological Problems," "Applied Research: Treatment," "Applied Research: Diagnosis," "Applied Research: Negative Side Effects," "Applied

Research: Conclusions," "Basic Research," "Premature Application," and "Conclusion." The research reveals that: (1) drug efficacy on learning and behavior remains unproven; (2) any positive effects may be attributed to physiological rather than psysiological mechanisms; (3) there is no satisfactory research on long-term negative side effects; (4) much drug therapy is premature, inappropriate, and dangerous; and (5) further research is imperative.

719 Barkley, Russell A. "Review of stimulant drug research with hyperactive children." J Child Psychol Psychiatry 18(2): 137-65, April, 1977. (159 References).
Summarizes studies concerning the use of stimulant drugs with hyperactive children. In general, drugs appear to energize the CNS of hyperactive children and aid in concentration, impulsivity, and other areas. Most children show improvement; a small percentage do not. Although side effects do occur, most are transitory. Perhaps the most persistent side effect is suppressed weight and height gain. Even though the efficacy of CNS stimulants seems apparent, the long-term prognosis of hyperactive children in terms of social and emotional adjustment is essentially unaffected by stimulant drug treatment.

720 ————. "Stimulant drugs and academic performance in hyperactive children." Ann Neurol 3(4): 376, April, 1978. (6 References).
Letter to editor.

721 ————. "Using stimulant drugs in the classroom." Sch Psychol Dig 8(4): 412-25, Fall, 1979. (60 References).
Reviews the research on the effects of stimulant drugs on the classroom behavior and academic achievement of hyperactive children. Although most studies indicate that these drugs are very effective at improving attention span, on-task behavior, activity level, and disruptive behavior in hyperactive children, a review of eighteen studies using fifty-five objective measures of scholastic achievement and productivity revealed that drug effects were found on less than 17 percent of these measures. Combined with the results of six long-term follow-up studies, these drug studies indicate that the stimulant drugs do not appreciably improve the academic achievement or outcome of hyperactive children. Reasons for this paradox, implications for the use of stimulants in the classroom, and the role to be played by school psychologists in drug therapy are briefly discussed.

Bosco, James J., ed.
see The hyperactive child and stimulant drugs. (Item No. 744).

722 Bosco, James J., and Robin, Stanley. "The hyperactive child and stimulant drugs: definitions, diagnosis, and directions: an introduction." Sch Rev 85(1): 1-4, November, 1976. (0 References).
This article introduces a special issue of School Review which is primarily devoted to the philosophical, social, and scientific perspectives of the hyperkinetic syndrome. The ten papers are briefly described. Contributors include physicians, psychologists, sociologists, educators, school administrators, government officials, philosophers, and psychobiologists. For the contents of this issue refer to Item No. 744.

723 Brodie, H. Keith H. "CNS activating drugs in the treatment of the hyperactive child: comment." In: Controversy in psychiatry. Edited by John P. Brady and H. Keith Brodie. Philadelphia, Pennsylvania: Saunders, 1978. 277-78. (0 References).

Comments on studies by Dennis P. Cantwell (Item No. 724) and Mark A. Stewart (Item No. 982).

724 Cantwell, Dennis P. "CNS activating drugs in the treatment of the hyperactive child." In: Controversy in psychiatry. Edited by John P. Brady and H. Keith Brodie. Philadelphia, Pennsylvania: Saunders, 1978. 237-68. (130 References).
Evaluates the role of CNS activating drugs in treating hyperactive children. The chapter deals with eight basic questions: (1) Should CNS activating drugs be used at all in the treatment of hyperactive children? (2) Which CNS activating drugs are effective? (3) What functions do CNS activating drugs effect in hyperactive children? (4) What are the long-term positive effects of the use of CNS activating drugs? (5) What are the side effects and possible detrimental effects? (6) Do all hyperactive children respond positively to CNS activating drugs? (7) Are CNS activating drugs more or less effective than other treatment modalities? and (8) What is the optimal management of the hyperactive child and what role do drugs play in this optimal management? For a commentary on this study refer to Item No. 723.

725 Cantwell, Dennis P., and Carlson, Gabrielle A. "Stimulants." In: Pediatric psychopharmacology: the use of behavior modifying drugs in children. Edited by John S. Werry. New York, New York: Brunner/Mazel, 1978. 171-207. (Bibliography).
Reviews the use of CNS stimulants (primarily amphetamine, methylphenidate, and pemoline) to alleviate a number of target symptoms, including hyperactivity. Considered are: pharmacology, clinical effects, predicting clinical response, side effects, drug interactions, clinical indications, clinical use, and social and ethical considerations.

726 Carpenter, Robert L., and Sells, Clifford J. "Measuring effects of psychoactive medication in a child with a learning disability." J Learn Disabil 7(9): 545-50, November, 1974. (10 References).
Describes three types of behavioral measurement: (1) direct measurement of behavior; (2) formal psychometric testing; and (3) rating scales. Because little information exists which shows that specific psychoactive medications generally have predictable effects on children with learning disabilities, simple but objective methods are needed to determine the efficacy of the drugs on behavior. The suggested techniques are applied to a four-and-one-half-year-old girl placed on psychoactive medication in a double-blind placebo-controlled program. The three techniques were then used to measure the child's progress. The obtained data did not demonstrate any drug effects on the behaviors for which the medication was prescribed.

727 Cline, F. W. "Stimulants and their use with hyperactive children." Nurse Pract 2(2): 33-34, November-December, 1976.

728 Clinical use of stimulant drugs in children. Edited by C. Keith Conners. Amsterdam: Excerpta Medica, 1974. 238p. (Bibliography). (International Congress Series, No. 313).
This volume is a collection of nineteen papers presented at a symposium held at Key Biscayne, Florida, March 5-8, 1972. Most papers address the ramifications of the use of drugs in children with academic and behavior problems.

Contents: Diagnosis of Minimal Brain Dysfunction and Hyperkinetic Syndrome (Klein and Gittelman-Klein - Item No. 491); Differences Between

Normal and Hyperkinetic Children (Douglas - Item No. 1198); Some Characteristics of Children with Minimal Brain Dysfunction (Bernstein, Page, and Janicki - Item No. 288); The Clinical Psychological Assessment of Minimal Brain Dysfunction (Clements - Item No. 484); Psychological Tests (Dykman, Ackerman, Peters, et al. - Item No. 563); The Special Neurological Examination (Peters, Dykman, Ackerman, et al. - Item No. 537); Follow-up Studies of Children Who Present with Symptoms of Hyperactivity (Weiss and Minde - Item No. 1947); Five Hundred Children Followed from Grade 2 Through Grade 5 for the Prevalence of Behavior Disorder (Huessy, Marshall, and Gendron - Item No. 1913); Electrodermal Studies in Minimal Brain Dysfunction Children (Satterfield, Atoian, Bradshears, et al. - Item No. 1812); A Multi-clinic Trial of Pemoline in Childhood Hyperkinesis (Page, Bernstein, Janicki, et al. - Item No. 840); A Double-blind Clinical Study of Pemoline in MBD Children: Comments on the Psychological Test Results (Dykman, McGrew, and Ackerman - Item No. 1743); Methylphenidate in Hyperkinetic Behavior: Relation of Response to Degree of Activity and Brain Damage (Millichap and Johnson - Item No. 1860); Experimental Psychology and Stimulant Drugs (Sprague, Christensen, and Werry - Item No. 1220); The Effect of Pemoline and Dextroamphetamine on Evoked Potentials Under Two Conditions of Attention (Conners - Item No. 1561); Levoamphetamine's Changing Place in the Treatment of Children with Behavior Disorders (Arnold and Wender - Item No. 876); Pilot Clinical Trial of Imipramine in Hyperkinetic Children (Gittelman-Klein - Item No. 847); NIMH-PRB Support of Research in Minimal Brain Dysfunction in Children (Lipman - Item No. 2008); Drugs in Maladaptive School Behavior (Zike - Item No. 771); Psychometric Assessment of Stimulant-induced Behavior Change (Knights - Item No. 747).

Author and subject indexes complete the collection.

729 Cohen, Michael W., and Comerci, George D. "Comments on Dr. Kinsbourne's paper." Pediatrics 54(2): 254, August, 1974. (2 References).
Letter to editor.

730 Cole, Jonathan. "Introduction." In: Clinical use of stimulant drugs in children. Edited by C. Keith Conners. Amsterdam: Excerpta Medica, 1974. xi-xii. (0 References). (International Congress Series, No. 313).
Presents introductory comments to the proceedings of a symposium held at Key Biscayne, Florida, March 5-8, 1972. (See Item No. 728).

731 Cole, Sherwood O. "Hyperkinetic children: the use of stimulant drugs evaluated." Am J Orthopsychiatry 45(1): 28-37, January, 1975. (35 References).
Critically appraises the use of stimulant drugs in the treatment of hyperkinetic children. The behavioral characteristics associated with the syndrome are outlined. It is reported that hyperkinesis is mainly a problem of young children and is usually terminated by adolescence. Because hyperkinetic children constitute a social and educational problem of major proportion, their treatment must merit careful consideration, especially in the use of stimulant drugs. Although evidence is seen to support the normalizing effects of stimulant drugs, far too little attention has been paid to potential side effects. A broader program of clinical evaluation is called for--one which assesses drug effects on appetite and the cardiovascular system, as well as on behavior. The sociological impact of drug use by children is also to be considered.

732 Conners, C. Keith. "Learning disabilities and stimulant drugs in children: theoretical implications." In: The neuropsychology of learning disorders: theoretical approaches. Edited by Robert M. Knights and D. J. Bakker. Baltimore, Maryland: University Park Press, 1976. 389-401. (Bibliography).
Discusses the variety of changes in behavior, cognition, and perceptual-motor functions which can be produced by stimulants. Information is provided as to which classes of children will be effected by this class of drugs and in what way.

Conners, C. Keith, ed.
see Clinical use of stimulant drugs in children. (Item No. 728).

733 Conners, C. Keith, and Wells, Karen C. "Method and theory for psychopharmacology with children." In: Hyperactivity in children: etiology, measurement, and treatment implications. Edited by Ronald L. Trites. Baltimore, Maryland: University Park Press, 1979. 141-57. (4 References).
Outlines a theory of how one class of drugs, stimulants, acts to produce changes in one class of childhood behavior disturbance--the hyperkinetic reaction of childhood. Two case studies are cited which illustrate some of the applications of the theory. Implications for future research are discussed. For a commentary on this study refer to Item No. 746.

734 Council on Child Health. "Medication for hyperkinetic children." Pediatrics 55(4): 560-62, April, 1975. (13 References).
Emphasizes the need for physicians to use great caution when prescribing stimulant drugs for the management of hyperkinetic children. Proper dosage, adequate trial periods, knowledge of side effects, and appropriate selection of patients are among the factors considered essential in successful drug treatment. Although the overall management of school failure is a multidisciplinary venture, the responsibility for drug therapy rests with the physician.

735 Cronin, John P. The use of psychopharmaceutical stimulants for the control of childhood hyperkinesis. 1975. 15p. (ED 126 654).
Reviews the literature and research on the use of drugs for control of hyperkinesis.

736 Denhoff, Eric. "Minimal brain dysfunction and stimulant drugs: indications, dosage, and side effects." Hosp Formul 11: 328-31, June, 1976.

737 Erenberg, Gerald. "Psychotropic drugs--harm or help." J Natl Med Assoc 66(3): 214-16, 218, May, 1974. (13+ References).
Summarizes the role of stimulant drug treatment for hyperkinetic children. It is pointed out that more than thirty diagnostic labels have been applied to children exhibiting behavioral abnormalities such as overactivity, short attention span, poor concentration, low frustration tolerance, distractibility, impulsiveness, and poor judgment. Before placing a child on a drug program, the physician must rule out the possibility of other contributing conditions--hunger, boredom in school, chronic illness, chaotic home situation, etc.--and try other treatment regimens. Only in those cases where an alternative therapy is unavailable should medication be considered. Then it should be prescribed with caution and as an adjunct to parental counseling, psychotherapy, and intensive educational planning. The paper was read at the 76th Annual Convention of the National Medical Association.

738 Fidone, George S. "Comments on Dr. Kinsbourne's paper." Pediatrics 54(2): 255, August, 1974. (0 References).
Letter to editor.

739 Fish, Barbara. "Stimulant drug treatment of hyperactive children." In: Cantwell, Dennis P., ed. The hyperactive child: diagnosis, management, current research. New York, New York: Spectrum Publications, distributed by John Wiley and Sons, 1975. 109-127. (14 References). (Series on Child Behavior and Development, Volume I).
Considers some of the main issues surrounding the use of stimulant drugs to treat hyperactive children. Topics covered include: (1) the definition of the syndrome; (2) how stimulants work; (3) when medication should be given; and (4) how to determine a drug's appropriateness for the child.

740 Golinko, Barry E. "Hyperactive child syndrome: system to improve treatment with psychoactive medication." For a summary see: Diss Abstr Int 38B(11): 5567-68, May, 1978. (0 References).

741 Grossman, Herbert J. "Mental retardation, school failure, and hyperactivity." In: Green, Morris, and Haggerty, Robert J., eds. Ambulatory pediatrics. Volume II.: Personal health care of children in the office. Philadelphia, Pennsylvania: Saunders, 1977. 271-93. (15 References).
Mental retardation, school failure, and hyperactivity are covered separately in this chapter. The discussion of hyperactivity focuses on clinical manifestations, diagnostic procedures, and drug management--the drugs of choice being methylphenidate, dextroamphetamine, and pemoline.

742 Halpern, Werner I. "The medication clinic in the spectrum of children's services." Dis Nerv Syst 38(9): 687-90, September, 1977. (22 References).
Reports on how a multidisciplinary child guidance clinic centralized its drug treatment program to better monitor children receiving stimulant medication. Observations are presented from a three-year study of sixty-nine children (ages two to twelve years) who had received medication for hyperactivity. Fifty of the children had no significant side effects; nineteen had side effects requiring changes in kind of drug and dosage levels. Some children continued to display behavior disturbances of moderate intensity.

743 Hechtman, Lily, and Weiss, Gabrielle. "The hyperkinetic child." In: The role of drugs in the treatment of behavioural disorders in children. Proceedings of a symposium held during the VIth World Congress of Psychiatry, Honolulu, Hawaii, August, 1977. Edited by G. Nissen. Bern, Switzerland: Hans Huber, 1978. 16-24. (24 References).
Offers a brief clinical picture of the hyperactive child and lists seven requirements for a comprehensive evaluation. It is concluded that although controlled trials show stimulant drugs improve behavior at home and at school, decrease restlessness, improve concentration, decrease impulsivity, and improve performance on tasks of motor functioning and rote memory, they have little demonstrated effect on the prognosis of the condition. Many children continue to have serious problems which may require other measures such as family counseling, behavior modification, remedial education, psychotherapy, and training in cognition and socialization skills.

744 The hyperactive child and stimulant drugs. Edited by James J. Bosco and Stanley S. Robin. Chicago, Illinois: University of Chicago Press, 1977. 191p. (Bibliography).
Presents ten contributed chapters relating to the medical, pharmacological, educational, social, and future implications of the use of stimulant drugs in treating hyperactive children. The book is a reprint of the November, 1976 issue of School Review (Item No. 722), and is directed toward the nonspecialized, educationally oriented readership rather than for medical personnel or child development researchers.

Contents: Minimal Brain Dysfunction, Hyperactivity, and Learning Disorders: Epidemic or Episode (Freeman - Item No. 151); Is Hyperactivity Abnormal? and Other Unanswered Questions (Stewart - Item No. 262); Ideological, Political, and Moral Considerations in the Use of Drugs in Hyperkinetic Therapy (Broudy - Item No. 1975); Choosing a Middle Path for the Use of Drugs with Hyperactive Children (Havighurst - Item No. 40); Developing School Policy for Use of Stimulant Drugs for Hyperactive Children (Johnson, Kenney, Davis - Item No. 1017); The Teacher and the Social Worker in Stimulant Drug Treatment of Hyperactive Children (Renstrom - Item No. 1481); The Role of the Teacher in Drug Treatment (Sprague and Gadow - Item No. 1507); The Social Context of Stimulant Drug Treatment for Hyperkinetic Children (Robin and Bosco - Item No. 757); Future Threats or Clear and Present Dangers? (Eisenberg - Item No. 2001); Neurobiology and the Future of Education (McGaugh - Item No. 2009).

Both subject and author indexes are included.

745 Kinsbourne, Marcel. "Reply to Drs. Wender, Cohen, Comerci, Fidone, Mutti, and Sterling." Pediatrics 54(2): 254, August, 1974. (0 References).
Letter to editor.

746 Kløve, Hallgrim. Discussion of "Method and theory for psychopharmacology." In: Hyperactivity in children: etiology, measurement, and treatment implications. Edited by Ronald L. Trites. Baltimore, Maryland: University Park Press, 1979. 158-59. (0 References).
Comments on a study by C. Keith Conners and Karen C. Wells (Item No. 733).

747 Knights, Robert M. "Psychometric assessment of stimulant-induced behavior change." In: Clinical use of stimulant drugs in children. Edited by C. Keith Conners. Amsterdam: Excerpta Medica, 1974. 221-31. (5 References). (International Congress Series, No. 313).
Interprets the results of a detailed literature review of the selection and utilization of psychological tests in studies of stimulant-induced behavior change in children. An attempt was made to locate tests most sensitive to drug-induced behavior change. The survey revealed that: (1) no existing single test, test battery, or tests of a particular ability consistently show drug effects; and (2) teacher and parent behavior ratings have a much higher sensitivity to the effects of drugs than do psychological test results. Six standards for reporting drug study data (which are shown to vary greatly) are proposed for future studies. General discussion follows the article.

748 Kolata, Gina Bari. "Childhood hyperactivity: a new look at treatments and causes." Educ Horiz 57(1): 19-21, Fall, 1978. (0 References).
Briefly reviews some recent studies dealing with the role of stimulant drugs in treating hyperactive children. Also cited are studies which

attempt to clarify the etiology of this poorly defined and often misunderstood disorder.

749 Krippner, Stanley; Silverman, Robert; Cavallo, Michael; et al. "Stimulant drugs and hyperkinesis: a question of diagnosis." Read World 13(3): 198-222, March, 1974. (57 References).
Comprehensively reviews the literature on stimulant drugs for hyperactive children. Details are provided for a study which compared two groups, drug and nondrug, on tests of mental ability, creativity, and mental health in an effort to support the hypothesis that the drug group would do less well on tests used to detect MBD. Results show that the two groups did not differ significantly on tests for MBD; they did, however, differ significantly on tests for mental ability, creativity, and mental health. The problem of overuse of drugs for hyperkinesis is discussed.

750 Lambert, Nadine M.; Windmiller, Myra; Sandoval, Jonathan; et al. "Hyperactive children and the efficacy of psychoactive drugs as a treatment intervention." Am J Orthopsychiatry 46(2): 335-52, April, 1976. (77 References).
Discusses the hyperactive child in terms of: (1) characteristics of children with this disorder; (2) previous research concerning the etiology of the syndrome; (3) drug effects studies; (4) drug treatment; and (5) unresolved issues. Individual differences in hyperactive children should form the basis for a treatment program, rather than simply treating groups of children under the rubric "hyperactivity."

751 Loney, Jan, and Ordoña, Truce T. "Using cerebral stimulants to treat minimal brain dysfunction." Am J Orthopsychiatry 45(4): 564-72, July, 1975. (18 References).
Considers questions raised during a study of the medical records of a group of MBD boys treated for hyperactivity with CNS stimulants. The medical case histories covering five-year periods of 135 boys (ages six to twelve years) were used for the study at the University of Iowa. In order to identify factors which would predict response to methylphenidate, data were collected on familial, perinatal, developmental, psychological, educational, neurological, and psychiatric variables. The questions discussed include: (1) Do physician factors contribute to child diagnosis, treatment choice, and clinical improvement? (2) What is improvement? (3) What kind of side effects occur and with what frequency? and (4) When should drugs be used? Answers are provided in the text.

752 Long, Thomas J. "Dealing with common classroom behavior problems." In: Principles of pediatrics: health care of the young. Editor-in-Chief Robert A. Hoekelman. New York, New York: McGraw-Hill, 1978. 549-52. (References).
Briefly describes symptomatology and criteria for diagnosis. Comments are also made on stimulant medication and family management.

753 Murray, Joseph N. "Drugs to control classroom behavior?" Educ Dig 39(5): 13-15, January, 1974. (0 References).
Addresses some frequent questions and issues concerning the use of psychoactive drugs to modify the behavior of overactive children. These questions are: (1) Why are some youngsters medicated while others are not? (2) Who should receive medication? (3) What are the possible causes of hyperkinesis? and (4) What drugs are most frequently used to control hyperkinesis? This researcher feels that medication should be given only when other treatment modalities fail, and only after careful reviewing by parents and family physician.

754 Mutti, Margaret, and Sterling, Harold M. "Comments on Dr. Kinsbourne's paper." Pediatrics 54(2): 254, August, 1974. (0 References).
Letter to editor.

755 Neisworth, John T.; Kurtz, P. David; Ross, April; et al. "Naturalistic assessment of neurological diagnoses and pharmacological intervention." J Learn Disabil 9(3): 149-52, March, 1976. (10 References).
Points out some of the inappropriate uses and shortcomings which commonly occur in prescribing and supervising stimulant drugs for children's behavior disorders. To combat this, certain minimal standards are proposed: (1) translation of the clinical diagnosis into measurable naturalistic behaviors; (2) collection of data by parents and teachers to determine the severity of the syndrome; (3) situational validation or disconfirmation of the clinical diagnosis; and (4) assessment of drug treatment when indicated. An example is included which applies these principles.

756 "Psychoactive medication and learning problems in children." RI Med J 58(4): 159-60, 170-71, April, 1975.

Robin, Stanley S., ed.
see The hyperactive child and stimulant drugs. (Item No. 744).

757 Robin, Stanley S., and Bosco, James J. "The social context of stimulant drug treatment for hyperkinetic children." Sch Rev 85(1): 141-54, November, 1976. (24 References).
Analyzes the obstacles to effective collaboration of educators, parents, and physicians in the diagnosis and stimulant drug treatment of hyperkinesis since their roles are not always congruent. Members of the three systems view the child from different perspectives and have different goals, and the lack of articulation among the systems leads to controversy. Three approaches to solutions are proposed: (1) development of agencies that bring the systems together for the purpose of addressing the problem; (2) development of constructive law and policy governing the roles of the systems; and (3) changing roles of system members or creating new roles to meet the situation. There are constraints and difficulties surrounding each approach; nevertheless, it is necessary to develop a coherent social context for the treatment of hyperkinetic children. For a reprint of this study refer to Item No. 744.

758 Simpson, R.; Reece, C. A.; Kauffman, R. E.; et al. The effects of central nervous system stimulants in classroom behavior of hyperactive children. Kansas City, Kansas: University of Kansas Medical Center, 1975.
Unpublished manuscript.

759 Sleator, Esther K., and Sprague, Robert L. "Pediatric pharmacotherapy." In: Principles of psychopharmacology. 2nd ed. Edited by William G. Clark and Joseph del Guidice. New York, New York: Academic Press, 1978. 573-91. (35 References).
Provides a brief guide to the appropriate use of psychotropic drugs for a number of children's behavior disorders, including hyperactivity and MBD. Comments are made on diagnosis, stimulant drug treatment, side effects of stimulant drugs, and long-term aspects of stimulant drug therapy.

760 Solow, Robert A. "Stimulants and hyperkinesis." West J Med 129(6): 488-89, December, 1978. (3 References).

Presents a very brief summary statement of the role of drugs as one therapeutic method available for treating hyperactive children.

761 Sprague, Robert L., and Sleator, Esther K. "What is the proper dose of stimulant drugs in children?" Int J Ment Health 4(1-2): 75-104, Spring-Summer, 1975. (58 References).
Reviews previous literature on the use of stimulant medication with hyperactive children. The thrust of the article centers on various criteria which should be used for determining correct dosage of stimulants. These points are argued: (1) dose-response relationships are important to the clinician as well as to the more theoretically oriented researcher; (2) dose-response relationships differ for different target behaviors; and (3) the titration method uses social behavior as the main criterion for determining dosages of stimulant medication. The titration method is questioned since there is evidence that the dosage levels considered with this method are well above the optimal range for cognitive performance. For a reprint of this study refer to Item No. 688.

762 "Stimulant drugs for hyperactive children." Drug Ther Bull 15(6): 22-24, March 18, 1977.
Briefly summarizes various stimulants currently being used to treat hyperactive children.

763 Taylor, E. "The use of drugs in hyperkinetic states: clinical issues." Neuropharmacology 18(12): 951-58, 1979. (42 References).
Evaluates the use of stimulant drugs in hyperactive children. The main points of the presentation are: (1) there is continuing confusion about the nature of the condition; (2) there is nothing paradoxical about the action of stimulant drugs; and (3) stimulant drugs do not reverse any specific pathology, rather, they exert multiple, independent effects on different aspects of a child's behavior and cognition.

764 Treegoob, Mark, and Walker, Kenneth P. "The use of stimulant drugs in the treatment of hyperactivity." Sch Psychol Dig 5(4): 5-10, Fall, 1976. (25 References).
Briefly summarizes the salient characteristics of the hyperkinetic syndrome and describes some of the most popular stimulants presently being used to control its symptoms. Drugs are not the only effective or best treatment and should be prescribed only after careful diagnostic procedures have taken place.

765 ————. "The use of stimulant drugs in the treatment of hyperactivity." Devereux Forum 12(1): 40-45, Summer, 1977.
Reprints an article from the School Psychology Digest 5(4): 5-10, Fall, 1976. (Item No. 764).

766 Wender, Esther H. "Comments on Dr. Kinsbourne's paper." Pediatrics 54(2): 253, August, 1974. (3 References).
Letter to editor.

767 Whalen, Carol K., and Henker, Barbara. "Psychostimulants and children: a review and analysis." Psychol Bull 83(6): 1113-32, November, 1976. (113 References).
The use of psychostimulant medication for children with hyperkinesis is reviewed. Three areas are covered: motor activity, attention and cognition, and social-adaptive behavior. Prevailing misconceptions about these drugs and the children who take them are examined as well as the dispari-

ties between findings on short- and long-term effects. Also discussed are the psychological concomitants of stimulant medication. Recent research on causal attributions is reviewed, and a set of hypotheses and research strategies is developed, centering on the proposition that stimulant medication is a powerful source of attributional change in both the child and others. Predicting and enhancing medication effects may depend on understanding and modifying the social and cognitive sequelae of drug intervention.

768 White, James H. "The hyperactive child syndrome." Am Fam Physician 15(4): 100-104, April, 1977. (0 References).
Defines hyperkinesis as a constellation of symptoms: increased motor activity, distractibility, short attention span, restlessness, impulsiveness, sometimes antisocial behavior, and, often, learning disabilities. Management involves counseling, behavioral therapy, and drugs--especially methylphenidate, pemoline, imipramine, dextroamphetamine, and thioridazine. These agents are very successful when used according to strict principles, i.e., minimum doses for short durations, careful scheduling, and close supervision.

769 ————. "Psychotropic drugs in child and adolescent psychiatry." In: Current psychiatric therapies. Volume 17. Edited by Jules H. Masserman. New York, New York: Grune & Stratton, 1977. (25 References).
Suggests guidelines for administering psychotropic drugs for a number of target symptoms including hyperactivity. Suggestions include: (1) identifying a target symptom before medicating; (2) selecting a drug to which the particular symptom is most likely to respond; (3) monitoring the child; (4) keeping the drug treatment program as short as possible; and (5) broadening the treatment program to include environmental changes and/or psychotherapy.

770 Wolraich, Mark L. "Stimulant drug therapy in hyperactive children: research and clinical implications." Pediatrics 60(4): 512-18, October, 1977. (34 References).
Although many aspects of drug treatment for hyperactive children remain controversial, this author believes that research has discovered some consistent results. Among these are: (1) there is a definite, positive, short-term effect of stimulant medication on school behavior; (2) methylphenidate and dextroamphetamine seem equally effective; (3) tolerance to drugs can occur; (4) long-term benefits are still unknown; (5) the placebo effect is evident in a number of cases; and (6) there should be close communication between pediatricians and teachers.

771 Zike, Kenneth. "Drugs in maladaptive school behavior." In: Clinical use of stimulant drugs in children. Edited by C. Keith Conners. Amsterdam: Excerpta Medica, 1974. 214-20. (16 References). (International Congress Series, No. 313).
Outlines a method of monitoring the use of psychoeffective drugs prescribed for maladaptive school behavior and points out cautions regarding their use. The method employed was a direct observational, double-blind sampling of specific parameters of school behavior. Studies of three children in an experimental education unit are documented in detail. Each child's dosage schedule and response to medication were carefully monitored. Selection of drugs and cautions regarding their use are discussed within this chapter.

ii. Amphetamine

772 Brown, Gerald L.; Ebert, Michael H.; Hunt, Robert D. "Plasma d-amphetamine absorption and elimination in hyperactive children." Psychopharmacol Bull 14(3): 33-35, July, 1978. (26 References).
Uses a single oral dosage of d-amphetamine to measure absorption and elimination of the drug in hyperactive children. The study group of sixteen children was selected. Urinary pH was monitored, hourly behavioral ratings both on and off drugs obtained, and blood samples drawn. Findings include: (1) there is an apparent elimination of half life of d-amphetamine (6.8 ± 0.5 hours); and (2) behavioral and motor activity response relate temporally to the absorption phase but do not correlate with actual plasma levels of d-amphetamine.

773 Brown, G. L.; Ebert, M. H.; Hunt, R. D.; et al. "Amphetamine blood levels, behavior and activity in minimal brain dysfunction." Paper presented at the American Psychological Association, Toronto, 1977.

774 Brown, Gerald L.; Hunt, Robert D.; Ebert, Michael H.; et al. "Plasma levels of d-amphetamine in hyperactive children: serial behavior and motor responses." Psychopharmacology 62(2): 133-40, April, 1979. (87 References).
Studies the pharmacokinetics of amphetamine in sixteen hyperactive boys. Peak plasma levels during absorption and elimination are detailed.

775 DiTullio, William M. "The use of amphetamines in treating children manifesting hyperactive behavior." In: Saunders, Bruce T., ed. Approaches with emotionally disturbed children. Hicksville, New York: Exposition Press, 1974. 94-115. (48 References). (An Exposition-University Book).
Provides an historical framework and perspective for the use of amphetamines in treating children with hyperactive behaviors and evaluates the use of amphetamines and their derivatives in this treatment. Also discussed are: (1) definitional problems of hyperactivity; (2) the place of amphetamines within the context of a total treatment program; and (3) the importance of differential diagnosis in successful management.

776 Firemark, H. M.; McIntyre, H. B.; Bodner, L.; et al. "Amphetamine metabolism in hyperactive children." Neurology 27(4): 400, April, 1977. (0 References).
Abstract of a conference paper presented at the 29th annual meeting of the American Academy of Neurology.

777 Gordon, Donald A.; Forehand, Rex; Picklesimer, D. Kris. "The effects of dextroamphetamine on hyperactive children using multiple outcome measures." J Clin Child Psychol 7(2): 125-28, Summer, 1978. (9 References).
Explores the effects of dextroamphetamine on a group of children using multiple outcome measures. Fifteen hyperactive children (ages eight to eleven years) participated in the study. While children who received the drug showed more positive behavior and less out-of-group behavior than those who received a placebo, they exhibited no change in negative behavior. The students were perceived by teachers as showing less hyperactivity and exhibiting less inattentive and impulsive behavior. No differences were found between drug and placebo conditions for three individually administered performance tests.

778 Grinspoon, Lester, and Singer, Susan B. "Amphetamines in the treatment of hyperkinetic children." In: The rights of children. Cambridge, Massachusetts: Harvard Educational Review, 1974. 241-81. (99 References). (Reprint Series, No. 9).
Consists of a literature review on use of drugs in hyperactive children. Early research on the use of amphetamines for the syndrome is cited, and the mechanism of amphetamine action is reported.

779 ———. "Amphetamines in the treatment of hyperkinetic children." In: Chess, Stella, and Thomas, Alexander, eds. Annual progress in child psychiatry and child development, 1974. New York, New York: Brunner/Mazel, 1975. 417-56. (99 References).
Reviews research on the effects of amphetamines on children, particularly hyperactive children in the classroom. It is pointed out that there is no clear evidence these drugs should be presented as often as they are. The "hyperkinetic syndrome" remains vague both in its diagnosis and its etiology, and the mechanism of amphetamine action is unclear. The assumption that amphetamines have a paradoxical, calming effect on hyperactive children, unlike the stimulating effect they exert on adults, may accurately describe the apparent effects of the drugs on attention and other aspects of socially accepted classroom behavior, but it does not justify the interpretation that amphetamine effects are qualitatively different for children than for adults, without the same potential for harm. The authors conclude that the possible adverse effects of these drugs and their unknown long-term risks require that we consider the present policy of amphetamine administration in the schools.

780 ———. "Amphetamines in the treatment of hyperkinetic children: a note of caution." In: Psychopharmacology of childhood. Edited by D. V. Siva Sankar. Westbury, New York: PJD Publications, 1976. 209-70. (150 References).
This lengthy review article details the use of amphetamines in the treatment of hyperkinetic children. Topics covered include: (1) early investigations (since Bradley); (2) the development of the syndrome; (3) the "paradoxical" effect of stimulant drugs; (4) the site of action of amphetamines; (5) amphetamine abuse; (6) long-term effects; and (7) alternatives to drug therapy.

781 ———. "Commentary on the Sleator article." Sci Am 231(3): 8, 12, September, 1974. (0 References).
Letter to editor.

782 Maletzky, Barry M. "d-Amphetamine and delinquency: hyperkinesis persisting?" Dis Nerv Syst 35(12): 543-47, December, 1974. (20 References).
Investigates the efficacy of the stimulant drug, d-amphetamine, in controlling the delinquent behavior of adolescents and demonstrates an association between hyperkinesis of childhood and delinquency of adolescence. Fourteen pairs of boys (ages thirteen to eighteen years), who had been referred for psychiatric outpatient care because of antisocial behaviors, served as subjects. The boys were administered a behavior rating scale and assigned either d-amphetamine or placebo for a three-month period. Through sequential analysis and follow-up scales, a significant improvement was seen in the d-amphetamine group. Few side effects such as tolerance, withdrawal, or euphoria could be detected. Also discussed are: (1) the similarities between the delinquent's response to d-amphetamine and the response usually observed in hyperactive children to stimulant medi-

cations; and (2) the link between a history or presence of hyperactive traits and a clinical response to d-amphetamine.

783 ————. "d-Amphetamine and delinquency: hyperkinesis persisting?" In: Progress in psychiatric drug treatment. Volume 2. Edited by Donald F. Klein and Rachael Gittelman-Klein. New York, New York: Brunner/Mazel, 1976. 433-43. (20 References).
Reprints an article from Diseases of the Nervous System 35(12): 543-47, December, 1974. (Item No. 782).

784 May, Deborah. "Amphetamine therapy with hyperactive children." AVISO 9-13, June, 1974.
Concedes that although much is understood about amphetamine's effect on the CNS of hyperactive children, potential intervening variables have been largely overlooked in research studies. These include parental attitudes, inconsistent administration of the drug, seasonal variations in behavior, and teacher, parent, and therapist expectation. In a literature review of 1,100 drug studies, only 210 are reported as having adequate controls. Other studies present subjective evidence only. It is recommended that future research clarify methodological questions and provide objective data on drug effects.

785 Montagu, J. D., and Swarbrick, Linda. "Effect of amphetamines in hyperkinetic children: stimulant or sedative? A pilot study." Dev Med Child Neurol 17(3): 293-98, June, 1975. (15 References).
Six hyperactive children were used to study the effects of two kinds of amphetamines on hyperkinetic behavior. Dextroamphetamine and levoamphetamine were administered in single equal doses, and the effects on motor activity and palmar skin admittance were measured. Results show that only the l-isomer resulted in a significant decrease in motor activity. Both isomers resulted in a significant decrease in skin admittance--the l-isomer having the greatest effect. The hypothesis that hyperkinetic children are underaroused cannot be substantiated by this study. The authors conclude that the beneficial effects of amphetamines are due to their apparent sedative action.

786 Oettinger, Leon, Jr. "The use of amphetamines in hyperactivity." Dev Med Child Neurol 17(1): 117, February, 1975. (0 References).
Letter to editor.

787 Sleator, Esther K. "Discussion of Grinspoon's and Singer's article." Sci Am 231(3): 8, September, 1974. (0 References).
Letter to editor.

788 Stein, Michel D. "Dextroamphetamine therapy in hyperactive children." West J Med 120(4): 327-28, April, 1974. (0 References).
Letter to editor.

iii. Caffeine

789 Conners, C. Keith. "The acute effects of caffeine on evoked response, vigilance, and activity level in hyperkinetic children." J Abnorm Child Psychol 7(2): 145-51, June, 1979. (11 References).
Studies the effects of caffeine on several variables on seventeen hyperkinetic children who had previously responded to sympathomimetic amines. The children were given three different dosages of caffeine in counterbalanced order (placebo, and low and high doses equivalent to one and

three cups of coffee). One hour following ingestions they were tested on measures of visual evoked response, alpha time, vigilance, and activity level. There was a significant effect on evoked response. The behavioral measures tended to be affected in a dose-related manner but not to a statistically significant degree. It is concluded that although centrally active, caffeine does not show the congruence between behavioral and central effects that other stimulants useful in behavioral management have shown.

790 ————. "A placebo-crossover study of caffeine treatment of hyperkinetic children." Int J Ment Health 4(1-2): 132-43, Spring-Summer, 1975. (1 Reference).
Examines the efficacy of caffeine on several measures in eight hyperkinetic children who had been successfully treated with either dextroamphetamine or methylphenidate. Parent, teacher, and clinical observations were employed at baseline and three weeks after the two treatment regimes. Measures of attention, activity level, and language function were also obtained at these times. Only one case showed some possible clinical benefits from caffeine. Two factors may account for the apparent failure of this stimulant: (1) the dosage level was fixed, and the minimal side effects suggest the possibility that adequate dosage levels were not reached; and (2) it is possible that only certain types of children are responsive to caffeine. On the basis of these findings the use of caffeine is not recommended for hyperkinesis until further research is undertaken. For a reprint of this study refer to Item No. 688.

791 "Coffee breaks for the hyperkinetic child." Hum Behav 3(4): 33, April, 1974. (0 References).
Briefly reports on a study of Robert C. Schnackenberg which compared the effects of CNS stimulants versus caffeine in eleven hyperactive children. The trials, each lasting three weeks, showed both approaches to be equally effective in controlling hyperactive behavior. However, undesirable side effects were eliminated with the coffee treatment.

792 Degraff, Arthur C. "Treating hyperactive children with coffee." Am Fam Physician 9(6): 145-46, June, 1974. (0 References).
Letter to editor.

793 Firestone, Philip; Poitras-Wright, Hélène; Douglas, Virginia. "The effects of caffeine on hyperactive children." Res Relat Child 41: 113, March, 1978-August, 1978. (0 References).
Abstracts a report of research in progress or recently completed research. Data are provided on: name of investigator(s), purpose of the study, number and kind of subjects used, methodology, principal findings, duration of research, cooperating group(s), and availability of publication(s). Research Relating to Children is compiled by the ERIC Clearinghouse on Early Childhood Education.

794 ————. "The effects of caffeine on hyperactive children." J Learn Disabil 11(3): 133-41, March, 1978. (25 References).
Investigates the effects of caffeine on the behavior of hyperactive children. Twenty boys (ages five to twelve years) were selected for the study and tested during a double-blind two-week trial period. The children received either caffeine or placebo. All were rated by parents and teachers on various psychological, physiological, and behavioral measures. Data analyzation shows: (1) caffeine did not significantly improve reaction times and psychological test scores; and (2) caffeine did improve

impulsivity and general behavior both in the home and in the classroom. A discussion and interpretation of these findings accompanies the article.

795 Gross, Mortimer D. "Caffeine in the treatment of children with minimal brain dysfunction or hyperkinetic syndrome." Psychosomatics 16(1): 26-27, First Quarter, 1975. (0 References).
This investigation sought to verify a pilot study by R. C. Schnackenberg (American Journal of Psychiatry 130: 796-98, 1973) which reflected improved behavior of hyperactive children as a result of drinking coffee. The present study used twenty-five hyperkinetic children to compare the effects of placebo, caffeine, and three other drugs. The regimen lasted five weeks: the first week placebo was administered; the second week the children received caffeine; the third week methylphenidate was given; dextroamphetamine was used for the fourth week; imipramine was administered during week five. Written reports were obtained from parents and teachers for each week. Tabulated results indicate that caffeine, at an average dose of two cups of coffee a day, showed an average improvement of -0.8. In contrast to previous studies, not one child's behavior improved as a result of caffeine administration.

796 Harvey, D. H. P., and Marsh, R. W. "The effects of decaffeinated coffee versus whole coffee on hyperactive children." Dev Med Child Neurol 20(1): 81-86, February, 1978. (12 References).
Compares the effects of whole and decaffeinated coffee on the behavior of hyperactive children. Twelve children (eight boys and four girls, mean age 7.26 years), referred to a psychology department for behavior disorders, served as subjects in the double-blind crossover design. Reactions, taken at the end of the seven-week period, were assessed by a variety of tests and scales. Whole coffee proved to be superior to decaffeinated coffee on all measures. It is suggested that whole coffee may be a useful initial measure in dietary management.

797 Powers, Hugh W. S., Jr. "Caffeine, behavior and the LD child." Acad Ther 11(1): 5-19, Fall, 1975. (16 References).
Studies the relationship of high sugar and carbohydrate intake and large amounts of caffeine intake to LD children with multiple nervous system complaints. Not only does caffeine reduce drowsiness, but its excitatory effects may adversely affect newly acquired motor skills and accurate timing. Tactile discrimination and acoustic associations are adversely affected by caffeine in excess of 250 mg. The combination of caffeine and sugar found in soft drinks may possibly increase insulin secretion, thereby explaining restlessness and inattention in some children with learning problems. Cases are presented in which regulation of sugar and caffeine in the diet was linked with decreases in nervous system irritability, though not necessarily with decreased learning problems. Tables are presented showing the sugar and caffeine contents of selected foods.

798 Schnackenberg, Robert C. "Caffeine therapy for hyperkinetic children." Curr Psychiatr Ther 15: 39-44, 1975. (9 References).
Reports on an experiment which tested the efficacy of caffeine in treating hyperactive children. Because some hyperactive children develop side effects to the Schedule II stimulants widely used to treat their hyperactive behavior, caffeine, in the form of one cup of coffee at breakfast and one at lunch, was administered to sixteen hyperactive children. The children, who had all been receiving methylphenidate, were taken off this drug for three weeks and were then given coffee for three weeks. Teachers, unaware of the change in treatment, were asked to rate the children by

the Davids method on three occasions. Mean scores for the children showed methylphenidate and caffeine to be approximately the same; however, no apparent side effects occurred with the latter. The place of caffeine in the treatment management of the hyperactive child is discussed.

799 Schwartz, Merny. "The use of caffeine for controlling the symptoms of hyperkinesis in children." For a summary see: Diss Abstr Int 38B(2): 916, August, 1977. (0 References).

800 "A surprising effect of coffee." Fam Health 6: 16, January, 1974. (0 References).
Briefly reports on the research of Dr. Robert C. Schnackenberg, a Columbia, South Carolina psychiatrist. The doctor accidently discovered that a large number of his young hyperkinetic patients drank coffee, which was found to have a soothing effect on the children. This form of treatment, if proven reliable by further testing, would be less expensive and more healthful than the medications presently being used to treat the symptoms of the hyperkinetic syndrome.

801 Young, S. R.; Ross, I. A.; Burns, J. F. "A cytogenetic study of children treated with caffeine for hyperactivity." Clin Res 24(1): A66, January, 1976. (0 References).
Abstract of paper presented at the annual meeting of the Southern Society for Pediatric Research.

iv. Deanol

802 Coleman, Nathan; Dexheimer, Patric; DiMascio, Alberto; et al. "Deanol in the treatment of hyperkinetic children." Psychosomatics 17(2): 68-72, April-June, 1976. (11 References).
Tests the efficacy of the drug deanol acetamidobenzoate in the treatment of the hyperactive behavior disorder in children. Twenty-five moderately disturbed hyperactive children (ages six to twelve years) were administered 300-500 mg of deanol per day for twelve weeks while twenty-five hyperactive children received only a placebo during this time. Behavioral changes were rated by a psychiatrist, a psychologist, physicians, teachers and parents using various rating scales and tests. The drug group was seen to show the most improvement by all persons concerned, although the difference was small in the teachers' ratings. A twelve-week test period may not be sufficient to show appreciable drug effects in some areas.

803 Knobel, Mauricio. "Approach to combined pharmacologic therapy of childhood hyperkinesis." PDM 5(9-12); 6(1-8): 56-59, January-December, 1974. (27 References).
Reports on the use of 2-dimethylaminoethanol (deanol) to treat the hyperkinetic behavior disorder, especially that which has a known organic etiology. Thirty hyperactive children (ages five to ten years) served as subjects and received 300 mg of deanol per day and a magnesium salt of dipropylacetic acid (DAP). Results at the end of the two-month period showed marked improvement in seventeen of the children and moderate improvement in six cases. The beneficial association of different anticonvulsants is discussed, as well as the undesirable side effects which might accompany the use of this type of drug.

804 ———. "Approach to a combined pharmacologic therapy of childhood hyperkinesis." Behav Neuropsychiatry 6(1-12): 87-90, April, 1974-March, 1975.

Reprints an article from PDM 5(9-12); 6(1-8): 56-59, January-December, 1974. (Item No. 803).

805 Lewis, James A., and Lewis, Barbara S. "Deanol in minimal brain dysfunction." Dis Nerv Syst 38(12, pt. 2): 21-24, December, 1977. (14 References).
Considers the complexities and controversies of MBD and reviews the use of deanol in its treatment. The role of deanol is still unclear because of the difficulties of identifying appropriate patients in terms of levels of arousal and appropriate measures of response. Further investigation of deanol is deemed justified.

806 Oettinger, Leon. "Pediatric psychopharmacology: a review with special reference to deanol." Dis Nerv Syst 38(12, pt. 2): 25-31, December, 1977. (81 References).
Comprehensively reviews the use of drugs to treat MBD with emphasis on deanol. The following conclusions are reached: (1) MBD is a syndrome with multiple etiologies and varying symptoms; (2) although drug therapy has been proven to be effective and practical, adjunct psychological and environmental controls are also necessary; (3) deanol is probably an effective drug with potential usefulness in treating MBD; and (4) urgency is needed for a diagnostic method which can give a better expectation of correctly choosing an effective drug on the first trial.

v. Methylphenidate

807 Barkley, Russell A., and Cunningham, Charles E. "Stimulant drugs and activity level in hyperactive children." Am J Orthopsychiatry 49(3): 491-99, July, 1979. (36 References).
Studies existing evidence and presents additional data on the effects of stimulants on activity level and exploratory behavior in activity-eliciting free field settings. Fourteen hyperactive boys served as subjects. Results indicate that activity and attention span appear to be affected by methylphenidate even in highly stimulating, informal settings. Comparison of the hyperactive boys with a group of fourteen normal controls suggests that this drug-induced reduction of activity and inattentiveness is not a "normalizing" effect. Implications of the findings are discussed.

808 Baxley, Gladys B., and Ullmann, Rina K. "Psychoactive drug effects in a hyperactive child: a case study analysis of behavior change and teacher attention." J Sch Psychol 17(4): 317-24, Winter, 1979. (25 References).
Investigates the effects of methylphenidate on the behavior and teacher interactions of one hyperactive child. A nine-year-old girl was observed under drug and placebo conditions. The teacher's ratings were also obtained. Ratings showed that when the subject was receiving methylpenidate she engaged in task-related activities a greater percent of the time, had a higher percent of teacher interactions that were instructional in quality, and received lower behavior ratings by the teacher than when she was receiving a placebo. It is suggested that the use of medication may enable the hyperactive child to profit both behaviorally and academically.

809 Broad, James. Assessing stimulant treatment of hyperactivity by Bristol Social Adjustment Guides. 13p. 1979. (ED 180 175).
Analyzes the effects of Ritalin on social behavior as measured by global rating scales. Eighteen hyperactive boys participated in the trial.

Behavior ratings by parents and teachers improved significantly when the boys were given Ritalin. The Bristol Social Adjustment Guides were deemed superior to Conners' Abbreviated Teacher Rating Scale for clinical evaluation of treatment efficacy.

810 Brown, Ronald T., and Sleator, Esther K. "Methylphenidate in hyperkinetic children: differences in dose effects on impulsive behavior." Pediatrics 64(4): 408-11, October, 1979. (35 References).
Tests the hypothesis that in hyperactive children a low dose of methylphenidate (0.3 mg/kg) would produce scores superior to those with a high dose (1.0 mg/kg) or placebo on the Matching Familiar Figures Test, a primary index of impulsivity. The hypothesis was based on an earlier finding that the highest percentage of correct responses on a short-term memory task were found in hyperactive subjects who were receiving 0.3 mg/kg of methylphenidate whereas at 1.0 mg/kg the percentage correct returned to the placebo level. The hypothesis was upheld by this research. For a commentary on this study refer to Item No. 830.

811 Charles, Linda; Zelniker, T.; Schain, R. J. "Dose dependent effects of methylphenidate on hyperactive children." Pediatr Res 12(4, pt. 2): 369, April, 1978. (0 References).
Presents an abstract of a paper read at the annual meeting of the American Pediatric Society and the Society for Pediatric Research.

812 Conners, C. Keith. "Controlled trial of methylphenidate in preschool children with minimal brain dysfunction." Int J Ment Health 4(1-2): 61-74, Spring-Summer, 1975. (2 References).
This research attempts to determine the safety and efficacy of the use of methylphenidate with a group of younger children. Fifty-three children (age six years) were administered a battery of tests. Medical and perinatal histories and visual and auditory cortical evoked responses were obtained. Evidence is provided for the following findings: (1) clinical improvement of children on the drug was apparent with a relatively small average dose of the drug; (2) objective measures of intelligence and visual-motor integration showed significant enhancement in children given the drug compared with those receiving a placebo; (3) measures of vigilance, seat activity, and impulsivity did not show significant enhancement by the drug, even though gains were always greater than in the placebo group; (4) parents noted a significant degree of reduction in restless and disturbing behavior in their ratings of children receiving the drug rather than a placebo; (5) the drug enhanced the cortical evoked responses in the left parietal area; (6) side effects of the drug were generally minimal, and there was no significant weight loss during the study. Implications of methylphenidate administration for younger children are given. For a reprint of this study refer to Item No. 688.

813 Ellis, M. J.; Witt, Peter A.; Reynolds, Ronald; et al. "Methylphenidate and the activity of hyperactives in the informal setting." Child Dev 45(1): 217-20, March, 1974. (13 References).
Although the ingestion of methylphenidate has been proven to have beneficial effects on the classroom behavior of hyperactive children in past studies, data from two preliminary studies reported here suggest that methylphenidate does not alter the behavior of hyperactive children in an informal setting such as play activity. Nine hyperactive and antisocial children (ages eight to ten years) were used as subjects and were brought to a play research laboratory and administered varying amounts of methylphenidate or placebo. Their play behavior was then observed and

recorded by camera. Since no discriminable effects were seen, it is concluded that methylphenidate's ability to reduce extraneous activity in a formal setting does not extend to the informal setting. It is suggested that methylphenidate does not directly affect the energy expenditures of the child; rather, it subtly alters attentional mechanisms so the hyperactive child can respond more appropriately to his surroundings.

814 Henker, Barbara; Whalen, Carol K.; Collins, Barry E. "Double-blind and triple-blind assessments of medication and placebo responses in hyperactive children." J Abnorm Child Psychol 7(1): 1-13, March, 1979. (21 References).
Hyperactive boys taking psychostimulant medication were studied using a randomized, placebo-controlled, crossover design. Behavior ratings and medication guesstimates were obtained for the boys when they were given methylphenidate (Ritalin) and when they were given a placebo. The ratings showed positive medication-related changes, and the guesses, done by independent judges, were significantly better than chance. The pattern of ratings for double-blind and triple-blind raters was identical. These results imply that positive psychostimulant effects are not attributable to rater sensitization or expectancy. The medication-placebo differences were highly reliable for the group comparisons and were in the predicted direction of twenty-one of twenty-two individuals, but the magnitude of the change for many individuals was not dramatic. Implications for child psychopharmacology research and differences between clinical and experimental significance are discussed.

815 Hoffman, Stanley P.; Engelhardt, David M.; Margolis, Reuben A.; et al. "Response to methylphenidate in low socioeconomic hyperactive children." Arch Gen Psychiatry 30(3): 354-59, March, 1974. (17 References).
Studies the efficacy of methylphenidate on the hyperkinetic behavior of a group of ghetto children. Sixty-two children from economically deprived urban areas served as subjects and were evaluated before and after the twelve-week program by parents, teachers, social worker, and child psychiatrist. Tests included the WISC, Wide Range Achievement Test, Marianne Frostig Development Test of Visual Perception, and motor inhibition and body boundaries tasks. Data analyzation reveals: (1) methylphenidate was as effective with this select population as it has been reported with other groups; (2) improvement was noted in many areas of the child's functioning; (3) weight loss was the most generalized side effect; and (4) variability in the teacher's weekly classroom hyperactivity ratings could be used as a means of dichotomizing the sample of children.

816 Humeid, M. S. "The hyperactive child." Can Med Assoc J 112(7): 803, April, 1975. (0 References).
Letter to editor.

817 Hungund, B. L.; Perel, J. M.; Hurwic, M. J.; et al. "Pharmacokinetics of methylphenidate in hyperkinetic children." Br J Clin Pharmacol 8(6): 571-76, December, 1979.
Investigates the metabolism and pharmacokinetics of methylphenidate use in children. Four hyperactive and behaviorally disturbed children served as subjects. Results show that: (1) the drug is metabolized to ritalinic acid with an apparent plasma half life of 2.5 h; (2) the variability in magnitude of plasma concentration seems to be due not to its metabolism to ritalinic acid but to the variability in the apparent volume of distri-

bution; (3) the brief half life of methylphenidate which parallels the short duration of action of methylphenidate in behaviorally disordered children may be explained in part by its low protein binding which results in high percentage of free drug being made available for metabolism to pharmacologically inactive metabolites.

818 Klein, Donald F., and Gittelman-Klein, Rachel. "Methylphenidate effects in children with learning disabilities." Res Relat Child 34: 61, March, 1974-August, 1974. (0 References).
Abstracts a report of research in progress or recently completed research. Data are provided on: name of investigator(s), purpose of the study, number and kind of subjects used, methodology, principal findings, duration of research, cooperating group(s), and availability of publication(s). Research Relating to Children is compiled by the ERIC Clearinghouse on Early Childhood Education.

819 Leary, P. M.; Arens, Leila; Marshall, Sheila. "Clinical experience with methylphenidate." S Afr Med J 55(10): 374-76, March 10, 1979. (5 References).
Outlines the indications for the use of methylphenidate and examines its effect on a large group of children. Two hundred and fifty children (ages three to fourteen years) participated in the study and were administered varying dosages of methylphenidate. The test showed that concentration improved or hyperactive behavior diminished in 89 percent of the children with normal IQs, in 72 percent of the children with cerebral palsy, and in 68 percent of the children with subnormal intelligence. In children with emotional disturbance, response to methylphenidate was seldom satisfactory. Side effects were nonsignificant.

820 Lerer, Robert J., and Lerer, M. Pamela. "The effects of methylphenidate on the soft neurological signs of hyperactive children." Pediatrics 57(4): 521-25, April, 1976. (13 References).
Reports findings of repeat neurological examinations in hyperactive children before and after treatment with methylphenidate and placebo. Forty children (thirty-four boys and six girls, mean age 8.9 years), who had been referred because of severe behavioral difficulties, distractibility, and short attention span, served as subjects. This group showed three or more neurological abnormalities at the initial consultation. After sixty days of treatment with methylphenidate, twenty-nine (72.5 percent) of the children showed marked improvement, especially in behavioral and motoric functions. Implications of these findings are discussed, and the value of the repeat examination following drug therapy is recommended.

821 ————. "Response of adolescents with minimal brain dysfunction to methylphenidate." J Learn Disabil 10(4): 223-28, April, 1977. (12 References).
Tests the efficacy of methylphenidate on behavior and academic achievement in a group of adolescents. Twenty-seven MBD boys served as subjects and were administered methylphenidate for a sixty-day trial period. Findings indicate that sixteen adolescents showed improvement in behavior, improvement in performance on the Bender-Gestalt, and improvement in academic achievement. The subjects also increased their ability to concentrate while anxiety and nervousness decreased. A trial of methylphenidate therapy is therefore recommended for MBD adolescents with a history of hyperactivity.

822 Levin, W. J. "Methylphenidate (Ritalin)." S Afr Med J 55(13): 494, March 24, 1979.
Letter to editor.

823 Loney, Jan, and Ordoña, Truce T. "Cerebral stimulants and minimal dysfunction: some questions, some answers, and some more questions." Am J Orthopsychiatry 44(2): 243-44, March, 1974. (0 References).
Discusses numerous questions raised during a large-scale search for predictors of children's response to Ritalin. The questions reviewed are: (1) Do physician factors contribute to diagnosis and treatment choice: (2) What is meant by improvement? (3) What kinds of side effects are said to occur and how frequent are they? and (4) When should cerebral stimulants be used? Brief answers are included.

824 "Methylphenidate (Ritalin) and other drugs for treatment of hyperactive children." Med Lett Drugs Ther 19(13): 53-55, July 1, 1977. (0 References).
Summarizes the effectiveness, dosage, interactions, and adverse effects of methylphenidate. Reference is made to alternative drugs used to treat hyperkinesis, e.g., dextroamphetamine, pemoline, imipramine, and deanol.

825 Saxon, Samuel A.; Magee, John T.; Siegel, David S. "Activity level patterns in the hyperactive Ritalin responder and non-responder." J Clin Child Psychol 6(3): 27-29, Winter, 1977. (11 References).
Tests the response to Ritalin by measuring the activity level of a group of young schoolchildren. Ten hyperactive children (ages four to ten years) participated in the experiment. Five children who were Ritalin responders became increasingly less active in the confines of a small, bare playroom, while five nonresponder children became increasingly more active under the same circumstances. Findings added support to Satterfield's psychophysiological model of hyperactivity.

826 Schain, Richard J., and Reynard, Carol L. "Effects of methylphenidate on children with hyperactive behavior." Pediatr Res 9(4): 384, April, 1975. (0 References).
Presents an abstract of the authors' research project. Full text of the article appears in Pediatrics 55(5): 709-16, May, 1975. (Item No. 827).

827 ————. "Observations on effects of a central stimulant drug (methylphenidate) in children with hyperactive behavior." Pediatrics 55(5): 709-16, May, 1975. (29 References).
Evaluates the efficacy of methylphenidate in a double-blind trial with ninety-eight hyperactive children (ages six to twelve years). Results show: (1) 79 percent of the children responded favorably to methylphenidate at the end of the sixteen-week trial period; (2) only 20 percent responded to placebo; (3) a wide range of dosage was required for optimal drug effect; (4) overweight children did not respond well to medication; and (5) children characterized by "developmental hyperactivity" (hyperactivity without other evidence of neurological or emotional disturbance) responded best. Based on these findings, it is concluded that a trial of stimulant drugs is indicated for hyperactive children, accompanied by close attention from teachers and parents.

828 Schleifer, Michael, and Weiss, Gabrielle. "Hyperactivity in preschoolers and the effect of methylphenidate (Ritalin)." Res Relat Child 34: 88, March, 1974-August, 1974. (0 References).

Abstracts a report of research in progress on recently completed research. Data are provided on: name of investigator(s), purpose of the study, number and kind of subjects used, methodology, principal findings, duration of research, cooperating group(s), and availability of publication(s). Research Relating to Children is compiled by the ERIC Clearinghouse on Early Childhood Education.

829 Schleifer, Michael; Weiss, Gabrielle; Cohen, Nancy; et al. "Hyperactivity in preschoolers and the effect of methylphenidate." Am J Orthopsychiatry 45(1): 38-50, January, 1975. (19 References).
Details the effect of methylphenidate (Ritalin) on the behavior of a group of preschool children. Twenty-eight hyperactive children of normal intelligence and twenty-six matched controls served as subjects. Observations of nursery behavior, tests of cognitive style and motor impulsivity, and psychiatric interviews with mothers provided the data. Analyzation reveals: (1) hyperactive preschoolers were more aggressive than controls; (2) both groups showed similar rates of impulsivity; and (3) there were no significant differences in family pathology between true and situational hyperactives. In further testing, twenty-six members of the hyperactive group were observed for three weeks, rated, and tested under two conditions--Ritalin and placebo. Ritalin was found to reduce hyperactivity at home, but it did not improve nursery behavior or psychological functioning. Because of unwanted side effects, Ritalin is seen to be less useful in management at the preschool level.

830 Schowalter, John E. "Paying attention to attention deficit disorder." Pediatrics 64(4): 546-47, October, 1979. (14 References).
Comments on studies by R. T. Brown and E. K. Sleator (Item No. 810) and L. Charles, et al. (Item No. 1560).

831 Sleator, Esther K., and Sprague, Robert L. "Dose effects of stimulants in hyperkinetic children." Psychopharmacol Bull 10(4): 29-31, October, 1974. (9 References).
Traces the effects of methylphenidate on hyperactive children in a series of experiments using a double-blind technique, placebo, and within-patient design. Twenty-three school-age children served as subjects and were administered various dosages of methylphenidate. The effects of the different doses on quantified parent and teacher rating scales, performance on a picture recognition task, seat movement, and heart rate were studied. Results indicate: (1) seventeen of the twenty-three subjects responded favorably to the drug; (2) of these seventeen, only three were placed on medication twice a day after the study period ended; (3) all dosage combinations were better than placebo without any significant differences between dosage combinations; (4) larger doses than necessary are often prescribed; (5) hyperactive children should be given only one dose per day initially; and (6) because teacher observations were highly reliable, physicians should consult the teacher before altering stimulant dosage.

832 Sleator, Esther K., and von Neumann, Alice W. "Methylphenidate in the treatment of hyperkinetic children: recommendations on diagnosis, dosage, and monitoring." Clin Pediatr 13(1): 19-24, January, 1974. (12 References).
Offers some practical clinical lessons on how to use stimulant medications more safely and effectively. Areas discussed include: (1) need for careful prescribing; (2) when to try stimulant medication; and (3) results and recommendations. In these studies, methylphenidate was found to be useful

in over 70 percent of forty-six hyperactive children. Emphasis is placed on the importance of obtaining the teacher's impression as an indicator of the drug's effectiveness.

833 Weiss, Gabrielle. "The hyperactive child." Can Med Assoc J 112(7): 803-5, April, 1975. (0 References).
Letter to editor.

834 ————. "The natural history of hyperactivity in childhood and treatment with stimulant medication at different ages: a summary of research findings." Int J Ment Health 4(1-2): 213-26, Spring-Summer, 1975. (21 References).
Reports on an observation study conducted with twenty-eight hyperactive preschool children and twenty-six matched controls. Observations were made during free play and during half-hour periods of structured play. After three weeks, half of the hyperactive children were given a three-week trial of methylphenidate; the other half was given an identical-looking placebo in a crossover design. Three weeks later, children on the active drug were given the placebo and vice versa. Results show great variability in the hyperactive children. Methylphenidate was found to be superior to the placebo in reducing hyperactivity. However, the drug proved no more useful for the "true" hyperactives than for the "situational" ones. Furthermore, the homes were more pathological for the true than for the situational hyperactives. It is concluded that there is considerable heterogeneity in the phenomenology of preschool hyperactives. For a reprint of this study refer to Item No. 688.

835 Werry, John S., and Sprague, Robert L. "Methylphenidate in children--effect of dosage." Aust NZ J Psychiatry 8(1): 9-19, March, 1974. (26 References).
Studies the effect of varying dosages of methylphenidate on clinical efficacy. The experiment also attempted to ascertain which of a large range of measures of drug effects are useful, and to note side and mood effects of the drug. The study was carried out at a United States childrens' research center and a department of psychiatry at a New Zealand university using two groups of hyperactive children (twenty in the United States and seventeen in New Zealand). All children were evaluated by neurological examination and IQ tests and were administered methylphenidate in a double-blind, placebo-controlled, crossover type design for four four-week periods. Among other conclusions it is shown that: (1) methylphenidate was superior to placebo for about two-thirds of the children; (2) there was little difference in effectiveness between different dosage levels, especially once 0.3 mg/kg was attained; (3) mild side effects were common at higher dosages; (4) teacher and physician ratings were the most sensitive to drug effects; and (5) methylphenidate was a useful treatment, but doses may be too high and side effects more common than generally recognized.

836 Whalen, Carol K.; Henker, Barbara; Collins, Barry E.; et al. "A social-ecology of hyperactive boys: medication effects in structured classroom environments." J Appl Behav Anal 12(1): 65-81, Spring, 1979. (31 References).
Investigates the sociability and other variables of three groups of boys under three conditions: (1) hyperactive boys on methylphenidate; (2) hyperactive boys on placebo; and (3) control boys. All boys were observed in the classroom setting. Quiet versus noisy conditions and self-paced versus other-paced activities were monitored. Compared to their peers,

hyperactive boys on placebo showed lower rates of task attention and higher rates of gross motor movement, regular and negative verbalization, noise-making, physical contact, social initiation, disruption, and acts that were perceived as energetic, inappropriate, or unexpected. Self-paced activities resulted in increased rates of verbalization, social initiation, and high-energy episodes. High ambient noise levels reduced task attention and increased the rates of many other behaviors including verbalization, physical contact, gross motor movement, and high-energy acts. Medication-by-situation interactions emerged for both classroom dimensions, with hyperactive boys on placebo being readily distinguishable from their peers under some classroom conditions and indistinguishable under other conditions. Implications of these findings are elucidated.

837 Whitehouse, Dennis. "CIBA Ritalin Study." Res Relat Child 38: 95, September, 1976-February, 1977. (0 References).
Abstracts a report of research in progress or recently completed research. Data are provided on: name of investigator(s), purpose of the study, number and kind of subjects used, methodology, principal findings, duration of research, cooperating group(s), and availability of publication(s). Research Relating to Children is compiled by the ERIC Clearinghouse on Early Childhood Education.

vi. Pemoline

838 Andresen, Brian D., and Weitzenkorn, Dan E. "Synthesis of pemoline-d5: a metabolic probe for hyperactivity." J Labelled Compo Radiopharm 15: 469-78, October, 1978. (18 References).
Provides information on the newest member of a group of drugs used to treat learning-disabled and hyperactive children. Considerable controversy exists in the literature regarding the effectiveness of pemoline, a drug which is chemically different from amphetamine, caffeine, and methylphenidate. Research into the use of the drug indicates that it appears suitable for metabolism studies in which new metabolites can be identified by mass spectrometry, as well as for use as an internal standard while monitoring blood levels of the parent drug in body fluids by various computer techniques.

839 Knights, Robert M., and Viets, Celia A. "Effects of pemoline on hyperactive boys." Pharmacol Biochem Behav 3(6): 1107-14, November-December, 1975. (9 References).
Explores the efficacy of the CNS stimulant, pemoline, on the activity level of children. Thirty hyperactive boys (ages six to twelve years) with normal intelligence participated in the study. The boys were rated as hyperactive by their teachers and parents and were administered pemoline or placebo in a double-blind design for a nine-week period. Ratings on the Conners scale showed significant improvement in the drug group according to teachers, but not by parents and physician. Side effects with pemoline were minimal. Although pemoline was effective in improving general behavior, no significant improvement occurred on psychological tests. Also discussed is an eighteen-month long-term phase for fourteen of the above children.

840 Page, John G.; Bernstein, Joel E.; Janicki, Robert S.; et al. "A multi-clinic trial of pemoline in childhood hyperkinesis." In: Clinical use of stimulant drugs in children. Edited by C. Keith Conners. Amsterdam: Excerpta Medica, 1974. 98-124. (16 References). (International Congress Series, No. 313).

This chapter reports on a controlled, double-blind study of pemoline and placebo in the management of hyperkinetic behavior. Two hundred and thirty-eight children (216 boys and 22 girls) participated in the trial and were assigned to drug or placebo groups. Observations were made by physician, teacher, parent, and psychologist at the end of a nine-week period. Some children were also seen in a long-term follow-up study. Significant benefits were noted from pemoline treatment as compared to placebo. For this reason pemoline should be considered a highly useful clinical alternative to some of the more commonly used drugs. General discussion follows.

841 Page, John G.; Janicki, Robert S.; Bernstein, Joel E.; et al. "Pemoline (Cylert) in the treatment of childhood hyperkinesis." J Learn Disabil 7(8): 498-503, October, 1974. (7 References).
Describes a controlled, double-blind study using placebo and pemoline, a mild CNS stimulant, in the management of hyperkinetic behavior. The study used 413 children (ages six to twelve years) previously diagnosed as having a hyperkinetic behavior disorder due to MBD. All 413 children were evaluated in terms of safety effects of the drug; 238 were rated on the efficacy of the drug. Global ratings, parent and teacher questionnaires, psychological tests, and physical and laboratory measurements were used to evaluate the results during the nine-week drug administration period. Impressive improvement was noted in gross behavior; few side effects were present. It is concluded that pemoline is a highly useful and safe clinical alternative to the amphetamines and methylphenidate in the management of hyperkinetic behavior.

842 "Pemoline (Cylert) for minimal brain dysfunction." Med Lett Drugs Ther 18(2): 5-6, January 16, 1976. (0 References).
Briefly discusses the central nervous system stimulant, pemoline (Cylert), which was recently approved by the U. S. Food and Drug Administration for treatment of MBD in children.

vii. Piracetam

843 Bereen, F. J. "Piracetam in management of minimal brain dysfunction." S Afr Med J 50(28): 1082, July 3, 1976. (1 Reference).
Letter to editor.

844 Leary, P. M. "Piracetam in management of minimal brain dysfunction." S Afr Med J 50(34): 1312, August 7, 1976. (4 References).
Letter to editor.

845 Leary, P. M.; Arens, L. J.; Rabkin, J. "Piracetam and pyrithioxine." S Afr Med J 49(31): 1236, July 19, 1975. (2 References).
Letter to editor.

b. Tranquilizers

i. Imipramine

846 Engelhardt, D. M.; Hoffman, S. P.; Polizos, P.; et al. "Outpatient treatment of hyperactive school children with imipramine." Am J Psychiatry 131: 587-91, May, 1974. (14 References).
Evaluates the effects of imipramine in a group of nineteen hyperactive boys. Behavioral improvement was noted, although side effects of anorexia and insomnia occurred in some cases.

847 Gittelman-Klein, Rachel. "Pilot clinical trial of imipramine in hyperactive children." In: Clinical use of stimulant drugs in children. Edited by C. Keith Conners. Amsterdam: Excerpta Medica, 1974. 192-201. (2 References). (International Congress Series, No. 313).
Analyzes the efficacy of imipramine on the behavior of hyperactive children as reported by their teachers and mothers. It is concluded that: (1) high doses are relatively well-tolerated; (2) the clinical course is not typically stable with increments of improvements and eventual leveling off of functioning over long periods of time; and (3) methylphenidate is not regularly efficacious when imipramine fails. Case summaries and a table of side effects are given. A brief general discussion is appended.

848 Saraf, Kishore R.; Klein, Donald F.; Gittelman-Klein, Rachel; et al. "EKG effects in imipramine treatment in children." J Am Acad Child Psychiatry 17(1): 60-69, Winter, 1978. (28 References).
Reports on the use of the electrocardiogram (EKG) to test the side effects of imipramine in a group of children receiving this medication. Twenty-five hyperactive and eight school-phobic children (mean age 9.3 years) participated in the study. Results indicate that children on doses of imipramine of 3.5 mg/kg or more are likely to show an increase in PR interval of .02 seconds or more and that such increases are more likely to occur in patients with a small pretreatment PR interval. In seven children the PR interval prolongation was above the rate-corrected norm. EKG monitoring is seen to be a desirable procedure when children are maintained on 3.5 mg/kg or more of imipramine.

849 ————. "Imipramine side effects in children." Psychopharmacologia 37(3): 265-74, 1974. (30 References).
Compares the incidence, range, and severity of side effects of imipramine with those of placebo. Sixty-five boys and girls (ages six to fourteen years) received imipramine while thirty-seven matched controls received placebo. Findings indicate that minor side effects occurred in 83 percent of the imipramine group and 70 percent of the placebo group. Approximately 5 percent of the imipramine group showed significant side effects, although there may be serious individual reactions to this drug. (One death occurred during the course of this study.) The research indicates that imipramine, if given in the proper dosage, is a relatively innocuous agent.

850 Solow, Robert A. "Drug treatment of affective illness in children." West J Med 129(6): 489-90, December, 1978. (3 References).
Briefly alludes to the role of two drugs, imipramine and lithium carbonate, in treating some of the symptoms of depression including hyperactivity, enuresis, temper tantrums, etc.

851 Waizer, Jonas; Hoffman, Stanley P.; Polizos, Polizoes; et al. "Outpatient treatment of hyperactive school children with imipramine." Am J Psychiatry 131(5): 587-91, May, 1974. (14 References).
Tests the efficacy of a long-acting antidepressant, imipramine, on a group of hyperactive children. Nineteen hyperactive boys (ages six to twelve years), who had been referred to the outpatient clinic of the Psychopharmacology Research Unit of Kings County Hospital Center in Brooklyn, New York, served as subjects. They were treated with imipramine for eight weeks, followed by four weeks of placebo. The subjects were then evaluated by psychiatrists, parents, and teachers using a variety of rating scales and psychological tests. Data interpretation points

out: (1) fourteen children were much improved in hyperactivity as well as in defiance, inattentiveness, and sociability; (2) two children showed minimal improvement; (3) thirteen of these children deteriorated on placebo, while only three retained their improved ratings. Although side effects of anorexia and insomnia were reported, they were not of a serious nature. The unique effect of imipramine in reducing hyperactivity in this population of schoolchildren is discussed.

ii. Lorazepam

852 Walters, Anne; Singh, N.; Beale, I. L. "Effects of lorazepam on hyperactivity in retarded children." NZ Med J 86(600): 473-75, November 23, 1977. (12 References).
Reports on a study to test the efficacy of lorazepam (Ativan) in a double-blind trial. Seven mentally retarded, institutionalized hyperactive children served as subjects and were given varying dosages of lorazepam and placebo. Results show that in this sample lorazepam not only did not improve hyperactivity, but, in some cases, actually increased hyperactivity. Side effects of various dosage levels are given.

iii. Phenothiazine

853 Solow, Robert A. "The use of phenothiazines in children." West J Med 129(6): 489, December, 1978. (3 References).
Briefly outlines the use of chlorpromazine, thioridazine, and fluphenazine to treat a variety of illnesses, including hyperactivity.

c. Antipsychotic

i. Haloperidol

854 Barker, Philip. "Haloperidol." J Child Psychol Psychiatry 16(2): 169-72, April, 1975. (12 References).
Evaluates the use of the drug, haloperidol, to treat hyperkinesis, tics, and stuttering in children. Although the drug, first produced in 1958, was originally used for various psychotic illnesses in adults, it has more recently been recommended for emotionally disturbed children. Dosage, side effects, and toxic effects are described. Haloperidol appears effective in treating behavior disorders, is safe when properly used, and should be used in combination with other treatment methods.

855 Ishishita, Kyoko, and Hachijima, Yuko. "Therapy for hyperactivity seen in minimal brain dysfunction." Psychiatr Neurol Japonica 78(8): 574-75, 1976.
Abstract.

d. Anticonvulsants

i. Carbamazepine

856 Kuhn-Gebhart, V. "Behavioural disorders in non-epileptic children and their treatment with carbamazepine." In: Epileptic seizures, behaviour, pain. Edited by Walther Birkmayer. Bern, Switzerland: Hans Huber, 1976. 264-67. (1 Reference).
Various studies are cited which show good response to anti-epileptic drug treatment for children's behavior disorders. Comments are made on the use of carbamazepine alone and in combination with other medications.

857 Puente, R. M. "The use of carbamazepine in the treatment of behavioural disorders in children." In: Epileptic seizures, behaviour, pain. Edited by Walther Birkmayer. Bern, Switzerland: Hans Huber, 1976. 243-47. (3 References).
Focuses on the use of the drug, carbamazepine (Tegretol), in the management of the typical symptoms of several behavior disorders, including hyperkinesis. Two studies are reported involving Mexican children (ages three to thirteen years). The drug was found to reduce considerably the signs and symptoms of the children with behavioral disorders, thereby improving school performance, family relationships, and adaptation to the environment.

858 Remschmidt, H. "The psychotropic effect of carbamazepine in non-epileptic patients, with particular reference to problems posed by chemical studies in children with behavioral disorders." In: Epileptic seizures, behaviour, pain. Edited by Walther Birkmayer. Bern, Switzerland: Hans Huber, 1976. 253-58. (15 References).
Discusses pros and cons of carbamazepine usage in epileptic and nonepileptic children. Guidelines for the drug's use are given.

ii. Sulthiame

859 Al-Kaisi, A. H., and McGuire, R. J. "The effect of sulthiame on disturbed behaviour in mentally subnormal patients." Br J Psychiatry 124: 45-49, January, 1974. (7 References).
Describes a double-blind drug trial to assess the effect of sulthiame on the behavior of very disturbed mentally handicapped patients. Thirty-four male and female subjects (ages six to twenty-four years) were selected. They possessed an IQ below fifty and included epileptics and nonepileptics. A special rating scale represented four main fields: hyperactivity, aggressiveness, destructiveness, and antisocial behavior. Subjects were administered sulthiame for a period of twelve weeks. Results indicate that sulthiame was significantly effective in reducing the incidence of destructive behavior in general and hyperactivity in particular. Only trivial side effects were noted.

860 Grant, Richard H. E. "Sulthiame and behaviour." Dev Med Child Neurol 16(6): 821-24, December, 1974. (13 References).
Reviews data on the anticonvulsant drug sulthiame (Ospolot). The effects of sulthiame on seizure control, hyperkinesis, incidence of disturbed behavior, concentration, etc. have been investigated by numerous researchers, among them Ingram and Ratcliffe, Gordon, Stutte, Hajnsek and Sartorius, Haran, Kneebone, Liu, and Hunter and Stephenson. All of these studies are said to suffer from the defect of being largely uncontrolled observations based on subjective impressions, the two exceptions being the work of Moffatt (1970) and Al-Kaisi and McGuire (1974 - Item No. 859). It is concluded that although sulthiame has been on the market for twelve years, and the body of literature surrounding its use is fairly extensive, no solid evidence exists as to its effectiveness on disturbed behavior. Physicians are urged to seek this evidence from the producers before prescribing the drug.

e. Miscellaneous

861 Bowdan, Newton D. "Hyperactivity or affective illness?" Am J Psychiatry 134(3): 329, March, 1977. (0 References).
Letter to editor.

862 Goetzl, Ugo; Grunberg, Frederic; Berkowitz, Bernard. "Lithium carbonate in the management of hyperactive aggressive behavior of the mentally retarded." Compr Psychiatry 18(6): 599-606, November-December, 1977. (13 References).
Investigates the effects of lithium carbonate on hyperactive and aggressive behavior in the residential setting. Three mentally retarded young adults (ages sixteen, nineteen, and twenty years) participated in the study and were administered lithium carbonate. In all three patients lithium carbonate was more effective in controlling aggressive behavior than the neuroleptics used for behavior control. Further studies are needed in the area.

863 Gross, Mortimer. "Improvement with L-dopa in a hyperkinetic child." Dis Nerv Syst 38(7): 556-57, July, 1977. (5 References).
The previously untried use of L-dopa to treat one hyperactive child is noted. A fourteen-year-old boy was placed on L-dopa because of the failure of more common medications to produce any behavior improvement. The boy showed significant improvement when treated with L-dopa. The theoretical and practical implications are commented upon.

864 Jackson, Richard T., and Pelton, E. W. "L-dopa treatment of children with hyperactive behavior." Neurology 28(4): 331, April, 1978. (0 References).
Abstract of a conference paper presented at the 30th annual meeting of the American Academy of Neurology.

865 Logue, G.; Nestadt, A.; Neumann, Yvonne. "The effects of pyrithioxine on the behaviour and intellectual functioning of learning-disabled children." S Afr Med J 48(54): 2245-46, November 9, 1974. (0 References).
Reports on a double-blind trial with pyrithioxine and placebo. The experiment was carried out for fifteen weeks with forty-five pairs of LD children, the pairs being equated in terms of certain variables. Results show that although both the trial and the control groups improved in reading and arithmetic, the trial group evidenced the greater improvement, especially in arithmetic. Eight of the pupils made dramatic gains in drive, alertness, and ability to concentrate on a task. The purpose, patients, methods, and results of the trial are given, and the action of Encephabol on the brain is outlined.

866 O'tuama, L. A.; Swisher, C. N.; Reichler, R. J.; et al. "Lack of effect of TRH in minimal brain dysfunction." Pediatrics 59(6): 955-56, June, 1977. (4 References).
Letter to editor.

867 Rapoport, Judith L., and Mikkelsen, Edwin J. "Antidepressants." In: Pediatric psychopharmacology: the use of behavior modifying drugs in children. Edited by John S. Werry. New York, New York: Brunner/Mazel, 1978. 208-33. (Bibliography).
Investigates the efficacy of antidepressant drugs for childhood psychopathological conditions, including hyperactivity. The authors conclude that the long-term beneficial effects of antidepressants on behavior and academic problems have not been demonstrated. Because long-term efficacy is questionable and side effects unknown, further investigation is necessary.

868 Rapoport, Judith L.; Mikkelsen, Edwin J.; Werry, John L. "Antimanic, antianxiety, hallucinogenic and miscellaneous drugs." In: Pedi-

atric psychopharmacology: the use of behavior modifying drugs in children. Edited by John S. Werry. New York, New York: Brunner/Mazel, 1978. 316-55. (Bibliography).
Considers the use of lithium for treating hyperactive children. Table I lists six controlled studies of lithium in psychiatric disorders of childhood and adolescence. It is concluded that lithium must be regarded as an interesting, though potentially toxic, experimental drug with several possible, but no firm, indications in pediatric psychopharmacology. The role of antianxiety drugs in hyperactivity is briefly discussed.

869 Simeon, J.; O'Malley, M.; Tryphonas, H.; et al. "Cromolyn DSG effects in hyperkinetic and psychotic children with allergies." Ann Allergy 42(6): 343-47, June, 1979. (27 References).
Evaluates the efficacy and safety of cromolyn in hyperkinetic and psychotic children presenting with symptoms of allergies. The preliminary findings of the open trial indicate that the medication is useful, safe, and well-tolerated. Further controlled studies are called for to confirm the drug's usefulness in child psychiatry.

870 Tiwary, Chandra M., and Rosenbloom, Arlan L. "Lack of effect of TRH in minimal brain dysfunction: reply." Pediatrics 59(6): 956, June, 1977. (1 Reference).
Letter to editor.

871 Tiwary, C. M.; Rosenbloom, A. L.; Robertson, M. F.; et al. "Effects of thyrotropin-releasing hormone in minimal brain dysfunction." Pediatrics 56(1): 119-21, July, 1975. (9 References).
Studies the effects of thyrotropin-releasing hormone (TRH) on two children of normal intelligence with MBD and hyperactivity. TRH was injected intravenously. The children's behavior was then observed and videotaped. Improved behavioral changes were apparent three to four hours after TRH injection. No side effects were noted. Since TRH is only available for use in children for study of thyroid disorders, this study has not been extended.

872 Výborová, L.; Náhunek, K.; Drtílková, I.; et al. "A controlled study of lisurid in hyperactive children." Act Nerv Super 20(1): 86-87, 1978. (0 References).
Evaluates the efficacy of lisurid on the hyperactive syndrome. Twenty hyperactive, primarily encephalopathic children (seventeen boys and three girls, mean age of eight years) participated in the double-blind crossover design. Lisurid (average minimum dose 17 microgr) was administered for fourteen days, followed by doctors' ratings after seven days and fourteen days. Although side effects were not notable, lisurid had a limited effect on the behavior of the children under study. Some selective uses of this preparation are offered.

873 Winsberg, Bertrand G., and Yepes, Luis E. "Antipsychotics (major tranquilizers, neuroleptics)." In: Pediatric psychopharmacology: the use of behavior modifying drugs in children. Edited by John S. Werry. New York, New York: Brunner/Mazel, 1978. 234-73. (Bibliography).
Reviews the use of antipsychotic agents in the management of a number of target symptoms, including hyperactivity. Although this class of drugs is very useful, their effect seems quasi-sedative rather than antipsychotic; many short- and long-term side effects are present. Careful clinical management is therefore a necessity.

3. COMPARISON OF DRUG TREATMENTS

874 Arnold, Eugene; Christopher, James; Huestis, Robert; et al. "Methylphenidate vs dextroamphetamine vs caffeine in minimal brain dysfunction: controlled comparison by placebo washout design with Bayes' analysis." Arch Gen Psychiatry 35(4): 463-73, April, 1978. (27 References).

Assesses the effects of three stimulants--methylphenidate, dextroamphetamine, and caffeine--on a group of children presenting symptoms of MBD. Twenty-nine such children (twenty-two boys and seven girls), who had been referred to a clinic, served as subjects for the double-blind crossover comparison. Results show that: (1) methylphenidate and dextroamphetamine were significantly better than placebo and caffeine, but not significantly different from each other; (2) placebo, caffeine, and ratings before drugs did not differ significantly; and (3) all three drugs caused significant weight loss and cardiovascular side effects.

875 Arnold, L. Eugene; Huestis, Robert D.; Smeltzer, Donald J., et al. "Levoamphetamine vs. dextroamphetamine in minimal brain dysfunction: replication, time response, and differential effect by diagnostic group and family rating." Arch Gen Psychiatry 33(3): 292-301, March, 1976. (19 References).

Compares the efficacy of two drugs, levoamphetamine and dextroamphetamine, as therapeutic agents for children presenting with MBD. Thirty-one previously diagnosed children served as subjects for the double-blind, crossover, randomized Latin square study. Findings reveal that: (1) both levoamphetamine and dextroamphetamine were more effective than placebo; (2) both drugs were not significantly different from each other, although dextroamphetamine was slightly superior; (3) certain subgroups responded best to levoamphetamine while others responded best to dextroamphetamine; (4) the efficacy of levoamphetamine is confirmed; and (5) parents' ratings, but not teachers' or psychiatrists' ratings, showed significant placebo effect.

876 Arnold, L. Eugene, and Wender, Paul H. "Levoamphetamine's changing place in the treatment of children with behavior disorders." In: Clinical use of stimulant drugs in children. Edited by C. Keith Conners. Amsterdam: Excerpta Medica, 1974. 179-91. (12 References). (International Congress Series, No. 313).

Reports on a study in which eleven hyperkinetic children were given placebo, dextroamphetamine, and levoamphetamine in a double-blind crossover trial. Each drug condition lasted three weeks. According to teachers' ratings, parents' ratings, and psychiatrists' ratings and rankings, both drugs were significantly better than placebo but not significantly different from each other. Based on these findings the authors conclude: (1) levoamphetamine should not be the first drug tried for a hyperkinetic child; and (2) unsocialized aggressive children seem to benefit most. The work of Samual Corson on hyperkinetic dogs is noted.

877 Campbell, Magda, and Shopsin, Baron. "A controlled study of lithium carbonate, chlorpromazine, and haloperidol in severely disturbed children, ages 6 to 12." Res Relat Child 39: 106, March, 1977-August, 1977. (0 References).

Abstracts a report of research in progress or recently completed research. Data are provided on: name of investigator(s), purpose of the study, number and kind of subjects used, methodology, principal findings, duration of research, cooperating group(s), and availability of publication(s).

Research Relating to Children is compiled by the ERIC Clearinghouse on Early Childhood Education.

878 Černý, L.; Kučerová, Z.; Šturma, J. "Pemoline in comparison with amphetamine and placebo in pedo-psychiatric practice." Act Nerv Super 17(4): 300-301, December, 1975. (0 References).
Compares the effects of the stimulant drug, pemoline, with amphetamine and placebo to treat the hyperkinetic behavior disorder. Thirty-seven hyperactive children, primarily boys, were used as subjects for the double-blind study and were administered the drugs. The children were rated according to a wide variety of characteristics including sleep, eating habits, motor activity, verbal production, attention, social adaptability, etc. Ratings by nurses and teachers showed that pemoline was not the most efficient drug in any of the parameters examined. Its effect was similar to that of amphetamine in aggression, lack of discipline and disturbed attention. Its effect was much less for verbal production, mood, and motor activity, and could not be distinguished from placebo.

879 Coleman, Mary; Steinberg, Grace; Tippett, Jean; et al. "A preliminary study of the effect of pyridoxine administration in a subgroup of hyperkinetic children: a double-blind crossover comparison with methylphenidate." Biol Psychiatry 14(5): 741-51, October, 1979. (30 References).
Pyridoxine, methylphenidate, and placebo are compared in this research. Six children participated. The children had had low whole blood serotonin levels and a history of previous responsiveness to methylphenidate. The results of the double-blind clinical evaluation showed trends suggesting that both pyridoxine and methylphenidate were more effective than placebo in suppressing the symptoms of hyperkinesis. Pyridoxine elevated whole-blood serotonin levels, methylphenidate did not. Clinical and laboratory evidence indicated that the pyridoxine effects persisted after the three-week period when the vitamin had been given in this experimental design.

880 Drtílková, I.; Náhunek, K.; Macháčkova, V.; et al. "Controlled comparison of the effect of dosulepin and diazepam in hyperkinetic children with phenylketonuria." Act Nerv Super 20(4): 247-48, 1978. (0 References).
Points out a relationship between children with phenylketonuria and accompanying hyperkinetic behavior and consequent drug treatment with diazepam and dosulepin. Twelve children (three boys and nine girls, mean age 10.25 years) participated in the double-blind, crossover seven-day study. The children received diazepam, dosulepin, or placebo. A psychiatric and psychologic examination was repeated weekly. Results show that although diazepam had the greatest tranquilizing effect, it also caused a decline in concentration of attention. For this reason dosulepin is the recommended choice of treatment.

881 Dykman, Roscoe A.; McGrew, Jeanette; Harris, T. Stuart; et al. "Two blinded studies of the effects of stimulant drugs on children: pemoline, methylphenidate, and placebo." In: Learning disability/minimal brain dysfunction syndrome: research perspectives and applications. Edited by Robert P. Anderson and Charles G. Halcomb. Springfield, Illinois: Thomas, 1976. 217-35. (23 References).
Two studies are documented which evaluated the efficacy of pemoline. Study one involved 105 children and compared pemoline, methylphenidate, and placebo. Study two used twenty children to compare pemoline and placebo. Pemoline is viewed a useful alternative to methylphenidate in the medical management of hyperactive children.

882 Eaton, Marie D.; Sells, Clifford J.; Lucas, Betty. "Psychoactive medication and learning disabilities." J Learn Disabil 10(7): 403-10, August-September, 1977. (3 References).
Reports on a double-blind placebo-controlled study designed to assess the effects of two stimulant drugs, Ritalin and Dexedrine, on academic and social behaviors. The subject was a seven-year-old emotionally disturbed boy. Most of the boy's academic and social behaviors were generally improved by the use of medication. Some undesirable side effects were noted with specific drug dosages. The importance of careful monitoring is stressed.

883 Firestone, P.; Davey, J.; Goodman, J. T.; et al. "Effects of caffeine and methylphenidate on hyperactive children." J Am Acad Child Psychiatry 17(3): 445-56, Summer, 1978. (46 References).
Studies the effects of caffeine and methylphenidate on a group of hyperactive children. Twenty-one subjects (ages six to twelve years) were administered either of the two regimens. Those receiving methylphenidate showed significantly improved behavior as rated by mothers and teachers. In addition, impulsivity and motor control improved. Children receiving caffeine showed only a slight improvement in some areas. Side effects of both drugs were found to be minimal.

884 Firestone, Philip; Goodman, John T.; Davey, Jean; et al. "The effects of caffeine and methylphenidate on hyperactive children." Res Relat Child 41: 112, March, 1978-August, 1978. (0 References).
Abstracts a report of research in progress or recently completed research. Data are provided on: name of investigator(s), purpose of the study, number and kind of subjects used, methodology, principal findings, duration of research, cooperating group(s), and availability of publication(s). Research Relating to Children is compiled by the ERIC Clearinghouse on Early Childhood Education.

885 Fras, Ivan. "Alternating caffeine and stimulants." Am J Psychiatry 131(2): 228-29, February, 1974. (1 Reference).
Letter to editor.

886 Fras, Ivan, and Karlavage, John. "The use of methylphenidate and imipramine in Gilles de la Tourette's disease in children." Am J Psychiatry 134(2): 195-97, February, 1977. (8 References).
Gilles de la Tourette's disease is described as "a triad of tics, explosive vocal utterances, and imitative phenomena." Two children presenting with this disease, and one child with Gilles de la Tourette's syndrome plus MBD were treated with methylphenidate. Although the symptoms of the two syndromes were exacerbated as a result of methylphenidate (imipramine was briefly used with one child with similar results), caution is to be used in treating patients with possible movement disorders. These findings lend support to the catecholamine hypothesis of the etiology of Gilles de la Tourette's disease.

887 Garfinkel, B. D.; Webster, C. D.; Sloman, L. "Individual responses to methylphenidate and caffeine in children with minimal brain dysfunction." Can Med Assoc J 113(8): 729-32, October 18, 1975. (25 References).
Compares the efficacy of two stimulants--methylphenidate hydrochloride and caffeine citrate--in the overall management of children with minimal brain dysfunction. Eight children were studied for their individual re-

sponses to the drugs in a double-blind crossover experiment. Four types of behavioral responses were observed: (1) four children responded favorably to both stimulants; (2) one child responded to methylphenidate alone; (3) two responded to the placebo; and (4) one child did not respond to either: his behavior worsened. Findings indicate that methylphenidate was superior to caffeine in reducing hyperactive and aggressive behavior. This drug is therefore recommended as an adjunct to other treatment regimens for MBD children.

888 ————. "Methylphenidate and caffeine in the treatment of children with minimal brain dysfunction." Am J Psychiatry 132(7): 723-28, July, 1975. (43 References).
This study compares the efficacy of methylphenidate, caffeine, and placebo in treating children with MBD. Two hypotheses were tested: (1) caffeine and methylphenidate are equally effective in treating the behavioral manifestations of MBD; and (2) caffeine and methylphenidate are superior to decaffeinated coffee and placebo in treating the behavioral manifestations of MBD. Eight boys participated in the double-blind crossover experiment. It was found that: (1) methylphenidate was superior to caffeine; and (2) methylphenidate alone was superior to decaffeinated coffee and placebo. Implications of the results are discussed.

889 Gittelman-Klein, Rachel, and Klein, Donald F. "Are behavioral and psychometric changes related in methylphenidate-treated hyperactive children?" Int J Ment Health 4(1-2): 182-98, Spring-Summer, 1975. (9 References).
Examines the relative efficacy of a placebo, methylphenidate, thioridazine, and a combination of methylphenidate and thioridazine. Thirty-nine hyperactive children (ages six to twelve years) participated in the study. Numerous psychological and behavioral measures were administered before and after treatment. Results indicate no relationship between psychometric and behavioral improvement after four weeks and a weak relationship after twelve weeks of treatment. Data fail to support the hypothesis that psychometric and behavioral changes occur together in hyperkinetic children treated with stimulants. The notion that a primary, unitary, CNS function is ameliorated by stimulants seems unlikely. Drug effects in this population appear more complex. For a reprint of this study refer to Item No. 688.

890 ————. "The relationship between behavioral and psychological test changes in hyperkinetic children." Psychopharmacol Bull 10(4): 34, October, 1974. (0 References).
Tests the hypothesis that there is a significant relationship between change in behavior and change on psychological test performance among hyperactive children treated with methylphenidate, a stimulant, and thioridazine, a tranquilizer. Seventy hyperactive children (mean ages eight to nine years) were used as subjects for a twelve-week period. Thirty-six children were administered methylphenidate while thirty-four received thioridazine. Improvement scores obtained from the mother, teacher, psychiatrist, and psychologist were correlated with changes in psychological test measures. Results indicate that there is some degree of association between behavior improvement and psychological improvement.

891 Gittelman-Klein, Rachel; Klein, Donald F.; Katz, Sidney; et al. "Comparative effects of methylphenidate and thioridazine in hyperkinetic children. I. Clinical results." Arch Gen Psychiatry 33(10): 1217-32, October, 1976. (19 References).

Compares various drugs--methylphenidate, thioridazine, methylphenidate/thioridazine combination, and placebo in the treatment of 140 hyperkinetic children. Active treatment lasted twelve weeks; placebo four weeks. Test results reveal that: (1) all treatments were superior to placebo as indicated by ratings of parents, teachers, and clinic staff; (2) methylphenidate alone and the methylphenidate/thioridazine combination were more effective than thioridazine alone; and (3) the methylphenidate/thioridazine combination produced greater improvement initially, but then was not superior to methylphenidate alone after twelve weeks of treatment. Side effects of the two drugs are noted.

892 Greenberg, Lawrence M.; Yellin, Absalom M.; Spring, Carl; et al. "Clinical effects of imipramine and methylphenidate in hyperactive children." Int J Ment Health 4(1-2): 144-56, Spring-Summer, 1975. (13 References).
The effects of imipramine and methylphenidate are examined in a double-blind crossover study. Forty-seven hyperactive children (ages six to thirteen years) who had responded well to methylphenidate were treated with imipramine, methylphenidate, or placebo. The comparison shows: (1) methylphenidate was slightly more efficacious than imipramine; (2) methylphenidate produced fewer side effects; and (3) methylphenidate treatment was associated with improved social relatedness and coordination.

893 Gross, Mortimer D. "A comparison of dextro-amphetamine and racemic-amphetamine in the treatment of the hyperkinetic syndrome or minimal brain dysfunction." Dis Nerv Syst 37(1): 14-16, January, 1976. (12 References).
Compares the effects of dextroamphetamine (Dexedrine) and racemic-amphetamine (Benzedrine) with each other and also with methylphenidate and placebo in the treatment of the hyperkinetic syndrome. Fifty children, previously diagnosed as hyperactive, were placed on the following regimen: a week each of dextroamphetamine, racemic-amphetamine at the same dose, methylphenidate at double dose, and placebo, in random order. Dextroamphetamine and methylphenidate were significantly superior to racemic-amphetamine, with side effects about the same. In some cases, though, racemic-amphetamine was superior to both dextroamphetamine and methylphenidate.

894 Hirst, Irene. "Effects of the psychoactive drug methylphenidate (Ritalin) on classroom disorders: hyperactivity, emotional disturbance." Paper presented at the 54th Annual International Convention, the Council for Exceptional Children, Chicago, Illinois, April 4-9, 1976. 25p. (ED 128 989).
Reviews research studies which compared the effects of methylphenidate, thioridazine, and amphetamine under various behavioral conditions and situations.

895 Huestis, Robert D.; Arnold, L. Eugene; Smeltzer, Donald J. "Caffeine versus methylphenidate and d-amphetamine in minimal brain dysfunction: a double-blind comparison." Am J Psychiatry 132(8): 868-70, August, 1975. (5 References).
Compares the efficacy of caffeine, methylphenidate, and d-amphetamine in an effort to locate a safer, but effective, medication for children with MBD. Eighteen children (twelve boys and six girls, mean age 8.5 years), who had been admitted to an outpatient psychiatric clinic, served as subjects. A double-blind crossover design was used to compare the

effects of the drugs. The dosage strengths were 80 mg of caffeine, 5 mg of d-amphetamine, and 10 mg of methylphenidate. Both prescription drugs resulted in significant behavioral improvement and were significantly superior to caffeine. The discrepancy between these findings and an earlier, more optimistic report on the efficacy of caffeine may stem from the use in this study of pure caffeine rather than whole coffee. This study is a preliminary analysis of the first half of the sample.

896 Klein, Donald F. "Comparative drug effects in hyperkinetic children." Psychopharmacol Bull 10(2): 62-63, April, 1974. (0 References).
Abstract.

897 Lewis, James A., and Young, Rosemarie. "Deanol and methylphenidate in minimal brain dysfunction." Clin Pharmacol Ther 17(5): 534-40, May, 1975. (52 References).
This study compares the efficacy of deanol, methylphenidate, and placebo in a three-month double-blind study. Seventy-four hyperactive and learning-disabled children served as subjects and were administered either 40 mg of methylphenidate, 500 mg of deanol, or placebo. Standard rating forms and tests were given before and after treatment. Results show that both drugs significantly improved performance on a number of the tests. Because of several unanswered questions concerning the action and side effects of deanol, further clinical studies are indicated.

898 ————. "Deanol and methylphenidate in minimal brain dysfunction." In: Progress in psychiatric drug treatment. Volume 2. Edited by Donald F. Klein and Rachel Gittelman-Klein. New York, New York: Brunner/Mazel, 1976. 444-53. (52 References).
Reprints an article from Clinical Pharmacology and Therapeutics 17(5): 534-40, May, 1975. (Item No. 897).

899 Rapoport, Judith L. "Comparative drug treatment on hyperactive children." Psychopharmacol Bull 10(2): 63-64, April, 1974. (0 References).
Abstract.

900 Rapoport, Judith L.; Quinn, Patricia O.; Bradbard, Gail; et al. "Imipramine and methylphenidate treatments of hyperactive boys: a double-blind comparison." Arch Gen Psychiatry 30(6): 789-93, June, 1974. (21 References).
Compares the effects of three treatments--methylphenidate, imipramine, and placebo--on the behavior of a group of hyperactive children. Seventy-six grade-school boys, referred to a clinic for distractibility, motor restlessness, and impulsivity served as subjects. Predrug behavior evaluation (Conners, etc.) was conducted. Following six weeks of drug treatment it is concluded that: (1) both drugs are superior to placebo; (2) methylphenidate is superior to imipramine; (3) psychologists' global estimates are the most likely of any clinic evaluation to predict teacher and parent reports; and (4) side effects are more prominent with imipramine.

901 Saletu, B.; Saletu, M.; Simeon, J.; et al. "Comparative symptomatological and evoked potential studies with d-amphetamine, thioridazine, and placebo in hyperkinetic children." Biol Psychiatry 10(3): 253-75, June, 1975. (54 References).

This study compares the efficacy of d-amphetamine, thioridazine, and placebo in a double-blind study. Sixty-two hyperkinetic children were selected and randomly assigned to eight weeks of treatment with one of the two drugs or placebo. Evidence is provided for the following conclusions: (1) d-amphetamine was significantly superior to placebo and thioridazine in decreasing hyperactive behavior; (2) overall clinical symptomatology improved with all three substances; (3) inattentive passive behavior was most improved by thioridazine; (4) thioridazine increased latencies and decreased amplitudes; (5) d-amphetamine also increased latencies, but augmented amplitudes; (6) the shorter the pretreatment latencies and the higher the amplitudes, the more disturbed the child; (7) good prognosis for the child was indicated by shorter pretreatment latencies, and small amplitudes with subsequent thioridazine treatment; and (8) good prognosis for the child was indicated by short latencies and high amplitudes with subsequent treatment with d-amphetamine.

902 Solomons, Gerald. "The role of methylphenidate and dextroamphetamine in hyperactivity in children." J Iowa Med Soc 61: 658-61, November, 1975. (11 References).
Briefly discusses drug treatment of hyperactive children according to: (1) problems of definition and methodology; (2) mode of action; and (3) therapeutic regimen. The administration of psychostimulant drugs is seen as a complex issue which must be thoroughly investigated before a drug program is initiated. Behavior modification techniques can reduce the need for drugs in some cases.

903 Sprague, Robert L., and Sleator, Esther K. "Drugs and dosages: implications for learning disabilities." In: The neuropsychology of learning disorders: theoretical approaches. Edited by R. M. Knights and D. J. Bakker. Baltimore, Maryland: University Park Press, 1976. 351-66. (Bibliography).
Reports on a series of psychotropic drug studies which experimented with varying doses of methylphenidate and dextroamphetamine to determine peak performance on different tasks. Inconsistent results are detailed.

904 Tate, Douglas L. "The effects of methylphenidate and thioridazine upon attention, arousal, and activity in mentally retarded youngsters." For a summary see: Diss Abstr Int 36B(12, pt. 1): 6424, June, 1976. (0 References).

905 Väisanen, K.; Kainulainen, P.; Paavilainen, M. T.; et al. "Sulpiride versus chlorpromazine and placebo in the treatment of restless mentally subnormal patients--a double-blind cross-over study." Curr Ther Res 17(2): 202-5, February, 1975. (4 References).
Documents the efficacy of two drugs, sulpiride and chlorpromazine, on the overactive behavior of a group of mentally subnormal patients. Sixty restless oligophrenics (ages eight to forty years, average age 19.4 and 18.1) were divided into two groups in a controlled double-blind crossover study. These patients had been resistant to previous drug therapy. Although no important side effects were observed, the behavioral effects of the drugs were found to be marginal.

906 Výborová, L.; Balastiková, B.; Drtílková, I.; et al. "Clonazepam and dithiaden in hyperkinetic children." Act Nerv Super 21(3): 155-56, 1979. (0 References).
Meeting.

907 Výborová, L.; Náhunek, K.; Balastiková, B.; et al. "Clozapin in psychomotor instability: a controlled study." Act Nerv Super 20(4): 274-75, 1978. (5 References).
Compares clozapin and chlorpromazine in a double-blind crossover study. Twenty-nine primarily encephalopathic children, hospitalized in the pediatric ward for hyperactive syndrome, served as subjects. Behavioral changes were assessed by rating scales, EEG, and psychological tests. Clozapin was found to reduce undesirable behavior more effectively than chlorpromazine. Side effects, though common, were not severe.

908 Výborová, L.; Náhunek, K.; Drtílková, I.; et al. "Controlled clinical comparative study of octoclothepin, propericiazine and placebo in hyperkinetic children." Act Nerv Super 17(4): 209-10, December, 1975. (12 References).
The effectiveness of octoclothepin (OC), propericiazine (PN), and placebo (PL) in the treatment of hyperkinesis is assessed. Twenty-four hospitalized children (ages five to fifteen years, mean age nine) served as subjects and were administered the compounds in a double-blind trial. The modified scale of Cerný was used for clinical assessment in seven-day intervals; EEG was recorded after fourteen days. Twelve patients were repeatedly examined with a battery of psychological tests. Results show that both neuroleptic drugs, (OC) and (PN), decreased psychomotor behavior, with (OC) having a more rapid onset of improvement. In other respects, the difference in the effects of the drugs was negligible.

909 Weiss, Gabrielle. "Child psychopharmacology." In: Psychopharmacology of childhood. Edited by D. V. Siva Sankar. Westbury, New York: PJD Publications, 1976. 123-37. (34 References).
Summarizes the effects of chlorpromazine, dextroamphetamine, methylphenidate, imipramine, haloperidol, and thioridazine with hyperactive children.

910 Werry, J. S.; Aman, M. G.; Lampen, E. "The effect of imipramine and methylphenidate in hyperactive aggressive children." Paper presented at the Annual Meeting of the Australian and New Zealand College of Psychiatrists, Brisbane, Australia, 1977.

911 ————. "Haloperidol and methylphenidate in hyperactive children." Acta Paedopsychiatr 42(1): 26-40, 1976. (22 References).
Three drug conditions(two doses of haloperidol and methylphenidate) and placebo were evaluated in a double-blind crossover study. Twenty-nine hyperactive children (ages five to ten years) were given the drugs for three weeks at a time. Through various tests and measures, all three drug conditions proved to be superior to placebo. Teachers preferred methylphenidate; parents preferred haloperidol. Side effects were more common with a high dose of haloperidol. In a related study, it was shown that while the low dose of haloperidol improved cognitive function, though to a lesser extent than methylphenidate, the high dose of haloperidol depressed it. There may thus be a conflict between demands for social and behavioral control and the needs of the child for optimum cognitive function. Haloperidol appears, however, to be a useful psychotropic drug for some children.

912 Winsberg, Bertrand G.; Press, Mark; Bialer, Irv; et al. "Dextroamphetamine and methylphenidate in the treatment of hyperactive/aggressive children." Pediatrics 53(2): 236-41, February, 1974. (22 References).
Compares the effectiveness of dextroamphetamine and methylphenidate on behavior disorders of eighteen children (fifteen boys and three girls, mean age 8.5 years). The two drugs were randomly administered. All children

were rated by teachers on a rating scale (BRS). Data reveal that both drugs attenuated hyperactive and aggressive behavior. Children who respond to one of the drugs may be expected to respond to the other. Side effects were modest and similar for both medications.

913 Yellin, Absalom M.; Spring, Carl; Greenberg, Lawrence. "Effects of imipramine and methylphenidate on behavior of hyperactive children." Res Commun Psychol Psychiatry Behav 3: 15-26, 1978. (7 References).
The efficacy of imipramine and methylphenidate in the treatment of hyperactive children is compared in a double-blind crossover study. Forty-seven children (forty boys and seven girls) previously diagnosed as hyperactive were randomly assigned to four treatment groups: placebo and methylphenidate, methylphenidate followed by placebo, placebo and imipramine, and imipramine followed by placebo. The Hyperactivity Rating Scale was used by parents and teachers to assess behavioral changes. Data reveal: (1) both methylphenidate and imipramine were superior to placebo in reducing hyperactive behavior; (2) methylphenidate was significantly more effective than imipramine; and (3) teachers were more sensitive to behavior changes than parents.

914 Yepes, L. E.; Balka, Elinor B.; Winsberg, Bertrand G.; et al. "Amitriptyline and methylphenidate treatment of behaviorally disordered children." J Child Psychol Psychiatry 18(1): 39-52, January, 1977. (35 References).
Compares the effects of two drugs, amitriptyline and methylphenidate, for treating hyperactive/aggressive behavior in children originally referred to a learning clinic. The effect of the two drugs on attention, short-term memory, and impulsivity was evaluated, and behavioral change was measured by teacher and parent ratings. Results show: (1) both drugs successfully reduced hyperactivity and aggression; (2) of the laboratory measures only attention was improved by both drugs; and (3) side effects were minor except for the sedation induced by amitriptyline. For this reason therapeutic trials with amitriptyline should be limited.

4. SIDE EFFECTS

915 Bremness, Andrew B., and Sverd, Jeffrey. "Methylphenidate-induced Tourette syndrome: case report." Am J Psychiatry 136(10): 1334-35, October, 1979. (8 References).
Reports the case of methylphenidate-induced Gilles de la Tourette syndrome in a nine-and-a-half-year-old boy referred for hyperactive/aggressive behavioral problems. After ten weeks on a 60 mg/day methylphenidate regimen, the boy developed all signs of Tourette syndrome. Cessation of methylphenidate treatment resulted in gradual symptom resolution for two weeks, followed by a reappearance of the full syndrome five weeks after discontinuation of methylphenidate. Results support the hypothesis of a catecholaminergic excess in the neuropathophysiology of Tourette syndrome.

916 Case, Quentin, and McAndrew, John B. "Dexedrine dyskinesia: an unusual iatrogenic tic." Clin Pediatr 13(1): 69, 72, January, 1974. (5 References).
Documents a case report which describes a dyskinesia associated with dextroamphetamine medication. An eight-year-old boy, as a result of receiving dextroamphetamine for extreme hyperkinesis, developed a movement disorder consisting of choreoathetoid movements of the mouth, tongue, and extremities. The movements ceased when the patient was given phenhydramine hydrochloride. Five weeks later dextroamphetamine was reintro-

duced, again producing dyskinesia, which was reduced by diphenhydramine hydrochloride. Also cited are cases of tardive dyskinesia associated with phenothiazine medication. Although cases such as these are rarely found cited in the literature, they should serve as a reminder that the differential diagnosis of movement disorders in children must include the side effects of drugs.

917 Chamberlin, Robert W. "Convulsions and Ritalin?" Pediatrics 54(5): 658-59, November, 1974. (0 References).
Letter to editor.

918 Denckla, Martha B.; Bemporad, Jules R.; MacKay, Mary C. "Tics following methylphenidate administration: a report of 20 cases." JAMA 235(13): 1349-51, March 29, 1976. (11 References).
Explores the relationship between tics and methylphenidate therapy, an usually rare occurrence. Patients were selected from a large population referred to physicians for MBD. Among the forty-five children receiving methylphenidate, tics developed in fourteen; in six children with preexisting tics, the tics became worse. Tics disappeared with the withdrawal of the medication in all but one case. The authors concluded that tics related to methylphenidate administration are rare and may be associated with a certain personality profile.

919 Farnham-Diggory, Sylvia. Learning disabilities: a psychological perspective. Cambridge, Massachusetts: Harvard University Press, 1978. 154p. (Bibliography). (The Developing Child Series).
Presents an overview of the learning-disabled child. Chapter 8 is devoted to the hyperactive syndrome. Emphasis is placed on treatment issues. The main points of the presentation are: (1) medication for hyperactivity may suppress physical growth; (2) the ingestion of amphetamine may be linked to forms of cancer; (3) the effects of medication on simple learning must be state-dependent; (4) the effects of medication on complex learning has not been determined; and (5) alternative methods of management exist. Comments are also made on the management of attention and the contributions of Porges and Meichenbaum.

920 Golden, Gerald S. "Gilles de la Tourette's syndrome following methylphenidate administration." Dev Med Child Neurol 16(1): 76-78, February, 1974. (10 References).
Documents a case study of a nine-year-old boy presenting with learning problems, hyperactivity, disruptive behavior, short attention span, and other symptoms of MBD. The boy was placed on 10 mg of methylphenidate twice a day. Although there was marked improvement in his behavior at home and in the classroom, he suddenly began to produce loud noises and uncontrolled tic movements of the face, arms, and body. The respiratory component and tic symptoms disappeared almost completely when methylphenidate was discontinued. Haloperidol (Haldol) was begun twice a day. Attempts to discontinue the drug lead to an exacerbation of the symptoms. It is suggested that methylphenidate stimulated an increase in dopamine turnover and may have triggered the onset of Gilles de la Tourette's syndrome in a vulnerable patient.

921 Goyer, Peter F.; Davis, Glenn C.; Rapoport, Judith L. "Abuse of prescribed stimulant medication by a 13-year-old hyperactive boy." J Am Acad Child Psychol 18(1): 170-75, Winter, 1979. (7 References).

Documents the case of a thirteen-year-old boy who abused the use of methylphenidate after two years of therapeutic treatment with the drug. During a research hospitalization the boy was administered methylphenidate in a double-blind placebo-controlled fashion to assess the mood changes induced by the drug and to verify expected therapeutic effects. The child met the research criteria of hyperkinesis and did demonstrate a therapeutic effect of methylphenidate. He did not, however, demonstrate the pattern of mood changes characteristic of adult stimulant users. Possible risk factors for later substance abuse in prepubertal patients on prescribed stimulant medication are discussed.

922 Greenberg, Lawrence M.; McMahon, Shirley A.; Deem, Michael A. "Side effects of dextroamphetamine therapy of hyperactive children." West J Med 120(2): 105-9, February, 1974. (6 References).
Reports on a double-blind, placebo-controlled, short-term comparative study of the effects of three drugs on the behavior of twenty-six school-age hyperactive boys. Dextroamphetamine was associated with significant personality deterioration in five of twenty-six treated cases. Discontinuance of the drug and, in some cases, substitution of others was followed by lessened symptoms of disorganization or of toxicity. It is concluded that children who are being treated with psychostimulants be kept under careful observation for undesirable reactions. Case studies of the five hyperactive boys showing severe side effects are documented in the text.

923 Greenblatt, David J., and Shader, Richard I. "Psychotropic drug overdose." In: Manual of psychiatric therapies: practical psychopharmacology and psychiatry. Edited by Richard I. Shader. Boston, Massachusetts: Little, Brown, 1975. 237-68. (16 References). (Basic Medical Sciences Series).
Pages 256-257 outline the etiology, manifestations, and five treatments of drug overdose of hyperactivity and agitation.

924 Gualtieri, C. Thomas, and Staye, Jeannette. "Withdrawal symptoms after abrupt cessation of amitriptyline in an eight-year-old boy." Am J Psychiatry 136(4A): 457-58, April, 1979. (10 References).
Reports the case of an eight-year-old hyperactive boy who suffered severe gastrointestinal symptoms when amitriptyline medication was stopped after a seven-month treatment period. Because of these withdrawal symptoms, the authors feel that amitriptyline should only be used for hyperkinesis if other drugs prove useless and that a child should not be abruptly withdrawn from the drug.

925 Hayes, Thomas A.; Panitch, Martha L.; Barker, Eileen. "Imipramine dosage in children: a comment on 'Imipramine and electrocardiographic abnormalities in hyperactive children'." Am J Psychiatry 132(5): 546-47, May, 1975. (18 References).
Refers to a previous study by B. G. Winsberg, et al. (Item No. 934) which found electrocardiographic (EKG) abnormalities in seven children (ages seven to ten years) receiving imipramine pharmacotherapy for behavior disorders. Questions are raised concerning: (1) whether the EKG abnormalities were, indeed, related to the administration of imipramine; (2) whether the children exhibited a peculiar sensitivity to cardiovascular effects of the drug; and (3) the reaction of the U. S. Food and Drug Administration to the findings.

926 Hooshmand, H. "Toxic effects of anticonvulsants: general principles." Pediatrics 53(4): 551-56, April, 1974. (36 References).

Describes some of the potential undesirable effects of anticonvulsant drugs. The toxicity may be due to: (1) dosage; (2) the size of the patient; (3) drug interaction; (4) drug specificity for the disease; (5) the nature of the disease for which the drug is used; and (6) the mode and frequency of medication. Drug toxicity can be mild or severe, acute or chronic. Drug-induced toxicity is not uncommon; approximately 7.3 percent of patients undergoing treatment with different drugs reveal some form of toxicity. Implications of the findings for the hyperactive child are discussed.

927 Huestis, R. D., and Arnold, L. E. "Possible antagonism of amphetamine by decongestant-antihistamine compounds." J Pediatr 85(4): 579, October, 1974. (2 References).
Documents a case report and comment of the possible interaction of over-the-counter remedies containing chlorpheniramine, with levoamphetamine (levamfetamine) in a twelve-year-old hyperactive boy. While receiving maintenance doses of levamfetamine the child, on separate occasions, received both Allerest and Contac, which contain phenylpropanolamine and chlorpheniramine with resultant ineffectiveness of the levamfetamine therapy. The possibility that chlorpheniramine side effects may have neutralized the levamfetamine effects is suggested. The need for alertness to possible drug interaction, not just among prescribed medications but also among over-the-counter remedies alone and with prescription drugs is stressed.

928 Kinsbourne, Marcel. "Dangers attending the stimulant therapy of hyperactive children." Spec Educ Can 53(3): 12-14, Spring, 1979.
Outlines the problems of stimulant therapy as to misuse, abuse, side effects, and exclusive use. Misuse causes personality changes and deterioration in performance. Abuse occurs when a drug is used by a person other than the one the drug was prescribed for, when the child becomes psychologically dependent, or when the child is predisposed to drug dependence. Side effects include loss of appetite and a rise in blood levels of liver enzymes. Exclusive use of drug therapy is unwise; most benefit can be obtained when drugs are used with behavioral therapies.

929 Lucas, Betty, and Sells, Clifford, J. "Nutrient intake and stimulant drugs in hyperactive children." J Am Diet Assoc 70(4): 373-77, April, 1977. (17 References).
Investigates the relationship between stimulant medication and nutrient intake. The growth data and food records of two boys (ages 7.5 and 10.5 years), placed on different types and dosages of stimulant drugs for hyperactive behavior, were examined over a twelve-month period. The data revealed that dextroamphetamine levels of 10 mg or more and methylphenidate levels of 30 mg or more significantly decreased caloric intake.

930 Ounsted, Christopher. "High activity and hyperactivity." Dev Med Child Neurol 16(5): 685, October, 1974. (5 References).
Letter to editor.

931 Renshaw, Domeena C. "Mentally retarded, hyperkinetic and psychotic." Dis Nerv Syst 38(7): 575-76, July, 1977. (0 References).
Presents a case study of a twenty-year-old hyperactive, retarded, and psychotic girl who suffered side effects as a result of the various medications prescribed for her conditions.

932 Rosenfeld, Alvin A. "Depression and psychotic regression following prolonged methylphenidate use and withdrawal: case report." Am J Psychiatry 136(2): 226-28, February, 1979. (5 References).
Cites a case report of a nine-year-old boy who suffered severe depression after the withdrawal of methylphenidate. The boy had been taking the drug for three years because of MBD and hyperactivity. Implications for diagnosis and treatment are given.

933 Sleator, Esther K. "Methylphenidate reaction." Pediatrics 55(6): 895-96, June, 1975. (0 References).
Letter to editor.

934 Winsberg, Bertrand G.; Goldstein, Stanley; Yepes, Luis; et al. "Imipramine and electrocardiographic abnormalities in hyperactive children." Am J Psychiatry 132(5): 542-45, May, 1975. (25 References).
Explores the relationship between the administration of imipramine, a tricylic antidepressant, and electrocardiographic (EKG) abnormalities in children. Seven children (ages seven to ten years) exhibiting behavior disorders served as subjects. Although other side effects of imipramine have been previously noted (drowsiness, dizziness, lethargy, tremors, sweating, nausea, seizures, and even death), abnormalities of EKG were found in these pediatric patients. Three of the children evidenced a first-degree atrioventricular block; the abnormalities were less pronounced in the other four children. Imipramine plasma levels during steady state were not found to be directly related to the extent of the electrocardiographic changes within the obtained plasma values. Careful monitoring of children receiving imipramine is necessary.

935 Wolf, Sheldon M., and Forsythe, Alan. "Behavior disturbance, phenobarbital, and febrile seizures." Pediatrics 61(5): 728-31, May, 1978. (8 References).
Studies the relationship of behavior disorders (especially hyperactivity) to the ingestion of phenobarbital. Three hundred and ninety-five children served as subjects. The children were receiving phenobarbital treatment for febrile convulsions. Data, based on parents' perceptions and observations of the children's behavior, indicated that 42 percent of the children showed behavior disturbance, usually hyperactivity, which appeared within several months and improved in all children when treatment was discontinued. Eighteen percent who received no phenobarbital developed behavior disorder, usually hyperactivity, which spontaneously disappeared in 52 percent of the cases.

5. "PARADOXICAL" EFFECTS

936 Brodemus, John, and Swanson, Jon C. "The 'paradoxical' effect of stimulants upon hyperactive children." Drug Forum 6(2): 117-25, 1977-78. (37 References).
Upholds the hypothesis that hyperactive children are actually understimulated rather than overstimulated. Therefore, amphetamines and other stimulant drugs are not causing "paradoxical" effects; rather, they are effective because they provide internal sources of stimulation. The need for external sources of stimulation is then reduced. This model, the Swanson-Brodemus model, predicts that several nondrug therapies could be effective if they provide external stimulation for the hyperactive child. The model allows integration of disparate theories of hyperactivity and concomitant therapies.

937 Millichap, J. Gordon. "The paradoxical effects of CNS stimulants on hyperkinetic behavior." Int J Neurol 10(1-4): 241-51, 1975. (19 References).
Investigates the relation of the degree of activity and brain damage to drug response and explores an experimental model for the development of new pharmacological therapies for hyperactivity. In the double-blind controlled trial, twenty-eight children (ages five to fourteen years) served as subjects. Motor activity was measured by means of an actometer before and during treatment with methylphenidate or placebo. Interpretation of the data reveals that: (1) suppression of activity by methylpenidate was observed in the patients with the higher level of activity; (2) a stimulant effect occurred in those patients with lower activity levels; and (3) children with the highest number of abnormal neurological signs tended to be the most active and also the most likely to benefit from methylphenidate. Implications for predicting response to medication are given as well as the animal model used for the study. Summaries in Spanish, French, and German complete the article.

938 Robbins, T. W., and Sahakian, B. "Paradoxical effects of psychomotor stimulant drugs in hyperactive children from the standpoint of behavioural pharmacology." Neuropharmacology 18(12): 931-50, December, 1979. (98 References).
Examines the hypothesis of a "paradoxical" drug response in hyperactive children. The article: (1) reviews the behavioral effects of stimulant drugs; (2) attempts to show from recent evidence and principles derived from behavioral pharmacology that the "paradoxical" effects of stimulants may be better understood as a normal behavioral action of psychomotor stimulants; and (3) discusses the implications of this conclusion both for clinical practice and animal models.

939 Sahakian, Barbara. "Hyperactive children and the drug paradox." New Sci 80(1127): 350-52, November 2, 1978. (0 References).
Uses a question-and-answer format to comment briefly on a few of the most common issues involving children with the hyperkinetic syndrome. The so-called "paradoxical" effect of certain drugs (amphetamine and methylphenidate), i.e., why these drugs stimulate adults, but seemingly decrease activity in children, is discussed.

940 Sahakian, B. J., and Robbins, T. W. "Are the effects of psychomotor stimulant drugs on hyperactive children really paradoxical?" Med Hypotheses 3(4): 154-58, July-August, 1977. (75 References).
Presents evidence, from both clinical and animal studies, in support of the hypothesis that the effect of amphetamines on hyperactive children is a normal reaction rather than the effect often called "paradoxical" by other researchers. These effects are often referred to in this manner because amphetamine-like drugs normally cause stimulation in adults; they "paradoxically" have a calming influence on certain behavior disorders in children. Amphetamine is seen to act in the normal dose-related manner in these children. Differences in response between normal and hyperactive children can be attributed to differences in baseline levels of activity in the nonmedicated state. Thus, caution is urged when medicating hyperactive children with amphetamine, as would be so if normal children were receiving the drug.

941 Yellin, Absalom M. "Recent advances in psychophysiology: psychophysiological studies in hyperkinesis." Res Commun Psychol Psychiatry Behav 3(3): 237-55, 1978. (50 References).

Discusses the "paradoxical" effects of psychostimulants on hyperactive children and the controversy concerning arousal levels of such children. It is noted that a substantial portion of the psychophysiological data accumulated to date supports the hypothesis of underarousal, with psychoactive medication having the effect of increasing arousal level. Both autonomic and cortical research data are summarized. Evidence is provided for these conclusions: (1) there is a subgroup of hyperkinetic children whose hyperkinesis is characterized by underarousal; (2) genetic involvement is unclear; and (3) medication may not be appropriate for children whose behavior does not appear to be related to arousal and attentional deficiencies.

942 Zentall, Sydney S., and Zentall, Thomas R. "Amphetamine's paradoxical effects may be predictable." J Learn Disabil 9(3): 188-89, March, 1976. (9 References).
Appraises the calming or depressant effects of the CNS stimulant, amphetamine, on normal adults and hyperactive children. It is suggested that the so-called paradoxical effects of the drug can be accounted for by the proposition that amphetamine will increase arousal when the initial level of arousal is low, but will decrease arousal when the initial level of arousal is high. This theory lends support to the hypothesis that hyperactive children suffer from underarousal rather than overarousal. The direction of change in arousal produced by amphetamine can be predicted if the prior level of arousal (or activity) is known.

6. LONG-TERM EFFECTS

943 Allen, Richard P., and Safer, Daniel J. "Long-term effects of stimulant therapy for HA children: risk benefits analysis." In: Drugs and the special child. Edited by Michael J. Cohen. New York, New York: Gardner Press, 1979. 189-201. (46 References).
Points out three benefits and four risks involved in the stimulant maintenance of therapy in hyperactive children.

944 Charles, Linda; Schain, R. J.; Guthrie, D. "Long-term use and discontinuation of methylphenidate with hyperactive children." Dev Med Child Neurol 21(6): 758-64, December, 1979. (14 References).
Describes the long-term effects of methylphenidate on the behavior and academic functioning of a group of hyperactive children. Thirty-six children having a positive response to methylphenidate entered a three-year follow-up study in which they were closely monitored physically, behaviorally, and psychometrically. Thirteen children discontinued medication during the trial period. The greatest improvement in performance occurred in the early months of treatment, but was only partially maintained during long-term therapy; little further change occurred after medication was discontinued. The findings indicate that sustained improvement is related to factors other than continued medication. Drug therapy should therefore be regarded as a short-term intervention until more positive social and school behavior can be established.

945 Cunningham. Constance P. "An exploratory study of the long-term effects of drug use in hyperkinesis." For a summary see: Diss Abstr Int 34A(9): 5752, March, 1974. (0 References).

946 Cunningham, Patricia A. "Long-term correlates of drug use in hyperkinesis." Psychopharmacol Bull 10(2): 61, April, 1974. (0 References).
Abstract.

947 Hontela, S. "Relative hyperactivity of brain centers." Can Med Assoc J 119(7): 689, October 7, 1978. (3 References).
Letter to editor.

948 Krager, John M.; Safer, Daniel; Earhart, Jane. "Follow-up survey results of medication used to treat hyperactive school children." J Sch Health 49(6): 317-21, June, 1979. (8 References).
Reports the results of a survey taken in Baltimore County, Maryland during 1975-1977. Items surveyed included: (1) kind of medicine prescribed for hyperkinesis; (2) trends in usage; (3) relationship between medium family income and medicine usage; (4) source of medical treatment; and (5) medication administration. This follow-up survey found that the use of medicine had increased only slightly since the first survey, but there was an increased use of stimulants as the drug of choice. Less affluent areas reported more cases at follow-up.

949 Quinn, Patricia O., and Rapoport, Judith L. "One-year follow-up of hyperactive boys treated with imipramine or methylphenidate." Am J Psychiatry 132(3): 241-45, March, 1975. (18 References).
Details the findings of a follow-up study which examined: (1) growth of children remaining on methylphenidate or imipramine; (2) the long-term pattern of use of medication; and (3) the behavior effect of continued drug treatment. Seventy-six hyperactive boys (96 percent) who had participated in an earlier comparative study of methylphenidate, imipramine, and placebo were examined one year later. Decreased growth was found with both medications. A resumption of behavior problems was associated with drug discontinuance.

950 Safer, Daniel J., and Allen, Richard P. "Stimulant drug treatment of hyperactive adolescents." Dis Nerv Syst 36(8): 454-57, August, 1975. (9 References).
Evaluates the characteristics and classroom behavior changes, in relation to age, of thirty-eight hyperactive school children who were treated with medication during the years 1969-1974. Fourteen children who began taking stimulants before age eight were compared with eleven children who began treatment at ages thirteen to sixteen. Next, thirteen children who continued stimulants into their teens were studied to compare their preteen with their teenage drug response. The primary results of the study show: (1) the child's response to stimulants did not change in the follow-up study; (2) the amount of stimulant needed to change behavior did not significantly increase with age; (3) the use of stimulants by young children did not lead to drug abuse among the hyperactive teenagers; (4) teenagers were more resistant to taking medication than were the younger children; and (5) teacher ratings showed teenage hyperactives had improved in aggression and restlessness, although inattentiveness remained a problem.

951 Sleator, Esther K.; von Neumann, Alice; Sprague, Robert L. "Hyperactive children: a continuous long-term placebo-controlled follow-up." JAMA 229(3): 316-17, July 15, 1974. (5 References).
This research reports on a long-term, continuous follow-up study of forty-two hyperactive children who had previously been subjects in an earlier study. All children had been receiving methylphenidate and were monthly rated by their teachers. Once each year placebo was inserted into the treatment program. Several patterns emerged from the follow-up data: (1) after two years of follow-up with forty-two children, 26 percent were able to function well without drugs; and (2) 40 percent still benefited

from medication and showed deterioration during the placebo month. On the basis of this study, it is recommended that physicians treating hyperactive children with stimulants should occasionally try drug-free periods during the school year.

952 Weiss, Gabrielle; Kruger, Elena; Danielson, Ursel; et al. "Effect of long-term treatment of hyperactive children with methylphenidate." Can Med Assoc J 112(2): 159-65, January 25, 1975. (23 References).
Assesses the results of a five-year follow-up study of three groups of hyperactive children. Some of these children had received methylphenidate while others received chlorpromazine; some had received no medication at all. No significant differences were found among the three groups on several measures of outcome: emotional adjustment, delinquency, WISC, Bender-Gestalt Visual Motor Test, and academic performance. Although methylphenidate was seen to be helpful for managing or controlling hyperkinetic behaviors at the time, the drug did not significantly effect outcome at follow-up.

953 ————. "Long-term methylphenidate treatment of hyperkinetic children." Psychopharmacol Bull 10(4): 34-35, October, 1974. (9 References).
Presents the results of a follow-up study of seventy-two hyperactive children who were diagnosed and evaluated in a Canadian children's hospital between 1962 and 1967. Three subgroups were selected on the basis of the treatment each group had received: group I was treated with methylphenidate; group II received chlorpromazine; group III had no medication. The three groups were then compared on various measures of outcome five years later--delinquency, emotional adjustment, hyperactivity, changes in scores on the Bender Gestalt Visual Motor Test, WISC, and school performance. No statistically significant differences were found on any of these measures of outcome for the three groups. Methylphenidate was found to be an efficacious drug in reducing the hyperactive behavior of children. However, as the sole method of treatment, it did not significantly affect the long-term prognosis of this group of children on the measures of outcome chosen in this study.

7. PREDICTIVE STUDIES

954 Barkley, Russell A. "Predicting the response of hyperkinetic children to stimulant drugs: a review." J Abnorm Child Psychol 4(4): 327-48, 1976. (55 References).
Examines thirty-six previous research reports involving over 1400 hyperkinetic children in an effort to determine which variables have proven useful in predicting which hyperkinetic children will respond favorably to stimulant drug therapy. The research is summarized under eight types of predictor variables: psychophysiological, neurological, familial, demographic/sociological, diagnostic category, parent/teacher/clinician ratings, psychological, and profile types. The results of the review indicate that: (1) the most useful predictor is the attention span of the child; and (2) CNS arousal may be an important factor. Problems of interpretation and suggestions for future research are included.

955 ————. "Predicting the response of hyperkinetic children to stimulant drugs: a review." In: Behavior therapy with hyperactive and learning disabled children. Edited by Benjamin B. Lahey. New York, New York: Oxford University Press, 1979. 77-91. (55 References).

Reprints an article from the Journal of Abnormal Child Psychology 4(4): 327-48, 1976. (Item No. 954).

956 ———. "The prediction of differential responsiveness of hyperkinetic children to methylphenidate." For a summary see: Diss Abstr Int 38B(6): 2842, December, 1977. (0 References).

957 Bhatara, Vinod; Arnold, L. Eugene; Knopp, Walter; et al. "A survey study of the use of electropupillogram in predicting response to psychostimulants." Psychopharmacology 57(2): 185-87, April 28, 1978. (11 References).
Evaluates the usefulness of the electropupillogram in predicting response to stimulant medication in order to confirm conclusions drawn by an earlier study. Data were analyzed from three prior and separate studies with hyperkinetic and LD children treated with stimulants. Changes in the extent of pupillary contraction after a test dose of stimulant drugs did not correlate significantly with actual rating change (with one exception out of fourteen correlations calculated). Problems and methodology, potential usefulness of the electropupillogram, and suggestions for follow-up research are discussed.

958 Callaway, E.; Halliday, R.; Naylor, H.; et al. "Prediction of response to methylphenidate in hyperkinetic children from visual event related potentials (VEP)." In: Biological psychiatry today, volume B: proceedings of the 2nd World Congress of Biological Psychiatry. Edited by J. Obiols, et al. Amsterdam: Elsevier North-Holland Biomed Press, 1979. 1356-59. (4 References). (Developments in Psychiatry, Volume 2).
Documents a study designed to extend and replicate a finding of a previous study (Item No. 959).

959 Halliday, Roy; Rosenthal, Joseph H.; Naylor, Hilary; et al. "Averaged evoked potential predictors of clinical improvement in hyperactive children treated with methylphenidate: an initial study and replication." Psychophysiology 13(5): 429-40, September, 1976. (27 References).
Reports on an attempt to predict drug response in hyperactive children and to identify those children who might benefit from stimulant medication. In two experiments certain measures of the visual evoked potential (VEP) were successful in discriminating between good and poor responders (as later judged by a pediatrician). Principal findings are: (1) with Ritalin, EP variability increased when responders went from a task requiring active attention (ATT) to one requiring passive observing (PAS). In contrast, EP variability decreased in nonresponders when they went from ATT to PAS; (2) the amplitude of the N140-P190 component in the ATT condition increased from placebo to Ritalin for the responders. It is suggested that the variability measure primarily reflects an abnormalizing effect of Ritalin on the nonresponder while the N140-P190 component represents an apparent deficit in responders that is normalized by Ritalin.

960 Itil, Turan M., and Simeon, Jovan. "Computerized EEG in the prediction of outcome of drug treatment in hyperactive childhood behavior disorders." Psychopharmacol Bull 10(4): 36, October, 1974. (0 References).
Uses computer EEG profiles to predict the efficacy of CNS stimulants on the hyperkinetic syndrome. In a double-blind, three-way study design, three treatments--dextroamphetamine, thioridazine, and placebo--were

given to a group of hyperkinetic children. Significant improvements were obtained in various areas with all the treatments, and similar alterations in brain function as determined by computer EEG profiles were found. The authors feel that the pretreatment computer EEG measurements can be used as predictors for the outcome of childhood behavior disturbances.

961 Loney, Jan; Prinz, Robert J.; Mishalow, Joel; et al. "Hyperkinetic/ aggressive boys in treatment: predictors of clinical response to methylphenidate. Am J Psychiatry 135(12): 1487-91, December, 1978. (25 References).
Attempts to identify factors that contribute significantly to variation in clinically rated improvement among hyperactive/MBD boys during a treatment trial of methylphenidate. Data on eighty-four hyperactive/MBD boys (ages six to twelve years), patients at a child psychiatry clinic, were analyzed. Results indicate that 25 percent of the variation in the children's response to methylphenidate is jointly predictable from age at referral, degree of perinatal complications, and score on the hyperactivity factor. Data were drawn from a comprehensive, longitudinal investigation called the Iowa HABIT project (Hyperkinetic Aggressive Boys in Treatment).

962 Margolin, David I. "The hyperkinetic child syndrome and brain monoamines: pharmacology and therapeutic implications." J Clin Psychiatry 39(2): 120-23, 127-30, February, 1978. (72 References).
Evidence is cited in support of the hypothesis that catecholamine hypoactivity plays a part in the pathopharmacology of the hyperactive child syndrome and that the reaction of the hyperactive child to analeptic therapy is therefore predictable rather than paradoxical. Topics covered include catecholamine metabolites, animal models, neurophysiological studies, neuroanatomical specificity, and therapeutic implications.

963 Omenn, Gilbert S. "Pharmacogenetic aspects of treating behavioral disorders in children with drugs." In: Psychopharmacology of childhood. Edited by D. V. Siva Sankar. Westbury, New York: PJD Publications, 1976. 29-44. (34 References).
Studies children's response to stimulant drugs and the factors which may influence a good or poor response. A four-step protocol is provided.

8. PROS AND CONS OF DRUG TREATMENT

964 Banks, William. "Drugs, hyperactivity and black schoolchildren." J Negro Educ 45(2): 150-60, Spring, 1976. (22 References).
Calls attention to the special concerns black children and parents have with psychoactive drugs. Emphasis is placed on the strategies needed to prevent abuse of black children through unwarranted drug administration, rather than by the use of necessary neurological and psychological examinations.

965 Berman, Steve. "How schools drug your children." Sci Dig 79(4): 72-77, April, 1976. (0 References).
Relates the experiences which one family encountered while having their daughter placed on medication for hyperactivity. Springfield, Massachusetts is the setting. The dangers of random prescribing are outlined.

966 Bosco, James. "Behavior modification drugs and the schools: the case of Ritalin." Phi Delta Kappan 56(7): 489-92, March, 1975. (11 References).

Appraises the use of Ritalin in schools to modify the behavior of hyperactive children and the educational, social, and ethical implications involved. Also discussed are the educational implications regarding the controversy surrounding drug usage; the role of school personnel; the legal and ethical responsibilities of the teacher; and ways in which the school may contribute to hyperactivity. Stress is placed on the need for further research. Six recommendations for improvement are included.

967 Box, Steven. "Hyperactivity: the scandalous silence." New Soc 42(791): 458-60, December 1, 1977. (0 References).
Disdains the use of "medical solutions" to school problems which are essentially moral, legal, and social. Hyperactivity has now reached epidemic proportions and, if untreated, can produce disastrous prognoses for both the individual and society. We need to examine the ideology which encourages us to view ourselves as surrounded by diseases (which can be cured by drugs), rather than moral, social, or political problems (in which social change would be required). Hyperactive children are receiving a form of psychological violence because physicians and educators refuse to come to grips with the real problem.

968 ————. "Hyperactivity: the scandalous silence." Am Educ 2(2): 22-24, 1978. (0 References).
Reprints an article from New Society 42(791): 458-60, December 1, 1977. (Item No. 967).

969 Cohen, Sanford N., and Cohen, Judith L. "Pharmacotherapeutics: review and commentary." Pediatr Clin North Am 21(1): 95-101, February, 1974. (23 References).
Discusses three common indications for drug therapy that may lead to dilemmas in the management of pediatric problems: fever, hyperactivity, and infection. Some of the potential difficulties arising from the treatment of these routine pediatric conditions--with commonly used pharmacological agents--are: (1) concern over toxic side effects; (2) cost of medications; and (3) ethics of medicinal drug use. Physicians are urged to reevaluate frequently their prescribing practices and to keep abreast of new developments in pediatric clinical pharmacology.

970 Cole, Sherwood O., and Moore, Samuel F. "Stimulants and hyperkinesis: drug use or abuse?" J Drug Educ 5(4): 371-78, 1975. (20 References).
The use of stimulants in the treatment of hyperkinesis is discussed in terms of: (1) the side effects and long-term consequences of drugs; (2) drugs as easy solutions to problems; and (3) the potential for abuse and addiction. Previous studies have shown the use of stimulants to be an effective means of controlling hyperactive behavior in children. However, a more intelligent and restrained use of stimulants is called for--one which stresses the total welfare of the child.

971 Fenichel, Gerald M. "Pros and cons of drug therapy in the management of the hyperactive child." Clin Proc Child Hosp 31(3): 49-51, March, 1975. (0 References).
Presents an overview of the hyperactive syndrome and summarizes various management approaches. Hyperactivity is seen as an environmental problem best resolved by behavior modification techniques. Drugs should be used only as an aid in making the child more amenable to behavior modification. Dexedrine is preferred because it is available as a sustained-release spansule. Children should rarely need to be medicated for more than two years.

972 Grinspoon, Lester, and Singer, Susan B. "Drugs for overactive schoolchildren: therapy or abuse?" Parents Mag 49(11): 52-53, 103-6, November, 1974. (0 References).
Despite the fact that almost no long-term studies have been undertaken concerning the effect of amphetamine in treating children's behavior disorders, strong proponents for the drug exist, especially among drug manufacturers and educators. Although many controlled and systematic studies have been conducted from 1937 through the late 1960s on the effects of drugs on the hyperkinetic syndrome, the authors contend that the findings are preliminary, inconclusive, contradictory, confusing, and methodologically incorrect. The main points of the presentation are: (1) alternatives to drug therapy for children's behavior disorders must be sought; (2) more research must be directed at discovering the causes underlying the symptoms of hyperactivity; and (3) extreme caution must be used in any decision involving amphetamine therapy for children.

973 Huessy, Hans R. "Chaining children with chemicals." Progressive 39(5): 45, May, 1975. (0 References).
Letter to editor.

974 "Hyperactivity and drugs." Sci Am 231(1): 47, July, 1974. (0 References).
Comments on research by Grinspoon and Singer (Item No. 972) which stresses the inappropriateness of administering amphetamines and other stimulants to treat all hyperactive children. It is suggested that the syndrome be treated as a social problem, rather than a physical disease.

975 Keiffer, Betsy. "The miracle that misfired." Good Housekeeping 178(1): 82-83, 111, 113-15, January, 1974. (0 References).
Although the practice of prescribing drugs for children with behavior problems has become commonplace in America over the last two decades, this is not a desirable or appropriate treatment for all children exhibiting hyperactivity. In order to eliminate the misuse of mood-altering drugs, careful monitoring of administration and follow-up is called for.

976 Offir, Carole W. "A slavish reliance on drugs: are we pushers for our own children?" Psychol Today 8(7): 49, December, 1974. (0 References).
Critically appraises the rising dependence on drugs in America and focuses on their use and abuse in treating hyperactive children.

977 "Should schools be allowed to force drugs on children?" Harper's Wkly 3148: 4, November, 1975.

978 Smith, Alexander, and Kronick, Robert F. "The policy culture of drugs: Ritalin, methadone, and the control of deviant behavior." Int J Addict 14(7): 933-44, 1979. (11 References).
Introduces various concepts relative to policy culture and the medicalization of deviant behavior. Two drugs, methadone and methylphenidate, are discussed within a framework which utilizes these concepts. The policy culture surrounding the introduction and use of these drugs is highly particularistic. This process in turn produces certain unintended consequences.

979 Smith, Altomease. "Social dangers of treating the hyperactive child." Urban League Rev 1(1): 30-34, Spring, 1975. (18 References).

Discusses problems of definition, diagnosis, treatments, the government's position, and implications for blacks with regard to behavior disorders prevalent in children from lower socioeconomic homes.

980 Stewart, Mark A. "Chaining children with chemicals." Progressive 39(5): 45-46, May, 1975. (0 References).
Letter to editor.

981 ———. "Hyperactive children." Sci Am 231(3): 12, September, 1974. (0 References).
Letter to editor.

982 ———. "The pros and cons of treating problem children with stimulant drugs: a dialogue." In: Controversy in psychiatry. Edited by John P. Brady and H. Keith Brodie. Philadelphia, Pennsylvania: Saunders, 1978. 269-76. (28 References).
Sets forth, in dialog fashion, the following points: (1) the hyperactive child suffers primarily from an attentional disorder with excessive motor activity as a secondary response; (2) few studies show that drugs enhance learning; (3) parents should play a greater role in child management; and (4) clinical subgroups need to be defined. For a commentary on this study refer to Item No. 723.

983 ———. "What are the problems of a hyperactive child?" Paper presented at the 83rd Annual Meeting of the American Psychological Association, Chicago, Illinois, August 30-September 2, 1975. 8p. (ED 120 598).
Criticizes drug treatment for hyperactive children. Rather than this mode of treatment, emphasis should be placed on multidisciplinary management and manipulation of the home and school environment.

984 Vonder Haar, T. A. "Chaining children with chemicals." Progressive 39(3): 13-17, March, 1975. (0 References).
Briefly discusses the hyperkinetic syndrome in terms of: (1) symptomatology; (2) etiology; and (3) dangers of drug treatment. Concern is expressed regarding side effects, addiction, and the over-prescribing of drugs for conditions which should be treated by other means.

985 ———. "Chaining children with chemicals." Progressive 39(5): 47, May, 1975. (0 References).
Letter to editor.

986 Watras, Joseph. "Sedation under glass." Intellect 103(2361): 181-82, December, 1974. (0 References).
Advises against the use of medical treatment for hyperkinesis or MBD for the sole reason of making the child receptive in the classroom. The medication of the child takes place "under glass"--insulated from outside criticism and evaluation. While the truly ill child should receive proper medical attention, the child labeled "behaviorally disturbed" should not fall within that category. Since the severity of behavior most often cannot be measured objectively, the child is often at the mercy of biased and undisputed opinions of those specialists who command his future. Open and free debate of the issues would help experts see their work more clearly and would help parents make a more informed choice about seeking medication for their child.

987 Weithorn, Corinne J. "Perspectives on drug treatment for hyperactivity." In: Drugs and the special child. Edited by Michael J. Cohen. New York, New York: Gardner Press, 1979. 85-98. (42 References).
Highlights some of the problems relating to stimulant drug treatment for hyperactivity.

988 Weithorn, Corinne J., and Ross, Roslyn. "Stimulant drugs for hyperactivity: some additional disturbing questions." Am J Orthopsychiatry 46(1): 168-73, January, 1976. (22 References).
Poses a number of questions of sociological, educational, and philosophical significance regarding the use of stimulant drugs to treat hyperactive children. The questions dealt with are: (1) Who is being medicated? (2) What are the bases for deciding drug treatment? (3) Are we relying too heavily on medications instead of education and other remedial treatments? (4) Are parents fully informed of all the ramifications of drug treatment? and (5) Are drug effects being made known to the physician who prescribed them? Continued professional recognition and concern are urged.

989 Werry, J. S. "Medication for hyperkinetic children." Drugs 11(2): 81-89, 1976. (66 References).
Examines the controversial issue of the use of medication in hyperactive children. Although the hyperkinetic syndrome is a symptom complex, none of the commonly used terms (hyperactivity, distractibility, impulsivity, etc.) have been objectively defined. Management of the disorder calls for the highest clinical skill and medical supervision. Comments are made relevant to the position set forth by the Council on Child Health in its 1975 report. Their conclusion that drugs do have a place in the management of children with hyperactive, attention, or impulsivity disorders is generally upheld, providing there is proper medical supervision.

990 "We've been asked about drugs for 'unruly' schoolchildren." US News 80: 68, April 5, 1976. (0 References).
Provides brief answers to some commonly asked controversial questions concerning the use of drugs to control unruly children.

C. PSYCHOTHERAPY

991 Ament, Aaron. "The learning-disabled or hyperactive child." JAMA 236(4): 344, July 26, 1976. (0 References).
Letter to editor.

992 ————. "Treatment of hyperactive children." JAMA 230(3): 372, October 21, 1974. (0 References).
Letter to editor.

993 Blau, Harold, et al. "Two year study of the effect of group therapy on teacher perceived classroom behavior of hyperactive children." Paper presented at the Conference of the New England Educational Research Organization, Inc., Sturbridge, Massachusetts, May, 1978. 20p. (ED 161 177).
Studies the effect of group therapy on the teacher-perceived classroom behavior of eighty-two hyperactive minority boys. Success with the therapy program is reported. Several appendices are included.

994 Brannigan, Gary G., and Young, Robert G. "Social skills training with the MBD adolescent: a case study." Acad Ther 13(4): 401-4, March, 1978. (0 References).
Describes a successful method of developing social skills in an adolescent with minimal brain dysfunction. A case study of a thirteen-year-old boy presenting with a variety of behavior problems (hyperactivity, inattentiveness, distractibility, and impulsivity) is cited. The boy also exhibited poor social adjustment, attention-seeking, poor emotional control, and nervous mannerisms. Weekly sessions with a therapist for a seven-month period reduced the boy's immature and inappropriate behaviors and improved his academic standing.

995 Gardner, Richard A. "The Mutual Storytelling Technique in the treatment of psychogenic problems secondary to minimal brain dysfunction." J Learn Disabil 7(3): 135-43, March, 1974. (7 References).
Child therapists frequently experience difficulty in eliciting conversation from their child patients. This is particularly true with the child with MBD because of hyperactivity, distractibility, inability to concentrate, perceptual deficiencies, and difficulty in abstracting and forming concepts. Involving the child in play activities facilitates his revealing his underlying psychodynamics. In the Mutual Storytelling Technique a self-created story is elicited from the child. The therapist surmises its psychodynamic meaning and retells the basic story introducing healthier adaptations than those of the child's story. The child is more receptive to this type of communication, as play is one of the child's natural modes of communication. Verbatim case material is included.

996 ————. "Psychotherapy in minimal brain dysfunction." In: Current psychiatric therapies. Volume 15. Edited by Jules H. Masserman. New York, New York: Grune & Stratton, 1975. 25-38. (19 References).
Emphasizes the importance of games as an aid in treating children, especially those with MBD. The games are designed as techniques to be used along with more traditional modalities. Games provide structure, interest, and involvement for the child and enable the therapist to gain insight into the psychogenic problems of the child. Many games are described in detail, along with clinical examples to facilitate their use.

997 ————. "Psychotherapy in minimal brain dysfunction." In: Current psychiatric therapies. Volume 14. Edited by Jules H. Masserman. New York, New York: Grune & Stratton, 1974. 15-21. (15 References).
Offers tips for successful psychotherapy with children presenting various symptoms of MBD. Suggestions include: (1) selecting the correct approach by the therapist; (2) keeping the mother in the session with the child, and having the parent tape-record the session; (3) structuring the therapeutic sessions; (4) using the Mutual Storytelling Technique; and (5) establishing a good relationship between the child and therapist.

998 ————. "Techniques for involving the child with MBD in meaningful psychotherapy." J Learn Disabil 8(5): 272-82, May, 1975. (19 References).
Describes various games used to engage the inhibited, uncooperative, or resistant child into meaningful psychotherapy. Emphasis is placed on the Mutual Storytelling Technique which elicits a self-created story from the child. The therapist surmises its psychodynamic meaning, selects one or two important themes, and then creates a story of his own intro-

ducing healthier resolutions and more mature adaptations. Verbalization and involvement on the child's part can aid in the therapeutic process.

999 Johansson, Mary A. "Evaluation of group therapy with children: a behavioral approach." For a summary see: Diss Abstr Int 34B(7): 3499, January, 1974. (0 References).

1000 Leeks, S. R. "Minimal brain dysfunction." NZ Med J 80(525): 315, October 9, 1974. (2 References).
Letter to editor.

1001 Lifshin, Joanne H., and Schultz, Myra. "Treatment of a constellation of perceptual and behavioral difficulties in a community mental health center: preliminary report." Psychol Sch 11(3): 333-37, July, 1974. (6 References).
Reports on a pilot study initiated to determine the prevalence of interacting perceptual-cognitive and behavioral difficulties in a child outpatient population and to evaluate the effectiveness of a treatment approach designed to modify these problems. Records of 155 children were reviewed and ten boys (ages eight to eleven years) were selected for the study. A battery of tests (Bender-Gestalt, WISC, Wepman Auditory Discrimination, and Wide Range Achievement Test) were administered and teachers' reports used to evaluate behavioral difficulties. The subjects were divided into two groups and administered a structured group program by trained therapists for a two-month period. Emphasis was placed on interpersonal relationships, group interactions, and training in perceptual motor skills and/or coping skills. Data are seen to be insignificant because of the small sample. The program, which emphasized the need to deal simultaneously with interacting behavioral and cognitive difficulties, should be explored on a broader basis.

1002 Schaefer, Jacqueline W.; Palkes, Helen S.; Stewart, Mark A. "Group counseling for parents of hyperactive children." Child Psychiatry Hum Dev 5(2): 89-94, Winter, 1974. (14 References).
Advocates the use of group therapy as an alternative or adjunct to individual psychotherapy, behavior therapy, and the use of stimulant drugs to treat hyperactive children. A procedure is described in which parents attend class to learn how to set up rules, enforce rules, and influence their children's behavior by using the principles of learning theory. Nine couples met weekly for ten sessions of group counseling and discussion. Teachers of hyperactive children can also play a role in this type of therapy.

1003 Zeifman, Israel. "Learning disorder and minimal brain dysfunction." In: Clinician's handbook of childhood psychopathology. Edited by Martin M. Josephson and Robert T. Porter. New York, New York: Aronson, 1979. 307-22. (9 References).
Covers etiology, diagnosis, and treatment of learning disabilities and MBD from a clinical child psychiatric point of view. The importance of expressing the diagnosis in behavioral terms is stressed.

D. CLASSROOM REMEDIATION

1004 Alabiso, Frank P., and Hansen, James C. The hyperactive child in the classroom. Springfield, Illinois: Thomas, 1977. 325p. (Bibliography).

Presents an overview of the hyperactive child in the classroom. An attempt is made to integrate medical, psychological, and educational knowledge for the benefit of the classroom teacher. The book encompasses standard studies on the subject, data from unpublished research articles, and European studies which have been disseminated in the United States. Chapter I describes the characteristics of the syndrome which is seen to be a subcategory of MBD. Chapter II includes a more comprehensive concept of hyperactivity, an overview of the major treatment modalities, and a section on etiology. The measurement, etiology, and behavioral control of activity level is considered in Chapter III. Chapter IV examines the attention-distractibility factor and behavior modification strategies. Chapter V, on cognitive dysfunction, covers cognitive abilities, memory abilities, learning set, and cognitive styles. The nature of impulsivity and treatments are considered in Chapter VI. Chapter summaries, references, and author and subject indexes are included.

1005 Bateman, Barbara D. "Educational implications of minimal brain dysfunction." Read Teach 27(7): 662-68, April, 1974. (6 References).

Reprints the text of a paper given at a conference of the New York Academy of Sciences. Major tenets of the article are: (1) the symptoms of MBD have not been clearly delineated; (2) etiological bases do not necessarily have educational implications; (3) direct CNS manipulations are beyond the domain of the educator; (4) medical classifications such as MBD are irrelevant to the educational setting; and (5) interdisciplinary communication is vital to the total well-being of the child. Steps toward the remedial process include selecting and establishing objectives, arranging the environment so that learning can occur, and assessing and monitoring the child's progress toward each objective. For the educator, then, the educational implication of MBD is that it prompts the question, "What does this child need to be taught?"

1006 Connor, James P. Classroom activities for helping hyperactive children. New York, New York: Center for Applied Research in Education, 1974. 61p. (Bibliography).

This handbook on classroom activities for hyperactive children is devoted to involving the child actively in the learning process. Following a brief section on the special needs of the hyperactive child are sections describing individual and group activities for various grade levels: primary, intermediate, and advanced. For each of the thirty-one activities listed, information is given in terms of educational objectives, time involved, directions for preparing needed materials, and a summary of the activity with possible variations.

1007 Consilia, Sister Mary. "USA in the '70s--a look at the learning-disabled child." Acad Ther 9(5): 301-8, Spring, 1974. (0 References).

Advocates the use of a special plan to assist the learning-disabled child in developing his potential. The plan, called USA (Understanding, Structure, Assimilation), involves: (1) understanding the LD child's strengths and weaknesses; (2) structuring guidelines, delineating tasks in small portions, and giving logical directions; and (3) assimilating or mainstreaming the LD child into the regular classroom, while individualizing his instruction to fit his strengths and weaknesses.

1008 Doerr, Andrea. "Help for the rural LD child." Am Educ 10(5): 26-29, June, 1974. (0 References).

Reports on a Nebraska education center designed to help the LD and hyperactive child. With the help of Dr. James C. Chalfant and a grant from the U. S. Office of Education, a program was begun to identify and provide educational remediation to the rural LD child.

1009 Flynn, Nona M., and Rapoport, Judith L. "Hyperactivity in open and closed traditional classroom environments." J Spec Educ 10(3): 285-90, Fall, 1976. (26 References).
Discusses a group of thirty boys (ages seven to thirteen years), previously diagnosed as hyperactive, who were observed in open and traditional classrooms in thirty different large metropolitan area public schools. The boys were compared for academic gains and hyperactive behaviors. Results show that the children in open classes were less distinctive and less disruptive than were the boys in the traditional classrooms. It is suggested that the findings be part of the total treatment for the hyperactive child. The limitations of the study are discussed.

1010 Forness, Steven. "Educational approaches with hyperactive children." In: Cantwell, Dennis P., ed. The hyperactive child: diagnosis, management, current research. New York, New York: Spectrum Publications, distributed by John Wiley and Sons, 1975. 159-72. (38 References). (Series on Child Behavior and Development, Volume I).
Sets forth three specific difficulties of hyperactive children: attentional deficits, impulse control, and motivation. These problem areas are defined, and behavioral approaches to classroom management are suggested. The chapter concludes: (1) the relevance of medical findings to the education of hyperactive children has not been demonstrated; (2) the level of a child's motor activity need not necessarily be an issue in school learning; (3) the potential usefulness of behavior therapy should be explored; and (4) better terminology is needed.

1011 Gearheart, Bill R. "Approaches for use with the hyperactive, learning disabled child." In: Gearheart, Bill R. Learning disabilities: educational strategies. 2nd ed. St. Louis, Missouri: Mosby, 1977. 112-22. (15 References).
The hyperactive child is analyzed in terms of: (1) identifying characteristics; (2) current etiological hypotheses; and (3) management approaches, including medicine, behavior modification, and environmental control. The research of Alfred Strauss, Laura Lehtinen, and William Cruickshank is discussed. Emphasis is placed on the environmental control approach as it relates to the classroom situation.

1012 Glennon, Claire A., and Nason, Doris E. "Managing the behavior of the hyperkinetic child: what research says." Read Teach 27(8): 815-24, May, 1974. (27 References).
Reviews research on the hyperkinetic syndrome relating to characteristics, educational management, and medical treatment. Various definitions are noted, and ways of educational management are offered to reduce distraction. Highlighted is the paradoxical effect of CNS stimulants and the Schenectady study, which investigated the effects of tutoring alone and tutoring together with medicine on the behavior and achievement of hyperactive children. Public concerns, limitations of medical treatment, and the possibility of drug dependency in later years are discussed.

1013 Guyer, Barbara P. "The Montessori approach for the elementary-age LD child." Acad Ther 10(2): 187-92, Winter, 1974-75. (9 References).

Discusses the applicability of the Montessori approach to the education of the primary school learning-disabled (LD) child. The particular self-teaching aspects of the Montessori approach can be applied to children with hyperactivity, short attention span, auditory and visual perception deficits, coordination problems, and language deficits. It is suggested that if LD children were taught from the beginning to progress systematically from concrete to semiabstract to abstract concepts using a multisensory approach, the number of school dropouts, juvenile delinquents, and school phobics might be vastly decreased.

1014 Hackett, Regina. "In praise of praise." Am Educ 11(2): 11-15, March, 1975. (0 References).
Reports on a program developed at the Center at Oregon for Research in the Behavioral Education of the Handicapped, one of four national centers funded by the Bureau of Education for the Handicapped, U. S. Office of Education. The program, Contingencies for Learning Academic and Social Skills (CLASS), was designed to change disruptive children's negative behaviors. This type of child is frequently acting-out, difficult to manage, and below grade level in academic skills. The CLASS program's basic principle is that behaviors are learned and maintained as a result of the presence of rewards or reinforcement and weakened in its absence. Details on procedures and difficulties of administering the program are outlined.

1015 Iowa. State Department of Public Instruction, Des Moines. Psychological intervention: case studies in school psychological services. Volume 3. 253p. 1979. (ED 175 220).
The book presents twenty-seven case studies illustrating psychological interventions with behavior problem schoolchildren. Studies usually introduce the target population, describe the method of psychological evaluation, report the results of treatment, and discuss the case's implications. Among cases reported are investigations of stimulant medication on hyperactive students, behavioral intervention for a depressed preschooler, a Gestalt approach to counseling an adolescent, the use of cognitive behavior modification, evaluation of hearing-impaired students, selective mutism, relaxation training with enuretic students, chronic absenteeism, treatment of encopresis, school phobia, dropouts, and group counseling with secondary school special education students.

1016 Jacob, Rolf G.; O'Leary, K. Daniel; Rosenblad, Carl. "Formal and informal classroom settings: effects on hyperactivity." J Abnorm Child Psychol 6(1): 47-59, March, 1978. (17 References).
Compares the behavior of two groups of children, hyperactive and controls, in two different classroom settings--formal and informal--to determine the most desirable setting for hyperactive children. The formal setting involved teacher specification of a small number of tasks and required the children to work quietly in their seats. The informal setting involved choice, a variety of tasks, and interrelationships with other children. Eight hyperactive children and sixteen controls served as subjects and were observed and rated. The study finds that: (1) there were significant differences between the hyperactive and control groups in the formal but not the informal setting; and (2) hyperactives displayed higher frequencies of behavior than did controls in both settings. Educational implications of the findings are discussed.

1017 Johnson, Richard A.; Kenney, James B.; Davis, John B. "Developing school policy for use of stimulant drugs for hyperactive children." Sch Rev 85(1): 78-96, November, 1976. (26 References).

Discusses the role of the public school in identifying and treating hyperkinesis, since schools deal directly with the issue in areas of local school policy and cooperation with the medical community. The problems of terminology, its prevalence, and the effects and side effects of drug treatment are presented, with the conclusion that choice of treatment is clouded by lack of concrete data. Several efforts to develop a policy governing drug treatments are described. General considerations in policy development are examined, and specific policy suggestions are given relating to coordination with other agencies, protection of student rights, and management. For a reprint of this study refer to Item No. 744.

1018 Johnson, Ross. "Hyperactivity: a classroom problem." Lutheran Educ 112(4): 210-14, March-April, 1977.
Sets forth the characteristics which the typical hyperactive child exhibits. Various forms of management available to parents and teachers are outlined.

1019 Kauffman, James M. Characteristics of children's behavior disorders. Columbus, Ohio: Merrill, 1977. 311p. (Bibliography).
This book, intended primarily as a text for an introductory course in special education for emotionally disturbed children, is divided into four major sections: (1) the problem and its history; (2) the origins of behavior; (3) the four facets of disordered behavior; and (4) implications for special education. Part I is an introduction to some of the major concepts and historical antecedents of special education; Part II discusses the origins of disordered behavior; Part III deals with the various types of disordered behavior; Part IV sets forth some of the implications of the behavior disorders for special education. Chapter VI (Part III) focuses on hyperactivity, distractibility, and impulsivity--problems of definition, etiology, and characteristics. Most of the chapter discusses current methods of controlling hyperactivity, e.g., medication, behavior modification, structured environment, self-instruction, modeling, and biofeedback. The techniques falling under the general rubric of behavior modification are seen to have the greatest value for the special educator. A long list of references, a glossary, and an index complete the volume.

1020 Krippner, Stanley. "An alternative to drug treatment for hyperactive children." Acad Ther 10(4): 433-39, Summer, 1975. (10 References).
Reports on the Churchill School, a special school in New York City which serves the educational needs of children diagnosed as "hyperactive," "brain-damaged," or "neurologically impaired," etc. The school offers three programs for its clientele: sensory-motor training, orthomolecular treatment, and open classroom instruction. Promising results in test scores were noted for the years 1972-1974. This type of school is advocated as an alternative to drug treatment for hyperactive children.

1021 ————. "The Churchill School: an alternative to drug treatment for hyperactive children." Paper presented at the 18th Annual Meeting of the College Reading Association, Bethesda, Maryland, October, 1974. 13p. (ED 103 751).
Calls attention to the progress of an alternative approach to treating hyperactive children. The educational program of the Churchill School is holistic in nature and utilizes three programs in its curriculum.

1022 Lall, Geeta R. "Hyperkinetic children: a synopsis of possible causes, treatments, and educational aspects." Sask J Educ Res Dev 7(1): 36-42, February, 1976.

Summarizes possible etiologies, available treatment modalities, and educational remediation for the hyperactive child.

1023 ————. Hyperkinetic children--a synopsis of possible causes, treatments, and educational aspects. 1976. 13p. (ED 123 857).
Consists of a brief overview of the etiology of hyperkinesis. Also presented is an analysis of various treatment methods, especially those focusing on educational remediation.

1024 ————. "Hyperkinetic children--a synopsis of possible causes, treatments, and educational aspects." Int J Early Child 9(1): 105-9, 1977. (9 References).
Points out the most significant differences between hyperkinetic children and normal children. Comments are also made concerning causes (psychiatric, neurochemical, or neurophysiological), drug therapy, and educational management. The latter includes: (1) individualizing instruction; (2) changing seating arrangements; (3) establishing some form of behavior modification system; (4) using physical activity and vigorous exercise in the school program; and (5) providing special classes and counseling for children who become emotionally disturbed as a result of their hyperactivity.

1025 ————. "Hyperkinetic children--a synopsis of possible causes, treatments, and educational aspects." Spec Educ Can 52(2): 21-23, Winter, 1978.
Discusses the hyperkinetic syndrome according to identifying characteristics, causes, and various treatment methods and techniques which can be used in dealing with the hyperactive child. Emphasis is placed on classroom remediation, such as providing a good physical education program. The role of drugs in the management therapy is discussed.

1026 Lasher, Miriam, et al. Mainstreaming preschoolers: children with emotional disturbance. A guide for teachers, parents, and others who work with emotionally disturbed preschoolers. 1978. 154p. (ED 164 108).
Consists of one of a series of eight manuals on mainstreaming preschoolers developed by Project Head Start. Chapters 4 and 5 discuss various types of emotional disturbance, including hyperactivity.

1027 LeBlanc, Percy H. "Learning problems." J Int Assoc Pupil Pers Work 20(3): 137-43, June, 1976.
Examines some of the problems parents and teachers face when dealing with hyperactive children. The paper was presented to the St. Amant Elementary Parent Teacher Organization, Louisiana, April, 1976.

1028 Lehtinen, Laura, and Cruickshank, William M. "Teaching the brain damaged child." In: Methods for learning disorders. Edited by Patricia A. Myers and Donald D. Hammill. 2nd ed. New York, New York: Wiley, 1976. 291-311. (Bibliography).
Surveys the multisensory systems of Lehtinen and Cruickshank. Suggestions are made concerning educational remediation for the hyperactive child.

1029 Levin, Alma J. "A comparison of the responses of selected educators on the effectiveness of specified procedures for reintegrating children with learning and behavioral disorders from special self-contained classes into regular elementary classes." For a summary see: Diss Abstr Int 35A(8): 5171, February, 1975. (0 References).

1030 Love, Harold D. Educating exceptional children in a changing society. Springfield, Illinois: Thomas, 1974. 255p. (Bibliography).

Chapter 9 briefly alludes to hyperactivity as one symptom of a symptom complex present in the learning-disabled child. A treatment plan of Sam Clements (1963) is reviewed.

1031 Reinert, Henry R. Children in conflict: educational strategies for the emotionally disturbed and behaviorally disordered. St. Louis, Missouri: Mosby, 1976. 205p. (Bibliography).

Concentrates on the theoretical aspects of the problem. Section I deals with definitions, theoretical constructs, background information, and placement. Section II covers classroom application and case studies. Section III outlines how theory can be integrated into practice. Although not concerned specifically with the hyperkinetic child, the text is teacher- and education-directed and has a broad range of application.

1032 Richey, David D., and McKinney, James D. "Classroom behavioral styles of learning disabled boys." J Learn Disabil 11(5): 297-302, May, 1978. (15 References).

Compares the classroom behavior of learning-disabled boys to those of their normal classmates as displayed in the same regular classroom. Also examined is the relationship between aspects of classroom environment and behavior patterns of learning-disabled children. Fifteen learning disabled and fifteen control third- and fourth-grade boys were observed in two elementary school classrooms using the SCAN system. Of twelve kinds of classroom behaviors examined, only one, distractibility, differentiated the two groups. There was no indication that learning-disabled children possess a cluster of negative symptoms (including hyperactivity) which has been traditionally associated with the syndrome. The influence of various settings on behavior is discussed.

1033 Ross, Alan O. "What can be done for the learning-disabled child?" In: Ross, Alan O. Learning disability: the unrealized potential. New York, New York: McGraw-Hill, 1977. 124-44. (8 References).

Studies effective methods of helping children with learning disabilities. Two approaches, cognitive and behavioral, are suggested as ways to aid the hyperactive and LD child.

1034 Routh, Donald K. "Activity, attention, and aggression in learning disabled children." J Clin Child Psychol 8(3): 183-87, Fall, 1979. (47 References).

Examines evidence concerning certain behavioral correlates (overactivity, attentional deficit, impulsivity, distractibility, and aggression) of specific learning disabilities in children and considers the implications of these behaviors for treatment. The report concludes that remediation of the academic problem, rather than directing all therapy toward the behavioral aspects, is needed. Thus, therapists should focus their efforts upon improving the child's academic skills, regarding hyperactivity and attention deficits as secondary problems.

1035 Sartore, Richard L. "The open school: designed to better accommodate children with problems." Thrust Educ Leadership 4(1): 21-22, October, 1974. (0 References).

Presents ten teacher-guided approaches that can be utilized in open school learning situations. The suggestions are designed to help minimize anxieties and frustrations for children with learning/behavior problems.

1036 Smith, S. K. "The hyperactive child in the classroom." Film News 35: 18-19, March-April, 1978.

1037 Valett, Robert. The psychoeducational treatment of hyperactive children. Belmont, California: Fearon, 1974. 113p. (Bibliography).

This book offers an overview of various treatment approaches. Emphasis is placed on educational management and instruction of the child at home and at school. Chapter 1 characterizes the hyperactive syndrome and how hyperactive children can best be identified. Sample rating scales and suggestions for their use are given. Chapter 2 is devoted to the causes as well as the behavioral and psychoeducational implications of hyperactivity. Psychoeducational approaches (autosuggestion, behavior modification, and biofeedback) are explored in Chapter 3. The following chapter covers psychosynthesis (teaching the child to "get it all together") and psychotherapy. Chapter 5 gives a programming schedule, followed by two chapters containing suggestions for parents.

1038 Williamson, Gary A. "The differentiation and treatment of two patterns of hyperkinesis in the classroom." For a summary see: Diss Abstr Int 39B(9): 4603-4, March, 1979. (0 References).

1039 Zeeman, Roger, and Martucci, Irene. "The application of classroom meetings to special education." Except Child 42(8): 461-62, May, 1976. (3 References).

W. Glasser's (1969) open-ended classroom meetings were initiated in a special education class for nine learning-disabled children (ages ten to eleven years). As the school year progressed, oral participation increased while impulsive behavior and hyperactivity decreased. These meetings were especially helpful in enabling socially isolated children to develop the "success identity" necessary to draw them into positive relationships with other children.

1040 Zupnick, Stanley M. "A new approach to disturbed children: the Medical College School Program." Psychiatr Q 48(1): 74-85, 1974. (11 References).

Advocates the use of a treatment-oriented day-school program as a remedial approach for emotionally disturbed children. While the principles and techniques of behavior modification have been successfully applied in the classroom and other clinical settings, few programs have been extended into the home. The present study outlines the daily routine emotionally disturbed children followed, the types of children served, and an analysis of the results of the training the children received at the Medical College School Program in Toledo, Ohio. A method of working with parents in the home is described. This program combines traditional psychotherapeutic principles with new behavioral techniques. A case example which illustrates the principles, procedures, and future directions of the program is included.

E. BEHAVIORAL TECHNIQUES

1. GENERAL

1041 Alabiso, Frank. "Operant control of attention behavior: a treatment for hyperactivity." Behav Ther 6(1): 39-42, January, 1975. (12 References).

Uses reinforcement training to modify the attention span, focus of attention, and selective attention of eight institutionalized hyperactive retardates (ages eight to twelve years). Span, focus, and selective attention were brought under operant control. Increased attention span was incompatible with the high rates of behavior usually associated with hyperactivity. Increases in focus of attention reduced distractibility, while increases in selective attention improved performance on discrimination tasks. Laboratory training in span, focus, and selective attention generalized to the classroom setting. It is suggested that reinforcement training in attention is a meaningful supplement to drug therapy in the treatment of hyperactive children.

1042 Becker, Robert A. "Non-medication management of hyperkinetic children in the classroom." For a summary see: Diss Abstr Int 36B(6): 3019, December, 1975. (0 References).

1043 Behavior therapy with hyperactive and learning disabled children. Edited by Benjamin B. Lahey. New York, New York: Oxford University Press, 1979. 260p. (Bibliography).
Presents a collection of twenty-six reprinted papers under the headings: I: Basic Concepts and Critical Issues; II: Behavior Intervention Strategies; and III: Behavior Therapy and Pharmacological Treatments.

Contents: Current Perspectives on Hyperactivity and Learning Disabilities (Lahey, et al. - Item No. 1074); Visual-Motor Processes: Can We Train Them? (Hammill, et al.); The Effectiveness of Psycholinguistic Training (Hammill, et al.); Organic Factors in Hyperkinesis: a Critical Evaluation (Dubey - Item No. 319); A Review of Treatment Approaches for Hyperactive Behavior (Brundage-Aguar, et al. - Item No. 1193); Psychotropic Medication with Children (Sulzbacher - Item No. 2017); Effects of Methylphenidate on Underachieving Children (Rie, et al. - Item No. 1751); Predicting the Responses of Hyperkinetic Children to Stimulant Drugs: a Review (Barkley - Item No. 955); Hyperactivity and Learning Disabilities as Independent Dimensions of Child Behavior Problems (Lahey, et al. - Item No. 162); Relationships Between Symptomatology and SES-Related Factors in Hyperkinetic/MBD Boys (Paternite, et al. - Item No. 474); Early Identification of Handicapped Children Through a Frequency Sampling Technique (Magliocca, et al.); Attention and Distractibility During Reading in Hyperactive Boys (Bremer, et al. - Item No. 1587); Current Medical Practice and Hyperactive Children (Sandoval, et al. - Item No. 1478); Behavioral Treatment of Hyperkinetic Children (O'Leary, et al. - Item No. 1085); Assessment of a Cognitive Training Program for Hyperactive Children (Douglas, et al. - Item No. 1056); The Effects of a Self-Instructional Package on Overactive Preschool Boys (Bornstein, et al. - Item No. 1154); Use of Biofeedback in the Treatment of Hyperactivity (Lubar, et al. - Item No. 1136); Treatment of Severe Perceptual-Motor Disorders in Children Diagnosed as Learning Disabled (Lahey, et al.); Remediating Academic Deficiencies in Learning Disabled Children (Stromer); The Use of Contingent Skipping and Drilling to Improve Oral Reading and Comprehension (Lovitt, et al); The Differential Effects of Reinforcement Contingencies on Arithmetic Performance (Smith); A Behavioral-Educational Alternative to Drug Control of Hyperactive Children (Ayllon, et al. - Item No. 1149); The Functional Independence of Response Latency and Accuracy: Implications for the Concept of Conceptual Tempo (Williams, et al.); Behavior Therapy and Withdrawal of Stimulant Medication with Hyperactive Children (O'Leary, et al. - Item No. 1085); The Relative Efficacy of Methylphenidate (Ritalin) and Behavior-Modification Techniques in the Treatment of a Hyperactive Child (Wulbert, et al. - Item No. 1228); Relative Efficacy of Methylphenidate and Behavior Modification in Hyperkinetic Children: an Interim Report (Gittelman-Klein, et al. - Item No. 1205).

1044 Benesch, Howard I. "Performance of hyperkinetic and normal children under two conditions of reinforcement." For a summary see: Diss Abstr Int 35B(12, pt. 1): 6064, June, 1975. (0 References).

1045 Bergman, Ronald L. "Treatment of childhood insomnia diagnosed as 'hyperactivity'." J Behav Ther Exp Psychiatry 7(2): 199-201, June, 1976. (13 References).
Documents a case of a seven-year-old boy who was having much difficulty in sleeping. He had also been diagnosed as hyperactive, and Ritalin had been recommended. The boy was brought to a behaviorally oriented therapist who derived a functional analysis of the problem behavior from an intensive history-taking session with the parents. Certain procedures were then explained to the parents; the most important was to keep the child in his own bed. Within two weeks of the procedure being implemented the child's insomnia had disappeared. A six-month follow-up indicated no evidence of sleeping disturbance; daytime activity level improved as well.

1046 Bidder, R. T.; Gray, O. P.; Newcombe, R. "Behavioral treatment of hyperactive children." Arch Dis Child 53(7): 574-79, July, 1978. (29 References).
Evaluates the benefit of behavioral treatment of young hyperactive children. Twelve children with multiple behavior problems were identified and treated during a three-month period. Six children were treated immediately and six were treated four to six weeks later. The children treated first were rated by parents, the home visitor, and videotaped recordings. Improvement was noted. The as yet untreated children showed no change, but later, with treatment, reflected the same improvement as the original group. It is concluded that even a short period of treatment may be sufficient for many hyperactive children to show beneficial changes in their behavior.

1047 Blackham, Garth J., and Silberman, Adolph. Modification of child and adolescent behavior. 2nd ed. Belmont, California: Wadsworth, 1975. 318p. (235 References).
The first six chapters of this book cover basic theory of management, methods, and the observation and recording of behavior. Chapters 7 through 9 deal with the specifics of changing behavior in various settings. Examples are included. Specific problems can be located through the glossary/index.

1048 Bugental, Daphne B., et al. "Differential effectiveness of two behavior change approaches with hyperactive children." Paper presented at the Biennial Meeting of the Society for Research in Child Development, New Orleans, Louisiana, March 17-20, 1977. 9p. (ED 149 512).
Assesses the effectiveness of a self-control program to reduce hyperactive behavior in two groups of hyperactive boys. The program produced significantly greater benefits than the traditional social reinforcement program for those students who had high perception of their own control and/or who were nonmedicated.

1049 Calhoun, George. "Hyperkinesis and chemotherapy." Acad Ther 15(2): 141-44, November, 1979. (3 References).

Reviews symptomatology and offers a number of nonmedical management suggestions to teachers and parents. A distinction is made between hyperactivity and hyperkinesis.

1050 Carter, Edwin N., and Reynolds, John N. "Imitation in the treatment of a hyperactive child." Psychother Theory Res Pract 13(2): 160-61, Summer, 1976. (1 Reference).
Details the successful use of token economies with a hyperactive child. One nine-year-old girl was given poker chip reinforcers whenever she did not behave as specified. Since this method proved ineffective, an oral cue was used followed by a token for correct imitation of behavior. Dramatic improvement, noted within two weeks, was sustained at a two-month follow-up.

1051 Copeland, Anne P. "Effects of modeling on hyperactivity-related behaviors." For a summary see: Diss Abstr Int 38B(5): 2357, November, 1977. (0 References).

1052 Cunningham, S. June, and Knights, Robert M. "The performance of hyperactive and normal boys under differing reward and punishment schedules." J Pediatr Psychol 3(4): 195-201, 1978. (34 References).
Two conditions, punishment and reward, were used to measure learning performance in two groups of children. Forty-eight hyperactive and forty-eight normal control boys were administered a discrimination learning task under feedback conditions of reward (marbles for correct answers) and punishment (loss of marbles for incorrect answers). In general, both groups learned more quickly under the punishment regimen and under continuous, rather than partial, feedback schedules. Other differences between the two groups are noted.

1053 DeFilippis, Nick A. "Application of a set of class-defining rules for the hyperkinetic reaction of childhood and the unsocialized aggressive reaction of childhood." For a summary see: Diss Abstr Int 37B(12, pt. 1): 6320, June, 1977. (0 References).

1054 Douglas, Virginia I. "Are drugs enough? To treat or to train the hyperactive child." Int J Ment Health 4(1-2): 199-212, Spring-Summer, 1975. (50 References).
Advocates the use of self-verbalization and modeling techniques to teach the hyperactive child problem-solving and inhibitory control. The work of A. R. Luria (1961), originator of the technique, is reviewed. For a reprint of this study refer to Item No. 688.

1055 Douglas, Virginia I.; Parry, Penny; Marton, Peter; et al. "Assessment of a cognitive training program for hyperactive children." J Abnorm Child Psychol 4(4): 389-410, 1976. (65 References).
Tests the effectiveness of a training program involving three behavior modification techniques on the cognition, academic progress, and social behavior of a group of hyperactive children. Eighteen hyperactive children took part in the training program; a control group of eleven children received no training. Numerous tests and measures were administered prior to training, at the end of the three-month training period, and again after another three-month period. The trained group showed significant improvement on several of the measures both at the time of posttesting and on the follow-up evaluation.

1056 ————. "Assessment of a cognitive training program for hyperactive children." In: Behavior therapy with hyperactive and learning disabled children. Edited by Benjamin B. Lahey. New York, New York: Oxford University Press, 1979. 138-51. (65 References).
Reprints an article from the Journal of Abnormal Child Psychology 4(4): 389-410, 1976. (Item No. 1055).

1057 Drabman, Ronald; Spitalnik, Robert; Spitalnik, Karen. "Sociometric and disruptive behavior as a function of four types of token reinforcement programs." J Appl Behav Anal 7(1): 93-101, Spring, 1974. (20 References).
Reports on an experiment which compared four different token economies as to their effectiveness in changing target behavior in a group of first-grade children. The children were divided into four groups, baseline measures determined, and the token economies introduced. The token economies were: (1) individual reinforcement determined by individual performance; (2) group reinforcement determined by the behavior of the most disruptive child; (3) group reinforcement determined by the behavior of the least disruptive child; and (4) group reinforcement determined by the behavior of a randomly chosen child. A number of factors including effectiveness, cost, ease of use, and preference by the targets were compared. All methods improved inappropriate behavior significantly, although there were differences in other areas.

1058 Drash, P. W. "Treatment of hyperactive two-year-old children." Paper presented at the 129th Meeting of the American Psychiatric Association, Miami Beach, Florida, May 10, 1976. 19p. (ED 136 543).
Examines the effectiveness of a behaviorally oriented treatment program. Five preschool boys participated in the study and were enrolled in a behavior modification class; their parents attended a parent training program. The success of the program in reducing hyperactive behavior is reported.

1059 ————. "Treatment of hyperactivity in the two-year-old child." J Pediatr Psychol 3(3): 17-20, Summer, 1975.
Reports on the use of various behavior modification techniques to reduce the hyperactive behavior of several very young children. Five children (ages one year, eleven months, to two years, six months) were involved in the program. Positive reinforcement, negative reinforcement (time-out), and parental training were successful in reducing hyperactive behavior. The main point of the presentation is that parents can and should be trained to act as primary therapists for their children.

1060 Drash, Philip W., et al. "Hyperactivity in preschool children as non-compliance: a new conceptual basis for treatment." Paper presented at the 29th Meeting of the Florida Psychological Association, Clearwater Beach, Florida, May 9, 1976. 15p. (ED 138 000).
Reports on the implementation of a multifaceted behavioral treatment program designed to reduce the hyperactivity of a group of five preschoolers. Parents were trained in methods of maintaining compliant behavior. The authors view this type of management as an effective means of remediating hyperactivity in preschool children.

1061 Edwards, Sally A. "Hyperactivity as passive behavior." Trans Anal J 9(1): 60-62, January, 1979. (11 References).
Hyperactivity is perceived as passive behavior indicative of a chronic unresolved problem. Although this problem may have various etiologies

(physiological, neurological, social, or emotional), the afflicted child adopts passive behavior in the form of agitation. A case study of a ten-year-old boy with both hyperactive and allergic symptoms is used to illustrate how transactional analysis can be used within an interdisciplinary framework to solve the problem.

1062 Farley, O. William; Edwards, Margie E.; Skidmore, Rex A. "A new program for hyperactive children." Health Soc Work 2(3): 67-86, August, 1977. (15 References).
Describes an interdisciplinary, clinic-based program for hyperactive children that used a social work model for intervention into the major systems of the child's life. Six children (ages six to ten years) participated in the ten-week experiment. Also involved were the children's parents, teachers, and physicians.

Fine, Marvin J., ed.
see Principles and techniques of intervention with hyperactive children. (Item No. 1091).

1063 Firestone, Philip. "The effects of reinforcement contingencies and caffeine on hyperactive children." For a summary see: Diss Abstr Int 35B(10): 5109, April, 1975. (0 References).

1064 Firestone, Philip, and Douglas, Virginia. "The effects of reward and punishment on reaction times and autonomic activity in hyperactive and normal children." J Abnorm Child Psychol 3(3): 201-16, 1975. (33 References).
Three reinforcement conditions (reward, punishment, and reward plus punishment) were used to compare the performance of hyperactive and control children on a delayed reaction-time task. Findings indicate that: (1) although reward was the most successful of the three reinforcement conditions in improving reaction time, it led to a significant increase in impulsive responses in the hyperactive group; and (2) reward also increased arousal to a greater extent than either punishment or reward plus punishment.

1065 Gardner, William I. Children with learning and behavior problems: a behavior management approach. 2nd ed. Boston, Massachusetts: Allyn and Bacon, 1978. 433p. (Bibliography).
Reviews basic social learning principles and related teaching and behavior management strategies for the LD child. A brief section in Chapter 13 offers eleven steps for modifying hyperactive behavior.

1066 Gilandas, Alex J., and Ball, Thomas. "Aversive conditioning as a means of reducing aggressive behavior." Aust Psychol 10(1): 45-49, March, 1975. (5 References).
Relates the use of aversive conditioning (electric shock) on a severely mentally retarded child. The hyperactive and aggressive behavior of one five-year-old boy improved as a result of the conditioning.

1067 Gittelman, Martin. "Behavioral intervention for hyperactive children." In: Harris, Gloria G., ed. Group treatment of human problems: a social learning approach. New York, New York: Grune & Stratton, 1977. 274p. (Bibliography).
The chapter introduces the application of behavior rehearsal to disruptive behavior of children. It is explained that children are initially seen in individual sessions in which the therapist uses role playing to elicit

the stress-causing situations and then begins to teach the child alternative behavior responses, building up from minor to major stress-causing situations. The child is then reported to become involved in group role-playing sessions. Six case studies illustrate the use of behavior rehearsal.

1068 Gray, Farnum. "Drugging for deportment." Nation 14(221): 423-25, November 1, 1975. (0 References).
Attempts to show how behavior modification techniques are superior to drugs in eliminating hyperactive behavior. Research by Teodora Ayllon, Dale Layman, and Henry Kandel is cited.

1069 Graziano, Anthony M. Child without tomorrow. Elmsford, New York: Pergamon Press, 1974. 290p. (Bibliography). (Pergamon General Psychology Series, PGPS-36).
Describes the development and dissolution of a group behavior modification program for emotionally disturbed children. The major points of the book are: (1) disturbed children can be taught complex, socially adaptive behavior; (2) parents and nonprofessionals can be trained to act as effective child behavior therapists; (3) the survival of a mental health program depends upon political realities; and (4) behavioral concepts and methods are sufficient to change behavior. Although not directed specifically toward the problems of the hyperactive child, the book is intended for wide readership.

1070 Kasner, Paul R. "The control of hyperactivity in neurologically-impaired children through behavioral-informational feedback procedures." For a summary see: Diss Abstr Int 40B(3): 1132, September, 1979. (0 References).

1071 Kent, Ronald N., and O'Leary, K. Daniel. "A controlled evaluation of behavior modification with conduct problem children." J Consult Clin Psychol 44(4): 586-96, August, 1976. (21 References).
Reports on a behavioral intervention program for children suffering both behavioral and academic difficulties. One hundred and four children were referred from fifty-three classrooms and were randomly assigned to treatment and a "no contact" control group. A standardized twenty-hour treatment program involved the child, his parents, and his teacher. Ph.D. clinical psychologists provided the treatment. At follow-up, treated subjects had better achievement scores and grades. Although not directed specifically at hyperactive behavior, the program might be effective in this area.

1072 Kozloff, Martin A. Educating children with learning and behavior problems. New York, New York: Wiley, 1974. 459p. (Bibliography).
Provides detailed instructions for parents, teachers, and allied health personnel on how to use behavioral methods to teach learning readiness skills, motor skills and imitation, and functional speech. A subject index is included.

Lahey, Benjamin B., ed.
see Behavior therapy with hyperactive and learning disabled children. (Item No. 1043).

1073 Lahey, Benjamin B.; Delemater, Alan; Kupfer, David L. "Behavioral aspects of learning disabilities and hyperactivity." Educ Urban Soc 10(4): 477-99, August, 1978. (63 References).

Presents a brief edited version of a chapter by the same authors that appears in: Behavior therapy with hyperactive and learning disabled children. (Item No. 1043).

1074 Lahey, Benjamin B.; Hobbs, Steven A.; Kupfer, David L.; et al. "Current perspectives on hyperactivity and learning disabilities." In: Behavior therapy with hyperactive and learning disabled children. Edited by Benjamin B. Lahey. New York, New York: Oxford University Press, 1979. 3-18. (80 References).
Serves as an introductory chapter to a collection of twenty-six papers which are mostly reprints from previous sources. (Item No. 1043).

1075 Maier, I., and Hogg, J. "Operant conditioning of sustained visual fixation in hyperactive severely retarded children." Am J Ment Defic 79(3): 297-304, November, 1974. (14 References).
Tests the effectiveness of operant procedures aimed at increasing the duration of visual fixation through the use of social and edible reinforcers. Ten hyperactive, institutionalized, severely retarded children (eight boys and three girls) served as subjects. The conditioning sessions took place in an experimental room. An increase in both total duration of fixation time and number of fixations was evident for most subjects. These findings replicate those of previous studies. This group of children also served as subjects for another study (Item No. 1605).

1076 Mash, Eric J., and Dalby, J. Thomas. "Behavioral interventions for hyperactivity." In: Hyperactivity in children: etiology, measurement, and treatment implications. Edited by Ronald L. Trites. Baltimore, Maryland: University Park Press, 1979. 161-216. (176 References).
Comprehensively reviews the literature relative to the application of behavioral interventions for hyperactive children and their families. Emphasis is placed on conceptual and methodological problems and interventions pertinent to a wide variety of problems and settings. The papers were presented at a symposium in Ottawa, Canada, February, 1978.

1077 Mesibov, Gary B., and Fontaine, Jim. "Use of token and response cost systems in sports activities with preadolescent boys." J Pediatr Psychol 3(3): 26-27, Summer, 1975.
Describes the use of a behavior modification technique to reduce inappropriate behaviors in a group of elementary schoolchildren. Intervention tactics were used in a football game involving nine learning-disabled or hyperactive boys (age twelve years). The boys earned points for appropriate behaviors and were penalized for inappropriate behaviors. A significant reduction in inappropriate behaviors is noted.

1078 Murphy, Michael J., and Zahm, David. "Effect of improved physical and social environment on self-help and problem behaviors of institutionalized retarded males." Behav Modif 2(2): 193-210, April, 1978. (25 References).
Examines the effects of treatment and environmental change on self-help skills and aggressive, hyperactive, and inappropriate behavior. Two studies are reported which involved severely and profoundly retarded hyperactive males. In study one significant skill gains were shown by the residents exposed to improved settings. Study two revealed no significant change without behavior modification training. These findings are indicative of the need for improved ward conditions.

1079 Murray, Michael E. "The use of concrete cues in controlling inappropriate behavior in public places." Behav Ther 8(4): 755-56, September, 1977. (0 References).
Advocates the use of the "black book" technique as an effective method of controlling unacceptable behaviors in public places. Parents carry a small black book and pen with them when they leave home with their child. The book represents home management contingencies. Parents are instructed to first use an oral warning and then to record the action in the book. Punishment or the withholding of privileges, if necessary, can take place when the family returns home.

1080 Nicholson, Elaine R. "The effects of differential feedback in the performance of multiple cue probability learning tasks by hyperkinetic children." For a summary see: Diss Abstr Int 39A(11): 6659-60, May, 1979. (0 References).

1081 O'Leary, K. Daniel; Pelham, William E.; Rosenbaum, Alan; et al. "Behavioral treatment of hyperkinetic children: an experimental evaluation of its usefulness." Clin Pediatr 15(6): 510-15, June, 1976. (19 References).
Tests the effectiveness of a ten-week home-based reward program on the hyperactive behavior of a group of children. Nine hyperactive children and eight controls participated in the program. Treatment effectiveness was assessed with the standardized Teacher Rating Scale and an individualized Problem Behavior Rating established for each child. Both groups were essentially equivalent prior to treatment but were significantly different by the end of treatment. The hyperactive groups showed considerable improvement.

1082 ————. "Behavioral treatment of hyperkinetic children: an experimental evaluation of its usefulness." In: Behavior therapy with hyperactive and learning disabled children. Edited by Benjamin B. Lahey. New York, New York: Oxford University Press, 1979. 133-37. (19 References).
Reprints an article from Clinical Pediatrics 15(6): 510-15, June, 1976. (Item No. 1081).

1083 O'Leary, Susan G. "Behavioral treatment of hyperactive children." Paper presented at the Annual Meeting of the Association for the Advancement of Behavior Therapy, Atlanta, Georgia, December, 1977.

1084 O'Leary, Susan G., and Pelham, William E. "Behavior therapy and withdrawal of stimulant medication in hyperactive children." Pediatrics 61(2): 211-17, February, 1978. (21 References).
Assesses the effectiveness of behavioral methods on several children who had been taken off stimulant medication. Seven hyperactive children (grades two through five) served as subjects and were given an initial behavioral assessment. Both the family and the teacher were instructed in various techniques and worked closely together in exchanging academic and social progress reports on a daily basis. Posttreatment assessment showed that the children's behavior improved both in the classroom and at home. This improvement equaled that of comparison children receiving medication and to the test children's own previous on-medication behavior. Behavior therapy was the more effective treatment in a highly structured environment. For a commentary on this study refer to Item No. 220.

1085 ————. "Behavior therapy and withdrawal of stimulant medication with hyperactive children." In: Behavior therapy with hyperactive and learning disabled children. Edited by Benjamin B. Lahey. New York, New York: Oxford University Press, 1979. 229-36. (21 References).
Reprints an article from Pediatrics 61(2): 211-17, February, 1978. (Item No. 1084).

1086 Orton, D. "Behavioural treatment of hyperactivity in a mentally handicapped child." Nurs Times 75(18): 758-60, May 3, 1979. (0 References).
Presents a case study of an eight-year-old boy who was admitted to a behavior modification unit at a hospital in Leicester. The boy's behavioral treatment is related in detail.

1087 Parry, Penny A. "The effect of reward on the performance of hyperactive children." For a summary see: Diss Abstr Int 34B(12, pt. 1): 6220, June, 1974. (0 References).

1088 Parry, Penny, and Douglas, Virginia I. "The effect of reward on the performance of hyperactive children." Paper presented at the Canadian Psychological Association Conference, Vancouver, 1974.

1089 Pelham, William E. "Behavioral treatment of hyperkinesis." Am J Dis Child 130(5): 565, May, 1976. (10 References).
Letter to editor.

1090 Pratt, Sandra J., and Fischer, Joel. "Behavior modification: changing hyperactive behavior in a children's group." Perspect Psychiatr Care 13(1): 37-42, January-March, 1975. (9 References).
Describes an operant reinforcement approach used to reduce the hyperactive behavior of one child. The subject, a nine-year-old boy, was unable to participate in group activities or to form satisfactory relationships with his peers. The program was used by a psychiatric nurse in an activity group of a child psychiatric unit. General principles of behavior modification were applied. The technique is viewed as an effective tool for psychiatric nurses to use when working with emotionally disturbed children.

1091 Principles and techniques of intervention with hyperactive children. Edited by Marvin J. Fine. Springfield, Illinois: Thomas, 1977. 314p. (Bibliography).
This book presents seven chapters which offer an overview of existing concepts and procedures with hyperactive children, including the application of transactional analysis and behavior modification techniques. Eleven professionals representing the fields of special education, psychology, child development, and medicine examine the hyperactive child in terms of educational, behavioral, and medical management.

Contents: Hyperactivity: Where Are We? (Fine - Item No. 34); Medical Management of the Hyperactive Child (Mira and Reece - Item No. 1523); A Behavioral Approach to the Management of Hyperactive Behavior (Rieth - Item No. 1094); Educational Management of Hyperactive Children (Dyck - Item No. 1160); Transactional Analysis and the Management of Hyperactivity (Wolf - Item No. 1108); Reflection-Impulsivity and Information-Processing from Three to Nine Years of Age (Wright and Vlietstra - Item No. 1697); The Measurement of Hyperactivity: Trends and Issues (Salkind and Poggio - Item No. 2013); The Hyperactive Child: Resources (Simpson - Item No. 11).

1092 Prinz, R. J., and Loney, J. "Modifying student behavior: what works and with whom?" Paper presented at the Annual Meeting of the American Psychological Association, 1974.

1093 Prout, H. Thompson. "Behavioral intervention with hyperactive children: a review." J Learn Disabil 10(3): 141-46, March, 1977. (39 References).
Reviews behavioral (nonmedical) approaches for the management and treatment of the hyperactive child. A variety of approaches is discussed, including both those interventions which have and have not been systematically evaluated. Suggested interventions include psychotherapy, operant procedures, self-regulation, and biofeedback. A critique of the current state of research in this area is offered with suggestions for future investigations.

1094 Rieth, Herbert J. "A behavioral approach to the management of hyperactive behavior." In: Principles and techniques of intervention with hyperactive children. Edited by Marvin J. Fine. Springfield, Illinois: Thomas, 1977. 77-114. (37 References).
Reviews and illustrates general and specific applications of behavioral modification with hyperactive children. The behavioral approach to the management of hyperactivity is based upon the assumption that, regardless of their etiology, hyperactive behaviors can be controlled by the application of general principles of learning theory; it entails the observation and measurement of these behaviors and the implementation of treatment. Emphasis is placed on reinforcement of appropriate behaviors. Nine case studies in the appendix illustrate the application of reinforcement, extinction, punishment, and antecedent events to modify hyperactive behaviors.

1095 Ross, Alan O. Psychological disorders of children: a behavioral approach to theory, research, and therapy. New York, New York: McGraw-Hill, 1974. 360p. (Bibliography). (McGraw-Hill Series in Psychology).
This book is a behaviorally oriented presentation of psychological disorders of children and their treatment through behavior therapy. The four main parts are: (1) principles of psychological disorders; (2) deficient behavior; (3) excess behavior; and (4) treatment of psychological disorders. Hyperactivity is briefly discussed in Chapter 5, "Learning Difficulties," and again in Chapter 14, "Treatment Approaches." A lengthy bibliography and an index complete the book, which is primarily directed toward those with some prior knowledge in the field.

1096 Schofield, Leon J., Jr.; Hedlund, Carol; Worland, Julien. "Operant approaches to group therapy and effects on sociometric status." Psychol Rep 35(1, pt. 1): 83-90, August, 1974. (42 References).
Four hyperactive, unsocialized boys were subjects for group therapy procedures. The boys, all living in a residential treatment center, showed increased attention to task and interacted more frequently with each other as a result of behavior modification techniques. However, the sociometric status of the subjects in their living groups showed no change. The difficulties in changing sociometric status are discussed, as is the value of a nonpublic school setting for the testing of operant techniques.

1097 Simmons, James Q., III. "Behavioral management of the hyperactive child." In: Cantwell, Dennis P., ed. The hyperactive child: diagnosis, management, current research. New York, New York:

Spectrum Publications, distributed by John Wiley and Sons, 1975. 129-43. (21 References). (Series on Child Behavior and Development, Volume I).

Advocates the use of several behavioral strategies to modify the behavior of hyperactive children. Five steps, representative of the behavioral approach to management, are outlined. Three case studies demonstrate the application of the behavioral principles.

1098 Spiegel, Elliot D. "The effects of self-observation on the social behavior of hyperactive children." For a summary see: Diss Abstr Int 38A(10): 6061, April, 1978. (0 References).

1099 Stoudenmire, John, and Salter, Leo. "Conditioning prosocial behaviors in a mentally retarded child without using instructions." J Behav Ther Exp Psychiatry 6(1): 39-42, April, 1975. (3 References).

Uses an operant conditioning procedure to increase prosocial behavior in a mentally retarded child. A three-and-one-half-year-old girl, referred to a psychology clinic because of life-endangering hyperactivity, served as the subject. Physical rewards, in the form of M&M candies, were used as reinforcers during the experimental sessions. No verbal instructions were given to the girl regarding expected behavior or possible rewards for such behavior. The instructionless conditioning program increased attention and decreased hyperactivity, thus indicating that it could be useful in training children who are unable to absorb oral instructions.

1100 Thomas, Diane S. "The effects of punishment on the activity level of hyperactive children." For a summary see: Diss Abstr Int 37B(5): 2531-32, November, 1976. (0 References).

1101 Varni, James W.; Boyd, Elizabeth F.; Cataldo, Michael F. "Self-monitoring, external reinforcement, and time-out procedures in the control of high rate tic behaviors in a hyperactive child." J Behav Ther Exp Psychiatry 9(4): 353-58, December, 1978. (14 References).

Studies the effect of self-monitoring, external reinforcement, and time-out on controlling a hyperactive child's multiple tic behaviors. A combination of a reversal design and a multiple-baseline design across settings and tic behaviors was employed. Tics, facial and otherwise, decreased in both home and clinic settings. A thirty-two-week follow-up showed maintenance of the treatment effects.

1102 Waldman, Lawrence S. "Effect of incentive on the cognitive and motor performance of hyperactive and normal boys." For a summary see: Diss Abstr Int 38B(5): 2389, November, 1977. (0 References).

1103 Weithorn, Corinne J., and Kagen, Edward. "Training first graders of high-activity level to improve performance through verbal self-direction." J Learn Disabil 12(2): 82-88, February, 1979. (16 References).

Uses a behavioral technique to improve performance of a group of elementary schoolchildren. Twenty-three impulsive, high-active first graders were trained to verbally mediate responses on a multiple choice task. On a standardized multiple choice test of perceptual matching ability, the children showed a significant pretest to posttest gain in comparison with an untrained control group of impulsive, high-active children and with both trained and untrained control groups of nonimpulsive, low-active children. Findings have implications for the validity of certain types of assessment materials for impulsive children and for the potential of verbal mediational training as a remedial technique.

1104 West, Mina G., and Axelrod, Saul. "A 3-D program for learning disabled children." Acad Ther 10(3): 309-19, Spring, 1975. (4 References).

Reviews numerous behavior modification techniques previously used to reduce disruptive behavior in problem students. Unfortunately, these techniques concentrated on narrow aspects of the total picture and were not concerned with the full spectrum of skills that lead to scholastic competence. The present study offers a three-phase plan designed to reduce hyperactive behavior, increase attending behavior, and aid academic achievement by combining behavior modification techniques and developmental principles. Seventy-seven learning-disabled children participated in the study. Details of each phase are given.

1105 Whitman, Thomas L.; Caponigri, Vicki; Mercurio, Joseph. "Reducing hyperactive behavior in a severely retarded child." In: Managing the severely retarded: a sampler. Edited by David Gibson and Roy I. Brown. Springfield, Illinois: Thomas, 1976. 210-16. (7 References).

Documents a study undertaken to determine whether the hyperactive behavior of a six-year-old SMR girl could be reduced through reinforcement of a more adaptive incompatible response. The girl's behavior disrupted all activities both at school and at home. A twenty-day training program was conducted which consisted of administering reinforcement for responses that led to the girl's seating herself. These responses, in turn, were incompatible with her hyperactive behavior. The average number of sitting commands given daily to the girl by the teacher during the pretreatment period was 17.8, in comparison with 2.8 for the posttreatment period. The response latencies were shortened as well. The results strongly suggest that hyperactivity can be reduced through appropriate reinforcement procedures.

1106 Willis, Thomas J., and Lovaas, Ivar. "A behavioral approach to treating hyperactive children: the parent's role." In: Learning disabilities and related disorders: facts and current issues. Edited by J. Gordon Millichap. Chicago, Illinois: Year Book Medical Publishers, 1977. 119-40. (67 References).

Advocates the use of a behavior therapy strategy to modify the maladaptive behavior of hyperactive children. A model parent training program, using an eight-year-old boy, outlines steps in teaching the mother ways of managing undesirable behaviors.

1107 Wolf, Clifton W. "Transactional analysis and the hyperactive child." Paper presented at the Annual Meeting of the American Psychological Association, New Orleans, August, 1974.

1108 ———. "Transactional analysis and the management of hyperactivity." In: Principles and techniques of intervention with hyperactive children. Edited by Marvin J. Fine. Springfield, Illinois: Thomas, 1977. 160-95. (20 References).

Presents basic transactional analysis (TA) theory and methods and illustrates the applications to both understanding the hyperactive child and to helping the child manage his own behavior. TA offers a treatment frame of reference which is consistent with other established forms of treatment and which can be used adjunctively with them. Examples are given of the use of TA in the classroom. One drawback to the use of TA with hyperactive children is the lack of controlled research studies reported in the literature.

1109 Wolraich, Mark L. "Behavior modification therapy in hyperactive children: research and clinical implications." Clin Pediatr 18(9): 563-70, September, 1979. (23 References).
Reviews one hundred and fifty-seven studies employing behavior modification in the management of hyperactive and disruptive children. The studies are analyzed against standards of scientific validity. The review finds: (1) behavior modification was effective in alleviating problem behaviors; (2) token programs were the most commonly used; (3) both positive reinforcement and punishment were effective; positive reinforcement, however, had the advantage of improving self-esteem; (4) behavioral problems occurring in the home most likely require a home-based program; (5) behavior modification and stimulant medication can be used simultaneously, often with additive effects; and (6) long-term benefits beyond one year have not been assessed.

1110 Workman, Edward A., and Dickinson, Donald J. "The use of covert positive reinforcement in the treatment of a hyperactive child: an empirical case study." J Sch Psychol 17(1): 67-73, Spring, 1979. (13 References).
Evaluates the effects of covert positive reinforcement (CPR) on the behavior of one student. A nine-year-old hyperactive boy served as the subject. CPR was conducted for six sessions over a three-week period to reduce out-of-seat behavior, excessive noisemaking, and rocking-in-chair behavior. There was an immediate improvement in three target behaviors following CPR implementation by the school psychologist. Potential applications of the method are discussed.

1111 Worland, Julien. "Effects of positive and negative feedback on behavior control in hyperactive and normal boys." J Abnorm Child Psychol 4(4): 315-26, 1976. (28 References).
Studies the hypothesis that hyperactive boys have relatively less response to negative feedback than to positive feedback. Sixteen hyperactive boys and sixteen controls were used as subjects and were compared on two tasks using different feedback conditions. The subjects were compared in amount of time on-task and on amount of work correctly completed. Results show that the control group responded equally to positive, negative, or no feedback. Hyperactives responded to negative feedback by better on-task performance, but negative feedback significantly decreased the accuracy of the work.

1112 ————. "Effects of reward and punishment on behavior control in hyperactive and normal boys." For a summary see: Diss Abstr Int 34B(12, pt. 1): 6227-28, June, 1974. (0 References).

1113 Yamaguchi, Kaoru. "Application of operant principles to the hyperactive behavior of a retarded girl." In: New developments in behavioral research: theory, method, and application. Edited by Barbara C. Etzel, Judith M. LeBlanc, and Donald M. Baer. Hillsdale, New Jersey: Lawrence Erlbaum, 1977. 389-402. (5 References).
Details the use of operant conditioning techniques to modify the hyperactive, distractible, and impulsive behavior of a mentally retarded four-year-old girl. In several experiments the girl was required to finish

a pegboard task in order to receive a reinforcer. It was necessary for her to carry out a given task as fast as possible, concentrating only on the task. At follow-up, the girl's concentration had substantially increased since baseline. She was subsequently placed in a regular class in elementary school.

2. BIOFEEDBACK

1114 Anchor, Kenneth, and Johnson, Lynda G. "The efficacy of EMG biofeedback in the treatment of hyperactivity." Behav Eng 4(2): 39-43, 1977. (24 References).
Reviews previous clinical and empirical literature describing the use of biofeedback instrumentation to treat hyperactive children. Pros and cons of drug therapies as well as EMG biofeedback intervention are considered. The authors conclude that: (1) EMG biofeedback strategies appear to present fewer risks than drugs; (2) EMG is a useful adjunct to drug therapy or a useful method by itself; and (3) EMG training is reported to increase self-confidence and self-concept while improving self-control.

1115 Anderson, Joy A. "Electromyographic feedback as a method of reducing hyperkinesis in children." For a summary see: Diss Abstr Int 36B(11): 5753, May, 1976. (0 References).

1116 Baldwin, Barbara G.; Benjamins, John K.; Meyers, Rose M.; et al. "EMG biofeedback with hyperactive children: a time series analysis." In: Proceedings of the Biofeedback Society of America, Ninth Annual Meeting, March 3-7, 1978, Albuquerque, New Mexico. Denver, Colorado: Biofeedback Society of American, 1978. 184-88. (8 References).
Evaluates the effectiveness of EMG biofeedback on hyperactive children using direct behavioral observations of hyperactivity and relaxation. Four boys (ages eight to twelve years), with the primary diagnosis of hyperactivity, served as subjects. The boys were evaluated at baseline and again after receiving frontalis EMG biofeedback for relaxation. Behavior observations revealed that EMG biofeedback is not an effective treatment procedure for hyperactivity.

1117 Braud, Lendell W. "The effects of EMG biofeedback and progressive relaxation upon hyperactivity and its behavioral concomitants." For a summary see: Diss Abstr Int 36B(1): 433, July, 1975. (0 References).

1118 ———. "The effects of EMG biofeedback and progressive relaxation upon hyperactivity and its behavioral concomitants." Paper presented at the Meeting of the Biofeedback Research Society, Colorado Springs, Colorado, 1975.

1119 ———. "The effects of EMG biofeedback and progressive relaxation upon hyperactivity and its behavioral concomitants." Bio-Feedback Systems, Inc., 1977.

1120 ———. "The effects of frontal EMG biofeedback and progressive relaxation upon hyperactivity and its behavioral concomitants." Biofeedback Self Regul 3(1): 69-89, March, 1978. (41 References).
Investigates whether hyperactive children possess higher muscular tension levels than normal children and if biofeedback and progressive relaxation therapy can reduce this muscular tension. Thirty children (fifteen hyperactive and fifteen controls) were compared on muscular tension levels.

The children were divided into groups and treated with biofeedback or relaxation therapy. Results show that both electromyographic biofeedback and progressive relaxation exercises were successful in reducing muscular tension, hyperactivity, and related symptoms. No differences were seen in the EMG improvement of drug and nondrug hyperactive children, since both groups made progress. A discussion of self-control techniques is included. The literature in the area is reviewed.

1121 Braud, Lendell W.; Lupin, Mimi N.; Braud, William G. "The use of electromyographic biofeedback in the control of hyperactivity." J Learn Disabil 8(7): 420-25, August-September, 1975. (11 References).

Reports on an experiment which used electromyographic biofeedback to reduce muscular activity and tension in a six-and-one-half-year-old boy with hyperkinesis. The experiment, which took place in eleven sessions, involved having the child turn off a tone which signaled the presence of muscular tension. Muscular activity and tension decreased at the time, was transferred to home and school, and remained stable at a seven-month follow-up. The beneficial effect of biofeedback on various test scores is discussed.

1122 ————. "The use of EMG (electromyographic) biofeedback in the control of hyperactivity." Paper presented at the 11th Annual International Convention for Learning Disabilities, Houston, Texas, February, 1974.

1123 Bryant, D. M., and Hunter, S. H. "Is biofeedback training really beneficial for attention-problem children?" Paper presented at the Meeting of the Association for the Advancement of Behavior Therapy, Atlanta, Georgia, December, 1977.

1124 Conners, C. Keith. "Application of biofeedback to treatment of children." J Am Acad Child Psychiatry 18(1): 143-53, Winter, 1979. (59 References).

Self-control over brain rhythms such as the sensorimotor rhythm and use of EEG feedback for altering hemispheric-specific activity are potentially applicable techniques for hyperactive, epileptic, and LD children. Other somatic control systems such as temperature regulation and electromyographic response have shown promise for regulation of stress responses, anxiety, and specific symptoms related to disturbances of autonomic or skeletal muscle systems in adults. It is proposed that in addition to their specific training effects, such methods may have potent side effects by altering the child's internal locus of control, thus affecting adjustment in a wide variety of stressful situations and correcting faulty learning histories.

1125 Dobbins, Ken M. "The effects of forehead EMG biofeedback training on the EEG and behavior of hyperactive children." For a summary see: Diss Abstr Int 40B(3): 1397-98, September, 1979. (0 References).

1126 Flemings, Danny G. "A study of electromyographic biofeedback as a method to teach hyperactive children how to relax within a public school setting." For a summary see: Diss Abstr Int 39A(11): 6693, May, 1979. (0 References).

1127 Gargiulo, Richard M., and Kuna, Daniel J. "Arousal level and hyperkinesis: implications for biofeedback." J Learn Disabil 12(3): 137-38, March, 1979. (17 References).
Letter to editor.

1128 Haight, Maryellen J., et al. "The response of hyperkinesis to EMG biofeedback." Paper presented at the 7th Annual Meeting of the Biofeedback Research Society, Colorado Springs, Colorado, March, 1976. 33p. (ED 125 169).
This study attempted to determine if electromyography (EMG) biofeedback training would reduce muscle tension and hyperactivity in eight hyperactive boys.

1129 Hampstead, William J. "The effects of EMG-assisted relaxation training with hyperkinetic children: a behavioral alternative." Biofeedback Self Regul 4(2): 113-25, June, 1979. (9 References).
Evaluates the effect of EMG-assisted relaxation training on the acquisition of self-regulatory skills to decrease hyperactive behavior. Six hyperactive children (ages six to nine years) participated in either of two experiments. The use of EMG-assisted relaxation training significantly reduced hyperactivity both during testing and at follow-up.

1130 ———. "The effects of EMG-assisted relaxation training with hyperkinetic children: an alternative to medication." For a summary see: Diss Abstr Int 38B(10): 5017, April, 1978. (0 References).

1131 Jeffrey, Timothy B. "The effects of operant conditioning and electromyographic biofeedback on the relaxed behavior of hyperkinetic children." For a summary see: Diss Abstr Int 37B(5): 2510, November, 1976. (0 References).

1132 ———. "The effects of operant conditioning and electromyographic biofeedback on the relaxed behavior of hyperkinetic children." In: Proceedings of the Biofeedback Society of America, Ninth Annual Meeting, March 3-7, 1978, Albuquerque, New Mexico. Denver, Colorado: Biofeedback Society of America, 1978. 192-94. (0 References).
Investigates the effects of operant conditioning and electromyographic biofeedback on the behavior of hyperactive children and examines the ability of hyperactive children to relax and remain relaxed. Twenty-seven hyperactive children (ages six to eleven years) participated in the study and received EMG biofeedback and a contingent reinforcement training program to reinforce the children for relaxed behavior. Results suggest that muscle tension can be reduced with biofeedback-induced relaxation training.

1133 Johnson, Basil M. "The use of electromyography and relaxation in the reduction of tension in families with identified hyperactive children: three case studies." For a summary see: Diss Abstr Int 39B(11): 5560, May, 1979. (0 References).

1134 Johnson, Wiley B. "An experimental study of the effect of electromyography (EMG) biofeedback on hyperactivity in children." For a summary see: Diss Abstr Int 37B(9): 4650-51, March, 1977. (0 References).

1135 Lubar, Joel F., and Shouse, Margaret N. "EEG and behavioral changes in a hyperkinetic child concurrent with training of the sensorimotor rhythm (SMR): a preliminary report." Biofeedback Self Regul 1(3): 293-306, September, 1976. (16 References).
Explores the potential application of sensorimotor rhythm (SMR) training to hyperkinesis in the absence of a seizure history. The data represent a progress report following several months of EEG biofeedback training with an eleven-year-old hyperactive boy. Changes in motor inhibition are indexed by muscular tension in the laboratory and by behavioral observations in the classroom. Results, given in detail, suggest the usefulness of SMR biofeedback training after medication has been withdrawn. This study represents a first attempt to explore the applicability of the technique to the problem of hyperkinesis independent of the epilepsy issue. A replication study is in progress.

1136 ————. "Use of biofeedback in the treatment of hyperactivity." In: Behavior therapy with hyperactive and learning disabled children. Edited by Benjamin B. Lahey. New York, New York: Oxford University Press, 1979. 161-78. (71 References).
Reprints an edited version of a chapter (by the same authors) that appears in Advances in Clinical Child Psychology. (Item No. 1137).

1137 ————. "Use of biofeedback in the treatment of seizure disorders and hyperactivity." In: Advances in clinical child psychology. Volume 1. Edited by Benjamin B. Lahey and Alan E. Kazdin. New York, New York: Plenum, 1977. 203-65. (85 References).
Defines biofeedback, gives a brief historical overview, and outlines areas of biofeedback application. The remainder of the chapter is devoted to the use of biofeedback methods in two areas: the control of epileptic seizures and the management of the hyperkinetic syndrome. Although studies are cited which show promising effects of sensorimotor rhythm (SMR), it is concluded that more research involving a larger population is needed for an adequate evaluation of the method.

1138 Martin, Larry L., and Hershey, Myrless. "An exploratory investigation of the effect of a biofeedback technique with hyperactive learning disabled children." Paper presented at the 54th Annual International Convention, the Council for Exceptional Children, Chicago, Illinois, April 4-9, 1976. 8p. (ED 126 640).
Studies the effects of biofeedback in reducing hyperactive behavior in five hyperactive and four nonhyperactive children. Success was reported following the eight-week test period.

1139 Moore, Craig L. "Behavior modification and electromyographic biofeedback as alternatives to drugs for the treatment of hyperkinesis in children." For a summary see: Diss Abstr Int 38B(6): 2872, December, 1977. (0 References).

1140 Moreland, Kevin L. "Stimulus control of hyperactivity." Percept Mot Skills 45(3, pt. 1): 916, December, 1977. (1 Reference).
Cites the use of a biofeedback procedure to control the hyperactive behavior of a four-year-old boy. Special equipment was employed to interrupt transmission from a videotape recorder to a videotape monitor, blanking out cartoons when the boy's behavior became too active. The boy received feedback via a meter on the back of a control box. Treatment took place once a week for eight weeks, after baseline had been established. The experiment suggests that hyperactive behavior can be significantly reduced by using this procedure.

1141 Patmon, Rozen, and Murphy, Philip J. "Differential treatment efficacy of EEG and EMG feedback for hyperactive adolescents." In: Proceedings of the Biofeedback Society of America, Ninth Annual Meeting, March 3-7, 1978, Albuquerque, New Mexico. Denver, Colorado: Biofeedback Society of America, 1978. 197-99. (0 References).
Compares the effects of three forms of EEG or EMG feedback with a no-training control on a comprehensive profile of physiological, cognitive, and behavior changes. Twenty-eight adolescents (twenty-three boys and five girls) were given a series of pretests and assigned to a treatment group. Outcomes of the various methods are given in detail.

1142 Shouse, Margaret N. "The role of CNS arousal levels in the management of hyperkinesis: management and EMG biofeedback training. For a summary see: Diss Abstr Int 37B(8): 4206-7, February, 1977. (0 References).

1143 "Turning off hyperactivity." Hum Behav 5(2): 22, February, 1976. (0 References).
Briefly reports on a pilot experiment by Lendell Braud, Mimi Lupin, and William Braud (Item No. 1121) which tested the effects of biofeedback on a six-year-old boy. The child was hooked to an electromyograph that monitored muscle tension and triggered a tone. The number of "tension seconds" was reduced by the fifth session and at follow-up seven months later. The advantages of behavior modification over drugs are outlined.

1144 Whitmer, Peter O. "EMG biofeedback manipulation of arousal as a test of the overarousal and underarousal theories of childhood hyperactivity." For a summary see: Diss Abstr Int 38B(7): 3423, January, 1978. (0 References).

3. CLASSROOM SETTING

1145 Anderson, Robert P., et al. "Modifying hyperkinetic behavior in the classroom." Paper presented at the Annual Meeting of the Southwestern Psychological Association, Albuquerque, New Mexico, April 29-May 1, 1976. 10p. (ED 141 725).
Documents an attempt to modify the attending on-task behavior of a group of hyperkinetic children in a naturalistic school setting.

1146 Ayllon, Teodoro; Layman, Dale; Kandel, Henry J. "A behavioral-educational alternative to drug control of hyperactive children." J Appl Behav Anal 8(2): 137-46, Summer, 1975. (27 References).
Reports on a token reinforcement procedure to control hyperactive behavior without inhibiting academic performance. Three learning-disabled children (ages eight to ten years) served as subjects. Using a time-sample observational method, hyperactive behavior was recorded during math and reading classes. Observations of hyperactive behavior and measures of academic performance were recorded for children with and without medication and before and after introduction of the reinforcement procedure. Data interpretation shows: (1) discontinuation of medication resulted in gross increase in hyperactivity from 20 percent to 80 percent; and (2) introduction of management techniques helped unmedicated children to perform, academically and behaviorally, at a level comparable to their performance when on drugs. Behavioral management techniques are suggested as a feasible alternative to medication for controlling hyperactive behavior.

1147 ————. "A behavioral-educational alternative to drug control of hyperactive children." In: Annual review of behavior therapy theory and practice, 1976. Edited by Cyril M. Franks and G. Terence Wilson. New York, New York: Brunner/Mazel, 1976. 459-74. (27 References).
Reprints an article from the Journal of Applied Behavior Analysis 8(2): 137-46, Summer, 1974. (Item No. 1146).

1148 ————. "A behavioral-educational alternative to drug control of hyperactive children." In: Child development: contemporary perspectives. Edited by Stewart Cohen and Thomas J. Comiskey. Itasca, Illinois: Peacock Publishers, 1977. 337-47. (27 References). (ED 139 539).
Reprints an article from the Journal of Applied Behavior Analysis 8(2): 137-46, Summer, 1975. (Item No. 1146).

1149 ————. "A behavioral-educational alternative to drug control of hyperactive children." In: Behavior therapy with hyperactive and learning disabled children. Edited by Benjamin B. Lahey. New York: Oxford University Press, 1979. 213-20. (27 References).
Reprints an article from the Journal of Applied Behavior Analysis 8(2): 137-46, Summer, 1975. (Item No. 1146).

1150 Ayllon, Teodoro, and Rainwater, Nancy. "Behavioral alternatives to the drug control of hyperactive children in the classroom." Sch Psychol Dig 5(4): 33-39, Fall, 1976. (11 References).
Cites previous studies which used behavior modification to increase academic performance and decrease hyperactive behavior. Behavioral approaches which are effective in dealing with hyperactivity are described: the application of structure and the reinforcement of correct performance. These are viewed as viable alternatives to drug therapy. The article is directed toward the classroom teacher.

1151 Ayllon, Teodoro, and Rosenbaum, Michael S. "The behavioral treatment of disruption and hyperactivity in school settings." In: Advances in clinical child psychology. Volume 1. Edited by Benjamin B. Lahey and Alan E. Kazdin. New York, New York: Plenum, 1977. 83-118. (61 References).
Reviews behavioral procedures currently employed to reduce the disruptive and hyperactive behavior of children in the classroom setting. The techniques focus on pinpointing and manipulating the consequences that follow classroom misbehavior. Topics covered include: (1) the role of teachers in controlling misbehavior; (2) the role of peers in controlling misbehavior; (3) the role of a token system in controlling misbehavior; (4) additional procedures: feedback, reinforcement schedule, free time as a reinforcer, self-regulation, time-out and home-based reinforcement instructions, modeling, and time limits; and (5) strengthening academic performance in normal and hyperactive children. It is concluded that the indirect approach, which focuses on academic performance by manipulating its antecedent and consequent stimuli, can reduce undesirable behavior. Structure, instructions and modeling, and reinforcement of academic performance are vital components in controlling disruptive behavior while improving academic performance.

1152 Bornstein, Philip; Hamilton, Scott B.; Quevillon, Randal P. "Behavior modification by long distance: demonstration of functional control over disruptive behavior in a rural classroom setting." Res Relat Child 39: 99, March, 1977-August, 1977. (0 References).

Abstracts a report of research in progress or recently completed research. Data are provided on: name of investigator(s), purpose of the study, number and kind of subjects used, methodology, principal findings, duration of research, cooperating group(s), and availability of publication(s). Research Relating to Children is compiled by the ERIC Clearinghouse on Early Childhood Education.

1153 Bornstein, Philip H., and Quevillon, Randal P. "The effects of a self-instructional package on overactive preschool boys." J Appl Behav Anal 9(2): 179-88, Summer, 1976. (46 References).
Reports on the application of a behavior modification technique to reduce the hyperactive behavior of a group of preschool children. Three overactive boys (age four) enrolled in Head Start were given a self-instructional program. The boys' progress at on-task behavior was eventually transferred from experimental tasks to the classroom. Treatment gains were maintained 22.5 weeks after baseline. A related study was completed by Friedling and O'Leary (Item No. 1164).

1154 ————. "The effects of a self-instructional package on overactive preschool boys." In: Behavior therapy with hyperactive and learning disabled children. Edited by Benjamin B. Lahey. New York, New York: Oxford University Press, 1979. 152-60. (46 References).
Reprints an article from the Journal of Applied Behavior Analysis 9(2): 179-88, Summer, 1976. (Item No. 1153).

1155 Bugental, Daphne B.; Collins, Susan; Collins, Leo; et al. "Attributional and behavioral changes following two behavior management interventions with hyperactive boys: a follow-up study." Child Dev 49(1): 247-50, March, 1978. (4 References).
Attempts to determine the extent to which two interventions carried out with hyperactive boys led to long-term changes in: (1) the child's perceptions of self-control; (2) behavioral indications of self-control; and (3) teacher perceptions of reduced hyperactivity. Follow-up measures were obtained on twenty of an initial sample of thirty-two boys. The six-month follow-up study showed different patterns of improvement on two types of manipulations: self-control and contingent social reinforcement. Each manipulation produced improvements in different areas of behavior, but both interventions produced stable changes in terms of decreased impulsivity.

1156 Bugental, Daphne B.; Whalen, Carol K.; Henker, Barbara. "Causal attributions of hyperactive children and motivational assumptions of two behavior-change approaches: evidence for an interactionist position." Child Dev 48(3): 874-84, September, 1977. (51 References).
Details a study designed to predict the extent to which children's causal-attribution systems would act as mediators of the differential effectiveness of two intervention programs. Thirty-six hyperactive boys (ages seven to twelve years) were tutored individually for two months in a classroom setting; half were instructed in self-controlling speech; the others were given contingent social reinforcement. Within each group, half the boys received Ritalin and half did not. Two measures were used to obtain the boys' perceptions of their reasons for their own academic success or failure. Significant interactions were found between interventions and child attributions and medication status.

1157 Cowin, Pauline. "Teaching the times tables to a hyperactive boy." Acad Ther 13(5): 569-77, May, 1978. (0 References).
Describes a highly structured teaching method used with an able, but hyperactive boy currently on Ritalin. Because of his difficulty with basic multiplication facts, he was assigned to a special tutor. Money (a bowl of nickels) and circles were used to help the boy come up with the correct arithmetic statement. A favorable response to the treatment is reported.

1158 Culbertson, Frances M. "An effective, low-cost approach to the treatment of disruptive school children." Psychol Sch 11(2): 183-87, April, 1974. (7 References).
Six highly disruptive kindergarten children were used to test the effectiveness of two methods of treatment on their disturbing behavior. A behavior modification model, first used alone, was later combined with a program of therapy that stressed the psychodynamic-relationship goals for treatment. Teacher reports show that the school behavior of all six children improved dramatically by the sixth week under the integrated approach, and, at the end of the two years, the children continued to show appropriate school and social behaviors. The children's rapport with the therapist is noted as a desirable corollary of the program.

1159 Davis, Jean E. Coping with disruptive behavior. 34p. 1974. (ED 096 256).
Suggests five methods for handling disruptive behavior in the classroom. A 104-item bibliography accompanies the booklet.

1160 Dyck, Norma J. "Educational management of hyperactive children." In: Principles and techniques of intervention with hyperactive children. Edited by Marvin J. Fine. Springfield, Illinois: Thomas, 1977. 115-59. (62 References).
Focuses on the educational management of a child when hyperactivity, distractibility, inattentiveness, or impulsivity appear to interfere with learning. Discussed first are several special class models (Strauss-Lehtinen-Cruickshank and Hewett) and their influence on the educational management of hyperactive children in the United States. The rest of the chapter is devoted to a discussion of the use of structure which is divided into five subgroups: structured environment, structured time, structured physical activity, structured rewards, and structured tasks. It is stressed that no single educational program or strategy is suitable for all hyperactive children. Rather, the educational management of each child must be determined by his or her strengths and weaknesses and social, emotional, physical, and cognitive needs.

1161 Edelson, Richard I., and Sprague, Robert L. "Conditioning of activity level in a classroom with institutionalized retarded boys." Am J Ment Defic 78(4): 384-88, January, 1974. (12 References).
Evaluates a method of controlling the attention and activity level of sixteen highly active, educable mentally retarded, institutionalized boys (mean age 12.7 years). The boys were brought into a classroom four at a time and shown filmstrips on which they were later tested. Stabilimetric cushions and behavioral relay equipment automatically counted and reinforced seat movement. There were five experimental periods comprising three baseline and two sequences of reinforcement contingency: first reinforcement for decreasing and then increasing movement, followed by order. The reinforcement contingencies significantly altered the boys' activity. The study indicates the possibility of mechanizing some behavior modification procedures.

1162 Fairchild, Thomas N., ed. Managing the hyperactive child in the classroom. Austin, Texas: Learning Concepts, 1977. 116p. (Mainstreaming Series).
Presents practical suggestions, in cartoon form, for managing the hyperactive child in the classroom. Part I focuses on four common characteristics of the syndrome: overactivity, distractibility, impulsivity, and excitability. Part II covers various theories of etiologies. The final section offers suggestions to the classroom teacher for managing the hyperactive behavior of their students. This is one of a series of eleven paperback books published in the Mainstreaming Series which provides a general overview on a number of current topics.

1163 Flynn, Nona M. "The effect of positive teacher reinforcement and classroom social structure on class behavior of boys diagnosed as hyperactive before and during medication." For a summary see: Diss Abstr Int 37A(4): 2109, October, 1976. (0 References).

1164 Friedling, Carol, and O'Leary, Susan G. "Effects of self-instructional training on second- and third-grade hyperactive children: a failure to replicate." J Appl Behav Anal 12(2): 211-19, Summer, 1979. (22 References).
Attempts to replicate a previous work by Bornstein and Quevillon (Item No. 1153). The present study uses a slightly older group of children (ages seven to eight years) to examine the effects of self-instructional training on on-task behavior. Eight hyperactive children were assessed according to on-task behavior in the classroom and performance measures in reading and arithmetic. The results of the earlier study were not replicated, although the subsequent introduction of a token program significantly increased on-task behavior.

1165 Goetze, Herbert, and Heinz, Neukater. "A structured, student-centered approach for teaching hyperactive, emotionally disturbed children." Paper presented at the 1st World Congress on Future Special Education, Stirling, Scotland, June 25-July 1, 1978. 10p. (ED 157 366).
Uses a self-control contingency management approach for teaching hyperactive, emotionally disturbed children. The basic plan involves a contingency between instructional activities and play time.

1166 Goodman, Gay, and Hammond, Brad. "Seat belts control hyperactivity." Acad Ther 11(1): 51-52, Fall, 1975. (0 References).
Because hyperactive children exhibit short attention span, distractibility, and impulsivity, they are often unable to remain seated in the classroom to complete school assignments. By means of "seat belts"--a long piece of string attached to the vertical rungs on the backs of the desk chairs and tied loosely around a child in front--constant oral reminders were reduced in a nonpunitive fashion. The "seat belts" served as a reminder to the child and were found to control extraneous movement and classroom disruptiveness. Subsequently, actual automobile seat belts were affixed to the chairs, allowing the child to fasten and unfasten his own belt. The belts were viewed as a piece of helpful classroom equipment rather than as a form of punishment.

1167 Hallahan, Daniel P., and Kauffman, James M. "Research on the education of distractible and hyperactive children." In: Cruickshank, William M., and Hallahan, Daniel P., eds. Perceptual and learning disabilities in children: Volume II. Research and theory.

Syracuse, New York: Syracuse University Press, 1975. 221-56. (148 References).
Reviews basic research pertinent to the problem and considers the effect of manipulation of environmental surroundings and teaching materials. The crucial role of behavior modification techniques as they relate to the treatment of attention deficits and motor skills is discussed, as well as the use of reward and punishment. Numerous suggestions using behavior modification are given which the teacher can employ to decrease hyperactive behavior in the classroom.

1168 Klosterman, Dale, and Frankel, Judith. "Tutoring effectively." Acad Ther 11(1): 107-10, Fall, 1975. (2 References).
Reports on the use of self-instructional techniques for hyperkinetic or learning-disabled children. Self-instructional techniques employ modeling to teach a child initially how to learn and how to control his behavior. These newly learned behaviors are "faded" from external control by the model to internal self-control through an oral mediation process. The concepts of modeling, self-verbalization, fading, a feedback type of reinforcement, and the recapitulation of oral to an internalized sequence are utilized in a five-step sequence for the child. Self-instructional techniques can: (1) provide an efficient method for learning a specific task; (2) transfer the responsibility to the child; (3) reinforce the student; (4) overcome self-defeating coping behavior; and (5) teach the child how to cope with his mistakes. A case is cited in which thirty-three hyperkinetic nine- and ten-year-old boys were exposed to self-instructional techniques by a special tutor in arithmetic. Favorable results are reported.

1169 Moore, Samuel F., and Cole, Sherwood O. "Cognitive self-mediation training with hyperkinetic children." Bull Psychon Soc 12(1): 18-20, July, 1978. (10 References).
Examines the efficacy of a behavior modification procedure in altering the attentional deficiencies of a group of hyperactive children. Fourteen boys and girls (ages eight to eleven years) selected from a residential special education facility for children with behavioral/educational problems served as subjects. A modeling procedure, cognitive self-instructional (CSI) training, was administered by six advanced undergraduate psychology majors. Training consisted of modeling appropriate task behaviors, selective cuing, and reinforcement. Effects were measured on a wide range of skills and abilities. On the basis of the experiment it is concluded that CSI training has excellent potential in modifying cognitive processes in hyperactive children.

1170 Munro, Barry C. "Control of disruptive behavior in an elementary classroom: two case studies." Can Couns 8(4): 257-71, October, 1974.
Two devices were used to increase appropriate in-class behavior of two children. Two hyperactive and uncooperative elementary schoolboys served as subjects. A signal device and a counter, making use of immediate reinforcement for appropriate behavior, were employed. Not only did on-task and inappropriate behavior improve, but gains were also made in social behaviors. Thus, the apparatuses are recommended as useful additions to the repertoire of school personnel for the modification of inappropriate classroom behaviors.

1171 Reiber, Joan L.; Goetz, Elizabeth M.; Baer, Donald M.; et al. "Increasing a Down's child's attending behavior with attention from teachers and normal preschool children." Rev Mex Anal Conducta 3(1): 75-85, June, 1977. (23 References).

Describes the modification of the attending (i.e., on-mat) behavior of a five-and-a-half-year-old hyperactive Down's syndrome boy. The boy participated in an individual activity time period when children engaged in independent activities on separate mats. An improvement of on-mat behavior was noted.

1172 Rollins, Howard A.; McCandless, Boyd R.; Thompson, Marion; et al. "Project Success Environment: an extended application of contingency management in inner-city schools." J Educ Psychol 66(2): 167-78, April, 1974. (24 References).

Reports on a study in which teachers were trained to use certain principles of behavior modification with their students. Sixteen black and white inner-city public schoolteachers and 730 Afro-American students (grades one to eight) served as subjects for the study. For one academic year the teachers applied a positive contingency management procedure to modify the disruptive behavior of the students. Compared with matched control teachers and classes, the experimental group showed: (1) higher incidence of positive reinforcement; (2) lower incidence of punishment; (3) accelerated academic improvement; and (4) more task involvement. Teacher morale was reported to be higher as well.

1173 Rosenbaum, Alan; O'Leary, K. Daniel; Jacob, Rolf G. "Behavioral intervention with hyperactive children: group consequences as a supplement to individual contingencies." Behav Ther 6(3): 315-23, May, 1975. (17 References).

Assesses the use of behavior modification techniques as a treatment approach for hyperactive children. Two groups of elementary school hyperactive children participated in the experiment and were rated four times daily on individually determined target behaviors. At the end of the school day the child received either an individual reward for himself or a group reward for himself and his classmates. Both systems were found to improve behavior, although the group reward system was more popular. It is concluded that behavioral intervention can be successfully applied to hyperactive children, producing changes in behavior similar to those reported with drug-related therapies.

1174 Shecket, Susan M., and Shecket, William C. Behaviors of children referred by classroom teachers as hyperactive. 1976. 9p. (ED 129 440).

Documents the use of a classroom observation technique to examine the behaviors of a group of teacher-referred hyperactive children in order to determine the frequency of specific behaviors exhibited. Also investigated were behavioral alternatives to drug therapy. It is suggested that behavioral intervention programs be implemented to decrease hyperactive behaviors.

1175 Snow, David L., and Brooks, Robert B. "Behavior modification techniques in the school setting." J Sch Health 44(4): 198-205, April, 1974. (55 References).

Reviews specific behavior modification techniques and aspects of the theory and procedures involved in this approach. Initial considerations include: designation of the behaviors that need to be modified; obtaining a baseline measure of that behavior; and developing an appropriate intervention program. A schedule of the reinforcement needed to change behavior, and ways of increasing appropriate and decreasing inappropriate behavior, must be derived. Social reinforcement, tangible reinforcement, and token reinforcement are discussed. Time out from positive reinforcement and punishment are cited with regard to their effectiveness in changing behavior. Modeling is described as a process in which more appropriate behavior is learned through observation of significant others.

1176 Starkey, Charles T. "An analysis of the components of a group contingency to control disruptive classroom behavior." For a summary see: Diss Abstr Int 34A(10): 6489, April, 1974. (0 References).

1177 Swift, Marshall S., and Spivack, George. "Therapeutic teaching: a review of teaching methods for behaviorally troubled children." J Spec Educ 8(3): 259-89, Fall, 1974. (78 References).
Focuses on teaching approaches to aid the performance of behavior problem children in the classroom and offers practical descriptions of procedures which teachers may use to increase behavior conducive to learning. Hyperactivity is discussed as one type of maladaptive behavior. Table I presents a summary of teaching techniques by problem behavior.

1178 Wasserman, Howard; Brown, David; Reschly, Dan. "Application of self-management procedures for the modification of academic and classroom behaviors of two 'hyperactive' children." SALT 7(1): 17-24, October, 1974. (10 References).
Recommends the use of self-management procedures to minimize the inappropriate behaviors of the hyperkinetic syndrome. Two elementary school hyperactive boys, members of a special education class, were selected from a larger population. A two-phase intervention plan was instituted for each child. Phase one involved the setting up of self-management procedures to modify the disruptive and noncooperative behaviors. Phase two used a shaping procedure in an attempt to place the boys in a regular classroom. After a six-week period dramatic changes were seen in target behaviors, and the boys were gradually returned to the regular classroom.

1179 Watson, Daniel L., and Hall, Deborah L. Self-control of hyperactivity. 1977. 48p. (ED 148 093).
Evaluates techniques for teaching children self-control of hyperactivity in the regular classroom setting and in special education classrooms. Eighty-six children were divided into three groups: control group, placebo-control group, and experimental group. The last received training in relaxation, biofeedback, and cognitive behavior modification. Favorable results are reported with the experimental group.

1180 Weissenburger, Fred E., and Loney, Jan. "Hyperkinesis in the classroom: if cerebral stimulants are the last resort, what is the first resort?" J Learn Disabil 10(6): 339-48, June-July, 1977. (22 References).
Examines the efficacy of behavior modification techniques in treating children with hyperkinetic behavior disorders. Three children (ages six to twelve years) were observed by a teacher. Between this initial test and a posttest the teacher was instructed to increase the number of approving encounters with the students. Most students' behavior improved as a result of contingency management.

4. DEVICES/APPARATUS

1181 Ball, Thomas S., and Irwin, Aubrey E. "A portable, automated device applied to training a hyperactive child." J Behav Ther Exp Psychiatry 7(2): 185-87, June, 1976. (4 References).

The use of a portable device to help modify the behavior of a twelve-year-old hyperactive boy is reported. The training device, worn by the subject, contained a mercury switch sensor that responded to a postural orientation consistent with in-seat behavior. It also utilized a timer-controlled buzzer which was automatically activated at the end of a two-minute period of correct sitting. This buzzer could be stopped and then reset by the boy who received a reward for each twenty-minute period of in-seat behavior. The apparatus, because of its portability, eliminated the need for experimental settings.

1182 Ryabik, James E. "A practical machine to measure and to reduce random movement of hyperactive and normal children." For a summary see: Diss Abstr Int 37B(7): 3627-28, January, 1977. (0 References).

1183 Schulman, Jerome L.; Stevens, Theodore M.; Kupst, Mary J. "The biomotometer: a new device for the measurement and remediation of hyperactivity." Child Dev 48(3): 1152-54, September, 1977. (7 References).

This article reports the development of an instrument designed to measure and modify hyperactive behavior. The instrument, the biomotometer, consists of a small electronic package worn at the child's waist. In addition to measuring activity level, the device allows the operator to monitor his own progress in biofeedback fashion. Twenty-five emotionally disturbed children were the subjects of two studies which concluded that the biomotometer is a reliable measure of activity level in the classroom. Comments on the actometer, an established measuring device, are included.

1184 Schulman, Jerome L.; Stevens, Theodore M.; Suran, Bernard G.; et al. "Modification of activity level through biofeedback and operant conditioning." J Appl Behav Anal 11(1): 145-52, Spring, 1978. (12 References).

Two studies are summarized. Study I involved an eleven-year-old boy. Material reinforcers were used to modify his hyperactive behavior below baseline during conditioning in the classroom setting. A return to baseline was noted when the child was no longer provided with feedback. Study II used the biomotometer, an electronic device that simultaneously measures activity and provides auditory feedback to the user. One ten-year-old hypoactive boy participated in the study. The boy's activity level increased. On the basis of these experiments, the biomotometer is viewed as a useful instrument for modifying activity level.

1185 Schulman, Jerome L.; Suran, Bernard G.; Stevens, Theodore M.; et al. "Instructions, feedback, and reinforcement in reducing activity levels in the classroom." J Appl Behav Anal 12(3): 441-47, Fall, 1979. (18 References).

The biomotometer, an electronic device which simultaneously measures motor activity and provides auditory feedback, was used in combination with material reinforcers in an experiment to reduce children's activity level in a classroom setting. Nine boys and two girls (ages nine to thirteen years), from a day hospital program for emotionally disturbed children, participated in the study. After five baseline trials, each child had five contingent reinforcement trials in which he/she received feedback "beeps" from the biomotometer and was given toy or candy rewards after each trial in which activity fell at least 20 percent below mean baseline level. Then five noncontingent reinforcement trials were run in which children received rewards for wearing the apparatus without the feedback attachment. The intervention strategies were successful in all five trials for eight of eleven children. Activity levels increased during the final noncontingent phase.

1186 Sueoka, Sarah, et al. Training of classroom relevant behaviors with the "Staats Box." Technical Report No. 9. 1974. 15p. (ED 158 836).
Reports on the use of a simple operant training apparatus with one hyperactive kindergarten boy. The apparatus, called a "Staats Box," requires that the child work alone with the teacher outside the classroom, sitting next to a partition containing a slot. Marbles are dropped into a container upon improvement of certain target behaviors.

5. COMPARISON STUDIES

1187 Axelrod, Saul, and Bailey, Sandra L. "Drug treatment for hyperactivity: controversies, alternatives, and guidelines." Except Child 45(7): 544-50, April, 1979. (32 References).
Discusses drug treatment and presents some alternatives to, and guidelines for, its use. Although drug therapy is an expedient and popular form of treatment for hyperkinesis, the authors cite evidence of overreliance on this form of therapy. Nine suggested guidelines for drug treatment, directed primarily toward the parent and teacher, are given. Also covered is the issue of potential teacher liability when giving medication to a child.

1188 Backman, Joan, and Firestone, Philip. "A review of psychopharmacological and behavioral approaches to the treatment of hyperactive children." Am J Orthopsychiatry 49(3): 500-504, July, 1979. (27 References).
Reviews recent studies that have investigated the relative effectiveness of behavior therapy and stimulant medication. From the accumulated evidence it is concluded that: (1) behavior therapy is much more expensive because it requires more time and effort from parents, teachers, and clinicians; (2) behavior therapy is not effective with all children; (3) medication is more useful in improving classroom and social behaviors and attentional processes; (4) behavior therapy has been demonstrated to be superior to stimulant medication in improving academic performance; and (5) effective treatment programs combine various therapeutic techniques such as medication, behavior therapy, family counseling, and educational intervention.

1189 Bower, K. Bruce, and Mercer, Cecil D. "Hyperactivity: etiology and intervention techniques." J Sch Health 45(4): 195-202, April, 1975. (44 References).
Delineates three theories of etiology of the hyperkinetic syndrome: pathophysiological, attentional and motivational, and environmental. Knowledge of the source of the hyperactivity should play an important role in the choice of treatments which include behavior modification, reduction of environmental distractions, and medical intervention. Alternatives to the last are stressed, and it is recommended that drugs be considered only when other intervention techniques fail. Modeling, oral mediation, stimuli arrangements, and contingency plans are offered as viable techniques for controlling hyperactive behavior.

1190 Bradbard, Gail S. "Minimal brain dysfunction with hyperactivity: a comparison of the behavioral and cognitive effects of pharmacological and behavioral treatments." For a summary see: Diss Abstr Int 35B(1): 496, July, 1974. (0 References).

1191 Brown, Ronald T. "A comparison of differential treatment approaches for impulsive responding of hyperactive children at two age levels." For a summary see: Diss Abstr Int 39A(7): 4176-77, January, 1979.

1192 Brundage-Aguar, Dian; Forehand, Rex; Ciminero, Anthony R. "A review of treatment approaches for hyperactive behavior." J Clin Child Psychol 6(1): 3-10, Spring, 1977. (105 References).
Generally reviews and discusses the pros and cons of various drug and nondrug treatment approaches for hyperactive children. Major problems in evaluating the effectiveness and desirability of the major treatment approaches are given. Chemotherapy and behavior modification have advantages and disadvantages as seen in the research.

1193 ————. "A review of treatment approaches for hyperactive behavior." In: Behavior therapy with hyperactive and learning disabled children. Edited by Benjamin B. Lahey. New York, New York: Oxford University Press, 1979. 49-60. (105 References).
Reprints an article from the Journal of Clinical Child Psychology 6(1): 3-10, Spring, 1977. (Item No. 1192).

1194 Childress, Robert N. "The effectiveness of EMG biofeedback training compared to Ritalin (methylphenidate) in the management of hyperkinesis." For a summary see: Diss Abstr Int 40B(2): 906, August, 1979. (0 References).

1195 Christensen, Donald E. "The combined effects of methylphenidate (Ritalin) and a classroom behavior modification program in reducing the hyperkinetic behaviors of institutionalized mental retardates." For a summary see: Diss Abstr Int 34B(11): 5671-72, May, 1974. (0 References).

1196 ————. "Effects of combining methylphenidate and a classroom token system in modifying hyperactive behavior." Am J Ment Defic 80(3): 266-76, November, 1975. (36 References).
Investigates the effects of combining two treatment modalities--pharmacotherapy and behavior therapy--into a single therapeutic procedure to modify hyperactive behavior. Specifically, methylphenidate (Ritalin) and a token reinforcement program were used to control the disruptive classroom behavior of sixteen hyperactive, institutionalized, retarded children. A within-subject, placebo-controlled, double-blind design was employed. Results show improved behavior when placebo and behavior therapy were combined. Few improvements were noted by the addition of medication to the program. Thus, findings suggest behavior modification to be a viable alternative to drug therapy for hyperactivity in retarded persons.

1197 Costello, William H. "The effectiveness of Ritalin and token economy in increasing hyperkinetic children's coloring behavior." For a summary see: Diss Abstr Int 35B(10): 5103, April, 1975. (0 References).

1198 Douglas, Virginia I. "Differences between normal and hyperkinetic children." In: Clinical use of stimulant drugs in children. Edited by C. Keith Conners. Amsterdam: Excerpta Medica, 1974. 12-23. (34 References). (International Congress Series, No. 313).
Discusses the hyperkinetic child in terms of: (1) problems of attention; (2) the value of behavioral approaches (feedback and reinforcement); (3) the concept of cognitive styles; and (4) the role of stimulant drugs.

1199 Dowrick, Peter W., and Raeburn, John M. "Video editing and medication to produce a therapeutic self model." J Consult Clin Psychol 45(6): 1156-58, December, 1977. (2 References).
Reports on the use of an edited videotape to enable a four-year-old hyperactive boy to role-play suitable behaviors. Both medication and self-modeling films had a beneficial influence on the boy's behavior.

1200 Firestone, Philip; Kelly, Mary Jo; Goodman, John T. "A comparison of behavior modification and methylphenidate with hyperactive children." Res Relat Child 41: 112, March, 1978-August, 1978. (0 References).
Abstracts a report of research in progress or recently completed research. Data are provided on: name of investigator(s), purpose of the study, number and kind of subjects used, methodology, principal findings, duration of research, cooperating group(s), and availability of publication(s). Research Relating to Children is compiled by the ERIC Clearinghouse on Early Childhood Education.

1201 Gittelman, Rachel. "Preliminary report of the efficacy of methylphenidate and behavior modification in hyperkinetic children." Psychopharmacol Bull 13(2): 53-54, April, 1977. (2 References).
Presents the preliminary results of an ongoing study designed to investigate the relative merits of methylphenidate, behavior therapy, and behavior therapy combined with methylphenidate in hyperactive children. Thirty-four children completed the eight-week study. Each child was randomly assigned to one of three experimental conditions: methylphenidate, behavior therapy and placebo, or behavior therapy and methylphenidate. Ratings were made by parents, teachers, and psychiatrists. Methylphenidate was superior to behavior therapy alone; no significant differences were noted with a combination of methylphenidate and behavior therapy.

1202 Gittelman-Klein, R.; Felixbrod, J.; Abikoff, H.; et al. "Methylphenidate vs. behavior therapy in hyperkinetic children." Paper presented at the 128th Annual Meeting of the American Psychiatric Association, Anaheim, California, 1975.

1203 Gittelman-Klein, Rachel, and Klein, Donald F. "Ritalin versus behavior therapy in hyperactive children." Paper presented at the Annual Meeting of the American Psychological Association, Washington, D.C., 1975.

1204 Gittelman-Klein, Rachel; Klein, Donald F.; Abikoff, Howard; et al. "Relative efficacy of methylphenidate and behavior modification in hyperkinetic children: an interim report." J Abnorm Child Psychol 4(4): 361-79, 1976. (28 References).
Compares two treatment approaches, methylphenidate and behavior therapy, in modifying the hyperactive behavior of a group of children. The children were randomly assigned to methylphenidate, behavior therapy and

placebo, or behavior therapy with methylphenidate for an eight-week period; rating scales were used to evaluate their behavior. Results indicate: (1) the participants' behavior improved with all treatments; (2) the methylphenidate group was superior to the group receiving behavior therapy and placebo; and (3) no significant differences between methylphenidate alone and methylphenidate combined with behavior therapy were noted.

1205 ————. "Relative efficacy of methylphenidate and behavior modification in hyperkinetic children: an interim report." In: Behavior therapy with hyperactive and learning disabled children. Edited by Benjamin B. Lahey. New York, New York: Oxford University Press, 1979. 247-57. (28 References).
Reprints an article from the Journal of Abnormal Child Psychology 4(4): 361-79, 1976. (Item No. 1204).

1206 Greenberg, I.; Altman, J. L.; Cole, J. O. "Combination of drugs with behavior therapy." In: Drugs in combination with other therapies. Edited by Milton Greenblatt. New York, New York: Grune & Stratton, 1975. 202p. (Bibliography). (Seminars in Psychiatry).

1207 Hersher, Leonard. "Treatment of disorders of learning in children." JAMA 229(9): 1167-68, August 26, 1974. (1 Reference).
Letter to editor.

1208 Hirst, Irene. "Removal of a student on a methylphenidate (Ritalin) prescription in an open classroom condition." Paper presented at the 54th Annual International Convention, Council for Exceptional Children, Chicago, Illinois, April 4-9, 1976. 5p. (ED 122 506).
Provides details of the successful withdrawal of a ten-year-old hyperactive boy from drug therapy. Behavior modification, an open classroom, and the assistance of five teachers aided the boy's academic and behavioral improvement.

1209 Jacobson, Ruth S. "A comparison of the relative efficacy of special class education and drug therapy for children with selected learning disabilities." For a summary see: Diss Abstr Int 35A(3): 1530-31, September, 1974. (0 References).

1210 Klein, Donald F., and Gittelman-Klein, Rachel. "Comparative effects of methylphenidate and behavior therapy in hyperkinetic children." Res Relat Child 34: 61, March, 1974-August, 1974. (0 References).
Abstracts a report of research in progress or recently completed research. Data are provided on: name of investigator(s), purpose of the study, number and kind of subjects used, methodology, principal findings, duration of research, cooperating group(s), and availability of publication(s). Research Relating to Children is compiled by the ERIC Clearinghouse on Early Childhood Education.

1211 Krause, Thomas R. "Psychophysiological changes in hyperactive and normal children as a function of medication and biofeedback training." For a summary see: Diss Abstr Int 38B(12, pt. 1): 6219, June, 1978. (0 References).

1212 Loney, Jan; Weissenburger, Fred E.; Woolson, Robert F.; et al. "Comparing psychological and pharmacological treatments for hyper-

kinetic boys and their classmates." J Abnorm Child Psychol 7(2): 133-43, June, 1979. (46 References).
This study compares the short-term effects of methylphenidate and of teacher consultation on the on-task behavior of hyperkinetic outpatient boys and controls. Statistically significant treatment effects were found for both drug-treated and behaviorally treated hyperkinetic boys; the size of these effects did not differ between the two types of treatment. Within the behavioral group, the treatment effect spilled over, so that there was also a significant treatment effect on overactive classmates of the behaviorally treated hyperkinetic children and a trend toward a significant treatment effect on their average classmates. Some implications of the findings are discussed.

1213 McDonald, James E. "Pharmacologic treatment and behavior therapy: allies in the management of hyperactive children." Psychol Sch 15(2): 270-74, April, 1978. (37 References).
Recommends that drug therapy be used in conjunction with other treatment modalities even though some of these have been proposed without sufficient empirical support. Behavior modification has demonstrated a favorable effect with hyperactive children especially in the areas of disruptive behaviors, self-concept, peer acceptance, and academic performance. Studies are summarized which provide empirical support for behavior therapy as an alternate or adjunctive treatment to drug therapy.

1214 Pelham, William E. "Withdrawal of a stimulant drug and concurrent behavioral intervention in the treatment of a hyperactive child." Behav Ther 8(3): 473-79, June, 1977. (23 References).
Outlines a treatment regimen in which behavioral intervention replaced methylphenidate in the case of one nine-year-old hyperactive boy. The boy, who had been receiving stimulants for eighteen months, could not be taken off the drug without a return of noncompliant and hyperactive behavior. In a two-phase program which established a behavioral intervention procedure while concurrently reducing the dose of methylphenidate, the boy was successfully withdrawn from the drug in seven months. During the last two months of the program there was no active therapist involvement.

1215 ————. "Withdrawal of a stimulant drug and concurrent behavioral intervention in the treatment of a hyperactive child." In: Annual review of behavior therapy theory and practice. Edited by Cyril M. Franks and G. Terence Wilson. New York, New York: Brunner/Mazel, 1978. 663-71. (23 References).
Reprints and article from Behavior Therapy 8(3): 473-79, June, 1977. (Item No. 1214).

1216 Renshaw, D. "Comprehensive management of the hyperkinetic child." Aust Fam Physician 5(9): 1289-90, 1293-94, passim, October, 1976.

1217 Shafto, Fay, and Sulzbacher, Stephen. "Comparing treatment tactics with a hyperactive preschool child: stimulant medication and programmed teacher intervention." J Appl Behav Anal 10(1): 13-20, Spring, 1977. (12 References).
Evaluates the efficacy of two treatment tactics on a four-and-one-half-year-old boy with learning disabilities and behavior problems. The two tactics--food and praise contingent on appropriate play, and the administration of methylphenidate--were monitored for possible side effects. Fewer free-play activity changes occurred during contingent reinforcement

phases, while medication had variable effects. Although attention to tasks increased with the medication, a higher dosage decreased intelligibility of speech and responsiveness to demands.

1218 Shouse, Margaret N., and Lubar, Joel F. "Management of the hyperkinetic syndrome with methylphenidate and SMR biofeedback training." Biofeedback Self Regul 2(3): 290, September, 1977. (1 Reference).
Abstract of a paper.

1219 Smith, Richard D. "Hyperactivity and medication." Am J Dis Child 133(12): 1287-88, December, 1979. (3 References).
Letter to editor.

1220 Sprague, Robert L.; Christensen, Donald E.; Werry, John S. "Experimental psychology and stimulant drugs." In: Clinical use of stimulant drugs in children. Edited by C. Keith Conners. Amsterdam: Excerpta Medica, 1974. 141-64. (26 References). (International Congress Series, No. 313).
Summarizes three recent studies in the field. Study I investigated the reduction of hyperactivity by conditioning procedures alone and combined with methylphenidate. The twelve children tested showed most improvement in the combined drug-behavior modification program. Study II examined normative data on the Conners' Teacher Rating Scale. There were 291 children in the sample. Results indicated the ability of teachers to correctly rate the children. Study III attempted to study the effect of varying dosage of methylphenidate in hyperactive children. Results and discussion complete the article.

1221 Stableford, William; Butz, Robert; Hasazi, Joseph; et al. "Sequential withdrawal of stimulant drugs and use of behavior therapy with two hyperactive boys." Am J Orthopsychiatry 46(2): 302-12, April, 1976. (34 References).
Investigates the effect of two treatment regimens in controlling the hyperactive behavior of two boys (ages eight and eleven years). The separate and combined effects of Ritalin and Dexedrine, placebo, and behavior modification were monitored. In each case, sequential replacement of drugs with placebo led to no changes in the boys' behavior. It is concluded that behavior therapy, by itself or combined with medication, is the most desirable and effective means for controlling hyperactive behavior.

1222 Thurston, L. P. "Comparison of the effects of parent training and of Ritalin in treating hyperactive children." Int J Ment Health 8(1): 121-28, 1979. (13 References).

1223 Trozzolino, Linda A. "Diagnostic indices of hyperactivity and an investigation of verbal mediation training as an alternative to pharmacotherapy." For a summary see: Diss Abstr Int 36B(1): 461-62, July, 1975. (0 References).

1224 Varni, James W. "A self-regulation approach to the treatment of the hyperactive child: interventions with and without stimulant medication." For a summary see: Diss Abstr Int 37B(6): 3100-3101, December, 1976. (0 References).

1225 Willoughby, Robert H. "Using behavior therapy in conjunction with pharmacotherapy in treating hyperactive children." Pediatr Res 11(4): 384, October, 1977. (0 References).

Abstract of a conference paper presented at the American Pediatric Society and the Society for Pediatric Research.

1226 Wolraich, Mark; Drummond, Thomas; Salomon, Marion K.; et al. "Effects of methylphenidate alone and in combination with behavior modification procedures on the behavior and academic performance of hyperactive children." J Abnorm Child Psychol 6(1): 149-61, March, 1978. (20 References).
Tests the effects of two management approaches, methylphenidate alone and methylphenidate and behavior modification combined, on the behavior/learning problems of a group of hyperactive children. Twenty hyperactive children (ages six to nine years) were studied in a half-day laboratory classroom during a two-week period using a baseline-treatment-reversal design for behavior modification. Half the children were then given Ritalin and half placebo. During the group period, behavior modification was successful in many areas while medication only decreased fidgeting. During the individual period, medication produced the most change in target behaviors, while behavior modification affected two academic measures.

1227 Wulbert, Margaret, and Dries, Robert. "The relative efficacy of methylphenidate (Ritalin) and behavior-modification techniques in the treatment of a hyperactive child." J Appl Behav Anal 10(1): 21-31, Spring, 1977. (21 References).
Compares the efficacy of drugs and contingency management in the treatment of a hyperactive third-grade student, using several criteria behaviors in two different settings--clinic and home. Both approaches were found to be situation-specific; no interaction effects were found. The criteria behaviors were unaffected by medication within the clinic but were significant within the home setting. A multiple-baseline design incorporating contingency reversals showed the reinforcement contingencies to be the crucial variable controlling behavior in the clinic.

1228 ————. "The relative efficacy of methylphenidate (Ritalin) and behavior-modification techniques in the treatment of a hyperactive child." In: Behavior therapy with hyperactive and learning disabled children. Edited by Benjamin B. Lahey. New York, New York: Oxford University Press, 1979. 237-46. (21 References).
Reprints an article from the Journal of Applied Behavior Analysis 10(1): 21-31, Spring, 1977. (Item No. 1227).

F. PARENTAL MANAGEMENT

1229 Adams, Elizabeth. "The mother is the first to know." Acad Ther 9(5): 373-76, Spring, 1974. (0 References).
Relates a mother's personal account of her attempts at home management of her hyperactive son.

1230 Berlin, Irving N. "Familial management of minimal brain dysfunction." In: Current psychiatric therapies. Volume 16. Edited by Jules H. Masserman. New York, New York: Grune & Stratton, 1976. 33-37. (17 References).
Offers suggestions to the physician as to how he can involve the family in the management of the MBD child. The family is seen to be either the physician's greatest ally or an obstacle to the child's improved functioning. A case study of a five-and-one-half-year-old hyperactive boy is presented. The boy's behavior improved as a result of psychiatric counseling of both the boy and his parents.

1231 ———. "Minimal brain dysfunction: management of family distress." JAMA 229(11): 1454-56, September 9, 1974. (17 References).
Urges the early involvement of parents in understanding the diagnosis of hyperactivity and its implications for management of the hyperactive child. The physician should aid the parents in this management.

1232 Bittinger, Marvin L., ed. Living with our hyperactive children: parents' own stories. Danvers, Massachusetts: BPS Books, 1977. 199p.

1233 Bourcier, Marilyn, et al. You are not alone: a parent discussion of hyperactive children and the group process. 1974. 30p. (ED 117 924).
Consists of two booklets providing general information for parents of hyperactive children.

1234 Cragg, Sheila. Tantrums, toads, and teddy bears. Scottdale, Pennsylvania: Herald Press, 1979. 221p.

1235 Crook, William G. Can your child read? Is he hyperactive? Rev. ed. Jackson, Tennessee: Professional Books, 1977. 224p. (Bibliography).
This manual for parents is divided into six sections: Section I gives general information about hyperactivity, learning disorders, allergies, and possible interrelationships between diet and/or academic and/or behavior problems. Section II offers suggestions for a management program organized in three phases: forms, systems and materials, and an illustrative case history. Examples are given of various health records, inventories, and tests. Section IV provides more information on school readiness, allergy, nutrition, megavitamins, vision, etc. Section V summarizes the major tenets of the book. References and other sources of information are given in Section VI. A list of organizations and an index complete the volume.

1236 Dahlin, I.; Engelsing, E. L.; Henderson, A. T. "Directive family therapy for hyperkinetic children." Paper presented at the CIBA Medical Horizons Symposium on Minimal Brain Dysfunction, Columbus, Ohio, The Ohio State University, 1975.

1237 Dubey, Dennis R. "Training parents of hyperactive children in child management: a comparative outcome study." For a summary see: Diss Abstr Int 37B(11): 5828, May, 1977. (0 References).

1238 Dubey, Dennis R., and Kaufman, Kenneth F. "Home management of hyperkinetic children." J Pediatr 93(1): 141-46, July, 1978. (22 References).
Describes six clinical programs and one controlled experimental program in which parents of hyperkinetic children were trained to alleviate behavior problems in the home. Eighty-seven families were enrolled in the program which consisted of ten-week workshops in behavior modification and child management. Ph.D. psychologists and doctoral interns conducted the sessions. Research indicates that parents were able to achieve significant reductions in their children's hyperactivity and in the severity of behavior problems. These gains were maintained at follow-up, pointing to the effectiveness of parental training workshops.

Disease	Girls	Boys		
			473	921
			474	924
216	115	116	475	949
		117	526	961
302	1113	122	530	1032
		150	606	
345	1680	226	607	
		231	836	
886		451	839	
		472	900	

Drugs						
40	677	763	964	1054	1510 ✓	~~2017~~
~~218~~	680	824	965	1139	1515 ✓	
613	681	868	970	1206	~~1575~~	
~~646~~	684	869	972	~~1240~~	~~1576~~	
646	701	903	974	~~1333~~	~~1581~~	
650	704	939	976	~~1369~~	1638 ✓	
~~651~~	723	945	977	1388 ✓	1875 ✓	
669	724	946	978	~~1483~~	1975 ✓	
674	753	963	990	~~1499~~	~~1990~~	

Cause	Etiology
253 ✓	~~42~~
~~257~~	
258 ✓	~~150~~
~~330~~	
~~362~~	~~256~~
~~370~~	
373 ✓?	435 ✓
~~417~~	
~~662~~	~~457~~
~~748~~	
~~1022~~	1189 ✓
~~1023~~	
~~1024~~	~~1378~~
~~1026~~	

treatment method - educational remediation

Diet

373 ✓	~~409~~	~~1333~~	1~~385~~
374 ✓	~~616~~	1343 ✓	1388 ✓
~~390~~	~~1278~~	~~1344~~	~~1441~~
~~391~~	~~1298~~	1~~351~~	
~~395~~	1301	~~1352~~	Cylert
~~396~~	1~~302~~	1357 ✓	841 ✓ ; ~~842~~
~~397~~	1~~306~~	1~~362~~	Cure
~~399~~	1314 ✓?	~~1362~~	~~218~~ ; ~~651~~
~~402~~	~~1310~~	1~~369~~	Definition
403 ✓	1378 ✓	~~1380~~	

1239 Dubey, D. R.; Kaufman, K. F.; O'Leary, S. G. "Behavioral and reflective parent training for hyperactive children: a comparison." Paper presented at the 85th Annual Convention of the American Psychological Association, San Francisco, California, 1977.

1240 Eisenpreis, Bettijane. "Drugs and the family." In: Drugs and the special child. Edited by Michael J. Cohen. New York, New York: Gardner Press, 1979. 111-27. (10 References).
Covers the subject of drugs and the special child in the context of the child's natural habitat, his or her family. The role of the parent in all phases of drug treatment is highlighted.

1241 Evans, Jean. "How to tell if your child is hyperactive and what to do about it." Redbook 147(6): 24ff., October, 1976. (0 References).
Presents a question-and-answer interview with Melvin Levine, Assistant Professor of Pediatrics at Harvard Medical School. Dr. Levine responds to several frequently asked questions concerning the hyperactive child.

1242 Feighner, Ann. "Videotape training for parents as therapeutic agents with hyperactive children." In: Cantwell, Dennis P., ed. The hyperactive child: diagnosis, management, current research. New York, New York: Spectrum Publications, distributed by John Wiley and Sons, 1975. 145-57. (42 References). (Series on Child Behavior and Development, Volume I).
Outlines a multimodality treatment program and discusses the use of videotape techniques in training parents to be effective behavior modifiers of their hyperactive children. The objectives of the program are to help parents reduce his child's maladaptive behaviors, reduce family tensions, and help correct long-standing communication problems. The advantages of videotaping for the child, parent, and therapist are discussed, as are the details of a taping session.

1243 Firestone, Philip, et al. Differential effects of parent training and stimulant medication with hyperactives: a progress report. 1979. 37p. (ED 181 615).
Assesses and follows forty-three hyperactive children and their parents during a three-month intervention program. Three regimens were used: (1) parent training in behavior modification with the child on placebo; (2) parent training in behavior modification with the child on Ritalin; and (3) Ritalin only without parent intervention. All groups improved at home and at school, but only those children receiving Ritalin improved academically as well as behaviorally. There was no evidence that parent training aided improvement.

1244 Firestone, Philip, and Kelly, Mary Jo. "Are fathers necessary for parent training groups?" Res Relat Child 39: 119, March, 1977-August, 1977. (0 References).
Abstracts a report of research in progress or recently completed research. Data are provided on: name of investigator(s), purpose of the study, number and kind of subjects used, methodology, principal findings, duration of research, cooperating group(s), and availability of publication(s). Research Relating to Children is compiled by the ERIC Clearinghouse on Early Childhood Education.

1245 Fisher, Johanna. "The hyperactive child." In: Fisher, Johanna. A parents' guide to learning disabilities. New York, New York: Scribner, 1978. 73-92. (Bibliography).

Through the use of four case studies, the major characteristics and treatment methods for hyperkinesis are summarized. Comments are made on behavior modification techniques, and five recommendations are offered to parents who wish to aid their children. A subject index is included.

1246 Frazier, James R., and Schneider, Henry. "Parental management of inappropriate hyperactivity in a young retarded child." J Behav Ther Exp Psychiatry 6(3): 246-47, October, 1975. (6 References).
Describes a procedure used by the parents of a three-year-old boy to eliminate inappropriate hyperactive behavior at mealtime and after meals. The technique involved a multiple baseline procedure, contingent attention, and time-out. A sharp decrease in inappropriate behaviors was reported; further, the behaviors remained at a low rate for approximately five weeks after treatment. This case illustrates the utilization of a successful home management program.

1247 Freeman, Stephen W., and Adler, Sol. "Hyperactivity: the Jekyll and Hyde syndrome." In: Freeman, Stephen W., and Adler, Sol. Does your child have a learning disability? Questions answered for parents. Springfield, Illinois: Thomas, 1974. 19-28. (Bibliography).
This book provides answers to questions parents frequently have on the identification and management of the LD child. Chapter III, devoted to hyperactivity, covers a wide range of topics including behavior patterns and the use of medication. Other sections offer guidelines for managing the LD child, specific training procedures and activities for parents and teachers, and a list of appropriate materials. Some case histories are documented. A glossary and subject index complete the volume.

1248 Fremont, Theodore S., and Seifert, David. "What you should know about hyperactivity." MH 60(2): 10-13, Summer, 1976. (0 References).
The use of drug agents in the treatment of hyperkinesis is discussed. Although necessary in some cases, CNS stimulants should be given a secondary role, with possible alternatives being vigorous exercise, rewards, and behavior conditioning techniques. The roles of parents and teachers in the implementation of these techniques are examined.

1249 Friedman, Delores L. "Your child: energetic or hyperactive?" Essence 9(6): 24, October, 1978. (0 References).
Points out that hyperactivity is a symptom, rather than a disease. Proper diagnosis is vital if the child is suspected of being hyperactive. Brief comments are made on various management approaches.

1250 Gordon, Neil. "Hyperkinesis: the overactive child makes the whole family suffer." Nurs Mirror 147(15): 35-36, October 12, 1978. (5 References).
Briefly discusses characteristics, causes, drug treatment, and other methods of management which can involve the whole family.

1251 Grounds, Anne. The hyperkinetic child. Specific Learning Difficulties Association (SPELD) NSW, P. O. Box 94, Mossman, New South Wales 2088. [n.d.] 10p.
The mother of a hyperactive child discusses various characteristics of and treatment methods for hyperactivity. Hyperkinetic children are reported to hear things more acutely than others, see dozens of objects at once, absorb things faster than other children, become stimulated with fatigue, and have poor concentration because of overreaction to stimuli.

Also covered are the effect of medication in slowing down behavior, the hyperactive child's need for firmer handling than other children, and the difference between behavior resulting from hyperactivity and behavior which is the result of other causes.

1252 Heiting, Kenneth. When your child is hyperactive. St. Meinrad, Indiana: Abbey Press, 1978. 96p.
This book is intended for parents of hyperactive children. Characteristics of the hyperactive child are described, and some theories of the causes of the condition are reviewed (including neurological and biochemical theories). The Feingold diet is discussed, along with the impulsivity and attention correlates of hyperactivity. The role of medication in the treatment of hyperactivity is covered. The chapter on education focuses on such aspects as mainstreaming, resource rooms, self-contained classrooms, the parent-teacher relationship, educational testing, and the special learning requirements of hyperactive children. Practical tips for dealing with such children at home are offered, such as discipline and the need for positive reinforcement rather than punishment. A directory of organizations offering assistance to parents of hyperactive children is included.

1253 Living with our hyperactive children. Danvers, Massachusetts: Two Continents Publishing Group, BPS Books, 1977.

1254 Loney, Jan; Comly, Hunter H.; Simon, Betty. "Parental management, self-concept, and drug response in minimal brain dysfunction." J Learn Disabil 8(3): 187-90, March, 1975. (7 References).
Compares three groups of elementary schoolboys in order to test several hypotheses concerning the type of management the boys had received. Boys with MBD were divided into two groups based on quality of parental management and compared with a group of normal controls. Self-esteem and impulse control were determined for all boys. Results suggest that parental management can influence both the self-esteem and the child's response to stimulant drugs. Significantly more well-managed MBD children responded positively to medication than did poorly managed children.

1255 McKay, Dixie. Parent handbook: for parents of children who learn in different ways. 1975. 15p. (ED 112 589).
Provides suggestions to parents for recognizing the symptoms of a learning disability. Information is also provided on child management techniques and activities which parents can use to help their child learn. Hyperactivity is included in the discussion.

1256 O'Leary, K. D., and Kent, R. N. "A behavioral consultation program for parents and teachers of children with conduct problems." Paper presented at the American Psychopathological Association, Boston, 1974.

1257 Pinkston, Elsie M. "Parents as behavioral therapists for their children." For a summary see: Diss Abstr Int 35B(9): 3660, March, 1975. (0 References).

1258 Q's and A's on child mental health: an interview with Dr. Berry Brazelton. 1977. 18p. (ED 143 174).
Reprints an interview with Dr. Brazelton who discusses some of the aspects of child mental health, including the hyperkinetic syndrome. Guidelines are given for parental management.

1259 Ritterman, Michele K. "Outcome study for family therapy, Ritalin, and placebo treatments of hyperactivity: an open systems approach." For a summary see: Diss Abstr Int 39B(12, pt. 1): 6138-39, June, 1979. (0 References).

1260 Schmitt, Barton. "Guidelines for living with a hyperactive child." Pediatrics 60(3): 387, September, 1977. (0 References).
Letter to editor.

1261 Schoenrade, Joyce L. "Help means hope for Laurie." J Learn Disabil 7(7): 414-16, August-September, 1974. (0 References).
Relates a mother's account of the frustrations and difficulties involved in raising her bright but hyperactive daughter. With the help of medication, counseling, and changes in parental strategy, the child will, it is hoped, develop into a competent and well-adjusted adult.

1262 Sugerman, Gerald I., and Stone, Margaret N. Your hyperactive child: a doctor answers parents' and teachers' questions. Chicago, Illinois: Regnery, 1974. 152p.
Intended for parents and teachers, this book was written by a pediatric neurologist. Topics include: (1) diagnosis; (2) etiology; (3) school factors (including suggested teaching strategies; (4) treatment approaches (including home management and medical assistance; (5) drug therapy (including dosage and possible side effects; and (6) future life considerations. The first of four appendices provides a listing by state of where to get help for the hyperactive child. Also included in the appendices are approximately fifty references on the topic, definitions of approximately forty terms, and sample forms and questionnaires used with hyperactive children.

1263 Tymchuk, Alexander J. Behavior modification with children: a clinical training manual. Springfield, Illinois: Thomas, 1974. 133p. (Bibliography).
This book is included as an example of the many books directed toward the parent as well as education and psychology students. Major principles of behavior modification are reviewed; each chapter contains examples and assignments which could be applied to a wide variety of problem behaviors.

1264 Wender, Paul H., and Wender, Esther H. The hyperactive child & the learning disabled child: a handbook for parents. Rev. ed. New York, New York: Crown, 1978. 138p. (0 References).
This update of the 1973 book, The Hyperactive Child, discusses the syndrome in terms of: (1) characteristics; (2) causal factors; (3) development and outcome; (4) treatment approaches; and (5) description and recommendations for the LD child. Since learning disabilities frequently accompany hyperactivity, the authors have added considerable material in this area. The volume is directed toward the parent and concerned layman.

1265 "What exactly is wrong with your child?: a parent's guide to hyperkinesis." Drug Ther 5: 58-60, September, 1975. (0 References).
Briefly outlines differences between hyperactive and normal children, how the diagnosis is made, and the treatment (medical and/or special education) which can be administered.

1266 Wiese, Nancy E. "The nightmare." Acad Ther 10(2): 245-48, Winter, 1974-75. (0 References).
Relates a mother's account of her six-year-old daughter's sleeping difficulties, hyperactivity, and learning problems. Four years later, through diagnostic tests, medication, and cooperation of teachers and parents, the girl has made satisfactory adjustment.

1267 Wiltz, N. A., and Gordon, S. B. "Parental modification of a child's behavior in an experimental residence." J Behav Ther Exp Psychiatry 5(1): 107-9, July, 1974. (11 References).
Describes an experiment in which a schizophrenic hyperactive nine-year-old boy and his parents were trained in the application of behavioral principles. The entire family spent five consecutive days in an apartment-like setting with observational facilities. The parents received training through instructional materials, prompting, modeling, and feedback. The family returned home and follow-up was maintained by telephone. An improvement in the child's deviant behavior and rate of noncompliance was observed.

G. ALTERNATIVE INTERVENTIONS

1. ART/MUSIC

1268 Carrington, Fredrick M. "The effects of music therapy on the attention span of hyperactive mental retardates." For a summary see: Diss Abstr Int 34A(7): 3864, January, 1974. (0 References).

1269 Geier, Annette F. "The effects on hyperkinetic behavior of a high stimulus arts intervention (Project MOPPET) in a school setting as measured by pre- and post-scale attainment (Conners' Teacher Behavior Rating Scale)." For a summary see: Diss Abstr Int 38A(5): 2867, November, 1978. (0 References).

1270 Guinter, William J. "The use of creative arts and behavior modification in a special treatment designed to increase academic achievement and social behavior in learning and behavior disorder pupils." For a summary see: Diss Abstr Int 35A(5): 2804-5, November, 1974. (0 References).

1271 Michielutte, Robert. "The use of music with exceptional children." In: Second review of special education. Edited by Lester Mann and David Sabatino. Philadelphia, Pennsylvania: JSE Press, 1974. 251-71. (74 References). (JSE Press Series in Special Education).
Focuses on the educational and therapeutic uses of music with emphasis on speculative and empirical aspects, rather than on activities in the classroom. A review of the literature summarizes positive benefits and indicates that music can be an effective method for controlling behavior and aiding in the development of social skills. Music appears useful in establishing communication, regulating physical activities, improving task performance, and controlling negative behavior. Several studies detailing the effect of music on hyperactive behavior are cited.

1272 O'Connell, Thomas S. "The musical life of an autistic boy." J Autism Child Schizophr 4(3): 223-29, September, 1974. (2 References).
A hyperactive eight-year-old boy with exceptional musical ability and absolute pitch was given music lessons two or three times a week for

four years. He not only learned to play the piano, but also improved in behavior and ability to concentrate.

1273 Reid, Dennis H.; Hill, Bonnie K.; Fawers, Robert J.; et al. "The use of contingent music in teaching social skills to a nonverbal, hyperactive boy." J Music Ther 12(1): 2-18, Spring, 1975.
Documents the use of contingent music in teaching social skills. One eight-year-old nonverbal hyperactive boy participated in three experiments. Experiment I employed a multiple baseline design in researching effects of contingent music on appropriate walking and showed an increase of 20-40 percent appropriate walking. Experiment II used a reversal design in investigating effects of music on appropriate car-riding and showed a 15-20 percent increase. Experiment III demonstrated the utility of a novel remote-control device for rapidly presenting contingent music.

1274 Simpson, Seymour A. "The influence of background music on the behavior of brain-injured children." Isr Ann Psychiatry 14(3): 275-79, September, 1976. (6 References).
Attempts to assess the effect of soft, continuous background music on the behavior and learning ability of brain-injured children and to test the hypothesis that music could have a salutary effect on distractible and hyperactive behavior. Six children attending a school for brain-injured children in Tel Aviv served as subjects and were rated on eight behavioral variables over a two-and-one-half-month period. Analysis of the data shows that background music tended to contribute to hyperactive behavior. At the same time, however, task performance increased. The possibility is suggested that background music might facilitate learning success by creating a state of arousal while blocking out other types of distractors.

1275 Walker, Barbara C. "The relative effects of painting and gross-motor activities on the intrinsic locus-of-control of hyperactivity in learning disabled elementary school pupils." For a summary see: Diss Abstr Int 38A(8): 4743, February, 1978. (0 References).

1276 Windwer, Catherine. "An investigation of the relationship between an ascending musical stimulation cycle and activity in hyperactive children." Res Relat Child 41: 115-16, March, 1978-August, 1978. (0 References).
Abstracts a report of research in progress or recently completed research. Data are provided on: name of investigator(s), purpose of the study, number and kind of subjects used, methodology, principal findings, duration of research, cooperating group(s), and availability of publication(s). Research Relating to Children is compiled by the ERIC Clearinghouse on Early Childhood Education.

2. DIET

1277 Abrams, B. F., et al. "Perspectives in clinical research: a review of research controversies surrounding the Feingold diet." Fam Community Health 1: 93-113, February, 1979.

1278 "Additive-free diet doesn't correct behavioral problems." Am Fam Physician 20(6): 145-46, December, 1979. (0 References).
Reports on a study which failed to substantiate the theories of Dr. Benjamin Feingold.

1279 Adler, Sol. "Behavior management: a nutritional approach to the behaviorally disordered and learning-disabled child." J Learn Disabil 11(10): 651-56, December, 1978. (8 References).
Explores the potential use of nutrition therapy as a treatment approach for children exhibiting behavioral disorders, including hyperkinesis. Nutrition programs, implemented by the physician or nutritionist, can be successfully used with behavior modification and psychopharmacological treatment. Table I reprints an elimination diet.

1280 Barr, M. "Feingold diet." Med J Aust 1(6): 234, March 24, 1979. (6 References).
Letter to editor.

1281 Bell, S. K. "Feingold diet: new hope for the hyperactive child." Can Consum 6: 4-5, October, 1976.

1282 Bierman, C. Warren, and Furukawa, Clifton T. "Food additives and hyperkinesis: are there nuts among the berries?" Pediatrics 61(6): 932-34, June, 1978. (6 References).
Comments on two studies appearing in this issue of Pediatrics (Harley -- Item No. 1325 and Williams -- Item No. 1388), which refute Dr. Feingold's findings. These methodologically correct studies fail to confirm a relationship between food additives and adverse behavior in children.

1283 Billingsley, Felix. "Feingold diet." Med J Aust 2(13): 508, September 25, 1976. (8 References).
Letter to editor.

1284 Breakey, Joan. "Dietary management of hyperkinesis and behavioural problems." Aust Fam Physician 7(6): 720-24, June, 1978. (9 References).
Briefly reports on the clinical experiences of the Australian version of the Feingold K-P diet by a dietitian in private practice. Children of seventy-one families were placed on the K-P diet from two to sixteen months. Questionnaires were completed by families at monthly follow-up meetings. The children improved in several areas: hyperactivity, aggression, anxiety, socialization, and concentration. In addition, there were reports of a decrease in eczema, fewer upper respiratory tract infections, diarrhea, headaches, bed-wetting, and nightmares. These conclusions are reached: (1) the Feingold diet is not significantly different from other dietary regimens which may be managed without dietary supervision; (2) better results are obtained with individual help from a dietitian; and (3) the Feingold concept has broadened the base of diet therapy further into behavioral areas.

1285 ———. "Feingold diet." Med J Aust 2(13): 508-10, September 25, 1976. (2 References).
Letter to editor.

1286 Brenner, Arnold. "A study of the efficacy of the Feingold diet on hyperkinetic children." Clin Pediatr 16(7): 652-56, July, 1977. (12 References).
Traces the progress of a group of children placed on the Feingold diet, a low-salicylate, additive-free diet from the Kaiser Permanente Institute. Forty-four hyperactive children participated in the study. Of these, twelve discontinued the regimen because of unwillingness on the part of the child, peer group pressure, or lack of determination on the part of

the parents. Of the remaining thirty-two children, eleven had an excellent response and were able to discontinue medication. Other children showed no change or "probably improved." At follow-up six months later, three of the eleven children with excellent responses had discontinued the diet and showed a marked deterioration in academic performance.

1287 ————. "Trace mineral levels in hyperactive children responding to the Feingold diet." J Pediatr 94(6): 944-45, June, 1979. (10 References).
Measures trace mineral levels in hyperactive children to test the hypothesis that a biochemical difference may be present in children who appear to be affected by the additives. Two groups of children with the hyperkinetic/MBD syndrome were compared: group one consisted of twenty children whose parents noted a positive beneficial effect from the restricted, additive-free diet; group two consisted of fourteen children whose parents observed beneficial effect and who had fully complied with the vigorous restrictions of the diet. Findings show a significantly higher level of copper in the children who were reported to respond to the restricted diet compared to those children who apparently had no response. Implications of the findings are discussed.

1288 Broadston, Elizabeth. "Nutrition plan for the hyperactive child." Lets Live 42: 38-39, 41, May, 1974. (0 References).
Of the various approaches currently being used in the management of the hyperactive child, e.g., drugs and orthomolecular psychiatry, the salicylate-free diet of Dr. Feingold merits the attention of nutritionists and physicians. This diet, which is free of artificial colors and flavors, has brought normalcy to hyperactive children. Suggestions are given for the family's role in the administration of this diet.

1289 "A case history: sugar, fried oysters, and zinc." Acad Ther 11(1): 119-21, Fall, 1975. (0 References).
Cites a case history of an adopted eighteen-year-old girl with a background of learning problems, erratic and irritable behavior, immaturity, and a compulsion for sugar. Although various diet regimens had been prescribed (sugar-free, megavitamins, etc.), the dramatic improvement in the girl's behavior is attributed, by her mother, to the daily ingestion of one 200 mg zinc tablet.

1290 Colon, A. R. "Response of minimal brain dysfunction to dietary management." Pediatr Res 8(4): 462, April, 1974. (0 References).
Summarizes a research project in which an experimental protocol was designed to treat MBD by the elimination of common food allergens. The most common offending agents were found to be milk and wheat. Possible food allergy should be explored in children with MBD and motor speech disorders.

1291 Conners, C. Keith. "Double-blind studies of food additives and hyperkinesis." Paper presented at the 2nd ACA International Food Allergy Symposium, Mexico City, Mexico, October 16-20, 1978.

1292 ————. "Food additives and hyperkinesis: a continuation study." Paper presented at the Annual Meeting of the Nutrition Foundation, Palm Springs, California, January 11-14, 1977.

1293 Conners, C. Keith, et al. Food additives and hyperkinesis: a controlled double-blind experiment. 1975. 59p. (ED 117 877).

Reports on a pilot study to test the Feingold hypothesis. Fifteen hyperactive children participated. Although findings suggest that the K-P diet may reduce hyperkinetic symptoms, results should be viewed with caution. Included is a NIE staff critique.

1294 Conners, C. Keith; Goyette, Charles H.; Southwick, Deborah A.; et al. "Food additives and hyperkinesis: a controlled double-blind experiment." Pediatrics 58(2): 154-66, August, 1976. (15 References).
Compares two diet regimens, control and the Feingold or K-P salicylate-free diet, in a double-blind crossover trial involving fifteen hyperkinetic children. The children were rated by parents and teachers before and after treatment. Both parents and teachers reported improved behavior on the K-P diet as compared with the pretreatment baseline, although the control diet ratings remained the same as baseline. Due to problems of study methodology, results are to be viewed with caution. Appendix A gives the K-P diet listing unapproved foods.

1295 ————. "Food additives and hyperkinesis: preliminary report of a double-blind crossover experiment." Psychopharmacol Bull 12(2): 10-11, April, 1976. (4 References).
Investigates the efficacy of the Feingold K-P diet for children with the hyperkinetic syndrome. This diet eliminates artificial flavors and colors and natural salicylates. The reports of success of the diet are seen to be "purely anecdotal" and lack objective methods of assessment as well as controls or systematic follow-up. In the present study fifteen children (ages six to twelve years), who had been diagnosed as hyperkinetic based on social and medical history, questionnaires, and psychiatric evaluation, served as subjects. The children were randomly assigned the Feingold diet or a control diet in a double-blind crossover experiment for the three-month program. Preliminary data suggest differences in hyperkinetic symptom reduction between diets favoring the K-P diet, because children generally demonstrated a greater degree of improvement than while on the control diet. However, the changes during the K-P diet period were not as great as improvements observed after initial clinic contact. It is concluded that the K-P diet may be effective for some children, but that a more extensive design will be necessary before this can be proven.

1296 Cook, Peter S., and Woodhill, Joan M. "The Feingold dietary treatment of the hyperkinetic syndrome." Med J Aust 2(3): 85-88, 90, July 17, 1976. (7 References).
Outlines a treatment regimen following the Feingold diet. Results of its application to fifteen hyperactive Australian children are presented. The parents of ten children are "quite certain" and those of three others "fairly certain" that behavior improved as a result of the diet. Hyperactive behavior resumed with dietary infringements. Possible ecological implications of these findings are discussed.

1297 ————. "Food additives and hyperactivity." Med J Aust 1(6): 188-89, February 5, 1977. (13 References).
Replies to Dr. Werry's guest editorial on food additives and hyperactivity (Item No. 1383).

1298 Cooperman, Earl M. "Hyperactivity and diet." Can Med Assoc J 119(2): 113, 116, July 22, 1978. (15 References).
This editorial comments on the Feingold K-P diet.

1299 Crook, William G. "An alternate method of managing the hyperactive child." Pediatrics 54(5): 656, November, 1974. (9 References).
Letter to editor.

1300 ————. "The hyperactive child--the dietary approach." Hosp Pract 14(6): 18-19, June 23, 1979. (0 References).
Letter to editor.

1301 ————. "More on diet/hyperkinesis." Hosp Pract 14(7): 16, 17, July, 1979. (0 References).
Letter to editor.

1302 Divoky, Diane. "Behavior and food coloring: lessons of a diet fad." Psychol Today 12(7): 145-48, December, 1978. (0 References).
Examines the Feingold diet and other studies criticizing this approach to management of the hyperactive child. The K-P diet appeals to many parents because of its apparent wholesomeness and because it offers an alternative to drug treatment. Emphasis should be directed, however, to revising child-rearing practices, improving teaching methods, and changing basic societal beliefs.

1303 "Dr. Feingold's diet revolution." Nations Sch Coll 2(3): 24-25, March, 1975. (0 References).
Briefly summarizes the Feingold diet for hyperactive children. This diet emphasizes the elimination of foods which contain artificial coloring and flavoring from meals served to overactive children. Although the diet has met with success in preliminary studies in various parts of the country, it has been largely ignored by the medical community.

1304 Dumbrell, Susan; Woodhill, Joan M.; Mackie, Leila; et al. "Is the Australian version of the Feingold diet safe?" Med J Aust 2(12): 548, 569-70, December 2, 1978. (14 References).
Evaluates the nutritional adequacy of the Australian version of the Feingold diet. Sixteen hyperactive children (fourteen boys and two girls, ages four to eight years) and twenty-two controls served as subjects for the sixteen-week trial, of which the first six weeks are detailed here. Anthropometric and dietary intake data were collected on both groups. The children spent two weeks on their normal diet and four weeks on the elimination diet. Food logs were coded and analyzed by computer for energy and nutrient consumption. The mean intakes of all computed nutrients were above the recommended level in the Australian Dietary Allowance for both diets. Quality in the elimination diet was found to be superior to the normal diet. Thus, the elimination test diet is deemed to be safe for use in the treatment of hyperactive children.

1305 Dunn, R. H. "Food additives and hyperactivity." Med J Aust 2(21): 806, November 20, 1976. (0 References).
Letter to editor.

1306 Eich, W. F., et al. "Effect of the Feingold Kaiser Permanente diet in minimal brain dysfunction." J Med Assoc State Ala 49(4): 16-18, 20, October, 1979.

1307 Feingold, Ben F. "Behavioral disturbances linked to the ingestion of food additives." Del Med J 49(2): 89-94, February, 1977. (5 References).

Cites several previous studies which reported favorable results when using the Kaiser-Permanente (K-P) diet to manage hyperactive children. Two tables classify characteristics of hyperkinesis and MBD. Table III lists the etiologies of neurologic damage. Table IV outlines various types of additives. Foods to be avoided on the K-P diet are listed in Table V.

1308 ———. "Food additives and hyperkinesis: Dr. Feingold replies." J Learn Disabil 10(2): 122-24, February, 1977. (11 References).
Letter to editor.

1309 ———. "Hyperkinesis-learning difficulty linked to artificial colors and flavors." Ann Allergy 32(5): 283, May, 1974. (0 References).
Abstract of a paper presented to an ACA scientific congress. The paper summarizes various topics concerning the salicylate-free diet advocated by the author in the management of hyperkinesis.

1310 ———. Why your child is hyperactive. New York, New York: Random House, 1975. 211p. (0 References).
This book, directed toward parents of hyperactive children, discusses how hyperactivity relates to food additives. Eighteen chapters cover the following topics: the relationship between behavior and diet; the role of allergy; behavior linked to artificial colors and flavors; the use of drugs with four hyperactive boys; how diet controls hyperactivity; the diary of a mother whose child was put on diet therapy; patterns of hyperactivity; hazards of drug treatment; success and failure of the K-P (additive free) diet; the problem of food labeling; the problem of medications for children; excerpts from letters of parents with hyperactive children; the story of food colors; synthetic food flavors; the safeness of "safe" additives; genetics and behavior; the need for research; and ingested pollutants. Also included are the K-P diet, sample menus, and suggested recipes.

1311 Feingold, Ben F., and Feingold, Helene S. The Feingold cookbook for hyperactive children, and others with problems associated with food additives and salicylates. New York, New York: Random House, 1979. 327p.

1312 "The Feingold diet for hyperactive children." Med Lett Drugs Ther 20(12): 55-56, June 16, 1978. (0 References).
Briefly reviews the use of the Feingold diet in the United States and reports on some of the controlled and uncontrolled studies done in the area. From the accumulated data it is concluded that there is no convincing evidence that any diet is effective for the treatment of hyperkinesis. It is yet undetermined what effect food colorings have on this syndrome.

1313 "Feingold's regimen for hyperkinesis." Lancet 2(8143): 617-18, September 22, 1979. (14 References).
Comments on the Feingold diet and concludes that there are few, if any, indications for the use of a rigorous additive-free diet for the treatment of hyperkinesis.

1314 Grosek, Robert J. Failure of an additive-free diet to control hyperactivity: a case study. Technical Report 77-02. 1977. 17p. (ED 158 449).

Measures the effects of a diet eliminating artificial flavors, colors, and salicylates on the hyperactivity of one four-year-old boy. In this case diet was not instrumental in reducing hyperactive behavior.

1315 Harbert, Ruth. "Therapy for the L.D. child: some alternatives to pills." Child House 10(2): 10-13, Winter, 1978.
Advocates the use of the Feingold diet to treat hyperactive children. This diet eliminates artificial food additives (e.g., flavors and colors) and salicylates from the diets of children displaying overactive behavior. Areas covered include problems of labeling; toxic nonfood items; medicine additives; reactions to foods other than those of the diet; child and physician acceptance of the diet; and the use of the diet by other members of the family.

1316 Harley, J. Preston. "Diet and behavior in hyperactive children: testing the Feingold hypothesis." Paper presented at the Annual Meeting of the American Psychological Association, 1976.

1317 ————. An experimental evaluation of hyperactivity and food additives. Madison, Wisconsin: University of Wisconsin, 197-. 2v.

1318 ————. An experimental evaluation of hyperactivity and food additives. 1977--Phase II. 1977. 134p. (ED 154 588).
Presents Phase II of a three-phase study on the effectiveness of the Feingold diet for hyperactive children. Nine children were challenged with placebo and food items containing artificial colors while being maintained on the elimination (Feingold) diet.

1319 ————. "The Feingold hypothesis: current studies." J Med Soc NJ 76(2): 127-29, February, 1979.

1320 ————. "Food additives and hyperactivity in children." Paper presented at the Annual Meeting of the Nutrition Foundation, Naples, Florida, January 30, 1975.

1321 Harley, J. Preston, and Matthews, Charles G. "The Feingold hypothesis: current studies." Contemp Nutr 3(4): 1-2, April, 1978.
Comments on the diet regimen of Dr. Ben F. Feingold. Dr. Feingold has claimed that the use of the K-P diet, which eliminates artificial flavors, colors, and salicylates from the food of hyperactive children, results in dramatic behavioral improvement for children suffering from this disorder. However, when experimental studies on Dr. Feingold's hypothesis are reviewed, the evidence fails to support the dramatic clinical reports of behavioral change, either qualitatively or quantitatively. The discrepancy between the clinical reports and experimental findings is discussed.

1322 ————. "The hyperactive child and the Feingold controversy." Am Pharm 18(6): 44-46, June, 1978. (14 References).
Assesses previous studies in the area which are generally nonsupportive of the Feingold hypothesis. It is concluded that there may be a small subgroup of younger children who have food allergies. However, drastic changes in national food manufacturing and distribution practices are premature at this time.

1323 ————. "The Wisconsin Hyperkinesis Study--how it all ended." Paper presented at the Annual Meeting, Wisconsin Food Research Institute, Madison, Wisconsin, 1977.

1324 Harley, J. Preston; Matthews, Charles G.; Eichman, Peter. "Synthetic food colors and hyperactivity in children: a double-blind challenge experiment." Pediatrics 62(6): 975-83, December, 1978. (16 References).
Represents Phase II of an earlier study reported in Pediatrics (Item No. 1325). The goal of Phase II was to select those individual children who "best" responded to diet management in Phase I and to further challenge them with specified amounts of synthetic food colors (specially prepared cookies and candy bars) during a nine-week period in which they were otherwise maintained on the elimination diet. Nine hyperactive boys were selected and found, through various tests and scales, not to be adversely affected by the artificial color challenge materials. Although the Feingold hypothesis was not upheld, it is believed that a small subgroup of younger children may display reactions to particular food substances.

1325 Harley, J. Preston; Ray, Roberta S.; Tomasi, Lawrence; et al. "Hyperkinesis and food additives: testing the Feingold hypothesis." Pediatrics 61(6): 818-28, June, 1978. (25 References).
Details a study, using controlled conditions and objective laboratory and classroom observational data, to test the Feingold hypothesis. Thirty-six hyperactive children and thirty-four controls (ages six to twelve years) served as subjects. Numerous measures were obtained under experimental and control diet conditions. All data revealed no support for the Feingold hypothesis. Further studies are recommended, especially those which involve large numbers of younger children. For Phase II of this study refer to Item No. 1324.

1326 Harley, J. Preston; Tomasi, Lawrence; Ray, Roberta S.; et al. An experimental evaluation of hyperactivity and food additives: Phase I. 1977. 207p. (ED 152 019).
Presents Phase I of a three-phase study on the effect of the Feingold (additive-free) diet for hyperactive children. Forty-six families were involved in Phase I. Overall results did not provide convincing support for the efficacy of the experimental diet. For Phase II of the study refer to Item No. 1324.

1327 ————. "Hyperactivity and food additives." Paper presented at the Annual Meeting of the American Psychological Association, San Francisco, California, 1977.

1328 Harper, Patricia H.; Goyette, Charles H.; Conners, C. Keith. "Nutrient intakes of children on hyperkinesis diet." J Am Diet Assoc 73(5): 515-19, November, 1978. (28 References).
Alludes to previous studies relating to the Feingold hypothesis and attempts to determine, apart from the issue of effectiveness on hyperactive behavior, if this diet meets nutritional adequacy. Fifty-four children (ages three to twelve years), reported to have displayed hyperactive behavior for at least two years, served as subjects. Food records were kept for three days. It is concluded that a diet free of artificial colors and flavors does not significantly change the nutrient intakes of children and compares favorably with the Recommended Dietary Allowances.

1329 Hawley, Clyde, and Buckley, Robert E. "Food dyes and hyperkinetic children." Acad Ther 10(1): 27-32, Fall, 1974. (5 References).

Discusses medical procedures for detecting food allergic reactions, particularly food dye allergies, in hyperkinetic children. It is recommended that these children be placed on Dr. Ben Feingold's salicylate-free diet for a two-week period. Foods can then be reintroduced for tolerance. The Feingold diet is suggested as the simplest and most practical method of dealing with the overactive child. The article contains a list of foods, beverages, drugs, and miscellaneous items to be avoided on an elimination diet.

1330 Hindle, R. C., and Priest, Janelle. "Dietary management of hyperkinesis." NZ Med J 88(622): 344-45, October 25, 1978. (2 References).
Letter to editor.

1331 ————. "The management of hyperkinetic children: a trial of dietary therapy." NZ Med J 88(616): 43-45, July 26, 1978. (11 References).
This article reports on an experiment to test the efficacy of the Feingold diet on a group of New Zealand children. Ten children (eight boys and two girls), all attending a clinic for hyperkinetic children, were treated with a modified K-P diet. Although the response to dietary management varied, all children showed some improvement during the first two weeks. This improvement was maintained in five of the children.

1332 Hine, R. Jean. "Hyperkinesis and food additives: a review of current research." Bur Memo 17(3): 10-12, Spring, 1976.
Summarizes the research of Dr. Ben Feingold and others concerning the relationship of food additives and salicylates to hyperkinetic behavior in children. Improvement in behavior is reported in 50 percent of the subjects (according to Dr. Feingold) and about 33 percent of the subjects (according to C. Keith Conners). Additional reports documented include those of the National Advisory Committee on Hyperkinesis and Food Additives and other current studies.

1333 Hirsch, Betty. "From drugs to diet." Coronet 14: 78-82, March, 1976.

1334 Holborow, P., et al. "Feingold diet reply." Med J Aust 1(11): 524, June 2, 1979. (4 References).
Letter to editor.

1335 Johnson, Warren R. "Hyperkinesis: still unsolved and unresolved." Del Med J 50(9): 493, 495-96, September, 1978. (14 References).
Briefly reviews some of the nonmedical approaches to treating the hyperactive child. Discussed in particular are the works of Dr. Ben Feingold (K-P diet) in California, Dr. J. Preston Harley in Wisconsin, and Dr. J. Ivan Williams in Canada.

1336 Kolata, Gina B. "Food additives and hyperactivity." Science 199(4328): 515-17, February 3, 1978. (0 References).
Cites several studies which fail to confirm Dr. Feingold's claims that food additives cause hyperactivity and that 50 percent of hyperactive children dramatically improve while following his diet. Studies referred to are those by J. Preston Harley, Robert Sprague, C. Keith Conners, and Esther Sleator.

1337 Kraus, H. E. "Feingold diet." Med J Aust 1(7): 285-86, April 7, 1979. (1 Reference).
Letter to editor.

1338 Kraus, P. A. "Feingold diet." Med J Aust 1(11): 524, June 2, 1979. (1 Reference).
Letter to editor.

1339 Lane, Alan. "Food additives and hyperactivity." Med J Aust 2(19): 734-35, November 6, 1976. (0 References).
Letter to editor.

1340 Levine, Melvin D., and Liden, Craig B. "Food for inefficient thought." Pediatricts 58(2): 145-48, August, 1976. (7 References).
Comments on a study by C. Keith Conners, et al. (Item No. 1294) concerning the Feingold diet for hyperkinetic children. Discussed are interrelationships among central nervous system function, unwholesome diet, and the diagnosis and treatment of dysfunctioning children. Attention problems are seen to be the common underlying dysfunction. Evaluation of the effect of the Feingold diet upon regulating hyperkinesis needs further study and documentation before final conclusions can be drawn.

1341 ———. "Food for inefficient thought." Pediatrics 61(2): 328, February, 1978. (1 Reference).
Letter to editor.

1342 Levy, F. "Current status of the Feingold hypothesis." Paper presented at Congress of International Association of Child Psychiatry and Allied Professions, Melbourne, Australia, 1978.

1343 Levy, F.; Dumbrell, S.; Hobbes, G.; et al. "Hyperkinesis and diet: a double-blind crossover trial with a tartrazine challenge." Med J Aust 1(2): 61-64, January 28, 1978. (18 References).
This study was designed to meet some of the methodological criticisms of the Feingold diet by means of a double-blind crossover trial with a tartrazine-placebo challenge. Twenty-two hyperactive children (nineteen boys and three girls) were selected for the study and baseline data obtained. The children were tested before and after four weeks on the elimination diet, after a tartrazine and placebo challenge, and again after a four-week washout period on the diet. Results showed a significant improvement of behavior in mothers' ratings after the first four weeks of the diet--a finding not substantiated by objective tests. Other results are given in detail.

1344 Levy, Florence, and Hobbes, Gary. "Hyperkinesis and diet: a replication study." Am J Psychiatry 135(12): 1559-60, December, 1978. (7 References).
Attempts to replicate an earlier study which tested the effectiveness of the Feingold diet on the behavior of hyperactive children. Eight children (seven boys and one girl) met study criteria and were randomly given challenge or placebo cookies for fourteen days. Various scales and tests failed to show significant improvement. Thus, the study did not replicate the significant challenge effect found by Goyette and associates.

1345 Lew, Frances. "The Feingold diet, experienced." Med J Aust 1(6): 190, February 5, 1977. (0 References).

Points out a physician's personal difficulties in having his family follow the Feingold diet. Reiterated are problems involving time in food preparation, food eaten outside the home, less appetizing meals, and the focusing of additional, often unneeded attention, on the problems of one family member.

1346 Lipton, Morris A. "Nutritional fads and the search for mental health." Univ NC Sch Med Bull 21(4): 4-10, Fall, 1975.
Some current nonmedical treatments that have gained popularity in recent years are outlined. Emphasis is placed on: (1) the Feingold diet which advocates the removal of artificial flavorings and colorings in foods for hyperactive children; and (2) L. Pauling's orthomolecular psychiatry which promotes the use of large doses of vitamins for the treatment of mental illness. Although there is a lack of scientific evidence supporting these treatment modalities, the element of hope that the treatment presents can play an important role in the recovery of psychiatric patients.

1347 Mattes, Jeffrey, and Gittelman-Klein, Rachel. "A crossover study of artificial food colorings in a hyperkinetic child." Am J Psychiatry 135(8): 987-88, August, 1978. (8 References).
Reports on a study designed to maximize the likelihood of demonstrating a diet effect in one child whose history indicated clear behavioral improvement on an elimination diet. The child, a ten-year-old boy, was given both placebo cookies and active cookies (with artificial food colorings) for ten weeks in a double-blind multiple crossover design. The results fail to support the contention that artificial food colorings contribute significantly to hyperactive behavior.

1348 Minde, Klaus. "The hyperactive child." Can Med Assoc J 112(9): 1042, May 3, 1975. (1 Reference).
Letter to editor.

1349 National Advisory Committee on Hyperkinesis and Food Additives. Report to the Nutrition Foundation. 1975. 21p. (ED 140 512).
Reviews research on hyperkinesis, with emphasis on the Feingold diet. Guidelines for experimental design are offered, and ethical considerations in future studies are discussed.

1350 ———. Report to the Nutrition Foundation. New York, New York: Nutrition Foundation, 1975. 19p.

1351 ———. Statement summarizing research findings on the issue of the relationship between food additive free diets and hyperkinesis in children. National Advisory Committee on Hyperkinesis and Food Additives, 1977. 10p. (ED 166 890).
Summarizes research findings on the issue of the relationship between food additive-free diets and hyperkinesis in children. The evidence of several challenge studies refutes Dr. Feingold's claim that artificial colorings in the diet aggravate the behavior of children with hyperkinesis and learning disabilities.

1352 ———. Statement summarizing research findings on the issue of the relationship between food-additive-free diets and hyperkinesis in children. New York: The Committee, 1977. 9p.

1353 Neal, B. "Feingold diet." Aust Fam Physician 8(1): 93, 95, January, 1979.
Letter to editor.

1354 Noonan, Roberta L. Nutrition and its effects on a hyperkinetic child's behavior and learning: a case study. 1977. 41p. (ED 161 548).
Reviews literature related to diet, behavior, and learning and describes procedures and results of a change in the diet of an adolescent girl who had an extensive history of problems at home and at school. Treatment of the girl consisted of excluding from her diet foods containing sugar, artificial flavor and color, nitrates, salicylates, MSG, and all foods to which the girl was allergic. The treatment period was two weeks. A dramatic improvement was noted in both behavior and academic performance. A behavior checklist, treatment diet, and results are appended.

1355 Orr, Richard. "Hyperactive children." Nurs Care 9(5): 24-26, May, 1976. (0 References).
Advocates dietary changes, rather than drug treatment, for treating the symptoms of hyperactivity. Comments are made on the Feingold diet.

1356 O'Shea, J. "Sublingual immunotherapy of hyperkinetic children with food, chemical and inhalent allergens: a double-blind study." Paper presented at the 12th Advanced Seminar in Clinical Ecology, Key Biscayne, Florida, 1979.

1357 Palmer, Sushma; Rapoport, Judith L.; Quinn, Patricia O. "Food additives and hyperactivity: comparison of food additives in diets of normal and hyperactive boys." Clin Pediatr 14(10): 956-59, October, 1975. (16 References).
Reports on a comparison study of the consumption of food additives in a group of hyperactive children and their normal peers. Seventy-nine white, middle-class boys of average intelligence (ages six to twelve years) served as subjects. Fifty-six of the boys were patients participating in an outpatient study of hyperactive boys. The boys' parents were administered a dietary questionnaire which was designed to compare the intake of foods high in natural and synthetic salicylates as noted in the Feingold diet. Results of this study show no significant differences in the diet ratings between the hyperactive group and the control group. These findings are in contrast to those of Dr. Feingold. However, it is suggested that hyperactive behavior due to food allergy could be improved by dietary management.

1358 Panjwani, Harry K. "Hyperactive children--problems of coping: what parents, teachers, and doctors should know." Consum Res Mag 60(9): 21-22, September, 1977. (0 References).
Advocates dietary changes for childhood hyperactivity. Success is reported with the Feingold diet plan.

1359 Parnell, Patrick A. "A new breakthrough." Plain Truth 39(1): 36, January, 1974. (0 References).
Briefly describes the Kaiser-Permanente diet. Because hyperkinetic children are plagued with restlessness, short attention span, and poor impulse control, their learning ability at school can be greatly hampered. Traditionally, these children have been treated with drugs, although these can produce harmful side effects. An alternative to drug treatment has been advocated by Dr. Ben F. Feingold of the Kaiser-Permanente Medical

Center in San Francisco. Dr. Feingold reports positive results using a salicylate-free diet with hyperkinetic children.

1360 Powers, Hugh W. S., Jr. "Dietary measures to improve behavior and achievement." Acad Ther 9(3): 203-14, Winter, 1973-74. (10 References).
Explores the relationship between blood sugar and brain metabolism and advocates the use of nutritional modifications to improve behavior/academic performance. Data were gathered from 260 children and young adults. The group underwent a variety of laboratory tests, including a glucose tolerance test. Dietary adjustments in the form of carbohydrate intake and blood sugar were made as necessary. Nine case studies which show the efficacy of the method are cited.

1361 "Proof of the Feingold thesis." Prevention 27(12): 56-57, December, 1975. (0 References).
Reports on a study by C. Keith Conners which has confirmed that removing artificial colors and flavors from the diet of hyperactive children can improve their behavior.

1362 Rapp, Doris J. "A diet that could help the hyperactive child." Consultant 17(5): 33-35ff., May, 1977.

1363 ————. "Food allergy treatment for hyperkinesis." J Learn Disabil 12(9): 608-16, November, 1979. (50 References).
Evaluates food therapy as an alternative method to treat a group of hyperactive patients who responded favorably to dietary management. Eleven children were treated with a food extract after titration food allergy testing. Their behavior remained improved for one to three months while ingesting the foods to which they were sensitive. Five of eight patients completed a double-blind evaluation of the food extract and successfully differentiated the latter solution from two placebo solutions. Two of the three children who failed to identify correctly the food extract relapsed when food therapy was discontinued, then responded favorably when this therapy was resumed. Teachers are urged to be aware of changes in children's activity level after eating or exposure to certain substances.

1364 Roth, June S. Cooking for your hyperactive child. Chicago, Illinois: Contemporary Books, 1977. 271p.

1365 Russell, David G. "Food additives and hyperactivity." Med J Aust 2(17): 661, October 23, 1976. (0 References).
Letter to editor.

1366 Sabo, Ruth. "A therapy that's too simple." Prevention 30(10): 59-61, October, 1978.
Briefly discusses and outlines the major features of the Feingold diet for hyperactive children. The diet, while providing adequate nutrition, is reported often to result in a dramatic improvement in the child's behavior.

1367 Salzman, Louis K. "Allergy testing, psychological assessment and dietary treatment of the hyperactive child syndrome." Med J Aust 2(7): 248-51, August 14, 1976. (7 References).
Explores the efficacy of an elimination diet for the treatment of children with behavior problems and learning difficulties. Of the thirty-one children who were tested for allergic sensitivity to salicylates,

artificial colors, and flavors, eighteen showed a positive response. Fifteen of these children were administered the Australian version of the Feingold K-P diet. Results indicate that 93 percent of the subjects exhibited improved behavior in the areas of overactivity, distractibility, impulsiveness, and excitability.

1368 ————. "Food additives and hyperactivity." Med J Aust 2(15): 582, October 9, 1976. (3 References).
Letter to editor.

1369 Sinaiko, R. J. "Hyperkinesis: diet vs. drugs." Hosp Pract 14(4): 24, April, 1979.
Letter to editor.

1370 Smith, Lendon H. Improving your child's behavior chemistry. Englewood Cliffs, New Jersey: Prentice-Hall, 1976. 228p. (Bibliography).
Attributes early childhood behavior problems to chemical imbalances in the body. These biochemical disorders, when coupled with environmental stress, lead to a number of behavior problems including hyperactivity, distractibility, allergies, eating and sleeping problems, and school and learning disabilities. The outcome of untreated affected children is adult psychopathology. The aim of all treatment, then, is to alter the body chemistry. Suggestions for accomplishing this are outlined. The author also discusses the problem child and the society in which he lives.

1371 Spring, Carl, and Sandoval, Jonathan. "Food additives and hyperkinesis: a critical evaluation of the evidence." J Learn Disabil 9(9): 560-69, November, 1976. (23 References).
Evaluates the Feingold diet which links synthetic food colors and flavors to hyperactivity. Analyzation reveals that: (1) consensual data as to the incidence of hyperkinesis are lacking; (2) clinical trials and uncontrolled studies of the Kaiser-Permanente diet recommended by Feingold are potentially contaminated by placebo responses; and (3) results from controlled investigations of the treatment are equivocal. It is recommended that further public use be ceased until controlled research firmly establishes the efficacy of the diet.

1372 Stevens, Laura J.; Stevens, George E.; Stoner, Rosemary B. How to feed your hyperactive child. Garden City, New York: Doubleday, 1977. 240p.
This book was written to assist parents in preparing meals for their hyperactive children who are on the Feingold diet (an additive- and salicylate-free regimen). Recipes for all areas of average American cooking are given--sauces, soups, candies, cakes, vegetables, meats, breakfast foods, etc. Since tomatoes contain salicylate, two tomato-less recipes for catsup are included, as are plans for birthdays, holiday meals, and teen parties. Helpful appendixes include additive-free brands of food, a two-week menu plan, forbidden and permitted food, and a chart for behavior evaluation. The book is directed toward pediatricians and parents who are trying this treatment on their hyperactive patients and children.

1373 Stine, John J. "Symptom alleviation in the hyperactive child by dietary modification: a report of two cases." Am J Orthopsychiatry 46(4): 637-45, October, 1976. (15 References).
Documents case reports of two hyperactive preschool boys, one exhibiting severe cognition problems and one having emotional problems. The boys

were successfully treated with the Kaiser-Permanente elimination diet after other treatment methods proved unsuccessful. It is suggested that the effectiveness of the diet be further studied, especially for the child who is unresponsive to medication and who may exhibit other learning, developmental, and emotional problems.

1374 "Taking the rainbow out of kid's vitamins. Part II: Hyperkinetic children and the Feingold diet." J Pract Nurs 28(7): 15-16, July, 1979. (0 References).
Lists forbidden foods on the Feingold diet.

1375 "Testing the K-P cure." Hum Behav 6: 42ff., February, 1977.

1376 Tryphonas, Helen. "Factors possibly implicated in hyperactivity: Feingold's hypothesis and hypersensitivity reactions." In: Hyperactivity in children: etiology, measurement, and treatment implications. Edited by Ronald L. Trites. Baltimore, Maryland: University Park Press, 1979. 93-102. (36 References).
Comments on studies conducted to test the Feingold hypothesis as well as other research supporting allergies as causes of hyperactivity. Problems of existing studies are outlined.

1377 Wacker, John A. "Eliminating the additives." Tex Key 12(4): 1-3, December, 1976.
Cites several case studies in support of the hypothesis of Dr. Ben Feingold concerning the effect of salicylates on the hyperactive behavior of children. A possible link between food additives and increased crime is suggested.

1378 Wender, Esther H. "Food additives and hyperkinesis." Am J Dis Child 131(11): 1204-6, November, 1977. (8 References).
Reviews previous studies of dietary treatment of hyperactive children with particular reference to the Feingold diet method. Generally, the studies refute the claims made by Feingold and his followers. As long as favorable behavioral change is noted the diet can be followed, but it should not be utilized to the exclusion of other methods if they appear necessary.

1379 ————. "Food additives and hyperkinesis: in reply." Am J Dis Child 132(8): 820, August, 1978. (0 References).
Letter to editor.

1380 ————. "Hyperactivity and the food additive free diet." J Fla Med Assoc 66(4): 466-70, April, 1979.

1381 ————. "More on food additives and hyperkinesis: reply." Am J Dis Child 133(10): 1081, October, 1979. (0 References).
Letter to editor.

1382 ————. "New findings on food additives and hyperkinesis." Am J Dis Child 132(11): 1149, November, 1978. (1 Reference).
Letter to editor.

1383 Werry, John. "Food additives and hyperactivity." Med J Aust 2(8): 281-82, August 21, 1976. (0 References).
The efficacy of the Feingold diet for hyperactive children is questioned in this editorial.

1384 Werry, John S., and Aman, M. G. "Dietary control of hyperkinesis." NZ Med J 88(621): 297-98, October 11, 1978. (2 References).
Letter to editor.

1385 Williams, J. Ivan, and Cram, Douglas M. "Diet in the management of hyperkinesis: a review of the tests of Feingold's hypothesis." Can Psychiatr Assoc J 23(4): 241-48, January, 1978. (26 References).
Reviews studies in support of and against the Feingold hypothesis, which claims a 30-50 percent success rate. Clinical studies have produced mixed results. Four recent sets of experimental studies are cited which do not support the hypothesis, although some younger children may respond favorably to a diet free of artificial flavors and colors. Additional research should be conducted in the area.

1386 Williams, J. Ivan; Cram, Douglas M.; Tausig, Frances T.; et al. Determining the relative effectiveness of dietary and drug management of hyperkinesis. Working Paper Series, Health Care Research Unit, The University of Western Ontario, London, Ontario, Canada, July, 1976.

1387 ————. "Examining the relative effectiveness of dietary and drug management of hyperkinesis." Paper presented at the Annual Meeting of the Food and Nutrition Liaison Committee of the Nutrition Foundation, Palm Springs, January, 1977.

1388 ————. "Relative effects of drugs and diet on hyperactive behaviors: an experimental study." Pediatrics 61(6): 811-17, June, 1978. (12 References).
Reports on a study to test Feingold's hypothesis that food additives and salicylates contribute to hyperactive behavior in children. Twenty-six children (ages five to twelve years), previously diagnosed as hyperactive and on stimulant medication, were selected as participants. For fourteen weeks they were randomly assigned to various treatment conditions: active or placebo medications in combination with challenge cookies containing artificial flavors and colors or control cookies with no additives. Each child received each treatment. Assessments were made through teacher and parent checklists. Results show stimulant medications clearly more effective than diet in reducing hyperactive behavior. Some evidence indicated that three to eight children could be diet-responsive. Further studies are required to pinpoint subtypes or special populations who might be good responders to a diet free of artificial flavors and colors.

1389 Wire, June E. "Nutrition helped our hyperactive son." Lets Live 42: 38, March, 1974. (0 References).
Relates a mother's report on the success of a special diet in the treatment of her preschool, hyperactive son. The child, exhibiting symptoms of hyperactivity since birth, was treated variously with Atarax, Ritalin, Stelazine, and Dilantine. After the child was placed on a special diet of megavitamins and protein supplement for five months, the mother reports that psychostimulants were no longer needed to control her son's behavior.

1390 Wolf, Alison. "Hyperactive children give food for thought." Times Educ Suppl 3112: 17, January 17, 1975. (0 References).

Comments on the work of Dr. Benjamin Feingold, a California allergist. Instead of prescribing drugs, Dr. Feingold places hyperactive children on a special additive-free diet--a diet designed to eliminate artificial colors and flavors and foods high in salicylates. Dr. Feingold reports that changes in children's behavior are immediate and dramatic, but can be reversed with additive-laden meals. Success is claimed with more than half the patients treated. A list of forbidden foods is included.

1391 Woodhill, Joan M.; Mackie, Leila; Glasheen, Valda. "Doctors' opinions of the Feingold diet." Med J Aust 2(3): 115-16, July 29, 1978. (0 References).

3. MEGAVITAMIN

1392 Adler, Sol. "Megavitamin treatment for behaviorally disturbed and learning disabled children." J Learn Disabil 12(10): 678-81, December, 1979. (17 References).
Reviews literature that gives results of research in megavitamin (or orthomolecular) nutritional therapy. The results primarily portray the treatment as a valid biochemical alternative to other means of therapy.

1393 Arnold, L. Eugene; Christopher, James; Huestis, Robert D.; et al. "Megavitamins for minimal brain dysfunction: a placebo-controlled study." JAMA 240(24): 2642-43, December 8, 1978. (6 References).
Attempts to determine the effects of vitamin supplementation in children with MBD. Previous research of A. Cott is cited. Thirty-one children (twenty-three boys and eight girls) with MBD who had been seen at a child psychiatry clinic served as subjects. They were randomly given either placebo or a megavitamin combination for a two-week period. Results show that only two children (both of the placebo group) responded so well that stimulants were not considered necessary. In general, the difference between placebo and megavitamin groups was not significant. Hyperkinetic behavior was one variable which might have shown some improvement, depending on interpretation. Vitamin therapy is recommended for MBD only if dietary history, certain symptoms, or biochemical findings suggest a specific vitamin deficiency.

1394 Hoffer, A. "Children with learning and behavioral disorders." J Orthomol Psychiatry 5(3): 228-30, 1976.
Advocates the use of vitamin therapy with children suffering from learning disorders, hyperactivity, MBD, and behavior problems. Vitamin B has been found to be particularly successful. Therapy includes vitamin B supplementation and the elimination of sucrose, allergens, and mineral excesses from the diet.

1395 Lall, Geeta Rani. Orthomolecular approach to the treatment of schizophrenia, childhood psychoses, and allied disorders such as: hyperactivity, autism, hypoglycemia and subclinical pellagra. 1976. 15p. (ED 123 858).
Supports the orthomolecular approach to treatment of hyperkinesis. This therapy involves the administration of megavitamins (following a study to determine biochemical needs), proper diet, exercise, and psychotherapy. Advantages of this method are outlined.

1396 Levinson, Michael B. "Megavitamin therapy and hyperactive children." J Am Optom Assoc 46(1): 69-72, January, 1975. (11 References).

Reports on the relatively recent use of vitamins in massive quantities to treat ailments such as schizophrenia, alcoholism, and hyperactivity. Particular attention is paid to the research of Dr. Allan Cott in treating hyperactive children with orthomolecular therapy. This form of treatment concerns optometry due to the many children seen in daily practice and those referred for learning disabilities. Optometrists are urged to keep abreast of future articles and developments in this field.

1397 Nichols V. "The orthomolecular treatment of low blood sugar, hyperkinesis and learning disabilities." In: Cookbook and eating guide. (Available from Virginia Nichols, 3350 Fair Oaks Drive, Xenia, Ohio 45385).

1398 Shaywitz, Bennett A.; Siegel, Norman J.; Pearson, Howard A. "Megavitamins for MBD: a potentially dangerous therapy." JAMA 238(16): 1749-50, October 17, 1977. (9 References).
Provides documentation for the case of a four-year-old boy who suffered a dangerous reaction to megavitamin therapy for MBD. Vitamin A intoxication, found through an abnormal bone scan, had caused irritability, bone pain, fissuring of the lips, and hepatomegaly. Implications are discussed.

1399 Thiessen, Irmgard, and Mills, Laura. "The use of megavitamin treatment in children with learning disabilities." J Orthomol Psychiatry 4(4): 288-96, 1975.
Outlines a treatment regimen using various amounts of vitamins with a group of twenty-four learning-disabled children. After megavitamin therapy these children were compared with nine dyslexic children who had received no treatment. Results of a battery of psychological tests showed no differences between the two groups in spelling and reading. However, children receiving megadoses of vitamins C, B3, pantothenic acid, and B6 (plus a high-protein, low-carbohydrate diet) did show a decrease in hyperkinetic behavior, sleep disturbance, and nystagmus, and an increase in perceptual abilities and basic language skills.

4. PHYSICAL EDUCATION/RECREATION

1400 Clift, John E., et al. "Therapeutic recreation with hyperactive children." Ther Recreat J 11(4): 165-71, 1977.
Therapeutic recreation produced positive results in six hyperactive children except in the area related to their perception of hyperactivity, which remained negative. The project involved the participation of the parents as well as the children; utilized recreational activities, verbal discussions, and behavioral reinforcement techniques; and included follow-up evaluations on how well individual and group goals were attained.

1401 Green, Paul A., et al. "The comparative motor and affective benefits of three physical education programming techniques used with emotionally impaired children." Paper presented at the 59th Annual Meeting of the American Educational Research Association, Chicago, Illinois, April, 1974. 12p. (ED 091 905).
Assesses the efficacy of three physical education programming techniques for improving physical performance and reducing undesirable behavior of ninety-six emotionally impaired hyperactive boys. The study took place in an eight-week summer camp setting. Specific coordination procedures yielded superior performance on the motoric measures, but little change in affective aspects was noted among the various treatments.

1402 McPherson, Irene T. "Control of hyperactive children in recreational activities." Ther Recreat J 11(2): 59-65, 1977. (34 References).
Examines hyperactivity and present methods for its control in recreational activities. Discussed are manipulation of the environment, development of self-control, and effective controlling techniques for the recreation leader. Music and other auditory stimulation, as well as certain visual stimuli, can reduce hyperactivity. "Sense relaxation exercises" (deep breathing, relaxing muscles, and self-directed oral commands) have been found to improve a child's performance. Techniques for use by the recreation leader include reinforcing positive behavior, ignoring disruptive behavior, being friendly to the child, and remaining calm, firm, and consistent.

1403 Mann, Lester; Burger, Robert M.; Proger, Barton B. "Physical education intervention with the exceptional child." In: Second review of special education. Edited by Lester Mann and David A. Sabatino. Philadelphia, Pennsylvania: JSE Press, 1974. 193-250. (87 References). (JSE Press Series in Special Education).
Comprehensively reviews research dealing with the effects of physical education upon physical, cognitive, affective, social and sundry variables. One study by Mann, et al. (1973) is cited on pages 222-23 and involves a hyperactive population. The program reported sought to devise a physical education curriculum which would direct undesirable physical/emotional behavior into purposeful physical activities for several groups of exceptional children. Four groups of twenty-four subjects each (eight aggressive, eight hyperactive, and eight withdrawn) were assigned to four treatments: controls, physical fitness, general coordination, and specific coordination. Results show that regardless of treatment, aggressive children were superior in physical performance to hyperactive children who, in turn, were superior to withdrawn children.

1404 Shoom-Kirsch, Donna. "The effects of a perceptual-motor programme and a physical education-type programme on hyperactive children." For a summary see: Diss Abstr Int 37B(9): 4707, March, 1977. (0 References).

1405 Stein, Julian U. "What research and experience tell us about physical activity, perceptual-motor, and recreation programs for children with learning disabilities." Am Correct Ther J 28(2): 35-41, March-April, 1974. (0 References).
Although this article does not deal specifically with the hyperactive syndrome, it outlines some problems and paradoxes related to the area. Topics include problems of semantics and terminology, research studies that present diametrically opposite findings, conclusions and recommendations, and society's inability to recognize individual differences. A return to basic concepts of various disciplines for programs, procedures, methods, and techniques is urged. Suggestions for reforms are included.

5. RELAXATION TRAINING/BREATHING

1406 Abbie, Margaret. "Treatment of 'minimal brain dysfunction'." Physiotherapy 60(7): 203-7, July, 1974. (36 References).
Stresses the importance of motor training programs to foster academic skills in clumsy learning-disabled children. Attention is focused on the role of the physiotherapist in this treatment.

1407 Bhatara, Vinod; Arnold, L. Eugene; Lorance, Tom; et al. "Muscle relaxation therapy in hyperkinesis: is it effective?" J Learn Disabil 12(3): 182-86, March, 1979. (8 References).
Reviews literature on two forms of muscle relaxation training in hyperkinesis: electromyographic (EMG) biofeedback and progressive muscle relaxation. The authors provide evidence for the following conclusions: (1) conflicting results are reported in the literature; (2) there is insufficient evidence to support the clinical efficacy of EMG biofeedback; and (3) muscle relaxation may have a place in the multimodality treatment of hyperactivity.

1408 Brown, Ray H. "An evaluation of the effectiveness of relaxation training as a treatment modality for the hyperkinetic child." For a summary see: Diss Abstr Int 38B(6): 2847, December, 1977. (0 References).

1409 Cratty, Bryant J. "Hyperactivity: evaluation and remediation." In: Cratty, Bryant J. Remedial motor activity for children. Philadelphia, Pennsylvania: Lea & Febiger, 1975. 253-83. (33 References). (Health Education, Physical Education, and Recreation Series).
Defines hyperactivity and hypoactivity and reviews theories of etiology (developmental, environmental, neurologically based, etc.). Emphasis is placed on remedial strategies and interventions for parents and teachers to use with overactive children. Methods to reduce movement include: (1) altering the environment to reduce or enrich the amount of visual stimulation to which a child is exposed; (2) medication; (3) "movement" methods which encompass relaxation training, impulse-control activities, and strategies which encourage a child to prolong physical acts; and (4) social modeling.

1410 Griffiths, Anita N. "A new look at hyperactivity." Acad Ther 14(5): 597-602, May, 1979. (0 References).
Advocates the use of deep-breathing exercises and brief, strenuous exercise several times a day to help alleviate tension and overactivity in hyperactive children.

1411 Haynes, S. N.; Griffin, P.; Sides, H.; et al. "Relaxation training and electromyographic biofeedback in modification of specific psychophysiological disorders." Paper presented at the Annual Convention of the Association for Advancement of Behavior Therapy, Chicago, Illinois, November, 1974.

1412 "Hyperactive ventilation." Hum Behav 3(12): 36, December, 1974. (0 References).
Six boys (three experimental and three control) served as subjects for experiments demonstrating the influence of respiration on hyperactive behavior. Findings indicate that the children given breathing control and attention training improved in self-control, which, unfortunately, was not generally transferred to other settings, i.e., home and classroom. This method is recommended for use only in specific situations.

1413 Illovsky, Joseph, and Fredman, Norman. "Group suggestions in learning disabilities of primary grade children: a feasibility study." Int J Clin Exp Hypn 24(2): 87-97, April, 1976. (14 References).
Assesses the effectiveness of tape-recorded hypnotic suggestions on a group of schoolchildren. Forty-eight hyperactive children (ages six to

eight years) served as subjects and were taken to a special room for fifteen-minute sessions. During this time they listened to suggestions of relaxation, to ideas for coping with emotional problems, and to suggestions for modifying attitudes toward learning. Data show: (1) forty-five of the forty-eight children functioned better in school according to teachers' ratings; (2) the improvement ranged from decreased hyperactivity to better than average class performance; and (3) significant correlations occurred between percent of relaxation with increased attention span and number of sessions attended with increased self-confidence.

1414 Klein, Stephen A. "Relaxation and exercise for hyperactive, impulsive children." For a summary see: Diss Abstr Int 37B(12, pt. 1), 6334, June, 1977. (0 References).

1415 Klein, Stephen A., and Deffenbacher, Jerry L. "Relaxation and exercise for hyperactive impulsive children." Percept Mot Skills 45(3, pt. 2): 1159-62, December, 1977. (13 References).
Explores the effectiveness of a relaxation and large muscle exercise program in helping the hyperactive child improve cognitive performance. Twenty-four hyperactive third-grade boys were randomly assigned to one of four treatments: muscle relaxation, large muscle exercise, attention-placebo control, and no-treatment control. Treatment lasted three weeks. The Matching Familiar Figures Test and a shortened version of the Continuous Performance Task were administered. Test results show improved accuracy on the matching test, but not on the performance task, suggesting the potential of relaxation and exercise in treating hyperactive and impulsive children. Implications of this treatment are discussed.

1416 Lupin, Mimi; Braud, Lendell W.; Braud, William; et al. "Children, parents, and relaxation tapes." Acad Ther 12(1): 105-13, Fall, 1976. (7 References).
Examines the effectiveness of a treatment program utilizing parents and tape recordings to teach relaxation skills to thirteen hyperactive children. Six commercially prepared tapes for parents and six for children required twenty minutes a day for a three-month period. The tapes for the parents included subjects such as behavior modification and relaxation exercises. The children's tapes contained stories which stressed relaxation in the classroom and how to cope with criticism. The positive results of the program are summarized.

1417 Lupin, M.; Braud, W. G.; Duer, W. F. "Effects of relaxation upon hyperactivity using relaxation tapes for children and parents." Paper presented at the 11th Annual Convention for Learning Disabilities, Houston, Texas, February, 1974.

1418 McBrien, Robert J. "Using relaxation methods with first-grade boys." Elem Sch Guid Couns 12(3): 146-52, February, 1978. (7 References).
Advocates the use of relaxation training to improve hyperactive behaviors of first-grade boys. One case study and a sample outline of a training technique are included. This self-management technique can also be used with children presenting no problem behaviors.

1419 Mantione, Frank F. "A comparison of the effects of muscular relaxation and rest on the behavior of grammar school children described as hyperactive." For a summary see: Diss Abstr Int 36B(10): 5268, April, 1976. (0 References).

1420 Pereboom, Margaret G.; Creaghan, Sally; Meehan, Anne-Marie. "An evaluation of two educational treatment programs for hyperactive children." Dev Med Child Neurol 19(1): 111-12, February, 1977. (0 References).

Abstract of a conference paper presented at the annual meeting of the American Academy for Cerebral Palsy and Developmental Medicine.

1421 Putre, William; Loffio, Kathleen; Chorost, Sherwood; et al. "An effectiveness study of a relaxation training tape with hyperactive children." Behav Ther 8(3): 355-59, 1977. (13 References).

Compares a relaxation tape with a control tape for effectiveness in reducing muscle tension in a group of boys. Twenty hyperactive boys (ages seven to thirteen years) listened to either the relaxation tape (instructions for sequential tightening and loosening of muscles) or the control tape (adventure stories) daily for two weeks. Forehead muscle tension, measured periodically, significantly dropped for both groups. Thus, relaxation tapes may be no more effective than recorded stories for inducing a state of physical relaxation in children.

1422 Rivera, Edelwina. "An investigation of the effects of relaxation training on attention to task and impulsivity among male hyperactive children." For a summary see: Diss Abstr Int 39A(5): 2841, November, 1978. (0 References).

1423 Shaw, William J., and Walker, C. Eugene. "Use of relaxation in the short-term treatment of fetishistic behavior: an exploratory case study." J Pediatr Psychol 4(4): 403-7, December, 1979. (2 References).

Details the use of relaxation training to treat a child for inappropriate and excessive response in the presence of barefoot women. The eight-year-old boy suffered from phenylketonuria resulting in mild to moderate mental retardation and hyperactivity. Tape recordings were used for a six-month period. At follow-up, the boy's strange behavior had virtually been eliminated.

1424 Simpson, D. Dwayne, and Nelson, Arnold E. "Attention training through breathing control to modify hyperactivity." J Learn Disabil 7(5): 274-83, May, 1974. (26 References).

Reports on the use of a behavior modification technique to reduce the hyperactive behavior of a group of elementary schoolchildren. Six hyperactive boys (ages six to eight years), who were students at a school for children with learning disabilities, were participants in the experiment. Three children were assigned to a control group and three were assigned to the experimental group which received attention training through breathing control. The experimental group incorporated biofeedback and operant conditioning principles to help the child develop self-control over his inattentive behavior. Measures obtained before, during, and after training included respiration indices, attention and vigilance test performance scores, and teacher ratings of classroom behavior. Significant improvement of the experimental group supports the effectiveness and feasibility of using respiration recordings to reduce hyperactive behavior. More research in this area is called for.

6. SURGERY

1425 Breggin, Phyllis. "Is psychosurgery an acceptable treatment for 'hyperactivity' in children?" MH 58(1): 19-21, Winter, 1974. (0 References).

Examines the positive and negative effects of psychosurgery for the treatment of hyperactivity in children. Psychosurgery, an operation that destroys brain tissue for the control of behavior, has not been sanctioned or funded by the United States government, although it is performed there and in other parts of the world, especially India, Thailand, and Japan. It is concluded that this controversial technique of management should be discontinued because: (1) the operation is irreversible because damaged brain cells deteriorate rather than regenerate; (2) desired results are rarely obtained since the goal of control is not for the benefit of the child, but rather for adults around him; and (3) unwanted side effects occur, such as blunting personality, learning, and creativity. Since many other types of interventions are possible for the treatment of this syndrome, the trend toward psychosurgery must be halted.

1426 Heimburger, R. F.; Small, Iver F.; Small, Joyce G.; et al. "Stereotactic amygdalotomy for convulsive and behavioral disorders: long-term follow-up study." Appl Neurophysiol 41(1-4): 43-51, 1978. (7 References).

Reports on a retrospective study of patients treated with stereotactic amydalotomy for behavior disorders, including hyperactivity. Fifty-eight patients (ages eight to sixty-one years) whose convulsions and behavioral disorders did not respond to medication and psychotherapy, were treated with surgery between 1963 and 1973. A retrospective study was carried out by a psychiatric research team one to eleven years postoperatively. Using reliable objective methods of assessment, they found that 50 percent of the patients operated on primarily for seizures, 33 percent for uncontrolled conduct disorders, and 50 percent with both conditions seemed improved after surgery. Evidence of increased central nervous system damage was not found.

1427 Older, Jules. "Psychosurgery: ethical issues and a proposal for control." Am J Orthopsychiatry 44(5): 661-74, October, 1974. (52 References).

Briefly outlines the history of the use of psychosurgery which dates back to 1888. Although drugs and electroconvulsive shock have generally supplanted surgical techniques for many years, psychosurgery has undergone an international resurgence in the last decade. Even though proponents of the treatment claim much success, and psychosurgery has a strong and renewed appeal to many, serious ethical issues surround its use. Implications for the hyperkinetic child are given.

7. MISCELLANEOUS

1428 Arnold, L. Eugene; Barnebey, Norma; McManus, John; et al. "Prevention by specific perceptual remediation for vulnerable first-graders: controlled study and follow-up of lasting effects." Arch Gen Psychiatry 34(11): 1279-94, November, 1977. (17 References).

Uses two matched control groups in an experiment to determine which mode of intervention was most helpful. Eighty-six first-grade children, screened as vulnerable to academic failure and behavioral problems, were assigned to one of three groups: (1) channel-specific perceptual stimulation; (2) regular academic tutoring; and (3) no contact. On most measures Group I showed the most improvement. At follow-up one year later Group I continued to show even more dramatic improvement in reading, IQ, and three behavior scales. The value of channel-specific perceptual remediation is explored.

1429 Bhatara, V.; Clark, David L.; Arnold, L. Eugene. "Behavioral and nystagmus response of a hyperkinetic child to vestibular stimulation." AJOT 32(5): 311-16, May-June, 1978. (30 References).
Tests a five-year-old hyperkinetic boy for vestibular function both before and after a four-week regimen of controlled semicular canal stimulation. Results, measured by behavioral instruments, show an improvement in symptoms of hyperkinetic behavior.

1430 Cannon, Phyllis. "Drug therapy and hyperactivity. Should all hyperactive children have a trial course on Ritalin?" Spec Educ Can 53(1): 27-29, Fall, 1978.
Focuses on some of the alternative nondrug treatments available to relieve the symptoms of hyperactivity. Reference is made to professionals in the area such as S. Walker, R. Hall, and B. Feingold to support this viewpoint.

1431 Clark, David L.; Bhatara, V.; Arnold, L. E. "Vestibular-rotational stimulation in the treatment of hyperactive children." Res Relat Child 39: 98-99, March, 1977-August, 1977. (0 References).
Abstracts a report of research in progress or recently completed research. Data are provided on: name of investigator(s), purpose of the study, number and kind of subjects used, methodology, principal findings, duration of research, cooperating group(s), and availability of publication(s). Research Relating to Children is compiled by the ERIC Clearinghouse on Early Childhood Education.

1432 ———. "Vestibular function in hyperactive children." Ohio J Sci 79: 40, 1979. (0 References).
Abstract.

1433 Doman, Glenn J. What to do about your brain-injured child, or your brain-damaged, mentally retarded, mentally deficient, cerebral-palsied, emotionally disturbed, spastic, flaccid, rigid, epileptic, autistic, athetoid, hyperactive child. Garden City, New York: Doubleday, 1974. 291p. (Bibliography).
Reviews the treatment of brain-injured children since 1940. Emphasized is the Doman-Delacato method. Only a few references to hyperactivity are included.

1434 Krippner, Stanley. "An evaluation of NO procedures on children with brain dysfunction." Acad Ther 9(3): 221-29, Winter, 1973/74. (21 References).
Reports on certain therapeutic procedures carried out by Neurological Organization (NO) rehabilitationists. Neural patterns (e.g., crawling, creeping, response to sensory stimulation), which are felt to have been omitted from a child's development, are introduced in a therapeutic program. One such program designed to investigate the effects of the NO regimen on a sample of brain-damaged children is reported in detail. Methodology, measuring devices, and results of the study are given.

1435 Loney, J.; Langhorne, J. E.; Paternite, C. E.; et al. "The Iowa HABIT: hyperkinetic/aggressive boys in treatment." Paper presented at the Meeting of the Society for Life History Research in Psychopathology, Fort Worth, Texas, October 6-8, 1976.

1436 Minde, Klaus K. "The hyperactive child." Can Med Assoc J 112(2): 130-31, January 25, 1975. (6 References).

Briefly reviews the major areas of concern in the drug treatment of hyperactive children and stresses the importance of environmental manipulation in any therapeutic program. Drug therapy will help the hyperactive child to use more effectively the relationships offered to him by his environment.

1437 O'Gara, Mary J. "The child in the middle." J Learn Disabil 7(6): 353-58, June-July, 1974. (0 References).
Presents a case study of a sixteen-year-old LD boy, as told from the experiences and recollections of his mother. The boy, a seemingly bright child, was, at age twelve, doing poorly in school and creating strains on his family. After several years of searching for help from doctors, educators, psychologists, and clinics, the boy was finally diagnosed by a pediatrician as suffering from a specific learning disability. Further evaluations followed and a broad program of support involving school, physician, and home was initiated. Of particular help was the STAAR (Skills, Techniques, Academic Application and Remediation) organization which is devoted to developing a long-range program of identification, diagnosis, remediation, prevention, and research in the area of specific learning disabilities. The boy's success in school and at home is reported.

1438 Quirós, Julio B. de. "Significance of some therapies on posture and learning." Acad Ther 11(3): 261-70, Spring, 1976. (12 References).
Describes a group of symptoms which falls under the category "minimal cerebral dysfunction." Hyperactivity, the principal symptom, is elicited by external stimuli. Therapies must be directed to brain dysfunctions or to postural disorders and consist of correlating the child's anatomical symmetries with modifications of his environment. Principal therapies for posture (reflex activity of the body in relation to space) and learning are outlined.

8. CONTROVERSY

1439 Buckley, Robert. "Hyperkinetic aggravation of learning disturbances." Acad Ther 13(2): 153-60, November, 1977. (13 References).
Comments on a study by Robert Sieben (Item No. 1452).

1440 Cott, Allan. "Reply to Dr. Sieben." Acad Ther 13(2): 161-71, November, 1977. (15 References).
Comments on a study by Robert Sieben (Item No. 1452).

1441 "Diets and other unproved remedies: panel discussion." In: Learning disabilities and related disorders: facts and current issues. Edited by J. Gordon Millichap. Chicago, Illinois: Year Book Medical Publishers, 1977. 155-62. (0 References).
Lists twelve unproven treatments which are said to be investigational in nature. Included are: (1) orthomolecular and megavitamin therapy; (2) minerals and trace elements; (3) lithium carbonate; (4) coffee and caffeine; (5) hypoallergenic diets; (6) hypoglycemic diets; (7) additive- and salicylate-free diets; (8) patterning exercises; (9) visual training; (10) vestibular stimulation; (11) biofeedback alpha-wave conditioning; and (12) fluorescent daylight lighting. Discussion focuses on the additive-free diet.

1442 Doman, Robert J., and Delacato, Carl H. "Concern for the future." [A reply to Dr. Sieben]. Acad Ther 13(2): 215-16, November, 1977. (0 References).
Letter to editor.

1443 Feingold, Benjamin E. "A critique of 'Controversial medical treatments of learning disabilities'." Acad Ther 13(2): 173-83, November, 1977. (0 References).
Comments on a study by Robert Sieben (Item No. 1452). Dr. Feingold reaffirms his position concerning dietary intervention for hyperactive children.

1444 Getman, G. N. "Searching for solutions or perpetuating the problems?" Acad Ther 13(2): 185-96, November, 1977. (14 References).
Comments on a study by Robert Sieben (Item No. 1452).

1445 Harris, F. Gentry. "Support for new methods." [A reply to Dr. Sieben]. Acad Ther 13(4): 480-82, March, 1978. (0 References).
Letter to editor.

1446 Kratoville, Betty Lou. "A parent's view." [A reply to Dr. Sieben]. Acad Ther 13(4): 477-79, March, 1978. (0 References).
Letter to editor.

1447 Mann, Stuart M. "Further studies cited." [A reply to Dr. Sieben]. Acad Ther 13(4): 480, March, 1978. (0 References).
Letter to editor.

1448 Mayron, Lewis W. "Concern for the present." [A reply to Dr. Sieben]. Acad Ther 13(4): 469-76, March, 1978. (24 References).
Letter to editor.

1449 Powers, Hugh W. S., Jr. "A reply to Robert S. Sieben's critique." Acad Ther 13(2): 197-203, November, 1977. (8 References).
Comments on a study by Robert Sieben (Item No. 1452).

1450 Reger, Roger. "Support for Dr. Sieben." Acad Ther 13(4): 476-77, March, 1978. (0 References).
Letter to editor.

1451 Rosborough, Pearl M. "Would an open mind provide prevention?" [A reply to Dr. Sieben]. Acad Ther 13(4): 482-83, March, 1978. (0 References).
Letter to editor.

1452 Sieben, Robert L. "Controversial medical treatments of learning disabilities." Acad Ther 13(2): 133-47, November, 1977. (21 References).
Consists of a physician's criticisms of some of the medical treatments currently used to treat children with learning disabilities. The controversial therapies under attack include: (1) dietary treatments; (2) neurophysiological retraining or "patterning"; (3) sensory integrative therapy; and (4) optometric training. The author believes these areas, supported by anecdotal records rather than scientific testing, must be submitted to peers in the scientific community before being used to treat children with LD. Parents are cautioned not to use their children as guinea pigs for new therapies. The physician's role in diagnosing and treating LD is explored.

1453 ————. "Dr. Sieben responds." Acad Ther 13(2): 216-20, November, 1977. (12 References).
Letter to editor.

1454 Wunderlich, Ray C. "Restoring balance in science and humanism." Acad Ther 13(2): 205-14, November, 1977. (21 References).
Comments on a study by Robert Sieben (Item No. 1452).

H. ROLE OF THE PROFESSIONALS

1. DENTIST

1455 Adler, C. I. "The hyperactive child in the dental office." Bull Eleventh Dist Dent Soc 16(5): 10, May, 1978.

2. NURSE

1456 Anonsen, D. Carol. "The hyperkinetic child." Can Nurse 71(5): 27-29, May, 1975. (3 References).
The hyperkinetic child is described as being overactive, aggressive, rowdy, unable to sit still, disruptive, antisocial, excitable, and inattentive. His intelligence may be normal and neurological tests essentially negative. Children presenting these symptoms can benefit from careful management by parents, teachers, physicians, and the school health nurse.

1457 Barker, D. "Hyperkinesis and its treatment." Aust Nurse J 7(8): 25, March, 1978.

1458 Bolden, Billie. "The nurse practitioner and the child on the Feingold diet." Am J Nurs 75(5): 801, May, 1975. (0 References).
Considers the role the nurse practitioner can play in the successful administration of the Feingold diet. Initially, the nurse reviews the diet with parents and children and completes periodic follow-up evaluations until the dietary routine is established. If response is favorable, Group I foods (those with natural salicylates) may be introduced. Group II items remain excluded.

1459 Cantwell, D. P. "Recognition, evaluation and management of the hyperactive child." Pediatr Nurs 5(5): 11-22, September-October, 1979.

1460 Holmberg, Nola J. "Serving the child with MBD and his family in a health maintenance organization." Nurs Clin North Am 10(2): 381-91, June, 1975. (12 References).
Defines the syndrome of MBD and outlines its major characteristics. Various approaches to management--family education and counseling, medical, and psychotherapy--are outlined. A summary of nursing functions includes: assessment, coordination, counseling, education, referral, and case-finding.

1461 Hutchens, Charlotte. "Subtracting additives." J Pract Nurs 28(7): 13-14, July, 1979. (5 References).
Presents a case report of a nine-year-old hyperactive boy whose behavior improved by diet therapy carried out by a nurse.

1462 Rae, E. "The overactive child." Midwife Health Visit 15: 491-92, December, 1979.

1463 Witty, K., ed. "Problem children: managing the MBD child and his family." Patient Care 8(11): 124-26ff., June 1, 1974.
Highlights the nurse's role in drug therapy with hyperactive children.

1464 Woodard, Patricia B., and Brodie, Barbara. "The hyperactive child: who is he?" Nurs Clin North Am 9(4): 727-45, December, 1974. (14 References).
Discusses the hyperactive child in terms of: characteristics, etiology, diagnosis, and treatment with drugs. The roles of the family, school, and nurse are highlighted. The school nurse should be an active member of the therapeutic teaching team and an aid to the classroom teacher. The public health nurse often assumes the responsibility of the school nurse in some communities, especially during the summer. When it is necessary for the hyperactive child to be hospitalized, the hospital nurse can help keep the child busy, protect him from unsafe situations, and aid in his general supervision.

3. PHYSICIAN

1465 Chamberlin, Robert W. "Management of preschool behavior problems." Pediatr Clin North Am 21(1): 33-47, February, 1974. (40 References).
Summarizes common types of problem behaviors frequently occurring in the preschool population. Children of this age display a wide variety of behaviors that parents find troublesome; these conditions may lead to frequent parent-child conflicts and concern. Few of these preschool behavior problems are "internalized" and therefore most do not require psychotherapy. Management programs, aimed at reducing conflicts and concerns, should include: (1) education about stage-related behaviors and individual differences; (2) better screening methods; (3) an organized approach to data-collecting; and (4) the use of brief intervention techniques. The roles of physician and nurse practitioner are discussed.

1466 Cobrinik, Ralph. "Learning disabilities: the role of the pediatrician; evaluations of patients and families." In: Developmental disabilities of early childhood. Edited by Barbara A. Feingold and Caryl L. Bank. Springfield, Illinois: Thomas, 1978. 15-34. (71 References).
Defines the term"learning disability" and summarizes the role of the pediatrician in this disorder. MBD is discussed under the heading "Diagnostic Categories." The papers published in this book are based on the proceedings of a conference.

1467 Denhoff, Eric. "The responsibility of the physician, parent, and child in learning disabilities." Rehabil Lit 35(8): 226-30, 233, August, 1974. (13 References).
Outlines the role of the physician in the management of the LD child. The physician must have knowledge of neurodevelopment, political sensitivity, a background in pharmacology and the psychosocial aspects of medicine, and an ability to work with the educational system. Further, the physician has major responsibilities in the areas of: (1) advocacy (a principle which guarantees optimal developmental conditions for all children); (2) early identification (including the identification of high-risk infants during the first year of life); (3) the provision of high-quality health care, referral and coordination of professional services; (4) the use of discrimination regarding reliable test data;

and (5) interpretation of the results of the diagnostic-remediation survey to the family. The most serious complications of learning disabilities are the failure to develop the child's potential and the persistence of poor self-image on the part of the child. Included is the official definition of LD by the American Academy of Pediatrics as well as definitions of hyperkinesis and minimal brain dysfunction.

1468 Fearon, David. "Learning disabilities: the doctor's role in diagnosis and treatment." Rem Educ 9(1): 19-22, 1977.
Highlights the role of the physician in diagnosing and managing the child with a variety of learning, emotional, and behavior problems.

1469 Gordon, Neil. "Learning difficulties: the role of the doctor." Dev Med Child Neurol 17(1): 99-102, February, 1975. (5 References).
The role of the physician in managing the child with learning disabilities is discussed in terms of: (1) making the purely medical diagnosis of the child which takes into account vision and hearing disorders, perceptual-motor irregularities, secondary emotional disturbances, home life, and educational underachievement; (2) analyzing and assessing the child's difficulties while consulting other team members--psychologists, occupational therapists, speech therapists, and social workers; (3) seeing that a suitable program of intervention is implemented by parents, teachers, clinics, and special remedial educational facility; and (4) serving as coordinator for the various medical, educational, and parental factions involved.

1470 Haller, Jerome S., and Axelrod, Penny. "Minimal brain dysfunction syndrome: another point of view." Am J Dis Child 129(11): 1319-24, November, 1975. (37 References).
Reviews incidence, causes, characteristics, diagnostic methods, and educational ramifications of the MBD syndrome. Highlighted are the physician's duties: acquainting himself with the syndrome; understanding various diagnostic tests; providing communication with teachers, parents, and the child; and monitoring medications used in therapy. For a commentary on this study refer to Item No. 152.

1471 Hart, Zwi; Rennick, Phillip M.; Klinge, Valerie; et al. "A pediatric neurologist's contribution to evaluations of school underachievers." Am J Dis Child 128(3): 319-23, September, 1974. (11 References).
Focuses on the role of the neurologist in the assessment and identification of children with school problems. One hundred and twenty-nine underachieving children (ages six to eleven years), who had been referred from a variety of sources, and thirty normal children from a public elementary school served as controls. All children were given a battery of tests. Medical histories and neurological examinations were completed by project personnel. Data reveal: (1) gross neurological abnormalities were present in 4 percent of the experimental group; (2) abnormalities occurred six times more frequently in the experimental group; (3) the presence or absence of these signs did not closely relate to achievement or intelligence tests; and (4) no correlation existed between EEG abnormalities and neurological findings. A multidisciplinary approach, including pediatrician, neurologist, and psychologist with training in evaluating neurologically related problems, will most benefit the child with school problems.

1472 Katz, Sidney; Saraf, Kishore; Gittelman-Klein, Rachel; et al. "Clinical pharmacological management of hyperkinetic children." Int J Ment Health 4(1-2): 157-81, Spring-Summer, 1975. (11 References).
Discusses the etiology and treatment of the hyperkinetic syndrome. The syndrome is characterized as a multifaceted entity whose phenomenology and treatment remain unclear. Highlighted is the role of the physician who must maintain close contact with parents and teachers, constantly review treatment strategies, and realize that proper treatment of this syndrome is a time-consuming undertaking. Hyperactive children are best managed in a clinic which has staff available to render a variety of services. Guidelines are set forth for effective management. For a reprint of this study refer to Item No. 688.

1473 ————. "Clinical pharmacological management of hyperkinetic children." In: Progress in psychiatric drug treatment. Volume 2. Edited by Donald F. Klein and Rachel Gittelman-Klein. New York, New York: Brunner/Mazel, 1976. 413-32. (11 References).
Reprints an article from the International Journal of Mental Health 4 (1-2): 157-81, Spring/Summer, 1975. (Item No. 1472).

1474 Levine, Michael S.; Rauh, Joseph L.; Levine, Carolyn W.; et al. "Adolescents with developmental disabilities: a survey of their problems and their management." Clin Pediatr 14(1): 25-32, January, 1975. (8 References).
Calls attention to the special characteristics and problems of adolescents with developmental disabilities by describing a group of children studied at the Children's Hospital Medical Center in Cincinnati, Ohio. Highlighted is the role of the physician who must recognize the varieties of disabilities, be ready to deal with the high incidence of emotional problems, relate to the adolescent, and be aware of the wide range of services (special education, vocational education, legal counseling, etc.) that the adolescent is likely to need.

1475 Litt, Iris F. "The role of the pediatrician in management of secondary school behavior problems." J Res Dev Educ 11(4): 92-100, Summer, 1978.
Suggests ways in which educators, faced with student behavior problems, can learn from, and collaborate with, the pediatrician in management of these problems.

1476 Marsh, George E., II. "Medical practice and research in learning disabilities." In: Gearheart, Bill R. Learning disabilities: educational strategies. 2nd ed. St. Louis, Missouri: Mosby, 1977. 169-84. (70 References).
Clarifies the role of the medical specialist in helping the LD child. The physician must keep school personnel informed on medically related strategies. Emphasis is placed on drug therapy.

1477 Sandoval, Jonathan; Lambert, Nadine M.; Yandell, Wilson. "Current medical practice and hyperactive children." Am J Orthopsychiatry 46(2): 323-34, April, 1976. (7 References).
Analyzes the results of a survey of forty-eight physicians (twenty-one pediatricians) in a California metropolitan area. The physicians were asked to complete an extensive questionnaire detailing the medical and behavioral information they collect in forming a diagnosis of the conditions of which hyperactive behavior is a symptom. The survey's aim was

to elicit from physicians: (1) opinions about the value of diagnostic procedures used in identifying conditions which include symptoms of hyperactivity; (2) preferences for several commonly used diagnostic labels; and (3) preferred treatment procedures for children with these conditions. Survey results show that physicians made their diagnoses primarily on the basis of behavioral indicators and on data gleaned from the child's medical history, rather than from data collected during the physical examination. Further, it was found that of the three treatment interventions (medication, psychotherapy, or special education), medication (especially methylphenidate and dextroamphetamine) was the preferred treatment for childhood hyperkinesis.

1478 ————. "Current medical practice and hyperactive children." In: Behavior therapy with hyperactive and learning disabled children. Edited by Benjamin B. Lahey. New York, New York: Oxford University Press, 1979. 120-29. (7 References).
Reprints an article from the American Journal of Orthopsychiatry 46(2): 323-34, April, 1976. (Item No. 1477).

1479 Silver, Larry B. "Acceptable and controversial approaches to treating the child with learning disabilities." Pediatrics 55(3): 406-15, March, 1975. (56 References).
Reviews various treatment therapies and highlights the role of the physician in helping the child with learning disabilities. Although medications will minimize hyperactivity and distractibility, and psychotherapy may minimize the emotional effects of the disorder, the essential part of treatment rests with special educational therapy. The difficulties of parents, often caught in the middle, are outlined. The current state of knowledge relating to each treatment approach is given.

1480 Stein, Martin T. "Minimal brain dysfunction: a note of caution in management." Clin Pediatr 14(9): 840-41, September, 1975. (0 References).
Relates the personal experiences of a pediatrician working with learning-disabled children in a large urban Navy community. Although many patients showed improvement immediately with medication, it was discovered that a significant number of moderately severe emotional problems were not uncovered, or their severity realized, in the initial evaluation. It is suggested that pediatricians study MBD children within a psychosocial as well as a neurological framework and become more conservative in the use of medications for this syndrome.

4. SOCIAL WORKER

1481 Renstrom, Roberta. "The teacher and the social worker in stimulant drug treatment of hyperactive children." Sch Rev 85(1): 97-108, November, 1976. (0 References).
Describes a social worker's experiences with, and perceptions of, hyperactive children and the school personnel involved with them. Problems considered are: (1) identification; (2) referral; (3) expectations of the student; and (4) termination of medication. For a reprint of this study refer to Item No. 744.

1482 Stambaugh, Harriett M. "Patient care and family counseling. Social work considerations in audits of hyperkinetic reaction of childhood." QRB 3(7): 24, July, 1977. (0 References).

Emphasizes the importance of the social worker's role in assuring optimal care for the child with hyperkinesis. The multidisciplinary audit should include the social worker. Specific process criteria can be established to assess the psychosocial evaluation of the patient, inpatient social work treatment, and follow-up care. Collectively, these criteria provide a mechanism with which to measure psychosocial factors that contribute to hyperkinesis, improvement in the patient's condition, family responsiveness to patient needs, and the effectiveness of the social work department in carrying out its responsibility for treatment of hyperkinetic children.

5. TEACHER

1483 Algozzine, Bob, and Algozzine, Karen M. "Some practical considerations of hyperactivity and drugs." J Sch Health 48(8): 479-83, October, 1978. (20 References).

Presents a guide to psychoactive medication for the teacher and discusses the teacher's role in monitoring medication. Table I lists common drugs, dosage, effects, and side effects. Table II is a drug-monitoring chart for teachers and other professionals.

1484 Allen, K. Eileen, and Turner, Keith D. "Are experimental procedures and service obligations compatible in a preschool program for young handicapped children?" In: New developments in behavioral research: theory, method, and application. Edited by Barbara C. Etzel, Judith M. LeBlanc, and Donald M. Baer. Hillsdale, New Jersey: Lawrence Erlbaum, 1977. 139-50. (7 References).

Uses a case study of a preschool autistic boy with various behavior problems, including hyperactivity, to demonstrate that priorities of busy preschool teachers can be made compatible with those of the experimental behaviorist. Social reinforcement procedures were used to alter hyperactivity. Data are presented which suggest: (1) autistic children are less responsive than normals to principles of behavior modification; (2) teachers can collect reliable data; and (3) the priorities of the educator can be made compatible with an experimental analysis of behavior.

1485 Bosco, James J., and Robin, Stanley S. "Ritalin usage: a challenge to teacher education." Peabody J Educ 53(3): 187-93, April, 1976. (0 References).

Investigates the preparation teachers receive regarding the use of Ritalin in schoolchildren. It is noted that prospective teachers are given little instruction about Ritalin or the policy problems which accompany stimulant drug administration and usage. The need for such education is stressed. For a commentary on this study refer to Item No. 1491.

1486 Brannigan, Gary G., and Reimondi, Robert. "Psychoeducational strategy with the emotionally disturbed LD child." Acad Ther 15(1): 77-80, September, 1979. (2 References).

Documents a case study of a hyperactive eleven-year-old boy presenting social and academic problems. Treatment of the child consisted of helping him develop and maintain a personal relationship with his teacher, modeling appropriate behavior, and suggesting alternate ways of behaving. Social skills improved over a three-month period.

1487 Buchan, Barbara; Swap, Susan; Swap, Walter. "Teacher identification of hyperactive children in preschool settings." Except Child 43(5): 314-15, February, 1977. (4 References).

Uses an ecological approach to investigate the extent to which inappropriate behaviors and differences in attention span provoke teachers to differentiate between highly active and hyperactive children. Six children (three normal and three control, ages four to five years) served as subjects. Hyperactive children entered all subsettings with greater frequency than highly active children.

1488 Calhoun, George, Jr. "Helping the hyperactive child in school and at home without chemotherapy." J Spec Educ Ment Retarded 13(3): 191-94, Spring, 1977. (0 References).
Briefly defines and describes the salient features of the hyperactive syndrome. This syndrome is delineated from hyperkinesis which involves neurological disorders as well as psychological disturbances. In lieu of chemotherapeutic treatment, six suggestions for management are offered for classroom teachers; three tips are given for more effective parental management.

1489 ————. "Hyperactive emotionally disturbed and hyperkinetic learning disabilities: a challenge for the regular classroom." Adolescence 13(50): 335-38, Summer, 1978. (10 References).
Summarizes some of the problems posed to the regular classroom teacher by LD and emotionally disturbed children who are also hyperactive. Hyperactivity is pinpointed as being one of the most demanding problems facing educators today because it is extremely prevalent and difficult to categorize. A distinction is drawn between hyperactivity (resulting from psychological disturbance) and hyperkinesis (resulting from neurological disorders). The role of psychoactive drugs in the management of children displaying excessive activity is briefly discussed.

1490 Calhoun, Mary L. "Teachers' causal attributions for a child's hyperactivity: race, socioeconomic status, and typicalness." Percept Mot Skills 41(1): 195-98, August, 1975. (6 References).
Investigates the variables which might influence the types of causes which teachers infer to explain a child's hyperactive behavior. Eighty teachers and teachers-in-training responded to paragraphs describing a child as hyperactive, with the three factors systematically varied: the socioeconomic status of the child, the typicalness of the behavior in the classroom, and the race of the child. Responses were affected by the described typicalness but not by the described race or sex.

1491 "The fourth 'R'." Hum Behav 3(5): 33, May, 1974. (0 References).
Briefly comments on a study by Stanley S. Robin and James J. Bosco (Item No. 1485) which surveyed 114 elementary schoolteachers to determine their knowledge about Ritalin. Teachers' common misconceptions about the drug are outlined.

1492 Gadow, Kenneth D. "Psychotropic and anticonvulsant drug usage in early childhood special education programs. I. Phase One: a preliminary report: prevalence, attitude, training, and problems." Paper presented at the 54th Annual International Convention, the Council for Exceptional Children, Chicago, Illinois, April 4-9, 1976. 66p. (ED 125 198).
Reports on Phase I of a three-phase study designed to survey teachers and parents of children receiving psychotropic and anticonvulsant drugs for a number of pathological conditions, including hyperactivity. Among other findings it is noted that even though most early childhood special education teachers had received no formal training in the area, most had

had experience teaching children who were receiving drug therapy. There were 208 teachers surveyed.

1493 ———. "Psychotropic and antiepileptic drug treatment in programs for the trainable mentally handicapped." For a summary see: Diss Abstr Int 39A(5): 2866, November, 1978. (0 References).

1494 Greenberg, Jerrold S. "Hyperkinesis and the schools." J Sch Health 46(2): 91-97, February, 1976. (22 References).
Delineates four types of hyperkinesis (maternal deprivation, psychoactive, situational tension, and neurotic tension) and discusses the roles of school and teacher in diagnosis. It is concluded that the educator must be aware of additional social and mental problems which can outlive the syndrome.

1495 Hughes, Robert B. "A comparison of the classroom behavior of teachers with high, average and low referral rates for hyperkinesis." For a summary see: Diss Abstr Int 40B(3): 1370, September, 1979. (0 References).

1496 Johnson, Charles F., and Prinz, Robert. "Hyperactivity is in the eyes of the beholder: an evaluation of how teachers view the hyperactive child." Clin Pediatr 15(3): 222-28, 233-38, March, 1976. (32 References).
Reports on a survey of elementary schoolteachers to determine how they define and manage hyperactive behavior in their students. The survey indicated that teachers and physicians differ on the two items whether in a clinic or classroom setting. For the study 201 children (average age 8.8 years) referred to a child development center for evaluation were rated by teachers and physicians. The physicians rated the children much lower in hyperactive behavior. A questionnaire was also sent to 104 teachers to test their knowledge of hyperactivity. The child's amount of classroom movement was the important variable in labeling the child. The incidence of hyperactivity increased with the age of the teacher. Teacher-physician communication is stressed.

1497 Jones, Nancy M.; Loney, Jan; Weissenburger, Fred E.; et al. "The hyperkinetic child: what do teachers know?" Psychol Sch 12(4): 388-92, October, 1975. (17 References).
Discusses the hyperkinetic child in terms of the school's changing role, the classroom situation, and implications for the school. In an experiment, fifteen elementary schoolteachers were asked to identify the most hyperactive children in their classes. The teachers' scores closely matched those of a clinic. This expertise in identifying a hyperactive population can have advantages over drug treatment methods. Early identification enables behavioral intervention programs to begin early, perhaps avoiding medical referral and treatment for many children.

1498 Mooney, Claire, and Algozzine, Bob. "A comparison of the disturbingness of behaviors related to learning disability and emotional disturbance." J Abnorm Child Psychol 6(3): 401-6, September, 1978. (13 References).
Attempts to ascertain the relationships between a set of behaviors characteristic of emotional disturbance and a set of behaviors characteristic of learning disability and to analyze the relative amount of disturbance of the behaviors to the teacher. Thirty vocational education teachers participated in the study and were asked to complete two checklists.

Differences suggest that behaviors characteristic of emotional disturbance were rated as more disturbing than those characteristic of learning disabilities. Educational implications are discussed.

1499 Murray, Joseph N. "Drugs--classroom learning facilitators?" In: Drugs and the special child. Edited by Michael J. Cohen. New York, New York: Gardner Press, 1979. 63-83. (9 References).
Considers several topics related to the involvement of educators in the issuance of medication to schoolchildren. Areas covered include: (1) the medication concept and the educational system; (2) medication to improve cognition; (3) medication and behavior modification; (4) stimulants and the CNS; (5) the role of the teacher in chemotherapy; (6) a recommended plan for the teacher; and (7) medication guidelines for educators.

1500 ————. "Is there a role for the teacher in the use of medication for hyperkinetics?" J Learn Disabil 9(1): 30-35, January, 1976. (10 References).
Briefly reviews literature concerning stimulant drug therapy for hyperactive children. It is stressed that causal factors, whether organic or environmental in nature, should determine the type of intervention used. Organically based overactive children may benefit from drug therapy, whereas a change in the child's surroundings may be necessary for environmentally based overactivity. The role and special responsibilities of the teacher in dealing with the child, parents, and physician are outlined.

1501 Okolo, Cynthia; Bartlett, Sharon A.; Shaw, Stan F. "Communication between professionals concerning medication for the hyperactive child." J Learn Disabil 11(10): 647-50, December, 1978. (13 References).
Investigates the involvement of school personnel in the administration of medication for the hyperactive child. Data were gathered by means of questionnaires which inquired about the degree of communication between nurses and school personnel. For the study 138 teachers and nine nurses completed the form. Questionnaire data revealed that teachers were not generally aware of the initiation or evaluation of medication therapy for hyperactive children. Part of the communication problem was found to be within the school, between nurse and teacher.

1502 Pavy, Robert N., and Metcalfe, Jean V. The teacher's and doctor's guide to a practical approach to learning problems. Springfield, Illinois: Thomas, 1974. 70p. (0 References).
Provides general suggestions for the diagnosis and management of the hyperactive and learning-disabled child.

Contents: Definition of Learning Disability; The Situation which Poses the Disability; Medical Neurological Evaluation; Physician's Questions; the Teacher's Answers; The Physician as Consultant; Exploration of Learning Problem Behavior; Techniques for Resolution of the Problem; and Philosophy. A subject index completes the volume.

1503 Rich, H. Lyndall. "Teachers' perceptions of motor activity and related behaviors." Except Child 45(3): 210-11, November, 1978. (6 References).
Reports on a study to determine if teachers can accurately identify hyperactivity in their students. Seven teachers failed to correctly dif-

ferentiate among twenty-eight students who demonstrated high and low levels of actual motor activity. Results suggest that the visibility dimension of noncompliant behavior in the classroom is a significant variable in the identification of hyperactivity.

1504 Rodriguez, Alejandro, and Fernandopulle, Gregory C. "Teacher awareness of common psychiatric disorders in children." In: Medical problems in the classroom: the teacher's role in diagnosis and management. Edited by Robert H. Haslam and Peter J. Valletutti. Baltimore, Maryland: University Park Press, 1975. 305-19. (7 References).

Deals with some of the common emotional problems of children--hyperactivity, stealing, lying, cruelty, firesetting, speech problems, school phobia, and truancy. Treatment modalities, e.g., psychotherapy, behavior modification, and medication are briefly discussed. The role of the teacher in recognizing and managing some of these common emotional problems is highlighted.

1505 Scranton, Thomas R.; Hajicek, Joseph O.; Wolcott, George J. "The physician and teacher as team: assessing the effects of medication." J Learn Disabil 11(4): 205-9, April, 1978. (10 References).

Attempts to determine whether classroom teachers can reliably collect direct measurement data which measure educationally relevant tasks. The teacher was used as an information source by the physician to determine the effects of Ritalin on two learning-disabled and hyperactive eight-year-old boys receiving methylphenidate. Five tasks were administered by the teacher under both drug and placebo conditions. Results indicate that: (1) teacher-collected data were very reliable; (2) three of the five measures were sensitive to the effects of Ritalin; and (3) cooperation between teacher and physician is highly desirable.

1506 Small, Beverly J. "The hyperactive child." Todays Educ 63(1): 34-36, January-February, 1974. (6 References).

Briefly discusses the hyperkinetic syndrome in terms of definition, characteristics, possible etiologies, and treatment strategies for the classroom teacher. Specifically, a teacher can aid the hyperactive child by: (1) giving short, interesting assignments; (2) allowing periods of movement activity; (3) creating schedules and routines to help organize the child; (4) giving short and explicit oral directions; (5) providing a stimulus-free study area in the classroom; (6) employing behavior modification principles; and (7) establishing close communication between school and home. In spite of these techniques, specialized medical therapy may still be necessary to further aid the child.

1507 Sprague, Robert L., and Gadow, Kenneth D. "The role of the teacher in drug treatment." Sch Rev 85(1): 109-40, November, 1976. (92 References).

Summarizes the role of the teacher in diagnosing, monitoring, and treating hyperactive children. Several techniques for measuring drug effects are described. Few studies of actual teacher participation and attitudes in the drug regimen are available; these reveal that teachers, although knowledgeable about drug properties, are largely unaware of their utility. The role of the teacher is a passive one, even though the teacher is willing to be a more active participant. Prevalence rates of the number of children receiving drugs are estimated. For a reprint of this study refer to Item No. 744.

1508 Terry, K. "Active help for the hyperactive child." Teacher 96: 55, May-June, 1979.

1509 Weithorn, Corinne J., and Ross, Roslyn. "Who monitors medication?" J Learn Disabil 8(7): 458-61, August-September, 1975. (5 References).
The increase in the use of stimulant drugs to treat childhood hyperkinesis in the last decade has raised a number of major concerns: (1) possible side effects and potential addiction; (2) idiosyncratic patient reaction to various drugs; (3) lack of knowledge about etiology of the syndrome; (4) generalized beneficial effects that have not been demonstrated outside the laboratory; and (5) the lack of follow-up studies. Surveys show that existing programs for monitoring drug administration have been inadequate. Careful monitoring is necessary so that relevant information can be exchanged between physician and teacher. Teachers' perceptions of the appropriateness of activity level and attention span are significantly related to their involvement with the child's physician.

1510 Welsch, Ellen B. "You may not know it, but your schools probably are deeply into the potentially dangerous business of teaching with drugs." Am Sch Board J 161(2): 41-45, February, 1974. (0 References).
Comments on the role of the school official and teacher in the use of medication by hyperactive children. Because the teacher is often a primary source of information upon which the decision to administer drugs is made, it is imperative that the diagnosis be correct. Four suggestions are offered for the educational setting: (1) school boards should develop guidelines for the use of drugs within the school context; (2) the community and the schools should be informed about hyperkinesis and about the characteristics and uses of drugs to treat hyperkinesis; (3) school personnel should receive in-service training about hyperkinesis; and (4) teacher colleges should instruct prospective teachers about the characteristics of behavior modification drugs. Two additional sections are: "What school leaders should know about hyperkinetic school children" and "About teachers and Ritalin."

1511 Wilson, Nancy O. "An autumn letter to teacher." Early Years 8(1): 38, September, 1977. (0 References).
Letter to editor.

1512 Zukow, Arnold H. "Helping the hyperkinetic child." Todays Educ 64(4): 39-41, November-December, 1975. (9 References).
Defines the hyperkinetic syndrome and presents a case study of a six-and-one-half-year-old boy. Teachers can be important partners in identifying hyperkinetic children and in carrying out the proper therapy with them.

6. OTHER

1513 Shrier, Diane K. "Memo to day care staff: helping children with minimal brain dysfunction." Child Welfare 54(2): 89-96, February, 1975. (7 References).
Highlights the role of day-care personnel in the identification of children with LD and MBD. Two important aspects involve recognizing the emotional and psychological factors and counseling parents to aid the MBD child. Day-care personnel are urged to become familiar with signs of MBD, since they are frequently the first professionals to come in contact with children.

I. THE MULTIDISCIPLINARY APPROACH

1514 Ambrosino, Salvatore V. "MBD: its diagnosis and treatment." Med Times 103(9): 70-81, September, 1975. (0 References).
Defines minimal brain dysfunction and outlines its major symptoms and causes. The need for a multidisciplinary approach to successful management is stressed, and various therapeutic modalities are discussed.

1515 Browning, Diane H. "Before giving drugs for hyperkinesis." Drug Ther Bull 5: 42-45, 49, 52-53, September, 1975. (8 References).
The author discusses hyperkinesis in regard to its: (1) definition; (2) characteristics; (3) differential diagnosis; and (4) drug therapy. It is suggested that if it is necessary to administer stimulant drugs, they should be accompanied by remedial education, parental counseling, and psychotherapy when indicated. In addition, drug-free periods, periodic reevaluation, and careful follow-up are essential corollaries for successful treatment.

1516 Feighner, Anne C., and Feighner, John P. "Multimodality treatment of the hyperkinetic child." Am J Psychiatry 131(4): 459-63, April, 1974. (39 References).
Describes a comprehensive program for the diagnosis and treatment of the hyperkinetic child. Evaluation included developmental history, physical examination, and assessment of mental status, activity level, soft neurological signs, and family relations. Treatment was multidisciplinary and involved drug therapy (methylphenidate and dextroamphetamine), group education of parents and teachers, behavior modification, classroom and curricular counseling, and psychotherapy. The program allowed for progression at the child's pace in order to ensure continuity of both care and development. Long-term follow-up is recommended to statistically validate this treatment approach.

1517 Gensemer, Ira B. "Psychological aspects of hyperactivity." Paediatrician 3(6): 329-35, 1974. (23 References).
Emphasizes the importance of the multidisciplinary approach in treating the hyperactive child. Various assessment tools can aid the clinician in proper diagnosis. Psychotherapy, pharmacology, and remedial education are advocated as the most effective ways to manage this syndrome.

1518 Goldstein, Earl H. "A multidisciplinary evaluation of children with learning disabilities." Child Psychiatry Hum Dev 5(2): 95-107, Winter, 1974. (2 References).
Documents five clinical case studies of children with learning problems. The clinical application of the definition of the learning-disabled child is discussed in relationship to the cases. An informal educational evaluation for the physician in residency and in practice to recognize the learning-disabled child is outlined in detail. The role of the neurological examination and electroencephalogram in the field of learning disabilities is reviewed. A multidisciplinary approach is proposed for the evaluation and treatment of these children.

1519 Kappelman, Murray M. "Basis of learning disorders: management implications." Child Psychiatry Hum Dev 5(3): 166-73, Spring, 1975. (16 References).
Categorizes potential etiologies of learning disorders in order to formulate various management strategies. Both organic and functional causes are listed and explained. The physician must: (1) consider a number of

possibilities for impairments in learning; (2) use caution when labeling a child with specific entities, thus excluding the possibility of secondary and tertiary causes; and (3) become a functioning member of a professional diagnostic management team composed of teacher, school nurse, social worker, psychologist, speech and hearing clinician, and special educator.

1520 ————. "Management and chemotherapy of hyperactivity in children." Med Dig 13-17, January, 1976.
Reviews research on the use of drugs in the management of hyperkinetic children with minimal brain dysfunction. The most important aspect in diagnosis, evaluation, and treatment is seen to be the team approach—one involving professionals, parents, and the child himself. The use of cerebral stimulants, tranquilizers, and sedatives is discussed along with results of research studies.

1521 Laybourne, Paul C. "Psychiatric response to the minimal brain dysfunction child." In: Learning disability/minimal brain dysfunction syndrome: research perspectives and applications. Edited by Robert P. Anderson and Charles G. Halcomb. Springfield, Illinois: Thomas, 1976. 126-38. (8 References).
Defines the syndrome and stresses the importance of a multidisciplinary approach, including psychotherapy, in the management of the hyperkinetic child.

1522 Machanick, Sonia. "The management of a child with a learning disability." S Afr Med J 48(17): 753-56, April 13, 1974. (9 References).
After an accurate assessment has been made of a child with a learning disability, a carefully planned program of management must be designed. Ideally this program is carried out by a team which includes medical, paramedical, psychological, and educational professionals. The involvement of the parent is not only desirable but necessary to the child's improvement. Remedial after-school lessons and remedial classes or schools may be valuable in giving each child the help needed to reach an attainable goal.

1523 Mira, Mary, and Reece, Carol Ann. "Medical management of the hyperactive child." In: Principles and techniques of intervention with hyperactive children. Edited by Marvin J. Fine. Springfield, Illinois: Thomas, 1977. 47-76. (61 References).
This chapter describes an optimal program of medical management of hyperactive children and the rationale for such a program. Adequate medical management requires a broad spectrum of evaluation and treatment which uses a team of people willing to participate in the program. The team can assist in collecting data that will help in defining the child's problem (to ensure that the treatment program is being administered) and in updating information concerning the direction of the child's behavior change. Description and assessment of the child's problem include an investigation of his environment, measurement of the severity of the disorder, and constant monitoring. Medical management of the syndrome must always be a part of a broader spectrum of evaluation and treatment.

1524 Morrison, Thomas L., and Thomas, M. Duane. "Judgments of educators and child-care personnel about appropriate treatment for mentally retarded or normal, overactive or withdrawn boys." J Clin Psychol 32(2): 449-52, April, 1976. (6 References).

Investigates the effects of mental retardation on professionals' perceptions about appropriate treatment for a child with a behavior disorder. Special educators and child-care personnel ranked the appropriateness of various psychological treatments for a seven-year-old boy described either as withdrawn or overactive. The predicted IQ level by behavior interaction was found only for drug treatment. Drug treatment was ranked as relatively more appropriate for the retarded overactive child. Drug treatment and behavior modification were perceived as more suitable for the overactive child. For the withdrawn child, play therapy, family therapy, and no treatment were deemed more appropriate. Educators favored behavior modification and school consultation more than did child-care personnel.

1525 Newton, Jerry. "Minimal brain dysfunction: toward an understanding between school and physician." JAMA 235(23): 2524-25, June 7, 1976. (0 References).

This editorial comments on the necessity for close interdisciplinary teamwork between physician and educator in treating the child with minimal brain dysfunction.

1526 Ross, Roslyn P. "Drug therapy for hyperactivity: existing practices in physician-school communication." In: Drugs and the special child. Edited by Michael J. Cohen. New York, New York: Gardner Press, 1979. 99-109. (13 References).

Advocates the establishment and maintenance of structured communication among physician, school personnel, and parents. Structured and standardized teacher rating forms and reporting forms for physicians need to be developed.

1527 Rosser, Pearl L. "Minimal brain dysfunction in children." Compr Ther 4(9): 22-28, September, 1978. (15 References).

Discusses the MBD syndrome according to definitions, etiology, signs and symbols, diagnosis, and treatment. The main points of the presentation are: (1) the physician is important in identifying and treating children with MBD; (2) a multidisciplinary approach is necessary in both diagnosis and treatment; and (3) pharmacotherapy should be used only when indicated and only then after a complete diagnostic assessment.

1528 Satterfield, James H.; Cantwell, Dennis P.; Satterfield, Breena T. "Multimodality treatment: a one-year follow-up of 84 hyperactive boys." Arch Gen Psychiatry 36(9): 965-74, August, 1979. (24 References).

Reports first-year findings of a three-year study of the efficacy of the multimodality approach to the problem of hyperkinesis. Eighty-four hyperactive boys and a therapeutic team are involved in the study. Preliminary findings suggest that the combination of medication with appropriate psychological treatments will have a promising outcome.

1529 Schour, Marianne, and Clemmens, Raymond L. "Fate of recommendations for children with school-related problems following interdisciplinary evaluation." J Pediatr 84(6): 903-7, June, 1974. (13 References).

Surveys the extent to which medical recommendations were used by schools and parents. Ninety-four regular classroom elementary schoolchildren with learning and/or behavior problems were subjects for the study. Nine to fifteen months after the clinical evaluation, original recommendations were divided into recommendations to parents, mental health recommendations, and recommendations to the schools. Results of questionnaires revealed that 73 percent of the recommendations to the schools were implemented; 69 percent of the recommendations to parents were implemented. The sole factor associated with increased implementation was the relevance of the recommendation to the child's learning problem. Further studies are needed to determine whether multiple channel communications are beneficial to the child.

1530 Swidler, Howard J., and Walson, Philip D. "Hyperactivity: a current assessment." J Fam Pract 9(4): 601-8, October, 1979. (44 References).

Analyzes the hyperactive child relating to: (1) incidence; (2) etiologies; and (3) traditional and nontraditional therapies. The most important consideration in therapy is that of defining specific problem areas for each child and assuring that each is dealt with appropriately. The importance of the multimodal approach is stressed.

VI. Physiological, Psychological, and Related Research

A. ACTIVITY LEVEL

1. DRUG

1531 Post, Georgia R. "The differentiation of two types of hyperactive children by activity level and task performance with methylphenidate (Ritalin) and placebo." For a summary see: Diss Abstr Int 35B(5): 2444, November, 1974. (0 References).

1532 Wade, Michael G. "Effects of methylphenidate on motor skill acquisition of hyperactive children." J Learn Disabil 9(7): 443-47, August-September, 1976. (7 References).
Investigates motor performance of hyperactive children given methylphenidate or placebo, and compares these children's performance with that of a group of normal children. Subjects for the study, twelve hyperactive and twelve normal children (ages eight to twelve years), were tested on an experimental task which required them to maintain their equilibrium on a square platform. The platform rotated on a central axis. The task took two sessions of thirty thirty-second trials with a thirty-second intertrial interval. Hyperactive subjects first received methylphenidate at one session and a placebo at the second. Data indicate that the hyperactive children performed more like normal controls while receiving methylphenidate than when receiving placebo.

1533 Witt, P.; Ellis, M.; Sprague, R. "Methylphenidate and free range activity in hyperactive children." Urbana, Illinois: Children's Research Center, University of Illinois, 1974.
Unpublished paper.

2. NONDRUG

1534 Hamner, James D. "A behavioral and telemetric analysis of hyperactivity." For a summary see: Diss Abstr Int 37B(12, pt. 1): 6326, June, 1977. (0 References).

1535 Keogh, Jack. "Movement outcomes as conceptual guidelines in the perceptual-motor maze." J Spec Educ 12(3): 321-29, Fall, 1978. (6 References).
Proposes three types of outcomes as guidelines for understanding movement in relation to learning problem theories and programs for perceptually handicapped children. Two outcomes are viewed as direct: movement control and movement behavior. Interpretations and applications of skills, behaviors, and experiences are shown in relation to clumsiness, hyperactivity, and perceptual-motor problems.

1536 Montagu, J. D., and Swarbrick, Linda. "Hyperkinesis: the objective evaluation of therapeutic procedures." Biol Psychol 2(2): 151-55, 1974.

Describes two methods for measuring the unrestricted movements of a hyperkinetic child in an experimental room. One method makes use of an ultrasonic system which quantifies all motor activity. The second method monitors only locational changes: it employs a matrix of electric pressure mats under the carpet.

1537 Shaffer, D.; McNamara, Nancy; Pincus, J. H. "Controlled observations on patterns of activity, attention, and impulsivity in brain-damaged and psychiatrically disturbed boys." Psychol Med 4(1): 4-18, February, 1974. (46 References).

Investigates three aspects of hyperkinesis: (1) the psychiatric correlates of activity; (2) the neurological correlates of activity; and (3) the consistency of overactivity and inattention. Subjects were selected from among the five- to eight-year-old boys registered as outpatients at a hospital. Objective measurements, by means of the actometer and stabilimeter, were obtained over a three-month period. The following conclusions are reached: (1) overactivity is a function of psychiatric disturbance rather than of an abnormality of the central nervous system; (2) environmental conditions affect behavior; (3) a global concept of overactivity is of dubious validity; and (4) studies of the hyperactive child should include some form of objective observation technique in the original selection of subjects, rather than selection based solely on subjective reports.

1538 ————. "Controlled observations on patterns of activity, attention, and impulsivity in brain-damaged and psychiatrically disturbed boys." In: Annual progress in child psychiatry and child development, 1975. Edited by Stella Chess and Alexander Thomas. New York, New York: Brunner/Mazel, 1975. 281-300. (46 References).

Reprints an article from Psychological Medicine 4(1): 4-18, February, 1974. (Item No. 1537).

1539 Smith, Katharine C. "Behavioral correlates of motor impersistence in kindergarten children." For a summary see: Diss Abstr Int 34B(11): 5693-94, May, 1974. (0 References).

B. AROUSAL/UNDERAROUSAL

1. DRUG

1540 Barkley, Russell A., and Jackson, Thomas L. "Hyperkinesis, autonomic nervous system activity and stimulant drug effects." J Child Psychol Psychiatry 18(4): 347-57, September, 1977. (34 References).

Investigates the relationship of the resting level of autonomic arousal and hyperkinetic behaviors to stimulant drug responses. Twelve hyperactive boys (ages five to twelve years) and twelve normal controls served as subjects. The results of a double-blind placebo-controlled crossover study of methylphenidate indicate that: (1) there were no significant differences between hyperkinetic and normal boys in psychophysiological activity; (2) no consistent relationship existed between this activity and the objective behavioral measures in either normal or hyperkinetic boys; (3) the drug did not produce an important effect on autonomic activity; (4) no simple level-of-arousal hypothesis can account for hyperkinetic behavior; and (5) the level of arousal is not a reliable predictor of drug response in hyperkinetic children.

1541 Fehr, F. S., and Sprague, R. L. "The effects of methylphenidate on two flash thresholds and physiological arousal of behavioral problem children as a function of rest and distraction conditions." Paper presented at a meeting of the Society for Psychophysiological Research, Monterey, California.

1542 Ferguson, H. Bruce; Simpson, Suzanne; Trites, Ronald L. "Psychophysiological study of methylphenidate responders and nonresponders." In: The neuropsychology of learning disorders: theoretical approaches. Edited by Robert M. Knights and Dirk J. Bakker. Baltimore, Maryland: University Park Press, 1976. 89-97. (Bibliography).
Compares arousal levels of hyperactive good and poor responders to those of methylphenidate and nonhyperactive LD children. Heart rate and skin conductance were used to assess arousal level. No consistent pattern of group differences emerged, suggesting that theories proposing arousal level differences among various classes of children may be oversimplifications.

1543 Kohn, Herbert; Pipher, David; Contessa, Cynthia. "Underarousal in MBD hyperactivity?" In: Psychopharmacology of childhood. Edited by D. V. Siva Sankar. Westbury, New York: PJD Publications, 1976. 75-85. (18 References).
The hypothesis that methylphenidate administration would result in an increase of arousal level in hyperactive children is investigated. Eight boys (ages six to twelve years) were given EEGs under drug and no-drug conditions. Tracings obtained failed to support the hypothesis.

1544 Satterfield, James H., and Cantwell, Dennis P. "CNS function and response to methylphenidate in hyperactive children." Psychopharmacol Bull 10(4): 36-37, October, 1974. (6 References).
Briefly summarizes the findings of four of the authors' previous studies on hyperactive children. The central theme for all studies is that those hyperactive children who respond best to stimulant medication (usually methylphenidate) are the ones who have low central nervous system (CNS) arousal levels before treatment. The studies involved normal IQ boys (ages six to nine years). Also proposed is a neurophysiological model that is consistent for research studies with animals as well as children.

1545 Satterfield, James H.; Cantwell, Dennis P.; Lesser, Leonard I.; et al. "CNS arousal level and response to stimulant drug treatment in hyperactive children." In: Psychopharmacology of childhood. Edited by D. V. Siva Sankar. Westbury, New York: PJD Publications, 1976. 45-57. (25 References).
Reports findings of four studies of hyperactive children which suggest that children who respond best to stimulant medication have low central nervous system (CNS) arousal levels before treatment. A number of neurophysiological and clinical predictors of response to treatment are discussed.

1546 Satterfield, James H.; Cantwell, Dennis P.; Satterfield, Breena T. "Pathophysiology of the hyperactive child syndrome." Arch Gen Psychiatry 31(6): 839-44, December, 1974. (57 References).

Summarizes four previous studies of hyperactive children which suggest that hyperactive children who respond best to stimulant medication are those who have low central nervous system (CNS) arousal levels before treatment. All studies involved boys (ages six to nine years) referred to a children's clinic for evaluation and treatment. Following tests, a three-week treatment with methylphenidate was carried out and teacher ratings obtained. Results reported show that: (1) there is an identifiable subgroup of "good responder" hyperactive children who are found to have low CNS arousal; (2) the lower the CNS arousal level, the more pronounced are the child's problems; (3) stimulant medication increases CNS arousal level; and (4) those hyperactive children with greatest increases in CNS arousal level resulting from stimulant medication obtained the best clinical response as measured by teacher rating scales.

1547 ————. "Pathophysiology of the hyperactive child syndrome." In: Annual progress in child psychiatry and child development, 1975. Edited by Stella Chess and Alexander Thomas. New York, New York: Brunner/Mazel, 1975. 311-24. (57 References).
Reprints an article from the Archives of General Psychiatry 31(6): 839-44, December, 1974. (Item No. 1546).

1548 Shouse, Margaret N., and Lubar, Joel F. "Physiological basis of hyperkinesis treated with methylphenidate." Pediatrics 62(3): 343-51, September, 1978. (22 References).
Reports on a study to determine the primacy of physiological arousal or motor activation levels in predicting the number of developmental problems, current symptoms, and response to methylphenidate in two groups of children. Twelve medicated hyperactive boys (ages six to twelve years) and twelve unmedicated controls served as subjects. All children were tested on auditory evoked responses, galvanic skin conductance, arousal, and motor activation. Results, given in detail, indicate that physiological measures fail to distinguish hyperkinetic children, although four children were diagnosed as hypoactive. A discussion of the arousal hypothesis in relation to these findings is included.

1549 Spring, Carl; Greenberg, Lawrence; Scott, Jimmy; et al. "Electrodermal activity in hyperactive boys who are methylphenidate responders." Psychophysiology 11(4): 436-42, July, 1974. (9 References).
Analyzes the results of a study of which the objectives were to: (1) determine if the arousal level of drug responders is consistently lower, when their medication is withheld, than that of normal boys; and (2) determine the effect of methylphenidate on arousal level after extended periods of drug treatment. Two groups of hyperactive boys (ages nine to ten years) and one group of normal matched controls were tested. Electrodermal measures were recorded including basal resistance, frequency of nonspecific responses, specific response amplitude to an auditory signal, and number of trials to habituation. Among other results it is seen that: (1) normal and off-drug hyperactive groups differed significantly on specific response amplitude and trials to habituation; (2) frequency of nonspecific responses was significant; and (3) lower reactivity in the off-drug group was evident.

1550 Zahn, Theodore P.; Little, Betsy C.; Wender, Paul H. "Pupillary and heart rate reactivity in children with minimal brain dysfunction." J Abnorm Child Psychol 6(1): 135-47, March, 1978. (16 References).

Attempts to replicate and extend previous findings on autonomic arousal and responsivity in children with diagnoses of MBD. Thirty-two MBD and forty-five control children participated in the study and were tested on pupil size, heart rate, skin conductance, and skin temperature. The MBD group was tested both on and off stimulant medication using a crossover design. A higher arousal level was noted in drug-free MBD children. Although this finding is incompatible with the low arousal hypothesis of MBD, it is consistent, however, with a previous report of the effects of a stimulating environment on MBD children.

2. NONDRUG

1551 Altschuler, Ellen, and Farley, Frank H. "Hyperactivity as a function of intrinsic arousal level and stimulation-seeking." Paper presented at the Annual Meeting of the American Education Research Association, New York, New York, April, 1977. 14p. (ED 145 352).
Investigates physiological arousal and overt behaviors in hyperactive and normal children. The study further examined Farley's theory that hyperactive children would exhibit lower arousal and a stronger stimulation-seeking motive than what is normally seen in children. However, this was not generally shown to be true.

1552 Grüenwald-Zuberbier, E.; Grüenwald, G.; Rasche, A. "Hyperactive behavior and EEG arousal reactions in children." Electroencephalogr Clin Neurophysiol 38(2): 149-59, February, 1975. (27 References).
Studies EEG arousal reactions and parameters of spontaneous EEG activity in two groups of children. Eleven hyperactive children and eleven nonhyperactive children (median age 12.2 years) served as subjects. EEGs were recorded in three reaction-time experiments: a tone-light conditioning paradigm and two series with random stimulation. The main findings of the study are: (1) hyperactive children, in periods free from stimulation, have a lower state of EEG arousal; (2) the amplitude reduction to tone develops more slowly in the hyperactive group; (3) hyperactive children have shorter arousal responses to the light stimulus; (4) hyperactive children show longer latencies in reaction-time performance; and (5) although conditional changes in the arousal reactions to both stimuli are reliably demonstrated in all children, the groups show no difference in the corresponding measures.

1553 Hastings, James E., and Barkley, Russell A. "A review of psychophysiological research with hyperkinetic children." J Abnorm Child Psychol 6(4): 413-47, December, 1978. (85 References).
Comprehensively reviews and evaluates prior literature related to arousal theories concerning the hyperactive syndrome. Section I deals with psychophysiological differences between hyperactive and normal children on such variables as cardiovascular system, electrodermal measures, EEG, EEG abnormalities, and cortical evoked responses. Section II covers stimulant drug effects on these physiological measures in hyperactive children. Included are measures of the cardiovascular system, electrodermal, sleep studies, EEG responses to drugs, and cortical evoked responses. In general, it is concluded that hyperactive children do not typically differ from normal children in measures of resting average cardiac rate activity. Studies using CNS measures underscore the possibility of underarousability. Research to date finds stimulant drugs energizing rather than sedative on psychophysiological measures; drugs heighten the impact of stimulation to the nervous system. Theoretical implications and suggestions for future research are offered.

1554 Kleemeier, C. P. "A comparative evaluation of the theoretical relationship between arousal and learning as demonstrated by the hyperkinetic syndrome." Atlanta, Georgia: Department of Psychology, Emory University, 1974.
Unpublished comprehensive examination paper.

1555 Koester, Lynne S. "Arousal and hyperactivity in open and traditional education: test of a theory." For a summary see: Diss Abstr Int 37A(9): 5703-4, March, 1977. (0 References).

1556 Koester, Lynne S., and Farley, Frank H. "Arousal and hyperactivity in open and traditional education." Paper presented at the Annual Convention of the American Psychological Association, San Francisco, California, August 26-30, 1977. 11p. (ED 155 543).
Tests the prediction that open classrooms provide children possessing low arousal levels with enough external stimulation to reduce their overt seeking of stimulation. Ninety-eight children in three open and three traditional classrooms served as subjects. A discussion of Farley's theory and results of the study are included.

1557 Montagu, J. D. "The hyperkinetic child: a behavioural electrodermal and EEG investigation." Dev Med Child Neurol 17(3): 299-305, June, 1975. (12 References).
Ten hyperactive children were individually matched with a group of normal controls for age and sex. They were then compared on the basis of behavioral measurements, electrodermal recordings, and spectral analysis of the EEG. The behavioral measures differentiated the two groups in the predicted directions. The groups did not differ significantly in respect to the skin admittance level or the EEG alpha rhythm propagation time. The findings do not support the hypothesis that hyperkinetic children are underaroused.

C. ATTENTION/DISTRACTION/VIGILANCE

1. DRUG

1558 Bambrick, James R. "Effect of two levels of methylphenidate hydrochloride for hyperkinetic children on measures of attention and mother-child interaction." For a summary see: Diss Abstr Int 40B(4): 1876, October, 1979. (0 References).

1559 Barkley, Russell A. "The effects of methylphenidate on various types of activity level and attention in hyperkinetic children." J Abnorm Child Psychol 5(4): 351-69, December, 1977. (26 References).
Studies the effects of methylphenidate on various measures, in various settings, on a group of children. Eighteen hyperactive boys (ages five to twelve years) and eighteen controls participated in the experiment and were tested on three repeated occasions in free play, movie viewing, testing, and restricted play periods. Methylphenidate significantly reduced seat movement activity in the hyperactive children in all settings. Drug effects were less noted on measures of concentration or attention. Improvement was also seen in parent ratings of their children's activity levels. Despite positive drug effects, it is concluded that methylphenidate may have reduced the interest of some children in their environment.

1560 Charles, Linda; Schain, Richard J.; Zelniker, Tamar; et al. "Effects of methylphenidate on hyperactive children's ability to

sustain attention." Pediatrics 64(4): 412-18, October, 1979. (20 References).
Investigates the attentional characteristics of hyperactive children, the relationship of subjective and objective measures of these characteristics, and the effects of methylphenidate on these measures of attention. Forty-five hyperactive children (ages six to ten years) were entered into an eighteen-week study of the effects of methylphenidate on attention. Measures included rating scales completed by teachers and parents and a vigilance task. Results of these measures are given in detail. For a commentary on this study refer to Item No. 830.

1561 Conners, C. Keith. "The effect of pemoline and dextroamphetamine on evoked potentials under two conditions of attention." In: Clinical use of stimulant drugs in children. Edited by C. Keith Conners. Amsterdam: Excerpta Medica, 1974. 165-78. (5 References). (International Congress Series, No. 313).
Compares the effects of pemoline (Cylert), dextroamphetamine, and placebo on visual and auditory evoked response under attending and nonattending conditions. Seventy children (mean age 8.16 years) were randomly assigned to one of the three treatment groups for an eight-week period. Results, given in detail, suggest that Cylert may have more effect on selective attention than dextroamphetamine, while both drugs act to increase cortical arousal. General discussion follows.

1562 Douglas, Virginia I. "Perceptual and cognitive factors as determinants of learning disabilities: a review chapter with special emphasis on attentional factors." In: The neuropsychology of learning disorders: theoretical approaches. Edited by Robert M. Knights and Dirk J. Bakker. Baltimore, Maryland: University Park Press, 1976. 413-21. (Bibliography).
Discusses the attentional-impulsivity deficit in hyperactive children and the role of stimulant drugs on this deficit. Treatment methods should place more emphasis on attention and impulse control than on activity level. The effects of positive reinforcement are discussed.

1563 Fisher, Mary A. "Dextroamphetamine and placebo practice effects on selective attention in hyperactive children." J Abnorm Child Psychol 6(1): 25-32, March, 1978. (5 References).
Examines the effect of dextroamphetamine, a CNS stimulant, on selective attention. Nine boys (mean age 8.8 years) were chosen from a larger population of boys referred to a hospital study unit for evaluation and treatment of hyperactive behavior. The boys were divided into three groups and tested on a classification task involving selective attention while receiving either dextroamphetamine or placebo. It was found that: (1) dextroamphetamine decreases response times in general and reduces interference from orthogonally varying irrelevant information; (2) practice on placebo is more effective than practice on amphetamine; and (3) the improvement in selective attention that appears spontaneously with amphetamine therapy can also be achieved by extended practice on placebo.

1564 Freeman, Richard J. "The effects of methylphenidate on avoidance learning and risk-taking by hyperkinetic children." For a summary see: Diss Abstr Int 39B(9): 4576-77, March, 1979. (0 References).

1565 Gabrys, Jan B. "Methylphenidate effect on attentional and cognitive behavior in six- through twelve-year-old males." Percept Mot Skills 45 (3, pt. 2): 1143-49, December, 1977. (17 References).

Studies the effect of methylphenidate on attentional and cognitive behaviors. Eighty-four boys (ages six to twelve years), referred to a mental health center for various learning-behavior problems, were studied. Each child was given twenty-one measures including WISC Digit Span and Coding, Block Design, Picture Arrangement, Mazes, and Non-verbal IQ. The boys were studied before and after drug treatment. Most test scores showed improvement with methylphenidate, especially in tests requiring a high attentional component. These findings replicate studies of other researchers and have implications for the drug management of the learning-disabled child.

1566 Halliday, R.; Callaway, E.; Rosenthal, J.; et al. "The effects of methylphenidate dosage on the visual event related potential of hyperactive children." In: NATO Conference on Human Evoked Potentials, Constance, 1978. Human evoked potentials: applications and problems. Edited by Dietrich Lehmann and Enoch Callaway. New York, New York: Plenum, 1979. 153-67. (17 References). (NATO Conference Series 3: Human Factors, Volume 9).

Employs event-related potential (ERP) to study the interaction of attention and stimulants in hyperkinetic children.

1567 Halsey, Chandra V. "Attentional performance in hyperkinetic children: an investigation of the relationship between methylphenidate, stimulus exposure duration and inter-trial interval." For a summary see: Diss Abstr Int 40B(1): 452-53, July, 1979. (0 References).

1568 Hiscock, Merrill; Kinsbourne, Marcel; Caplan, Bruce; et al. "Auditory attention in hyperactive children: effects of stimulant medication on dichotic listening performance." J Abnorm Psychol 88(1): 27-32, February, 1979. (25 References).

Examines the performance of hyperactive children on a binaural rivalry task and investigates the effect of methylphenidate on several variables. Twenty hyperactive children (ages six to sixteen years) were administered dichotic digits tasks requiring free report and selective listening, respectively. The children received stimulant medication (methylphenidate) before two experimental sessions and a placebo before two control sessions. Although the stimulant did not improve free-report performance significantly, it facilitated or impaired performance, depending on how it affected the order in which stimuli were reported. Medication also had no effect on overall selective-listening performance, but it increased the difficulty of switching attention from one ear to the other. The results of both tasks demonstrate that stimulants may act to maintain selective attention and to inhibit channel switching.

1569 Humphries, Thomas; Swanson, James; Kinsbourne, Marcel; et al. "Stimulant effects on persistence of motor performance of hyperactive children." J Pediatr Psychol 4(1): 55-66, March, 1979. (23 References).

Assesses the effect of methylphenidate on the persistence of maze-tracking performance in a group of children. Twenty-four hyperactive children (mean age ten years) were tested under drug and placebo conditions using a double-blind design. Although methylphenidate was not successful in decreasing errors, it was effective in helping the children maintain their attention to a task.

1570 Klorman, R.; Salzman, L. F.; Pass, H. L.; et al. "Effects of methylphenidate on hyperactive children's evoked responses during passive and active attention." Psychophysiology 16(1): 23-29, January, 1979. (19 References).

Tests the evoked responses of two groups of boys (eighteen hyperactive boys receiving methylphenidate and placebo, and seventeen normal boys). Evoked potentials were recorded during a continuous performance test. Results confirm previous findings of attentional disturbance in hyperactivity and normalization by methylphenidate of these children's performance and electrophysiological activity during sustained attention.

1571 ————. "Effects of methylphenidate on hyperactive children's evoked responses during passive and active attention." In: NATO Conference on Human Evoked Potentials, Constance, 1978. Human evoked potentials: applications and problems. Edited by Dietrich Lehmann and Enoch Callaway. New York, New York: Plenum, 1979. 459. (0 References). (NATO Conference Series 3: Human Factors, Volume 9).

Abstract.

1572 Kozuch, Donna P. "The effects of methylphenidate on the attention span and learning performance of hyperactive children." For a summary see: Diss Abstr Int 38A(11): 6647, May, 1978. (0 References).

1573 Kupietz, Samuel S., and Balka, Elinor B. "Alterations in the vigilance performance of children receiving amitriptyline and methylphenidate pharmacotherapy." Psychopharmacology 50(1): 29-33, 1976. (16 References).

Presents an analysis of drug effects on the vigilance of hyperactive children. Twenty hyperactive/aggressive children received doses of amitriptyline (Elavil, 50-150 mg/day) and methylphenidate (Ritalin, 20-60 mg/day). Their attention spans were investigated using an auditory version of the Continuous Performance Test (CPT). Results show that over the course of this letter-detection task, correct detections tended to return to pretreatment levels under placebo but were maintained at significantly improved levels under amitriptyline and methylphenidate. Medications improved the level of vigilance leading to an increase in the number of correct detections. The findings seem to be contrary to reports by teachers and parents that drugs make children appear drowsy.

1574 Rapoport, Judith L.; Buchsbaum, Monte S.; Zahn, Theodore P.; et al. "Dextroamphetamine: cognitive and behavioral effects in normal prepubertal boys." Science 199(4328): 560-63, February 3, 1978. (20 References).

Investigates the effect of dextroamphetamine on attention and hyperactivity in a sample of children. Fourteen normal boys (ages six to twelve years) participated in the double-blind study. The study, occupying three mornings, contained a baseline session followed by drug or placebo sessions. Numerous measures were obtained: motor activity, reaction time, continuous performance test, verbal learning and memory test, and language tests. Data show that amphetamine, in comparison with placebo, caused a decrease in motor activity and galvanic skin response amplitude and an increase in attention. It is stressed that the responses of these normal children are similar to those of hyperactive/MBD children, refuting the hypothesis that hyperactive/MBD children have a clinically specific or "paradoxical" response to stimulants.

1575 Schain, Richard J. "Attentional behavior and drugs in hyperactive children." Res Relat Child 39: 107, March, 1977-August, 1977. (0 References).
Abstracts a report of research in progress or recently completed research. Data are provided on: name of investigator(s), purpose of the study, number and kind of subjects used, methodology, principal findings, duration of research, cooperating group(s), and availability of publication(s). Research Relating to Children is compiled by the ERIC Clearinghouse on Early Childhood Education.

1576 ————. "Attentional behavior and drugs in hyperactive children." In: The psychologist, the school, and the child with MBD/LD. Edited by Leon Oettinger, Jr. and Lawrence V. Majovski. New York, New York: Grune & Stratton, 1978. 75ff. (References).

1577 Seger, Eva Y., and Hallum, Gyda. "Methylphenidate in children with minimal brain dysfunction: effects on attention span, visual-motor skills, and behavior." Curr Ther Res 16(6): 635-41, June, 1974. (11 References).
Investigates the efficacy of methylphenidate on the academic accomplishments and hyperactive behavior of a group of elementary schoolchildren. Twenty-nine children (twenty-five boys and four girls, ages six to eleven years) with MBD participated in the study. The Digit Span and Coding subtests of the WISC and the Bender Visual Motor Gestalt Test were used to establish a baseline for the children. After eight weeks of administration of methylphenidate, the following improvements were noted: (1) significant increases in mean raw scores had occurred in the Digit Span and Coding subtests of the WISC as well as in the BVMGT; (2) twenty children on the Digit Span and nineteen on the BVMGT had improved; and (3) parent and teacher evaluations also showed improvement in social and learning situations after drug treatment. Only four minor side effects were noted. Judicious use of methylphenidate as part of a total treatment regimen is advocated.

1578 Thurston, Catherine M.; Sobol, Michael P.; Swanson, James; et al. "Effects of methylphenidate (Ritalin) on selective attention in hyperactive children." J Abnorm Child Psychol 7(4): 471-81, December, 1979. (39 References).
Investigates the effect of methylphenidate (Ritalin) on the selective attention of hyperactive children designated as favorable or adverse responders to stimulant medication. Using a type II incidental learning paradigm, researchers found that children in the drug condition recalled more central and less incidental stimuli than those children in the placebo condition. While no differential effects on recall were found for responder type, methylphenidate did affect the spontaneous overt labeling of central stimuli by the favorable responder group. Results are interpreted in terms of the role of methylphenidate in narrowing the focus of attention. Implications for the classification of hyperactive children as favorable and adverse responders are also discussed.

1579 Ullman, Douglas G.; Barkley, Russell A.; Brown, H. Wesley. "The behavioral symptoms of hyperkinetic children who successfully responded to stimulant drug treatment." Am J Orthopsychiatry 48(3): 425-37, July, 1978. (29 References).
Compares a group of children who had successfully responded to drug treatment with control children on a series of objective measures of activity and attentional problems. Eighteen hyperactive boys and eighteen controls

served as subjects. The children were individually evaluated during four consecutive experimental periods: free play, movie viewing, testing, and restricted play periods. Data, given in detail, showed that even though there were group differences on most measures, there were no indications that good responders were more homogeneous in their behavioral symptoms than the hyperkinetic population in general.

1580 Whalen, Carol K., et al. "Behavior observations of hyperactive children and methylphenidate (Ritalin) effects in systematically structured classroom environments: now you see them, now you don't." J Pediatr Psychol 3(4): 177-87, 1978. (33 References).
Uses a naturalistic summer school program to study in context the behaviors that distinguish hyperactive from normal boys and methylphenidate from placebo states. Three groups of sixty-two boys (hyperactive and normal) were observed on various measures. Findings indicate that: (1) compared to boys on methylphenidate, the placebo group showed lower rates of task attention and higher rates of motor activity and disruption; (2) there were no differences between hyperactive boys on medication and the normal group; and (3) group differences in specific behaviors varied with the two classroom dimensions (easy versus difficult materials and self-paced versus other-paced activities), pointing to the impact of medication by situation interactions. Discussion follows on issues concerning ecological validity and scientific precision.

1581 Zelniker, T.; Charles, L.; Schain, R. J. "Attentional behavior and drugs in hyperactive children." Clin Res 26(2): A169, February, 1978. (0 References).
Abstract of a conference paper presented at the 25th meeting of the Western Society for Pediatric Research.

2. NONDRUG

1582 Anderson, Robert P.; Halcomb, Charles G.; Gordon, Jr., William; et al. "Measurement of attention distractibility in LD children." Acad Ther 9(5): 261-66, Spring, 1974. (9 References).
Studies the vigilance task as a means of experimentally examining attentional deficits in children with learning disabilities. The research also attempts to determine if the vigilance task can be used as a measure of the effects of methylphenidate on the attention of LD children. Eighteen LD boys (ages six to twelve years), all regularly receiving a CNS stimulant while attending special classes, served as subjects. Each child was tested twice on the same vigilance task: once while on medication, and once while off medication. In general, attentional deficits can be modified by medication, especially the ability to sustain attention among primary grade hyperactive boys.

1583 Baldwin, Martha A. "Activity level, attention span, and deviance: hyperactive boys in the classroom." For a summary see: Diss Abstr Int 37B(10): 5341, April, 1977. (0 References).

1584 Blackwell, Scott L., et al. "Hyperactivity and cuing responsivity in learning disabled boys." Paper presented at the Southwest Society for Research and Human Development, Dallas, Texas, March 17, 1978. 11p. (ED 155 867).
Compares performance of four groups of boys on a visual search task. Findings and explanations for the attentional problems of the hyperactive groups are given.

1585 Bremer, David A. "Attention during reading in hyperactive boys: reactions to distracting stimuli and to rewards." For a summary see: Diss Abstr Int 34B(12, pt. 1): 6206-7, June, 1974. (0 References).

1586 Bremer, David A., and Stern, John A. "Attention and distractibility during reading in hyperactive boys." J Abnorm Child Psychol 4(4): 381-87, 1976. (15 References).
Attempts to determine if hyperactive children are less attentive, yet more distractible, than nonhyperactive children. Fifteen hyperactive and normal boys were given reading tasks under quiet and distracting conditions. During these tests the hyperactive group was found to be less attentive to task-relevant stimuli and more attentive to task-irrelevant stimuli than the normal controls. Results support previous laboratory findings and suggest that the hypothesis can be generalized to the school setting.

1587 ————. "Attention and distractibility during reading in hyperactive boys." In: Behavior therapy with hyperactive and learning disabled children. Edited by Benjamin B. Lahey. New York, New York: Oxford University Press, 1979. (15 References).
Reprints an article from the Journal of Abnormal Child Psychology 4(4): 381-87, 1976. (Item No. 1586).

1588 Bryan, Tanis S. "An observational analysis of classroom behaviors of children with learning disabilities." J Learn Disabil 7(1): 26-34, January, 1974. (26 References).
This study was designed to measure task-oriented and social behavior of a group of elementary schoolchildren. Five learning-disabled and five normal third-grade children served as subjects. Using an Interaction Process Analysis, the classroom behaviors of the children were coded for five days over a five-month period. The research indicates that: (1) there is a difference in attending behaviors of LD and normal children; (2) LD children are generally capable of greater work efforts than they expend in the nonspecialized classroom; (3) situational and environmental factors can have an important effect on the LD child; and (4) LD children have different interpersonal relations with teachers and peers than do comparison children.

1589 Callaway, Enoch. "Miscellaneous measures." In: Callaway, Enoch. Brain electrical potentials and individual psychological differences. New York, New York: Grune & Stratton, 1975. 112-31. (Bibliography).
Studies the relationships among attention, MBD, hyperkinesis, and auditory evoked potential (AEP).

1590 Callaway, E.; Halliday, R.; Naylor, H.; et al. "Locus of the attention defect in hyperkinetic children." Paper presented to the Society of Biological Psychiatry, Atlanta, Georgia, May, 1978.

1591 Cappella, Betty; Gentile, J. Ronald; Juliano, Daniel B. "Time estimation by hyperactive and normal children." Percept Mot Skills 44(3, pt. 1): 787-90, June, 1977. (9 References).
Compares normal and hyperactive children on time estimation, i.e., the capability of a child to estimate the amount of time spent at a task. Two studies, one involving twelve hyperactive children (ages seven to ten years) and twelve controls, and the other using twenty-five hyperactive

children (ages eight to twelve years) and seventy-five controls are reported. Children were asked to participate in several time-estimation tasks. The intervals to be estimated were seven, fifteen, and thirty seconds. The differences between estimated and elapsed time were larger for hyperactive children than for controls, the differences between the two groups increasing with the length of the interval to be estimated. Implications for attention problems in hyperactive children are discussed.

1592 Chess, Stella, and Hassibi, Mahin. "Hyperkinesis and attentional deficiencies." In: Chess, Stella, and Hassibi, Mahin. Principles and practice of child psychiatry. New York, New York: Plenum, 1978. 334-38. (12 References).
Describes the clinical features of hyperkinesis with emphasis on defects of attention. Comments are also made on etiology and treatment.

1593 Craggs, M. D.; Wright, J. J.; Werry, J. S. "The vigilance-related EEG in hyperactive children." Electroencephalogr Clin Neurol 44(6): 793, 1978. (0 References).
Abstract of a conference paper read at a meeting of the EEG Society, London, England, October 29, 1977.

1594 Denton, Claire L., and McIntyre, Curtis W. "Span of apprehension in hyperactive boys." J Abnorm Child Psychol 6(1): 19-24, March, 1978. (6 References).
Compares span of apprehension (a measure of the amount of information processed simultaneously from a brief visual display) of hyperactive and normal boys with a forced-choice letter-recognition task. Developed by W. K. Estes, this task provides an estimate of the span which is relatively insensitive to either memory or motivational influences. Thirty-eight boys (nineteen hyperactive and nineteen controls, mean age 8.0 years) participated in the experiment and were given various stimulus displays. Span size proved to be the same for both groups except in the presence of visual "noise" which decreased the span size of the hyperactive group. Explanations for this outcome are offered. (See Item No. 1614 for a related study).

1595 Doyle, Robert B. "The effects of distraction and attention deficits among children with learning disabilities on a vigilance task." For a summary see: Diss Abstr Int 34B(9): 4658-59, March, 1974. (0 References).

1596 Doyle, Robert B.; Anderson, Robert P.; Halcomb, Charles G. "Attention deficits and the effects of visual distraction." J Learn Disabil 9(1): 48-54, January, 1976. (15 References).
This study was designed to investigate the effects of a visual distractor on the vigilance task performance among groups of learning-disabled and normal children, thus providing quantitative measures of the attentional deficit prevalent in LD children. LD children were found to have a lower correct detection rate and a higher false alarm rate than normal controls. The effect of hyperkinetic behavior on test scores is discussed.

1597 Dykman, Roscoe A., and Ackerman, Peggy T. "The MBD problem: attention, intention and information processing." In: Learning disability/minimal brain dysfunction syndrome: research perspectives and applications. Edited by Robert P. Anderson and Charles G. Halcomb. Springfield, Illinois: Thomas, 1976. 27-93. (136 References).

Examines three problem areas of MBD: attention, memory, and concept attainment. Some comments are made on hyperactivity.

1598 Dykman, Roscoe A.; Ackerman, Peggy T.; Oglesby, D. Michael. "Selective and sustained attention in hyperactive, learning-disabled, and normal boys." J Nerv Ment Dis 167(5): 288-97, May, 1979. (17 References).
Surveys attentional deficits in three groups of boys: hyperactive, LD, and normal. Boys classified as nonhyperactive learning-disabled (LD), hyperactive but not LD, and normal in behavior and achievement were contrasted on a visual search task hypothesized to elicit differences in selective and sustained attention. Results are given in detail. Generally, the hyperactive boys' lack of "tolerance for a problem" is theorized to account for their poor performance, whereas the LD children's poor performance indicated defects in selective as well as sustained attention.

1599 Firestone, Philip, and Martin, Jaclynn E. "Analysis of the hyperactive syndrome: a comparison of hyperactive, behavior problem, asthmatic, and normal children." Res Relat Child 41: 113, March, 1978-August, 1978. (0 References).
Abstracts a report of research in progress or recently completed research. Data are provided on: name of investigator(s), purpose of the study, number and kind of subjects used, methodology, principal findings, duration of research, cooperating group(s), and availability of publication(s). Research Relating to Children is compiled by the ERIC Clearinghouse on Early Childhood Education.

1600 ————. An analysis of the hyperactive syndrome: a comparison of hyperactive, behavior problem, asthmatic and normal children. 1978. 30p. (ED 162 753).
Reports on a study to identify cognitive and behavioral deficits which might be unique to hyperactive children. Fifty children (ages five to twelve years) served as subjects and were given several tests measuring impulsiveness, attention, and motor inhibition. Hyperactive children were judged to be more inattentive, more impulsive, and more easily frustrated than normal children.

1601 ————. "An analysis of the hyperactive syndrome: a comparison of hyperactive, behavior problem, asthmatic, and normal children." J Abnorm Child Psychol 7(3): 261-73, September, 1979. (38 References).
Surveys four groups of children in an attempt to determine if certain behaviors associated with hyperactivity (inappropriate activity, short attention span, low frustration tolerance, and impulsivity) were prevalent in all the groups. Hyperactive children, when compared with normal children, did show deficits in the tested areas. However, when compared with the behavior problem and asthmatic groups, only the attentional deficits differentiated hyperactives from other children.

1602 Fisher, Mary A. "Dimensional interaction in hyperactive children: classification of computer-displayed stimuli." Bull Psychon Soc 10(6): 443-46, December, 1977. (5 References).
Assesses selective attention of hyperactive boys from their performance on a classification task using dimensions that are separable for adults. Three groups of three hyperactive boys each (ages five to seven years, seven to nine years, and nine to eleven years) served as subjects. A cathode ray tube was used to present the stimuli. The type of dimensional

interaction found in the two younger groups replicates earlier studies. Although younger boys processed the stimuli dimensionally, a failure of selective attention was evident.

1603 Friedman, Judith A. "A developmental study of selective attention in hyperactive children." For a summary see: Diss Abstr Int 38B(3): 1399, September, 1977. (0 References).

1604 Hallahan, Daniel P. "Distractibility in the learning disabled child." In: Cruickshank, William M., and Hallahan, Daniel P., eds. Perceptual and learning disabilities in children: II. Research and theory. Syracuse, New York: Syracuse University Press, 1975. 195-218. (62 References).
One part of this chapter considers the relationship between distractibility and hyperactivity in the LD child. Clinical evidence is cited which suggests a correlation between these two problems. A study is reported which investigated twenty-nine LD children on two behavioral-observation measures of activity, five behavioral-observation measures of motor activity, and a laboratory test of attention. The author stresses the need for further naturalistic studies focusing on the antecedent and consequent events of distractibility and hyperactivity.

1605 Hogg, J., and Maier, I. "Transfer of operantly conditioned visual fixation in hyperactive severely retarded children." Am J Ment Defic 79(3): 305-10, November, 1974. (4 References).
Investigates transfer, in a variety of situations, of conditioned visual fixation. Ten severely retarded hyperactive children, who had previously undergone operant conditioning of sustained visual fixation (Item No. 1075), served as subjects. The children were given a series of transfer tests: (1) a distracting testroom; (2) neutral stimuli; (3) experimenter replacement; (4) simple play tasks presented in the testroom and the classroom; (5) Seguin formboard; (6) bead manipulation; and (7) classroom assessment involving prescribed tasks. Findings indicate consistent improvement for most subjects in the majority of tests for frequency and duration of visual fixation.

1606 Kaspar, J. C. "Research in distractibility and activity level: a review." Paper presented at the 86th Annual Convention of the American Psychological Association, New Orleans, Louisiana, September, 1974.

1607 Keogh, Barbara K., and Margolis, Judith S. "A component analysis of attentional problems of educationally handicapped boys." J Abnorm Child Psychol 4(4): 348-59, 1976. (13 References).
Tests three components of attention: coming to attention, decision-making, and maintaining attention over time. Seventy-three educationally handicapped (EH) and seventy-eight normally achieving (NA) children (grades three to eight) were administered a variety of tests and rating scales designed to assess various measures of attention and behavior. Results are given in detail for the EH group (divided into hyperactives and nonhyperactives) and for the NA group.

1608 Kirchner, Grace L. "Difference in vigilance performance between highly active and normal second-grade males under four experimental conditions." For a summary see: Diss Abstr Int 36B(5): 2474, November, 1975. (0 References).

1609 ———. "Differences in the vigilance performance of highly active and normal second-grade males under four experimental conditions." J Educ Psychol 68(6): 696-701, December, 1976. (29 References).

The objective of this research was to determine if differences occurred between highly active and normal boys on a vigilance performance task. Sixty-four white, middle-class, second-grade boys served as subjects and were divided into two groups. All boys were tested on a forty-eight-minute vigilance task in which four conditions were used: (1) control; (2) feedback about signal occurrence; (3) an extraneous auditory stimulation; and (4) an oral reminder to pay attention. The highly active group performed more poorly than the control group on this task.

1610 Kistner, J. A. "Attentional deficits of hyperkinetic children." Paper presented at the Meeting of the Association for the Advancement of Behavior Therapy, Atlanta, Georgia, December, 1977.

1611 Kupietz, Samuel S. "Attentiveness in behaviorally deviant and nondeviant children: I. Auditory vigilance performance." Percept Mot Skills 43(3, pt. 1): 1095-1101, December, 1976. (16 References).

Examines vigilance performance and suggests that the vigilance paradigm might serve as a basis for a standardized test of continuous attention in children. Sixteen behaviorally deviant inpatient children and sixteen normal controls served as subjects. They were given an auditory vigilance task on two separate occasions, four days apart. Results, consistent with prior clinical studies, show that deviant children are less able to maintain a continuous level of attention.

1612 Loiselle, David L. "Electrophysiological and neuropsychological indices of attention in older hyperactive children." For a summary see: Diss Abstr Int 39B(4): 2001, October, 1978. (0 References).

1613 McIntyre, Curtis W., et al. Visual search in learning disabled and hyperactive boys. 1979. 19p. (ED 175 227).

Investigates selective attention in twelve learning-disabled, twelve learning-disabled hyperactive, and twelve hyperactive boys (ages six to eleven years). All boys were asked to search for a target letter embedded within a group of noise letters. Test results support the hypothesis that a deficit in selective attention is characteristic of learning-disabled boys but not of hyperactive boys.

1614 McIntyre, Curtis W.; Blackwell, Scott L.; Denton, Claire L. "Effect of noise distractibility on the spans of apprehension of hyperactive boys." J Abnorm Child Psychol 6(4): 483-92, December, 1978. (14 References).

Examines the influences of signal-noise similarity and noise redundancy upon the spans of apprehension of nineteen normal and nineteen hyperactive boys. Thirty-eight boys (ages six to ten years) participated in the experiment. Various arrays of letters made up the stimulus display. The effects of noise similarity and noise redundancy upon the spans of apprehension of all boys were compared to determine whether noise letters act as more potent distractors for the hyperactive group. The experiment found: (1) the average span of hyperactive boys was only about 83 percent as large as that of normal boys; and (2) the spans of both groups were effected equivalently by variations in signal-noise similarity and noise redundancy. Implications are discussed. (See Item No. 1594 for a related study).

1615 McIntyre, Curtis W., and Murray, Michael. "Attention mechanisms in hyperactive and learning disabled boys." Res Relat Child 39: 47, March, 1977-August, 1977. (0 References).
Abstracts a report of research in progress or recently completed research. Data are provided on: name of investigator(s), purpose of the study, number and kind of subjects used, methodology, principal findings, duration of research, cooperation group(s), and availability of publication(s). Research Relating to Children is compiled by the ERIC Clearinghouse on Early Childhood Education.

1616 Mack, Cary N. "The effects of different schedules of knowledge of results on the vigilance behavior of hyperactive learning disabled children." For a summary see: Diss Abstr Int 36B(12, pt. 1): 6389-90, June, 1976. (0 References).

1617 Ozolins, Delmar A. "The effects of knowledge of results on the vigilance performance of hyperactive and hypoactive children with learning disabilities." For a summary see: Diss Abstr Int 35B(10): 5128-29, April, 1975. (0 References).

1618 Peters, Kenneth G. Selective attention and distractibility in hyperactive and normal children. Montreal, Ontario, Canada: McGill University, 1977.
Doctoral thesis.

1619 Porges, Stephen W. Psychophysiological studies of attention during infancy and early childhood. Final report. 1977. 23p. (ED 142 306).
Calls attention to current research investigating the utility of physiological responses to predict attentional capacity and to monitor attentional responsivity. Most experiments assessed heart rates in newborns.

1620 Ricks, Nancy L. "Sustained attention and the effects of distraction in underachieving second grade children." For a summary see: Diss Abstr Int 35A(3): 1535-36, September, 1974. (0 References).

1621 Rosenthal, Ronald H. "A comparison of intra-task distractibility in hyperkinetic and non-hyperkinetic children." For a summary see: Diss Abstr Int 39B(11): 5582, May, 1979. (0 References).

1622 Rosenthal, Ronald H., and Allen, Terry W. "An examination of attention, arousal, and learning dysfunctions of hyperkinetic children." Psychol Bull 85(4): 689-715, July, 1978. (116 References).
Empirical studies are reviewed which support the hypothesis that hyperkinesis is a dysfunction of information processing. Data on measures of arousal, learning, attention, and performance were examined for hyperactive children receiving drugs, hyperactive children not receiving drugs, and normal children. Although some support is found for the hypothesis that hyperkinetic children exhibit low physiological arousal, several findings indicate the need for modifying this view. Suggestions for future empirical work in the area are offered.

1623 Stamm, John S., and Loiselle, David L. "Auditory evoked potentials indicate attentive dysfunctions in hyperkinetic adolescents (meeting)." In: NATO Conference on Human Evoked Potentials, Constance, 1978. Human evoked potentials: applications and problems. Edited by Dietrich Lehmann and Enoch Callaway. New York, New York: Plenum, 1979. 474. (0 References). (NATO Conference Series 3: Human Factors, Volume 9).

Abstract.

1624 Steinkamp, Marjorie W. "Relationships between task-irrelevant environmental distractions and task performance of normal, retarded hyperactive, and minimal brain dysfunction children." For a summary see: Diss Abstr Int 35A(12, pt. 1): 7730-31, June, 1975. (0 References).

1625 Tarver, Sara G., and Hallahan, Daniel P. "Attention deficits in children with learning disabilities: a review." J Learn Disabil 7(9): 560-69, November, 1974. (35 References).

Reviews twenty-one experimental studies of attention deficits in children with learning disabilities. Areas surveyed include distractibility, hyperactivity, impulsivity, vigilance, and intersensory integration. From the accumulated evidence, the following conclusions are drawn: (1) LD children are more easily distracted than controls on tasks involving embedded contexts; (2) hyperactive children with LD exhibit higher levels of activity in structured settings; (3) LD children are more impulsive than controls; and (4) attention deficits are notable in the LD group.

1626 Victor, James B., and Halverson, Charles F. "Distractibility and hypersensitivity. Two behavior factors in elementary school children." J Abnorm Child Psychol 3(1): 83-94, 1975. (24 References).

Relates the development of a modified problem checklist and reports on two factors: distractibility and hypersensitivity. One hundred normal elementary schoolchildren attending a predominantly white, middle-class, suburban school served as subjects. Convergent validity data are presented from peer judgments, in-class activity level, physical fitness measures, standardized achievement scores, and comparison with another teacher's judgment.

1627 Yekell, Howard S. "Distractibility and attention in MBD and normal children." For a summary see: Diss Abstr Int 35B(1): 530, July, 1974. (0 References).

1628 Zentall, Sydney S., et al. "Distraction as a function of within-task stimulation for hyperactive and normal children." Paper presented at the 55th Annual International Convention, the Council for Exceptional Children, Atlanta, Georgia, April 11-15, 1977. 25p. (ED 139 132).

Assesses the effects of distraction and task performance with or without within-task color. Twenty-five hyperactive children and twenty-two controls served as subjects and were tested on two visual-motor drawing tasks, one visual concentration task, and a combined visual-motor and visual concentration task. Results are included.

1629 Zentall, Sydney S.; Zentall, Thomas R.; Barack, Robin S. "Distraction as a function of within-task stimulation for hyperactive and normal children." Res Relat Child 38: 90, September, 1976-February, 1977. (0 References).

Abstracts a report of research in progress or recently completed research. Data are provided on: name of investigator(s), purpose of the study, number and kind of subjects used, methodology, principal findings, duration of research, cooperating group(s), and availability of publication(s).

Research Relating to Children is compiled by the ERIC Clearinghouse on Early Childhood Education.

1630 ———. "Distraction as a function of within-task stimulation for hyperactive and normal children." J Learn Disabil 11(9): 540-48, November, 1978. (28 References).
Studies task performance of hyperactive and normal children with and without within-task color while holding the complexity of the task constant. Twenty-five hyperactive children (twenty-three boys and two girls, ages six to ten years) and controls participated in the experiment which took place in a small room. Performance was measured on four tasks: two visual-motor drawing tasks, one visual-concentration task, and a combined visual-motor and visual-concentration task. Generally, hyperactives performed poorer than controls. Implications of the results are given.

D. BLOOD

1. DRUG

1631 Bhagavan, Hemmige N.; Coleman, Mary; Coursin, David B. "Distribution of pyridoxal-5-phosphate in human blood between the cells and the plasma: effect of oral administration of pyridoxine on the ratio in Down's and hyperactive patients." Biochem Med 14(2): 201-8, October, 1975. (28 References).
Studies the distribution of pyridoxal-5-phosphate (PLP) in blood between the cells and the plasma in hyperactive, Down's syndrome patients, and normal controls. PLP appeared equally distributed and concentrated in all three groups. However, when patients were treated with pyridoxine, PLP content of the blood rose sharply and became localized in the red cells. Implications of these findings are discussed.

1632 ———. "The effect of pyridoxine-hydrochloride on blood serotonin and pyridoxal phosphate contents in hyperactive children." Pediatrics 55(3): 437-41, March, 1975. (24 References).
Investigates the effect of pyridoxine on the blood of a group of hyperactive children. Eleven hyperactive children and eleven controls served as subjects. Blood samples revealed the contents of serotonin and pyridoxal phosphate (PLP). A significant decrease in serotonin content was found in blood samples of hyperactive children, although there were no differences in PLP between the two groups.

1633 Coleman, Mary; Greenberg, Alan; Bhagavan, Hemmige; et al. "The role of whole blood serotonin levels in monitoring vitamin B_6 and drug therapy in hyperactive children." Monogr Neural Sci 3: 133-36, 1976. (14 References).
This paper, presented at the Satellite Symposium on the Clinical Pharmacology of Serotonin, 6th International Congress of Pharmacology, examines the relationship between serotonin (5-HT) levels and vitamin B6 in hyperactive children. The data on 5-HT levels revealed in this study show: (1) low whole blood levels of 5-HT occur in 88 percent of hyperactive children with normal intelligence; (2) vitamin B6 in pharmacological doses can be used to elevate 5-HT; (3) drugs, e.g., methylphenidate and dextroamphetamine, usually given to hyperactive children, do not elevate serotonin; (4) pyridoxal phosphate (PLP) content of whole blood was also increased following B6 administration; and (5) in many cases an improvement in hyperactive behavior followed the elevation of whole blood levels. Additional studies involving larger numbers of patients are needed to

confirm or deny these findings, most of which support conclusions reached in previous research.

1634 Greenberg, Alan S., and Coleman, Mary. "Depressed 5-hydroxyindole levels associated with hyperactive and aggressive behavior: relationship to drug response." Arch Gen Psychiatry 33(3): 331-36, March, 1976. (21 References).
Studies and monitors 5-hydroxyindole (5-Hl) levels in the blood of a group of institutionalized mentally retarded patients. Thirty patients (ages four to thirty-nine years) participated in the experiment. The 5-hydroxyindole levels were measured before and after drug therapy. Depression of 5-Hl levels occurred in 83 percent of the hyperactive patients. Implications of these findings are discussed.

1635 Linnoila, Markku; Gualtieri, C. Thomas; Jobson, Kenneth; et al. "Characteristics of the therapeutic response to imipramine in hyperactive children." Am J Psychiatry 136(9): 1201-3, September, 1979. (10 References).
This pilot study investigates the relationship between plasma and red blood cells and imipramine and desipramine therapeutic response in a group of hyperactive children. Six children participated in the study. Findings indicate that a therapeutic response to imipramine among hyperactive children is associated with relatively low plasma and RBC levels of the drug and its active metabolite. Onset of action seems to be immediate, but a precise therapeutic level for hyperactive children needs further investigation.

1636 Milberg, R. M.; Rinehart, K. L., Jr.; Sprague, R. L.; et al. "A reproducible gas chromatographic mass spectrometric assay for low levels of methylphenidate and ritalinic acid in blood and urine." Biomed Mass Spectrom 2(1): 2-8, February, 1975. (13 References).
Reports on a rapid, sensitive method for analyzing methylphenidate and ritalinic acid in blood and urine in order to study the relationship of behavioral effects to blood and urine levels of the drug and metabolites. The method developed uses a gas chromatography mass spectrometry and selected ion monitoring for separation and detection. The methylphenidate is isolated by solvent extraction into chloroform; the ritalinic acid is isolated by salting out into isopropyl alcohol, followed by methylation and subsequent solvent extraction. Implications for the hyperactive child are given.

2. NONDRUG

1637 Goldman, Janice O.; Thibert, Robert J.; Rourke, Byron P. "Platelet serotonin levels in hyperactive children." J Pediatr Psychol 4(3): 285-96, September, 1979. (21 References).
Analysis of blood samples taken from a group of reportedly hyperactive children and nonhyperactive controls supports the possibility that some hyperactive children may have allergic responses that are related to maturation, changes in serotonin (5-hydroxytryptamine, 5-HT) metabolism, and symptoms of hyperactivity. Increased platelet 5-HT concentrations, if extrapolated to the neuronal level, indicate the possibility of raised neuronal levels of 5-HT that may lead to increased activity in serontonergic pathways, and possibly to decreased activity in other biogenic amine pathways through "false" neurotransmission by 5-HT.

1638 Langseth, Lillian, and Dowd, Judith. Glucose tolerance and hyperkinesis. 1977. 22p. (ED 149 557).
Details the results of a five-hour glucose tolerance test (GTT). It was found that: (1) hematocrit levels were low in 27 percent of the children; (2) eosinophil levels were abnormally high in 86 percent of the children; and (3) GTT results were abnormal in a majority of the children.

1639 ————. "Glucose tolerance and hyperkinesis." Food Cosmet Toxicol 16(2): 129-33, 1978. (16 References).

1640 Rapoport, Judith L.; Quinn, Patricia O.; Scribanu, N.; et al. "Platelet serotonin of hyperactive school age boys." Br J Psychiatry 125(8): 138-40, August, 1974. (12 References).
Monitors platelet serotonin content before and during treatment with methylphenidate and imipramine. Thirty-five hyperactive boys (ages six to twelve years) and nineteen normal controls served as subjects, the latter being matched for age with the patient group. The hyperactive boys were selected from a larger clinical study of the efficacy of methylphenidate and imipramine. Platelets were isolated from blood samples and serotonin content determined. Findings indicate that platelet serotonin content did not differ between the two groups. Imipramine treatment greatly reduced platelet serotonin, while methylphenidate had no similar effects. As both drugs were clinically effective, it seems unlikely that change in serotonin transport is closely related to the mechanism of actions of these drugs on hyperactive behavior.

1641 Takahashi, Saburo; Kanai, Hideko; Miyamoto, Yoshihiro. "Reassessment of elevated serotonin levels in blood platelets in early infantile autism." J Autism Child Schizophr 6(4): 317-26, December, 1976. (18 References).
Reports on an experiment examining blood platelet serotonin content in thirty children with early infantile autism, thirty age-matched normal children, and forty-five children with a variety of neurological and psychiatric disorders. Data reveal that: (1) serotonin levels in autistic children were elevated; (2) autistics under school age had higher concentrations than older autistics, although normal children did not show this pattern; and (3) elevated serotonin was also seen in some of the nonautistic pathological group, who were disturbed and hyperactive. It is suggested that elevated serotonin levels are not limited to autistic children.

1642 Uluitu, M.; Oancea, C.; Petec, G. H.; et al. "Determination of blood serum protein reactivity in children with behavior disturbances." Physiologie 12(2): 113-17, 1975. (21 References).
Attempts to determine if blood serum proteins in children with behavior disturbances differ from serum proteins of normal controls. Seventeen children (ages five to fifteen years) and six normal children were used as subjects. The serum cationic state was determined by an original method. Data reveal that serum proteins in children with behavior disturbances differ from those of normals, having: (1) a smaller number of serotonin-fixing sites; (2) higher strength interaction between the serotonin and proteins; and (3) lower resistance to the denaturant agents, with consequently an increase of cationic activity in the serum and an increased electrophoretic mobility. The need for future research is emphasized.

E. BONE AGE

1. NONDRUG

1643 Oettinger, Leon, Jr. "Bone age and minimal brain dysfunction." J Pediatr 87(2): 328, August, 1975. (3 References).
Letter to editor.

1644 Oettinger, Leon, Jr.; Majovski, Lawrence V.; Limbeck, George A.; et al. "Bone age in children with minimal brain dysfunction." Percept Mot Skills 39(3): 1127-31, December, 1974. (11 References).
Reports on a study in which bone-age determinations were done on a group of children to determine if bone age was retarded in minimal brain dysfunction. Fifty-three MBD children (forty-three boys and ten girls) were chosen from a larger study, and X rays of their left wrists and hands were taken for the determination of bone age. Since bone age for this group was significantly retarded as compared with the norms of the standard group, it is suggested that children diagnosed as having MBD may be physiologically retarded in their bone age. The concept of physiological immaturity should be considered by professionals when planning for the child with this syndrome.

1645 Safer, Daniel J., and Allen, Richard P. "Bone age and minimal brain dysfunction." J Pediatr 87(2): 329, August, 1975. (4 References).
Letter to editor.

1646 Schlager, G., et al. "Bone age in children with MBD." Can J Neurol Sci 5(3): 352-53, 1978. (0 References).
Abstract of a conference paper.

1647 Schlager, G.; Newman, D. E.; Dunn, H. G.; et al. "Bone age in children with minimal brain dysfunction." Dev Med Child Neurol 21(1): 41-51, February, 1979. (38 References).
Studies bone age in a group of sixty Caucasian Western-Canadian children with MBD. Ten percent of the children were found to have bone age below the normal mean for their chronological age. The bone age of fifty-eight of the children, when blindly reassessed, was found to be more than eight months lower than the mean chronological age. Further analyses of the data show that MBD children exhibited a significantly greater variance of bone age than the control children. It is therefore possible that a subgroup of MBD children with significant delay of bone age may prove to have special characteristics which are worthy of study, as they may shed some light on the control of skeletal maturation.

F. CARDIORESPIRATORY

1. DRUG

1648 Aman, M. G., and Werry, J. S. "The effects of methylphenidate and haloperidol on the heart rate and blood pressure of hyperactive children with special reference to time of action." Psychopharmacologia 43(2): 163-68, August 21, 1975. (23 References).
Briefly reviews previous literature relating to the effects of psychotropic drugs on children's behavior disorders. The present study used twelve hyperactive children in a double-blind crossover design with drug order (placebo, methylphenidate, and haloperidol) randomized across sub-

jects. Resting heart rates, blood pressures, and EKGs were obtained. Analysis of the data shows: (1) methylphenidate caused a small increase in heart rate; (2) methylphenidate caused a significant increase in blood pressure; (3) changes with haloperidol were minimal; (4) no EKG changes were noted with either drug; and (5) changes in heart rate were of a minimal nature as compared with those occurring with digestion, which tended to obscure drug effects.

1649 ————. "Methylphenidate in children: effects upon cardiorespiratory function on exertion." Int J Ment Health 4(1-2): 119-31, Spring-Summer, 1975. (16 References).
Examines the effect of methylphenidate and placebo on heart rate, respiratory rate, and work completed (pedal rotations) in a group of hyperactive, aggressive children. Ten hyperactive boys served as subjects in a double-blind crossover design. Methylphenidate (0.3 mg/kg) and an inert placebo were administered. Results show that: (1) methylphenidate increases heart rate, but this effect can be partially eliminated by exertion; and (2) methylphenidate can cause a reduction in oxygen expenditure during exercise. These results replicate those of other studies. For a reprint of this study refer to Item No. 688.

1650 Ballard, Joyce E. Duration of cardiovascular effects produced by methylphenidate in hyperactive children. Urbana-Champaign, Illinois: Institute for Child Behavior and Development, University of Illinois, 1976.
PHS Research Grant No. MH 18909.

1651 ————. "The effects of methylphenidate during rest, exercise, and recovery upon the circulorespiratory responses of hyperactive children." For a summary see: Diss Abstr Int 36A(1): 170-71, July, 1975. (0 References).

1652 Ballard, Joyce E.; Boileau, Richard A.; Sleator, Esther K.; et al. "Cardiovascular responses of hyperactive children to methylphenidate." JAMA 236(25): 2870-74, December 20, 1976. (15 References).
This study was designed to determine the effects of methylphenidate on the cardiovascular responses of hyperactive children during rest, exercise, and recovery from exercise. Twenty-three hyperactive children being treated with methylphenidate and twenty-three matched normal controls served as subjects and were rated with the Conners' Rating Scale. Measurements of heart rate, blood pressure, diastolic blood pressure, oxygen intake, volume of expired air, respiratory rate, and stepping rate were made under varying conditions. Findings indicate: (1) oxygen consumption did not change with methylphenidate; (2) heart rate and blood pressure increased significantly with methylphenidate; (3) there was a significant correlation between size of dosage and increase in heart rate and blood pressure; (4) no evidence of tolerance to drug effects was found; and (5) no ECG changes other than tachycardia were seen.

1653 Boileau, Richard A.; Ballard, Joyce E.; Sprague, Robert L.; et al. "Effect of methylphenidate on cardiorespiratory responses in hyperactive children." Res Q Am Assoc Health Phys Educ 47(4): 590-96, December, 1976. (15 References).
Assesses the effect of methylphenidate on cardiorespiratory responses during rest and exercise conditions. Twenty hyperactive children (ages

six to twelve years) served as subjects and were studied in medicated and placebo conditions. In measuring heart rate and oxygen consumption it was found that: (1) heart rate elevated at rest and during exercise with medication; (2) the increased heart rate was independent of the work output as reflected by the oxygen consumption of the walk; and (3) heart rate responses tended to increase with an increase in dosage.

1654 Butter, H. J., and Lapierre, Y. D. "The effect of methylphenidate on cardiovascular sensory differentiation on the hyperkinetic syndrome." Int J Clin Pharmacol Biopharm 11(4): 309-14, June, 1975. (11 References).
Studies the effect of methylphenidate on mean heart rate in eighteen hyperactive children (ages six to twelve years). The action of methylphenidate was observed while the children were attending to monosensory, bisensory, and trisensory stimuli presentations. During relaxation periods neither subjects receiving methylphenidate nor those receiving placebo showed a shift in tonic heart rate. However, while attending to sensory stimuli, heart rates were higher for subjects receiving placebo than for those receiving methylphenidate in all experimental conditions for the high and moderate levels of overactive behavior. For the mildly hyperkinetic subjects a drug reversal effect was noted.

1655 Conte, R.; Swanson, J. M.; Kinsbourne, M. "The effects of stimulant medication on cardiac activity during manual tracking in hyperactive children." Psychophysiology 16(2): 181, March, 1979. (0 References).
Abstract of a paper presented at the 18th annual meeting of The Society for Psychophysiological Research.

1656 Greenberg, Lawrence M., and Yellin, Absalom M. "Blood pressure and pulse changes in hyperactive children treated with imipramine and methylphenidate." Am J Psychiatry 132(12): 1325-26, December, 1975. (2 References).
Reports the results of a double-blind crossover study to evaluate the effects of imipramine and methylphenidate on blood pressure and pulse of hyperactive children. Forty-seven children (forty boys and seven girls, ages six to thirteen years) were involved in the eight-week experiment. Half the children received placebo followed by medication (imipramine or methylphenidate). Table 1 summarizes the precise medication sequence. Significant increases in systolic and diastolic blood pressure and pulse rate were found in the hyperactive children treated with imipramine. Although children treated with methylphenidate showed a weight loss, there were no significant changes in blood pressure or pulse. Since three children had to be taken off imipramine because of elevated diastolic blood pressure, caution should be used when prescribing this drug.

1657 Porges, Stephen W.; Walter, Gary F.; Korb, Robert J.; et al. "The influences of methylphenidate on heart rate and behavioral measures of attention in hyperactive children." Child Dev 46(3): 727-33, September, 1975. (26 References).
Reaction-time performance and heart-rate responses associated with attention were used to assess the hyperactive child's attentional deficit and his response to methylphenidate. Sixteen hyperactive children (ages six-and-one-half to twelve years) served as subjects. During trials with a race track apparatus, the subjects were monitored under placebo and methylphenidate conditions. Attentional deficits shown by long response latencies were reflected in heart-rate responses theoretically incompat-

ible with sustained attention. Children showing the greatest deficits in attention displayed the most favorable response to methylphenidate in both reaction-time performance and physiological measures. Subjects who showed the greatest improvement in social behavior showed the least improvement in reaction-time performance.

1658 Aman, Michael G. "Drugs, learning and the psychotherapies." In: Pediatric psychopharmacology: the use of behavior modifying drugs in children. Edited by John S. Werry. New York, New York: Brunner/Mazel, 1978. 79-108. (Bibliography).
Discusses cognitive deficits, ways in which these deficits are measured, and the effects of drugs on the deficits. The hyperactive child is characterized by attentional problems, perceptual difficulties of a visual nature, and a tendency toward high levels of impulsivity. Table I summarizes the effects of various drugs on cognitive tasks and tests; Table II lists various tests of cognitive function as measures of drug effects. Seven conclusions complete the chapter.

G. COGNITION/PERCEPTION

1. DRUG

1659 Butter, H. J., and Lapierre, Y. D. "The effect of methylphenidate on sensory perception and integration in hyperactive children." Int Pharmacopsychiatry 9(4): 235-44, 1974. (14 References).
Attempts to define the perceptual deficiencies frequently associated with hyperactive children and to determine if methylphenidate can improve performance. Thirty-two hyperactive Canadian boys and girls (ages six to twelve years) served as subjects. The Illinois Psycholinguistic Ability Scale was used as the basic psychometric measure. The IPAS revealed the hyperactive subjects were eighteen to twenty-four months less mature than normal controls, especially in the areas of tactile and auditory modalities. The latter improved with methylphenidate, indicating that the hyperactive child's maturational lag can be partly corrected by methylpenidate.

1660 ————. "The effect of methylphenidate on sensory perception in varying degrees of hyperkinetic behaviour." Dis Nerv Syst 36(6): 286-88, June, 1975. (6 References).
Reports on a study to determine the effectiveness of methylphenidate on visual, auditory, and tactile perception in a group of children with varying degrees of hyperkinesis. Subtests of the Illinois Test of Psycholinguistic Ability (ITPA) and other measures were used to assess performance. Results indicate that the children exhibiting the more marked hyperkinetic behavior showed the most improvement in sensory perception while on methylphenidate.

1661 Gittelman, Rachel, and Abikoff, Howard. "Cognitive training and stimulant medication in hyperactive children." Res Relat Child 42: 77, September, 1978-February, 1979. (0 References).
Abstracts a report of research in progress or recently completed research. Data are provided on: name of investigator(s), purpose of the study, number and kind of subjects used, methodology, principal findings, duration of research, cooperating group(s), and availability of publication(s). Research Relating to Children is compiled by the ERIC Clearinghouse on Early Childhood Education.

1662 Gittelman-Klein, Rachel, and Klein, Donald F. "Methylphenidate effects in learning disabilities." Arch Gen Psychiatry 33(6): 655-64, June, 1976. (10 References).
Focuses on a test to determine whether methylphenidate improves the cognitive performance and academic achievement of children with learning defects, but without noticeable behavior problems. Sixty-one children meeting these criteria participated in the study. The children received methylphenidate or placebo for a twelve-week period. Methylphenidate improved performance on psychological tests, but not on achievement tests. Implications for MBD and hyperactive children are included.

1663 Gordon, Norman G., and Kantor, Donald R. "Effects of clinical dosage levels of methylphenidate on two-flash thresholds and perceptual motor performance in hyperactive children." Percept Mot Skills 48(3, pt. 1): 721-22, June, 1979. (5 References).
Investigates the effects of clinical dosage levels of methylphenidate and its discontinuance on the two-flash thresholds and perceptual-motor performance of hyperactive children. Three groups of subjects--ten normal controls, ten hyperactive children on medication, and ten hyperactive children off medication--were administered eight perceptual-motor tasks. The normal controls were significantly superior in performance on three tasks in comparison with the hyperactives taken off methylphenidate; however, the controls were only superior on one task when compared to hyperactives on methylphenidate.

1664 Ives, Sara B. "Conceptual tempo, attention, and skin conductance in Ritalin-responsive hyperkinetic boys." For a summary see: Diss Abstr Int 38B(9): 4524-25, March, 1978. (0 References.)

1665 Kinsbourne, Marcel; Swanson, James; Kurland, Laura. "A dose response analysis of the effect of methylphenidate (Ritalin) on cognition of hyperactive children." Pediatr Res 12(4, pt. 2): 372, April, 1978. (0 References).
Abstract of a conference paper presented at the annual meeting of the American Pediatric Association and the Society for Pediatric Research.

1666 Merrill, Diedre M. "Cognitive effects of methylphenidate on hyperactive children." For a summary see: Diss Abstr Int 36B(3): 1446, September, 1975. (0 References).

1667 Mock, Karen R., et al. "Stimulant effect on matching familiar figures: changes in impulsive and distractible cognitive styles." Paper presented at the Annual Meeting of the American Educational Research Association, Toronto, Canada, March 27-31, 1978. 22p. (ED 160 189).
The effects of methylphenidate on cognitive style are investigated. Fifty-five hyperactive and LD children (ages seven to fifteen years) participated in the study and were administered Kagan's Matching Familiar Figures Test. It was found that Ritalin resulted in poorer MFFT performance for poor responders to the drug; it did, however, improve performance for the impulsive and distractible groups.

1668 Rapoport, Judith L.; Quinn, Patricia O.; Copeland, Anne P.; et al. "$ACTH_{4-10}$: cognitive and behavioral effects in hyperactive, learning-disabled children." Neuropsychobiology 2(5-6): 291-96, 1976. (18 References).

Tests the effect of $ACTH_{4-10}$, a peptide, on the cognition of hyperactive learning-disabled children. Twenty children (eighteen boys and two girls, ages seven to thirteen years) served as subjects. They were administered a single dose of $ACTH_{4-10}$ (30 mg im) or placebo. A battery of tests was given to the children: the Digit Span and Coding subtests of the Revised WISC, the Matching Familiar Figures Test, the Continuous Performance Test, Draw-A-Person test, a paired-associate learning task, and the State-Trait Anxiety Inventory. Findings show no significant drug effects on cognition or behavior. There was only a slight increase in pulse rate for the drug group as compared with the placebo group.

1669 Reichard, Catherine C., and Elder, S. Thomas. "The effects of caffeine on reaction time in hyperkinetic and normal children." Am J Psychiatry 134(2): 144-48, February, 1977. (30 References).
Attempts to show a relationship between caffeine and reaction time (RT) in hyperkinetic children. Using a double-blind design, six hyperkinetic children and six normal children (mean age 9.3 years) were used as subjects for the study. Topics investigated were: (1) the effect of caffeine on a choice RT task; (2) whether caffeine has different effects on simple reaction time and choice reaction time; and (3) whether its effects in the hyperkinetic compared with the normal group of children are best described by the law of initial values or as a "paradoxical effect." Testing reveals that caffeine produced an increase in the accuracy of stimulus identification and processing and a decrease in lapses of attention for hyperkinetic children. The law of initial values best represented the phenomena observed.

1670 Schupp, Robin R. "The effect of methylphenidate on cognitive and behavioral functioning in a selective population of hyperactive children." For a summary see: Diss Abstr Int 36B(12, pt. 1): 6399-6400, June, 1976. (0 References).

1671 Skorina, Jane K. "A study of the effects of Ritalin intervention upon the perceptual competencies of children diagnosed as giving evidence of psychoneurological learning disabilities." For a summary see: Diss Abstr Int 34A(11): 7055-56, May, 1974. (0 References).

1672 Spring, Carl; Yellin, Absalom; Greenberg, Lawrence. "Effects of imipramine and methylphenidate on perceptual-motor performance of hyperactive children." Percept Mot Skills 43(2): 459-70, October, 1976. (24 References).
Examines the effects of two drugs, imipramine (20 mg) and methylphenidate (50 mg), on the perceptual-motor performance of a group of hyperactive children. Forty-seven nine-year-old children participated in the double-blind study. The authors provide evidence for these findings: (1) methylphenidate improved performance on several tests; (2) no effects were found for imipramine; (3) improvement due to methylphenidate was not related to baseline scores; and (4) a digit-span test, which was not sensitive to methylphenidate, effectively discriminated hyperactive from normal children.

1673 Waddell, Kathleen J. "The effects of methylphenidate hydrochloride on psycholinguistic, motor and visual-perceptual abilities of hyperkinetic children with learning disabilities." For a summary see: Diss Abstr Int 35B(12, pt. 1): 6122, June, 1975. (0 References).

1674 Werry, John S., and Aman, Michael G. "Methylphenidate and haloperidol in children: effects on attention, memory, and activity." Arch Gen Psychiatry 32(6): 790-95, June, 1975. (37 References).
Compares the effects of four drug conditions on cognitive function of a group of hyperactive children. Twenty-four hyperactive or unsocialized-aggressive children served as participants in a double-blind crossover Latin square design. Each subject received methylphenidate, two dosage levels of haloperidol (0.25 and 0.05 mg/kg), and placebo. At the end of each eighteen-day trial period, attention, immediate recognition memory, reaction times, and seat activity were tested. Analysis of the data shows: (1) methylphenidate improved cognitive performance most; (2) the low dose of haloperidol improved cognitive performance to a lesser extent; (3) the high dose of haloperidol caused a slight deterioration in performance; and (4) the high dose of haloperidol improved behavior. The effects of drugs on cognitive function is viewed as a complex problem.

2. NONDRUG

1675 Abikoff, Howard. "Cognitive training interventions in children: review of a new approach." J Learn Disabil 12(2): 123-35, February, 1979. (49 References).
Reviews cognitive training studies which relate to children with behavioral, attentional, or cognitive problems. Cognitive training interventions include self-instructional, problem-solving, and component attentional skills training. Some studies lend support to the theory that cognitive training may enhance academic functioning. The effectiveness of the procedure in reducing classroom disruption has been equivocal. With hyperactive children, cognitive training has resulted in improved and sustained cognitive functioning, but it has had little impact on classroom behavior. The usefulness of the training as an adjunct to clinical management is discussed.

1676 Adams, Jerry. "Visual and tactual integration and cerebral dysfunction in children with learning disabilities." J Learn Disabil 11(4): 197-204, April, 1978. (8 References).
Compares performance on visual and tactual form-recognition tasks of two groups of children: seventy-four learning-disabled and hyperactive children with cerebral dysfunction and seventy-three similar children without cerebral dysfunction. All children were trained using either unisensory (visual or tactual) or bisensory (visual and tactual) input and tested through either the visual or tactual modality. Results, which replicate previous studies, demonstrate visual form-recognition to be more efficient than tactile form-recognition.

1677 Agnew, Patricia N. "Verbal mediation, cognitive tempo, and self-esteem in normal-active, high-active, and hyperactive boys." For a summary see: Diss Abstr Int 39B(11): 5531, May, 1979. (0 References).

1678 Agnew, Patricia N., and Young, Richard D. "Verbal mediation, cognitive tempo, and self-esteem in normal-active, high-active, and hyperactive boys." Paper presented at the Biennial Meeting of the Society for Research in Child Development, San Francisco, California, March 15-18, 1979. (ED 172 915).
Discusses three criteria (verbal mediation, cognitive tempo, and self-esteem) which can be used in identifying and understanding the hyperactive child.

1679 Becker, Laurence D. "Modifiability of conceptual tempo in educationally 'high risk' children." For a summary see: Diss Abstr Int 34A(11): 7072, May, 1974. (0 References).

1680 Burns, Rosemary. "Perceptual cognitive development and its relation to activity in adolescent girls." For a summary see: Diss Abstr Int 35B(3): 1400, September, 1974. (0 References).

1681 Butter, Hendrik J., and Lapierre, Y. D. "Intersensory perception and integration in hyperkinetic children." Psychiatr J Univ Ottawa 2(2): 78-83, July, 1977.

Studies the relationship between intersensory perceptual processing deficit and degree of hyperkinesis in a group of children. Thirty-two hyperactive children and eleven controls served as subjects for the study and were administered various visual, auditory, tactile, and intersensory integration tests. Significant intersensory differences emerged among degrees of hyperkinesis and modality presentation. Very active children perceived the bisensory and trisensory stimuli more poorly in a simultaneous modality presentation than in successive presentation.

1682 Campbell, S. B. "Cognitive styles and behavior problems of clinic boys: a comparison of epileptic, hyperactive, learning-disabled, and normal groups." J Abnorm Child Psychol 2(4): 307-12, 1974.

1683 Copeland, Anne P. "Cognitive behavior in hyperactive and impulsive children." Res Relat Child 41: 113-14, March, 1978-August, 1978. (0 References).

Abstracts a report of research in progress or recently completed research. Data are provided on: name of investigator(s), purpose of the study, number and kind of subjects used, methodology, principal findings, duration of research, cooperating group(s), and availability of publication(s). Research Relating to Children is compiled by the ERIC Clearinghouse on Early Childhood Education.

1684 Epstein, Michael H.; Hallahan, Daniel P.; Kauffman, James M. "Implications of the reflectivity-impulsivity dimension for special education." J Spec Educ 9(1): 11-25, Spring, 1976. (12 References).

Discusses individual differences of cognitive tempo, or the reflectivity-impulsivity concept of Jerome Kagan. Emphasis is placed on the antecedents, scanning strategy, and implications for the educational setting. Remedial suggestions are given for the modification of an impulsive tempo.

1685 Ferguson, Frances A. "Administrative data base for plant planning and utilization related to the cognitive gain of hyperactive male students in open-space and self-contained selected Texas public elementary classrooms." For a summary see: Diss Abstr Int 36A(5): 2531, November, 1975. (0 References).

1686 Freudman, Judith D. "Reflection-impulsivity and pupil attentive behavior in the classroom." For a summary see: Diss Abstr Int 34B(10): 5166, April, 1974. (0 References).

1687 Gordon, Michael. "The assessment of impulsivity and mediating behaviors in hyperactive and nonhyperactive boys performing on DRL." For a summary see: Diss Abstr Int 38B(8): 3878-79, February, 1978. (0 References).

1688 ———. "The assessment of impulsivity and mediating behaviors in hyperactive and nonhyperactive boys." J Abnorm Child Psychol 7(3): 317-26, September, 1979. (21 References).
Twenty boys (six to eight years) rated by their teachers as hyperactive and a matched sample of nonhyperactive boys performed a task that required them to withhold responding for a set time interval in order to be rewarded (Differential Reinforcement Low Rate Responding--DRL 6-second schedule). Half of each group worked on a one-button console while the other half was provided with additional collateral buttons. Results indicate that hyperactive children were relatively unable to perform efficiently on the task, and that this deficit endured regardless of age, IQ, or experimental condition. DRL was thus found to discriminate accurately between teacher-rated and parent-rated hyperactive and nonhyperactive children. Furthermore, a wide variety of self-generated mediating behaviors was observed, and it was determined that a child's DRL performance was related to the kind of mediating behaviors he displayed. Results are discussed in terms of the clinical assessment of hyperactivity and the training of impulsive children.

1689 Halverson, Charles F., Jr., and Waldrop, Mary F. "Relations between preschool activity and aspects of intellectual and social behavior at age 7½." Dev Psychol 12(2): 107-12, March, 1976. (15 References).
Studies the relationship between the intense, high-energy behavior of sixty-two preschoolers and differences in cognitive style and related social behavior of the same children five years later. For both boys and girls, vigorous, high activity showed considerable stability over five years. Vigorous, intense behavior expressed by high activity levels is negatively related to various measures of cognitive and intellectual performance at age seven-and-one-half. Vigorous, intense behavior as expressed in social participation is positively related to the same measures of intellectual performance. The activity level component is closely related to an index of minor physical anomalies, whereas the social component is not.

1690 Juliano, Daniel B. "Conceptual tempo, activity and concept learning in hyperactive and normal children." For a summary see: Diss Abstr Int 34A(8): 4875, February, 1974. (0 References).

1691 ———. "Conceptual tempo, activity, and concept learning in hyperactive and normal children." J Abnorm Psychol 83(6): 629-34, December, 1974. (15 References).
Reports on an experiment which examined the relationships among activity, conceptual tempo, and diagnostic categories on a concept learning and transfer task. Forty hyperactive boys (ages eight to eleven years) and eighty normal controls participated in the experiment. Results show: (1) a small but significant performance decrement by the hyperactive group on the learning task; (2) that this decrement did not carry over to the transfer task, in which a group difference was not found; (3) that activity and conceptual tempo were related to diagnosis, with the hyperactive group being more active and having a greater percentage classified as impulsive; and (4) that activity and conceptual tempo were not related to the performance tasks. Future research should focus on this area of study.

1692 Kuchta, John C. "The differential operation and modification of certain cognitive styles in hyperactive and nonhyperactive boys."

For a summary see: Diss Abstr Int 35B(12, pt. 1): 6098, June, 1975. (0 References).

1693 Marwit, Karen L. "Conservation ability in children with minimal brain dysfunction." For a summary see: Diss Abstr Int 39A(3): 1478-79, September, 1978. (0 References).

1694 Montgomery, Leslie E. "A comparison of the performance of emotionally disturbed and normal children on a measure of reflection-impulsivity." For a summary see: Diss Abstr Int 35B(5): 2441, November, 1974. (0 References).

1695 Sergeant, J. S.; Van Velthoven, R.; Virginia, A. "Hyperactivity, impulsivity and reflectivity: an examination of their relationship and implications for clinical child psychology." J Child Psychol Psychiatry 20(1): 47-60, January, 1979. (37 References).

By employing groups of children classified by the Matching Familiar Figures test and groups of children concordantly judged by two independent sources to be hyperactive, an evaluation was made of the relationship between perceived hyperactivity and the dimension of impulsivity-reflectivity. No significant relationship was found. Direct observational variables scored by observers blind to the group identity of the children gave substantial support to the group structure derived from ratings, but had only a moderate relationship to specified perceived symptoms. The need for developing a valid and reliable instrument for hyperactivity research is indicated.

1696 Weithorn, Corinne J., and Kagen, Edward. "Interaction of language development and activity level on performance of first graders." Am J Orthopsychiatry 48(1): 148-59, January, 1978. (32 References).

Compares fifty-nine first graders of high activity level with sixty-one classmates of low activity level in order to test the developmental theory that language may be a compensatory factor in the cognitive functioning of hyperactive children. Participants were selected on the basis of all first-grade teachers' responses to a questionnaire and were rated and tested. The overall results support the predictions that high language maturity can be an important factor in the performance of high-activity-level children, enabling them to function well despite their behavioral impulsivity. Implications for teaching such children are discussed.

1697 Wright, John C., and Vlietstra, Alice G. "Reflection-impulsivity and information-processing from three to nine years of age." In: Principles and techniques of intervention with hyperactive children. Edited by Marvin J. Fine. Springfield, Illinois: Thomas, 1977. 196-243. (156 References).

Presents research on cognitive tempo in children, focusing on the dimensions of impulsivity and reflectivity. Reflection-impulsivity describe the speed and accuracy of information processing more comprehensively than either style or ability alone and more effectively than the raw speed and accuracy data on which their diagnosis is based. While reflectivity may be both preferred by the dominant culture and correspondingly more useful than impulsivity for survival in that culture, it is still likely that certain important but educationally neglected forms of intellectual competence develop more fully within the impulsive mode. Each child should be helped to function in both modes, and any individualized program of instruction or remediation based on the diagnosis of stylistic nonconformity should emphasize these principles.

1698 Zahn, Thomas P. "Identification of sensory motor and perceptual limitation, potential learning disability and hyperkinetic behavior disorder in kindergarten children." For a summary see: Diss Abstr Int 36B(8): 4142-43, February, 1976. (0 References).

H. EYE MOVEMENT

1. NONDRUG

1699 Bala, Stanley P. "Eye movements of hyperkinetic children." For a summary see: Diss Abstr Int 37B(7): 3662, January, 1977. (0 References).

1700 Bala, Stanley; Cohen, Bernard; Morris, Ann G. "Eye movements of normal and hyperkinetic children." Neurology 25(4): 380, April, 1975. (0 References).
Presents an abstract of a paper examining eye movements of normal and hyperkinetic children. Eye movements were recorded by electrooculography to determine if they reflected the hyperactive children's motor overactivity. Results to date indicate that hyperactive children have several differences in comparison with their age-matched controls: (1) they cannot hold their eyes steady either in direct forward or in lateral gaze; (2) they use head movements to a later age; and (3) there is an increase in saccadic movements during pursuit. The implications of these findings for the differential diagnosis of hyperkinesis are outlined.

1701 Bala, Stanley P.; Morris, Anne G.; Cohen, Bernard. "Saccadic eye movements during visual pursuit and fixation in hyperactive and normal boys." Pediatr Res 12(4, pt. 2): 549, April, 1978. (0 References).
Abstract of a conference paper presented at the combined meeting of the American Pediatric Society and the Society for Pediatric Research.

1702 Cohen, Bernard, et al. "Do hyperactive children have manifestations of hyperactivity in their eye movements?" Paper presented at the Biennial Meeting of the Society for Research in Child Development, Denver, Colorado, April 10-13, 1975. 13p. (ED 112 601).
Tests the hypothesis that hyperactive children manifest the same type of hypermotility in their eyes as in the rest of their body. Eighteen children (ages three to twelve years) served as subjects. The hypothesis is generally upheld.

1703 Cohen, Bernard; Bala, S.; Morris, A. G. "Do hyperactive children have manifestations of hyperactivity in their eye movements?" Bull NY Acad Med 51(10): 1152, November, 1975. (0 References).
Abstract of a conference paper presented at a meeting of the Health Research Council and the Association of Career Scientists.

I. GROWTH

1. DRUG

1704 Aarskog, D.; Fevang, F. Ø.; Kløve, H.; et al. "The effect of the stimulant drugs, dextroamphetamine and methylphenidate, on secretion of growth hormone in hyperactive children." J Pediatr 90(1): 136-39, January, 1977. (9 References).

Compares the stimulant effect of L-dopa (125 to 500 mg) to dextroamphetamine and methylphenidate (15 and 20 mg respectively) on growth hormone secretion in children. Twenty hyperactive children (three girls and seventeen boys, ages six to thirteen years) were used as subjects for the study conducted in Bergen, Norway. All three stimulants were responsible for peak GH concentration in serum at sixty minutes after drug ingestion; there was no significant difference between the mean GH level at any time of sampling. Seven of the children were retested with L-dopa and dextroamphetamine after six to eight months of treatment with methylphenidate. After treatment, there was a tendency to higher zero time levels of GH, and to delayed and/or paradoxical response to dextroamphetamine. Since the findings indicate that drugs can effect the homeostasis of growth hormone, caution should be used when administering these agents.

1705 AvRuskin, Theodore W.; Lala, Vinod; Tang, Shiu-C.; et al. "Methylphenidate (Ritalin) and growth hormone secretion." Am J Dis Child 133(5): 553-55, May, 1979. (15 References).
Studies growth hormone secretion in five boys and three girls after methylphenidate administration. Results are given in detail.

1706 Barter, M., and Kammer, H. "Methylphenidate and growth retardation." JAMA 239: 1742-43, April 28, 1978. (3 References).

1707 Beck, Leah; Langford, William S.; MacKay, Mary; et al. "Childhood chemotherapy and later drug abuse and growth curve: a follow-up study of 30 adolescents." Am J Psychiatry 132(4): 436-38, April, 1975. (5 References).
Attempts to establish a relationship between treatment with methylphenidate in childhood and later drug abuse and growth in height. Thirty adolescents who had been previously diagnosed as MBD and who had received methylphenidate for at least six months were compared with thirty adolescents who had received no stimulant medications during childhood. Results of the study show no correlation between the ingestion of methylphenidate and later drug abuse or a significant suppression of growth over a period of time.

1708 Dickinson, Linda C.; Lee, Jason; Ringdahl, Irving C.; et al. "Impaired growth in hyperkinetic children receiving pemoline." J Pediatr 94(4): 538-41, April, 1979. (11 References).
Traces the effects of pemoline (Cylert) on height and weight as well as on growth hormone and plasma somatomedin concentrations. Twenty-two boys and two girls participated in the study and were placed on pemoline and followed for a period of twelve months. Results show that pemoline slowed growth; however, the drug had little effect on body weight, basal and stimulated growth hormone values, and plasma concentrations.

1709 Greenhill, Laurence L.; Puig-Antich, Joaquim; Sassin, Jon; et al. "Hormone and growth responses in hyperkinetic children on stimulant medication." Psychopharmacol Bull 13(2): 33-36, April, 1977. (10 References).
Studies growth patterns and human growth (HGH) hormone suppression and prolactin responses during sleep and insulin tolerance tests in a group of MBD children. The children were selected, started on d-amphetamine, and growth and HGH measured for two years. Data on hormone responses, sleep patterns, growth patterns, and behavior responses are presented for seven children.

1710 Gross, Mortimer D. "Growth of hyperkinetic children taking methylphenidate, dextroamphetamine, or imipramine/desipramine." Pediatrics 58(3): 423-31, September, 1976. (7 References).
Appraises the effects of four CNS stimulants on the long-term growth and height of hyperactive children. One hundred children who had been previously weighed and measured and treated with methylphenidate, dextroamphetamine, imipramine, or desipramine, served as subjects. The duration of treatment averaged five years. Weight and height at follow-up were normal; no correlations were found between dosage level and changes in weight and height. It is concluded that although there may be an initial slowing of growth with stimulant medications, the condition is temporary.

1711 Hechtman, Lily; Weiss, Gabrielle; Perlman, Terrye. "Growth and cardiovascular measures in hyperactive individuals as young adults and in matched normal controls." Can Med Assoc J 118(10): 1247-50, May 20, 1978. (20 References).
Reports on a study to determine if hyperactive young adults who had not taken stimulant medication during childhood showed any differences in growth from a normal population. Sixty-five hyperactive individuals (ages seventeen to twenty-four years) and thirty-nine matched controls participated in the survey. Height, weight, pulse rate, and blood pressure were measured. No significant differences in the physiologic measures between the two groups were noted. However, hyperactive young adults who had taken phenothiazines during childhood were significantly taller than those who had received no drugs.

1712 Kaffman, M., et al. "MBD children: variability in developmental patterns or growth inhibitory effect of stimulants?" Isr Ann Psychiatry 17(1): 58-66, March, 1979.

1713 McNutt, Barbara; Ballard, Joyce E.; Boileau, Richard. "The effects of long-term stimulant medication on growth and body composition of hyperactive children." Psychopharmacol Bull 12(2): 13-15, April, 1976. (5 References).
This study was designed to measure growth and body composition changes of hyperactive children while on medication. Twenty-six hyperactive children (seventeen boys and three girls on medication, and six boys off medication) served as subjects. All children were participants in a long-term follow-up study conducted at the University of Illinois Institute for Child Behavior and Development. These children had been receiving medication (mean dose 19.8 mg) for nine to forty-seven months with an average time of 30.3 months. Twenty-three normal children were used as controls and were matched for age. Statistics were kept on standing height, body weight, skinfold-pinch measurement, muscle girth, and skeletal widths. Multivariate (MANOVA) and univariate (ANOVA) analyses of variance were used to assess change. It is concluded that although hyperactive children receiving methylphenidate experienced the same amount of growth as the twenty-three normal control children, their body composition characteristics differed from the control group.

1714 McNutt, Barbara A.; Boileau, Richard A.; Cohen, Miye N.; et al. "The effects of long-term stimulant medication on the growth and body composition of hyperactive children." Psychopharmacol Bull 13(2): 36-38, April, 1977. (2 References).
Reports on the effect of methylphenidate on growth in height and weight of hyperactive children receiving this stimulant medication. Two groups

of children (some participants of a previous study, plus a new sample) were studied during the twenty-four-month period. Follow-up figures show no significant differences of growth between the medicated hyperactives and the controls, although there were some differences between the groups as to body composition characteristics. Demographic data are shown in Table I.

1715 Millichap, J. Gordon. "Growth of hyperactive children treated with methylphenidate: a possible growth stimulant effect." In: Learning disabilities and related disorders: facts and current issues. Edited by J. Gordon Millichap. Chicago, Illinois: Year Book Medical Publishers, 1977. 151-54. (5 References).
Examines the effect of methylphenidate on the growth of hyperactive children. Data reveal that relatively small doses of the stimulant given intermittently as an adjunct to remedial education are effective and do not cause growth suppression in hyperactive/MBD children.

1716 ————. "Growth of hyperactive children treated with methylphenidate." J Learn Disabil 11(9): 567-70, November, 1978. (7 References).
Reports on a study designed to obtain scientifically acceptable data on the effect of methylphenidate on the growth of hyperactive children. Thirty-six hyperactive boys (ages five to ten years) participated in the study. Methylphenidate was administered in daily doses of 10-20 mg for an average period of sixteen months. The author concludes that relatively small doses of methylphenidate, given intermittently as an adjunct to remedial education, are well-tolerated by the child and do not cause growth suppression.

1717 Millichap, J. Gordon, and Millichap, Martin. "Growth of hyperactive children." N Engl J Med 292(24): 1300, June 12, 1975. (2 References).
Letter to editor.

1718 Oettinger, Leon, Jr.; Gauch, Ronald R.; Majovski, Lawrence V. "Maturity and growth in children with MBD." In: Learning disabilities and related disorders: facts and current issues. Edited by J. Gordon Millichap. Chicago, Illinois: Year Book Medical Publishers, 1977. 141-49. (19 References).
Physiological immaturity in MBD children is studied. These conclusions are reached: (1) children with MBD are significantly more immature physiologically; (2) the long-continued use of stimulant drugs does not produce statistically significant loss in height; and (3) two studies suggest that MBD children will be taller than would be expected from their original heights. This does not, however, imply that drugs stimulate growth.

1719 ————. "Maturation and growth in children with MBD/LD before and after treatment with stimulant drugs." In: The psychologist, the school, and the child with MBD/LD. Edited by Leon Oettinger, Jr. and Lawrence V. Majovski. New York, New York: Grune & Stratton, 1978. 187ff. (References).

1720 Puig-Antich, Joaquim; Greenhill, Laurence L.; Sassin, Jon; et al. "Growth hormone, prolactin and corisol responses and growth patterns in hyperactive children treated with dextroamphetamine." J Am Acad Child Psychiatry 17(3): 457-76, June, 1978. (48 References).

Reports the preliminary findings of a study of the growth and hormone patterns of a group of hyperactive children. Fifteen hyperactive children participated in the study and were administered daily doses of dextroamphetamine and a control of phenothiazine. The study finds: (1) children treated with dextroamphetamine showed growth retardation and inhibition of mean sleep-related prolactin secretion; and (2) a significant correlation existed between loss of expected height percentile during the first year and decrease of mean sleep-related prolactin at six months. It is suggested that growth inhibition secondary to chronic dextroamphetamine administration in hyperactive children might be mediated by inhibition of prolactin secretion.

1721 Roche, Alex F.; Lipman, Ronald S.; Overall, John E.; et al. "The effects of stimulant medication on the growth of hyperkinetic children." Pediatrics 63(6): 847-50, June, 1979. (43 References).
Reviews the literature on possible growth-suppressing effects of stimulant medications in the long-term treatment of hyperkinetic children. From the accumulated evidence the following conclusions are drawn: (1) there is a temporary slowing of growth in stature; (2) there is no long-term effect on adult stature or weight; (3) the temporary effect on growth is present during the first few years of drug treatment; and (4) little is known of the growth-related effects of treatment extending past the prepubertal period.

1722 Safer, Daniel J., and Allen, Richard P. "Side effects from long-term use of stimulants in children." Int J Ment Health 4(1-2): 104-18, Spring-Summer, 1975. (36 References).
Considers the long-term side effects of dextroamphetamine and methylphenidate. Areas discussed are growth suppression and resting pulse evaluation while on medication. It is noted that when stimulant medication is abruptly withdrawn, a significant growth rebound follows. Cardiovascular changes are most notable with methylphenidate. For a reprint of this study refer to Item No. 688.

1723 Safer, Daniel J.; Allen, Richard P.; Barr, Evelyn. "Growth rebound after termination of stimulant drugs." J Pediatr 86(1): 113-16, January, 1975. (4 References).
Reports on a study to determine if the stimulants taken to control hyperactive behavior could suppress rate of growth and if a weight rebound occurred when the drugs were discontinued. Over a three-year period (1971-1973) a number of hyperactive students in a suburban, blue-collar, Caucasian area were examined. All students were receiving stimulant medication during the school year. Data revealed that those children whose stimulant medication was terminated at the start of summer subsequently grew in weight and height at a significantly greater rate than did children who continued to receive medication from June to September. Discontinuance of the medication resulted in a growth rebound for this period which was much above the age-expected increment.

1724 Salter, Anna C. "Children referred and treated for hyperactivity: a descriptive and control comparison study." For a summary see: Diss Abstr Int 38B(11): 5592, May, 1978. (0 References).

1725 Satterfield, James H.; Cantwell, Dennis P.; Schell, Ann; et al. "Growth of hyperactive children treated with methylphenidate." Arch Gen Psychiatry 36(2): 212-17, February, 1979. (12 References).

Reports a study of weight and height gain in a group of seventy-two hyperactive boys treated for one year and forty-eight hyperactive boys treated for two years with methylphenidate. The boys' height and weight measurements were obtained before treatment and at monthly intervals. Major findings are that methylphenidate produced an adverse effect on growth in height and weight in the first year of treatment, but not in the second year; the first-year height deficit was offset in the second year by a greater-than-expected growth rate. No clinical predictors of growth deficits are found; growth in height deficits was not related to total dosage or summer drug holidays, but weight deficits may be related to these factors. The temporary growth deficit of the first year were not considered to be significant.

1726 Sells, C. J.; Eaton, Marie; Lucas, Betty. "Central nervous system stimulants--their use in the 'non-classical' hyperkinetic syndrome: a case controlled study." Clin Pediatr 16(3): 279-83, March, 1977. (6 References).
Cites a case of a seven-year-old boy with a history of hyperkinesis, severe emotional problems, delayed use of language, and echolalic speech. An eleven-month trial with stimulant medication was begun, along with a double-blind placebo-control program to assess the effects of the therapy. Academic tasks, social behaviors, caloric intake, and height and weight were recorded. Although results show a marked improvement in academic and social behaviors, some undesirable side effects were observed in the areas of appetite and growth suppression. It is stressed that children on CNS stimulants merit careful supervision of their growth.

1727 Simeon, J. "Effects of psychotropic medication on heights and weights in children." Paper presented at the Meeting of the American College of Neuropsychopharmacology, Puerto Rico, December, 1975.

1728 Stahl, Monte L.; Orr, William C.; Griffiths, William J. "Nocturnal levels of growth hormone in hyperactive children of small stature." J Clin Psychiatry 40(5): 225-27, May, 1979. (15 References).
Examines sleep-related growth hormone secretion in a group of hyperactive children with short stature. Five such patients (ages six to twelve years) were compared with nine age-matched controls. The research revealed no differences in sleep patterns and growth hormone levels for the hyperactive group; both were within normal limits.

J. LATERALITY

1. NONDRUG

1729 Beaumont, J. G. "The cerebral laterality of 'minimal brain damage' children." Cortex 12(4): 373-82, December, 1976. (20 References).
Investigates lateral preference, unimanual motor speed, reaction time to lateralized stimuli, and dichotic ear advantage in a group of children. MBD children and their matched controls were assessed on a variety of tests. Findings show that: (1) MBD children were less extreme and stable in their lateral preferences; (2) MBD children were less lateralized in their motor performance; and (3) MBD children suffer from a partial disconnection syndrome which underlies their varied deficits.

1730 Davidson, E. M., and Prior, M. R. "Laterality and selective attention in hyperactive children." J Abnorm Child Psychol 6(4): 475-81, December, 1978. (29 References).

Uses a dichotic listening task to measure laterality and selective attention. Twenty hyperactive children (sixteen boys and four girls, ages six to ten years) and matched controls were selected and tested individually on free recall and selective attention. Results of the two experiments show no abnormalities in either hemisphere functioning or selective attention. It is concluded that the attentional problems of hyperactive children are situation- or task-specific and are aggrevated by more distracting settings such as a classroom.

1731 Sommers, Ronald K.; Moore, Walter H., Jr.; Brady, William; et al. "Performances of articulatory defective, minimal brain dysfunctioning, and normal children on dichotic ear preference, laterality, and fine motor skills tasks." J Spec Educ 10(1): 5-14, Spring, 1976. (27 References).
Attempts to test the importance of cerebral dominance on selected linguistic and perceptual tasks. Sixty children (ages 5.5 to 10.5 years) in four groups of fifteen children each comprised the sample: group I had normal articulation; group II possessed mild articulatory defectiveness; group III showed severe articulatory defectiveness; and group IV was diagnosed as having MBD. Three tests--a dichotic word task, a measure of fine-motor skills, and a test of laterality--were administered to the children. Test data revealed: (1) all children except group III had left cerebral dominance for speech on the dichotic word task; (2) a relationship was found between articulation errors and ear choices on the dichotic word task; (3) some relationship linked performances on the tests of motor skills to their dichotic ear choices; (4) a relationship was found between ear choices and numbers of articulation errors; and (5) traditional measures of laterality were not related to cerebral processing of speech.

K. LEARNING/ACADEMIC PERFORMANCE

1. DRUG

1732 Aman, Michael G., and Sprague, Robert L. "The state-dependent effects of methylphenidate and dextroamphetamine." J Nerv Ment Dis 158(4): 268-79, April, 1974. (19 References).
Evaluates the effects of methylphenidate and dextroamphetamine on learning and retention and the effects which might result when changes were made in the drug condition from learning to retention sessions. Eighteen hyperactive children (mean age 7.7 years) were assigned to one of three treatment regimens: placebo, methylphenidate, or dextroamphetamine. Testing was done on three tasks--a recognition task, a paired-associate task, and a maze task--in various sequences. Neither of the drugs significantly improved learning or retention performance; all tests for state-dependent effects were nonsignificant.

1733 Arnold, L. Eugene; Huestis, Robert; Wemmer, Douglas; et al. "Differential effect of amphetamine optical isomers on Bender Gestalt performance of the minimally brain dysfunctioned." J Learn Disabil 11(3): 127-32, March, 1978. (11 References).
Studies the effect of dextroamphetamine, levoamphetamine, and placebo on performance on the Bender Gestalt of a group of children. Thirty-one hyperactive minimally brain dysfunctioned children (twenty-six boys and five girls) were given the drugs as part of a double-blind crossover randomized Latin-square comparison. Results show that both isomers were significantly superior to placebo and roughly comparable to each other. These findings are discussed with illustrations.

1734 Barkley, Russell, and Cunningham, Charles E. "Do stimulant drugs improve the academic performance of hyperactive children?: a review of outcome studies." Clin Pediatr 17(1): 85-92, January, 1978. (51 References).
Reviews and discusses studies on the effects of stimulant drugs on the academic performance of hyperkinetic children, both in short-term use and in long-range follow-up. Table I summarizes the studies reviewed. It is concluded that: (1) stimulant drugs have little, if any, effect on the academic performance of hyperkinetic children; (2) stimulants do improve behavior, reducing overactivity and impulsivity; (3) objective measures must be used in evaluating a child's performance; and (4) stimulants should be used only when the goal of treatment is improved manageability.

1735 Baxley, Gladys B. "Effects of psychotropic drugs on the short-term memory of retarded children." For a summary see: Diss Abstr Int 34B(12, pt. 1): 6229, June, 1974. (0 References).

1736 Beal, Donald G. "The effect of methylphenidate hydrochloride on objective task learning, interpersonal learning and judgment behavior of hyperkinetic children." For a summary see: Diss Abstr Int 40B(2): 902, August, 1979. (0 References).

1737 Beal, Don, and Gillis, John S. "Methylphenidate hydrochloride and judgmental behavior in hyperkinetic children." Curr Ther Res 26(6): 931-39, December, 1979. (15 References).
Attempts to determine the effect of methylphenidate on the judgment behavior of children in support of the hypothesis that the drug would enhance judgment as well as attention and concentration. Forty-four hyperactive boys were randomly assigned to a drug or placebo group. The children were evaluated on a weekly basis. At the end of four weeks on their respective regimens, each child participated in a judgmental learning task. Results indicated that drug-induced differences in cognitive functioning did appear on the judgment tasks but in a direction contrary to expectations. Medication was associated with a decrease in complex learning relative to the placebo condition. It is suggested that these results are a function of the cognitive style facilitated by the medication.

1738 Bradley, Eunice. Academic, behavioral, and psychological responses of hyperactive children to stimulant medication. Chicago, Illinois: Northeastern University, 1975. 78p. (ED 116 419).
Master's thesis.

1739 Brandman, Edward S. "A test of the state dependent learning effects of methylphenidate in hyperactive children." For a summary see: Diss Abstr Int 36B(6): 3117, December, 1975. (0 References).

1740 Dalby, J. Thomas; Kinsbourne, Marcel; Swanson, James M.; et al. "Hyperactive children's underuse of learning time: correction by stimulant treatment." Child Dev 48(4): 1448-53, December, 1977. (18 References).
Investigates the effects of methylphenidate on hyperactive children's performance on a paired-associate learning task, and tests the hypothesis that a fixed amount of time is necessary to learn a fixed amount of material, regardless of the number of trials into which that time is divided. Twenty-eight hyperactive children (twenty-seven boys and one girl, mean age 9.8 years) served as subjects. They had previously been determined to be good responders to methylphenidate. In the double-blind

study eighty-four color slides of animals were used. Results show improved attention and improved use of learning time in the drug state and inattention in the placebo state, supporting the total-time hypothesis. Detailed results and comments on methodology are given.

1741 Douglas, Virginia I. "Effects of medication on learning efficiency research findings review and synthesis." In: Learning perspectives and minimal brain dysfunction syndrome: research perspectives and applications. Edited by Robert P. Anderson and Charles G. Halcomb. Springfield, Illinois: Thomas, 1976. 139-48. (19 References).
Discusses the hyperactive child in terms of: (1) terminology problems; (2) classification; (3) characteristics of the syndrome; (4) attention and performance problems; and (5) effect of medication on learning.

1742 Duchowney, Michael, and Leviton, Alan. "Stimulant drugs and academic performance in hyperactive children--reply." Ann Neurol 3(4): 376, April, 1978. (0 References).
Letter to editor.

1743 Dykman, Roscoe A.; McGrew, Jeanette; Ackerman, Peggy T. "A double-blind clinical study of pemoline in MBD children: comments on the psychological test results. In: Clinical use of stimulant drugs in children. Edited by C. Keith Conners. Amsterdam: Excerpta Medica, 1974. 125-29. (14 References). (International Congress Series, No. 313).
Reports on a clinical trial of pemoline. The experiment indicated that pemoline had a statistically significant effect on Performance IQ but not on Verbal IQ, a finding consistent with other studies.

1744 Fahrmeier, Edward D. "Stimulant drug therapy in control of on-task behavior: a case study." Psychol Rep 42(3, pt. 2): 1285-86, June, 1978. (2 References).
Outlines a simple procedure for school personnel to use to measure actual effects of stimulant drugs on academic behavior. Data are provided for an eight-year-old boy who was observed under drug and placebo conditions and then rated by the author. No significant differences were found between drug and no-drug conditions. Thus, further drug treatments were not recommended for the child.

1745 Garfunkel, J. M. "CNS stimulant therapy." J Pediatr 91(1): 133, July, 1977. (4 References).
Comments on a study by Robert J. Lerer (Item No. 1748).

1746 Kinsbourne, Marcel; Roberts, Wendy; Swanson, James. "Stimulant-related state-dependent learning in hyperactive children." Pediatr Res 10(4): 304, April, 1976. (0 References).
Abstract of a conference paper presented at the annual meeting of the American Pediatric Society and the Society for Pediatric Research.

1747 Lerer, Robert J.; Artner, Jeanne; Lerer, M. Pamela. "Handwriting deficits in children with minimal brain dysfunction: effects of methylphenidate (Ritalin) and placebo." J Learn Disabil 12(7): 450-55, August-September, 1979. (13 References).
Assesses the effects of methylphenidate on handwriting difficulties in a group of MBD children. Fifty such children were selected for the study and received either methylphenidate or placebo under double-blind condi-

tions. While placebo had little effect on the children's handwriting, twenty-six students (52 percent) showed improvement with methylphenidate. Reasons for this improvement are offered.

1748 Lerer, Robert J.; Lerer, M. Pamela; Artner, Jeanne. "The effects of methylphenidate on the handwriting of children with minimal brain dysfunction." J Pediatr 91(1): 127-32, July, 1977. (15 References).
Reports on a study to determine if methylphenidate could improve the handwriting skills of a group of children with MBD. Fifty children received methylphenidate or placebo in a double-blind four-week trial. The major findings include: (1) twenty-six children (52 percent) improved in handwriting; (2) handwriting tended to deteriorate promptly when the drug was discontinued; and (3) thirty-six children (72 percent) improved in attention and behavior, an improvement which did not always correspond with improvement in handwriting. Gains in handwriting were maintained for up to twenty-six months of follow-up in twenty-one children who received methylphenidate on a long-term basis. For a commentary on this article see Item No. 1745.

1749 Rie, Herbert. "The effects of methylphenidate on learning." Res Relat Child 39: 106-7, March, 1977-August, 1977. (0 References).
Abstracts a report of research in progress or recently completed research. Data are provided on: name of investigator(s), purpose of the study, number and kind of subjects used, methodology, principal findings, duration of research, cooperating group(s), and availability of publication(s). Research Relating to Children is compiled by the ERIC Clearinghouse on Early Childhood Education.

1750 Rie, Herbert E.; Rie, Ellen D.; Stewart, Sandra; et al. "Effects of methylphenidate on underachieving children." J Consult Clin Psychol 44(2): 250-60, April, 1976. (32 References).
Compares the effects of methylphenidate and placebo on the achievement and behavior of a group of primary grade children. Twenty-eight children participated in the double-blind, counter-balanced design, with each treatment regimen lasting for twelve weeks. A variety of medical and psychological measures, achievement tests, and behavior ratings revealed that although methylphenidate was effective in reducing hyperactivity, no substantial drug effects on achievement were found. Thus, it is suggested that methylphenidate be used to improve specific behavior disorders rather than to "treat" learning disorders. For a related study refer to Item No. 1752.

1751 ————. "Effects of methylphenidate on underachieving children." In: Behavior therapy with hyperactive and learning disabled children. Edited by Benjamin B. Lahey. New York, New York: Oxford University Press, 1979. 66-76. (32 References).
Reprints an article from the Journal of Consulting and Clinical Psychology 44(2): 250-60, April, 1976. (Item No. 1750).

1752 ————. "Effects of Ritalin on underachieving children: a replication." Am J Orthopsychiatry 46(2): 313-22, April, 1976. (28 References).
Reports on an experiment which replicates the findings of an earlier study by the authors (Item No. 1750). A new sample of eighteen academically deficient children was selected according to the original criteria, and the same methods were used for the follow-up study. The effects of

Ritalin were analyzed on the same dependent variables. The results confirm previous findings, i.e., while Ritalin is effective in reducing hyperactivity, it does not enhance scholastic achievement. Caution is recommended when prescribing this drug, which should only be used with other management techniques.

1753 Sprague, Robert L., and Sleator, Esther K. "Methylphenidate in hyperkinetic children: differences in dose effects on learning and social behavior." Science 198(4323): 1274-76, December 23, 1977. (22 References).
Studies the effect of various doses of methylphenidate on learning and social behavior of a group of children. Twenty hyperactive children (eighteen boys and two girls) participated in the study. Three drug conditions were used: placebo, 0.3 mg/kg methylphenidate, and 1.0 mg/kg methylphenidate, each given for a three-week period. The Abbreviated Conners Rating Scale was used to measure social behavior; a learning performance task was also administered. Data show a peak enhancement of learning with 0.3 mg per kilogram of body weight and a decrement in learning with 1.0 mg per kilogram of body weight, thus concluding that different target behaviors improve at different dosage levels. Implications of these findings are discussed.

1754 Stein, Claudia L. "The effects of medication and reading programs on the reading performance of hyperactive children." For a summary see: Diss Abstr Int 40B(4): 1917, October, 1979. (0 References).

1755 Swanson, James, and Kinsbourne, Marcel. "Stimulant-related state-dependent learning in hyperactive children." Bull Psychon Soc 6(4B): 421, October, 1975. (0 References).
Abstract of a conference paper presented at the 16th Annual Meeting of the Psychonomic Society.

1756 ————. "Stimulant-related state-dependent learning in hyperactive children." Science 192(4246): 1354-57, June 25, 1976. (21 References).
Discusses the phenomena of state-dependent learning and the fallacies of previous research. Thirty-two hyperactive children and sixteen controls (mean age 10.5 years) performed a learning task in two states: placebo and while taking methylphenidate. The learning task used photographs of forty-eight animals as stimuli and four familiar city names as responses. Each group was tested for retention of each class of learned material in both states. Symmetrical state-dependent learning was demonstrated in the hyperkinetic group, but not in the control group. The state-dependent effect was contingent on the presence of drug-induced facilitation during initial learning. This is apparently the first report on record of state-dependent learning with a drug agent that facilitates, rather than impairs, performance of human subjects.

1757 Swanson, James; Kinsbourne, Marcel; Roberts, Wendy; et al. "Time-response analysis of the effect of stimulant medication on the learning ability of children referred for hyperactivity." Pediatrics 61(1): 21-29, January, 1978. (41 References).
Outlines a method for obtaining behavioral time-response information on the effects of methylphenidate (Ritalin), a psychotropic drug widely used to treat hyperkinesis. Using a laboratory learning task for documentation, researchers found that methylphenidate exerts its maximum effect on learning ability in one or two hours after administration and then dis-

sipates within the same day. This rapid and transient effect of the drug allows the researcher to classify children in a single day as to those who will respond favorably and those who will not. Implications of these findings are discussed.

1758 Van Duyne, H. John. "Effects of stimulant drug therapy on learning behaviors in hyperactive/MBD children." In: The neuropsychology of learning disorders: theoretical approaches. Edited by Robert M. Knights and Dirk J. Bakker. Baltimore, Maryland: University Park Press, 1976. 381-87. (Bibliography).
The effects of methylphenidate on hyperactivity and learning are examined. Discussion centers on drug condition, training procedures, and complex behaviors. The research of various authors is cited.

2. NONDRUG

1759 Ando, Haruhiko, and Yoshimura, Ikuko. "Comprehension skill levels and prevalence of maladaptive behaviors in autistic and mentally retarded children." Child Psychiatry Hum Dev 9(3): 131-36, Spring, 1979. (10 References).
A statistical study on the comparison of the comprehension skill levels between the group with and the group without each maladaptive behavior of nine items was done for autistic and mentally retarded children. Results indicated that the group of autistic children with hyperactivity or withdrawal had slightly, but not significantly, lower comprehension skill levels than the group without each of these maladaptive behaviors. On the other hand, the correlation between the prevalence of hyperactivity or withdrawal and lower comprehension skill levels was seen more clearly, with statistically significant differences, among the mentally retarded children.

1760 Arbuckle, Norma J. "The effect of white noise on short- and long-term recall in hyperactive boys." For a summary see: Diss Abstr Int 39B(2): 1030-31, August, 1978. (0 References).

1761 Beck, Wilford W. "Response selectivity as a function of developmental activity level." For a summary see: Diss Abstr Int 37B(5): 2493, November, 1976. (0 References).

1762 Cantwell, Dennis P., and Satterfield, James H. "The prevalence of academic underachievement in hyperactive children." J Pediatr Psychol 3(4): 168-71, 1978. (10 References).
Investigates academic underachievement in a group of hyperactive elementary schoolboys. Ninety-four hyperactive boys (ages six to eleven years) and fifty-four matched controls were studied. "Predicted grades" were computed for each of the boys and actual grade levels then compared with the predicted grade levels. The hyperactive group was shown to be behind in reading, spelling, and arithmetic. In addition, they were behind in more different subjects and grade levels than normal controls.

1763 Coulter, Susan K. "Concept attainment in normal and hyperactive boys as a function of stimulus complexity and type of instructions." For a summary see: Diss Abstr Int 36B(4): 1913, October, 1975. (0 References).

1764 Das, J. P.; Leong, Che K.; Williams, Noel H. "The relationship between learning disability and simultaneous-successive processing." J Learn Disabil 11(10): 618-25, December, 1978. (21 References).

Compares two groups of children in two studies using simultaneous-successive tasks. Experiment I involved learning-disabled children who were subdivided into hyperactive, hypoactive, and balanced types. Although the LD group as a whole performed poorly on the tasks in comparison with normal controls, there were no significant differences among the various groups. Experiment II tested only those children who had demonstrated specific reading deficits. They also performed more poorly than controls on simultaneous-successive processing. Reasons for the poorer performance are attributed to the strategies that need to be chosen when the child is faced with a somewhat unfamiliar task.

1765 Dubey, Dennis R., and O'Leary, Susan G. "Increasing reading comprehension of two hyperactive children: preliminary investigation." Percept Mot Skills 41(3): 691-94, December, 1975. (20 References).

Examines the effects of oral reading on comprehension in hyperactive children. Two hyperactive children (one eight-year-old boy and one nine-year-old girl), who had displayed deficits in reading comprehension, served as subjects. Each child, in individual tutoring sessions, read four stories per session, two silently and two orally. Each reading was timed and the children were then questioned orally as to the content of the stories. Results show that the children made only half the comprehension errors with the oral readings than with the silent readings. Extended studies, examining whether oral readings can be generalized in the regular classroom, are required.

1766 Frey, William D. "The effects of knowledge of response on initial concept learning in hyperactive; non-hyperactive, impulsive; and non-hyperactive, non-impulsive third grade boys." For a summary see: Diss Abstr Int 37A(12, pt. 1): 7681-82, June, 1977. (0 References).

1767 Friedman, Barry C. "Didactic vs. discovery learning in hyperactive and non-hyperactive learning disabled children." For a summary see: Diss Abstr Int 40A(3): 1402-3, September, 1979. (0 References).

1768 Gupta, Swapna. "Development of a curriculum-oriented training program for short-term memory skills in language-delayed and hyperactive children." For a summary see: Diss Abstr Int 38A(4): 2042, October, 1977. (0 References).

1769 Kravetz, Richard J. "Comparison of discrimination learning characteristics of hyperkinetic disorder and normal children under non-reinforcement and reinforcement pretraining treatments." For a summary see: Diss Abstr Int 40A(6): 3233-34, December, 1979. (0 References).

1770 Lillesand, Diane B. "The effects of varying the information content of a distracting stimulus on discrimination learning in hyperactive and nonhyperactive children." For a summary see: Diss Abstr Int 35B(9): 4654, March, 1975. (0 References).

1771 Loney, Jan. "The intellectual functioning of hyperactive elementary school boys: a cross-sectional investigation." Am J Orthopsychiatry 44(5): 754-62, October, 1974. (15 References).

Attempts to test the hypothesis that hyperactive children have lower IQs than do normal children. Group intelligence test scores and behavior ratings were investigated for a group of hyperactive children along with classmate controls chosen from three second-grade and three fifth-grade classrooms in a small Midwestern college town. Deficits in intellectual functioning were found in the older hyperactive group, but not in the younger group. Both younger and older hyperactive children differed from controls in teacher ratings of impulse control, art proficiency, and general adjustment; older children showed significant deficits in self-esteem. It is concluded that hyperactive children do not differ from their peers in intellectual endowment, but only in intellectual functioning. This situation is attributed to repeated failures and repeated negative interactions between the child and his environment. The need for careful large-scale longitudinal studies is emphasized.

1772 Milich, Richard S., and Loney, Jan. "The factor composition of the WISC for hyperkinetic/MBD males." J Learn Disabil 12(8): 491-95, August-September, 1979. (8 References).
Assesses the intellectual functioning of ninety hyperkinetic/MBD boys at five-year follow-up. Statistical procedures were used to replicate and clarify research findings of attentional and memory deficits on the WISC. The results agree with and tend to replicate previous findings concerning the intellectual functioning of hyperkinetic, minimally brain-damaged children.

1773 Stein, Steven R. "Effect of print size and extraneous noise on reading acquisition for hyperactive and nonhyperactive children." For a summary see: Diss Abstr Int 38A(6): 3391, December, 1977. (0 References).

1774 Tant, Judy L. "Problem solving in hyperactive and reading disabled boys." For a summary see: Diss Abstr Int 39B(9): 4601, March, 1979. (0 References).

1775 Wallbrown, Fred H. "Shedd's formulations concerning the hyperkinetic syndrome--an empirical test of selected features." Percept Mot Skills 46(3, pt. 1): 809-10, June, 1978. (5 References).
Investigates Shedd's formulations which studied score patterns that hyperkinetic children had earned on different types of ability tests. Sixty-two hyperactive children (forty-seven boys and fifteen girls, ages eight to thirteen years) were used to test the Shedd hypothesis that hyperactive children would attain highest IQs on a picture vocabulary test, followed by the Wechsler Intelligence Scale for Children (WISC), and a drawing test. The hypothesis was confirmed by this study.

1776 Zentall, Sydney S.; Zentall, Thomas R.; Booth, M. E. "Within-task stimulation: effects on activity and spelling performance in hyperactive and normal children." J Educ Res 71(4): 223-30, March-April, 1978. (44 References).
Examines the effects of within-task stimulation on activity level and spelling. Four hyperactive and four normal first-grade children served as subjects and were given a set of spelling words with or without added color, movement, and increased size in a repeated measures design. The results support the view that the hyperactive group would have more difficulty in separating the relevant parts of a task from within-task stimulation. This condition led to more errors and interfered with learning.

L. NEUROLOGICAL

1. DRUG

1777 Andreasen, N. J. C.; Peters, Jon F.; Knott, John R. "CNVs in hyperactive children: effects of chemotherapy." In: International Congress on Event-related Slow Potentials of the Brain, 3rd, Bristol, 1973. The responsive brain: the Proceedings of the Third International Congress on Event-related Slow Potentials of the Brain. Edited by W. Cheyne McCallum and John R. Knott. Bristol, England: John Wright and Sons, 1976. 178-82. (Cumulative bibliography at the end of the volume).
Compares CNVs (contingent negative variation) in hyperactive children with learning disabilities while on and off medication and also compares CNVs in hyperactive children with an age-matched control group. CNVs were obtained from seven boys. As a result of the experiment it is concluded that: (1) cerebral stimulants appeared to normalize the CNV in hyperactive children with LD; (2) the more severe the symptoms of hyperactivity, the more questionable or absent were the CNVs; (3) no distinct age-related patterns emerged; (4) there was no demonstrable relationship between clinical EEG evaluation and CNV magnitude; and (5) future research into drug effects on the CNV is required.

1778 Goetz, Christopher; Kramer, Jeffrey; Weiner, William J. "Pharmacology of minimal brain dysfunction." In: Clinical neuropharmacology. Volume 3. Edited by Harold L. Klawans. New York, New York: Raven Press, 1978. 185-201. (157 References).
Presents a neuropharmacologic proposal for the pathophysiology of MBD. Preclinical and clinical data are discussed in four sections: (1) an analysis of centrally active drugs that are used therapeutically in MBD; (2) a review of neurotransmitter assays in MBD; (3) observations on physiologic alterations in children with MBD; and (4) possible animal models of MBD.

1779 Hall, R. A.; Griffin, R. B.; Moyer, D. L.; et al. "Evoked potential, stimulus intensity, and drug treatment in hyperkinesis." Psychophysiology 13(5): 405-18, September, 1976. (16 References).
Attempts to show a relationship between the averaged visual evoked potential (AVEP) and behavior. The responses of a group of hyperactive boys and controls to light flashes of four different intensities were measured with the AVEP. Tests were repeated in both drug (dextroamphetamine) and drug-free conditions. The data failed to support the hypotheses that: (1) hyperkinetic children show a small response to weak stimuli and a normal to increased response to strong stimuli or "hyperaugmentation"; (2) they show increased response to weak stimuli or "reduction" when they are treated with dextroamphetamine; and (3) behavioral responsiveness to this drug is related to the degree of augmentation.

1780 Klorman, Rafael. "Effects of methylphenidate on hyperactive children's evoked potentials." Res Relat Child 41: 115, March, 1978-August, 1978. (0 References).
Abstracts a report of research in progress or recently completed research. Data are provided on: name of investigator(s), purpose of the study, number and kind of subjects used, methodology, principal findings, duration of research, cooperating group(s), and availability of publication(s). Research Relating to Children is compiled by the ERIC Clearinghouse on Early Childhood Education.

1781 Kløve, H., and Bu, B. "The effect of Ritalin on electrodermal responses, blood serotonin, and behavior in hyperkinetic children." Paper presented at the International Neuropsychology Society Meeting, Toronto, Canada, February, 1976.

1782 McIntyre, H. B.; Firemark, H. M.; Cho, A.; et al. "Electrophysiological studies and amphetamine metabolism in hyperactive children." Electroencephalogr Clin Neurophysiol 43(4): 468, October, 1977. (0 References).
Abstract of a conference paper presented at the 9th International Congress of Electroencephalography and Clinical Neurophysiology.

1783 Millichap, J. Gordon. "Neuropharmacology of hyperkinetic behavior: response to methylphenidate correlated with degree of activity and brain damage." In: Drugs and the developing brain. Edited by Antonia Vernadakis and Norman Weiner. New York, New York: Plenum, 1974. 475-88. (17 References). (Advances in Behavioral Biology, Volume 8).
Reports on clinical and laboratory studies which sought to investigate the relation of the degree of activity and brain damage to drug response and to develop an experimental model for the development of new pharmacological therapies for hyperactivity. A close correlation was found between clinical and laboratory evaluations of methylphenidate. The positive effects of methylphenidate were found to be related to the level of motor activity before treatment and the incidence of abnormal neurological signs.

1784 Milstein, Victor, and Small, Joyce G. "Photic responses in 'minimal brain dysfunction'." Dis Nerv Syst 35(8): 355-57, August, 1974. (17 References).
Details a study designed to investigate the effects of magnesium pemoline on EEG recordings of hyperactive children. The study is based on the hypothesis of Shetty (T. Shetty. "Photic responses in hyperkinesis of childhood." Science 174: 1356-57, 1971) which states that the fundamental impairment in children with MBD is a disorder of inhibitory mechanism in the CNS. Twenty hyperactive children (ages six to twelve years) with normal IQs were matched for age, sex, and grade level with normal controls. Findings contradict Shetty's studies and suggest that drugs effective in the treatment of childhood hyperkinesis exert a stimulant effect upon the CNS.

1785 Prichep, Leslie S. "Attention and the auditory evoked potential in hyperkinetic children treated by methylphenidate and in normal children." For a summary see: Diss Abstr Int 35B(12, pt. 1): 6140-41, June, 1975. (0 References).

1786 Prichep, Leslie S.; Sutton, Samuel; Hakerem, Gad. "Evoked potentials in hyperkinetic and normal children under certainty and uncertainty: a placebo and methylphenidate study." Psychophysiology 13(5): 419-28, September, 1976. (42 References).
Investigates the differences between hyperkinetic and normal children and the effects of methylphenidate on the hyperkinetic group under conditions of differential attentional demands. Auditory average evoked potentials were recorded from vertex using a single/double click-guessing paradigm under conditions of certainty and uncertainty. The findings are believed to: (1) reflect the deficit in attention generally associated with hyperactivity; (2) support a model of hypoarousal in hyperactive children; and

(3) reflect the behavioral "normalization" observed in hyperactive children treated with methylphenidate.

1787 Ruthven, Courtney. "The effects of methylphenidate (Ritalin) on the neuropsychological status of learning-disabled-minimal brain dysfunction children." For a summary see: Diss Abstr Int 39B(1): 396, July, 1978. (0 References).

1788 Saletu, Bernd. "The evoked potential in pharmacopsychiatry." Neuropsychobiology 3(2-3): 75-104, 1977. (118 References).
Reviews research in which somatosensory, visual, and auditory evoked potentials (EP) were recorded in different psychiatric populations before and during psychotropic drug treatment. In hyperkinetic children EP measurements revealed that the shorter the latencies and the higher the amplitudes, the sicker the child. It is noted that amphetamines caused a latency increase. The "paradoxical" effects of amphetamines is explained.

1789 ————. "The utilization of evoked potentials in psychopharmacology and pharmacopsychiatry." In: NATO Conference on Human Evoked Potentials, Constance, 1978. Human evoked potentials: applications and problems. Edited by Dietrich Lehmann and Enoch Callaway. New York, New York: Plenum, 1979. 471. (0 References). (NATO Conference Series 3: Human Factors, Volume 9).
Abstract.

1790 Surwillo, Walter W. "Changes in the electroencephalogram accompanying the use of stimulant drugs (methylphenidate and dextroamphetamine) in hyperactive children." Biol Psychiatry 12(6): 787-99, December, 1977. (37 References).
Investigates the effect of stimulant drugs (methylphenidate and d-amphetamine) on cortical maturation in hyperactive children. Fifteen hyperactive boys (ages 5.6 to 10.6 years) served as subjects. EEGs were recorded during drug and no-drug conditions on a simple reaction task. Findings, given in detail, support the concept of a neurophysiological maturational lag in hyperactive children. The role of stimulant drugs in modifying this lag is discussed.

1791 Weber, Bruce A., and Sulzbacher, Stephen I. "Use of CNS stimulant medication in averaged electroencephalic audiometry with children with MBD." J Learn Disabil 8(5): 300-303, May, 1975. (5 References).
The use of averaged electroencephalic audiometry (AEA) with a group of MBD children is reported. In this technique a brief diphasic electroencephalic response at stimulus onset is utilized as an indicator of a child's response to sound. Twelve MBD children were tested on three separate days in a double-blind design under varying conditions: no-drug, placebo, and CNS stimulant. Lower thresholds were evidenced when the children were on medication. Thus, it is suggested that AEA can be enhanced by drugs. Implications of this suggestion are discussed.

1792 Zahn, Theodore P.; Abate, Frank; Little, Betsy; et al. "Minimal brain dysfunction, stimulant drugs, and autonomic nervous system activity." Arch Gen Psychiatry 32(3): 381-87, March, 1975. (26 References).
Investigates autonomic base levels and responsivity to stimuli in two groups of children. Fifty-four normal and minimally brain-dysfunctioned

children served as subjects and were measured on skin conductance, heart rate, skin temperature, and respiration rate under varying conditions (rest, at-task, and at presentation of tones). Data reveal that: (1) no significant differences in base levels were obtained between normal and MBD children who were not taking drugs; (2) stimulant medication increased skin conductance and heart rate and decreased skin temperature and reaction time; (3) MBD children were less reactive, autonomically, to all types of stimuli; and (4) stimulant drugs decreased electrodermal responsivity, which was predictable from concurrent changes in baseline skin conductance and skin temperature. It is concluded that MBD performance deficits are not related to lower autonomic responsivity or lower arousal levels.

1793 Zahn, T. P.; Rapoport, J. L.; Thompson, C. L. "Autonomic and behavioral effects of dextroamphetamine in normal and hyperactive prepubertal boys." Psychophysiology 16(2): 186, 1979. (0 References).
Abstract.

2. NONDRUG

1794 Bauer, Babetta A. "Tactile-sensitive behavior in hyperactive and nonhyperactive children." Am J Occup Ther 31(7): 447-53, August, 1977. (20 References).
Uses a checklist to measure tactile-sensitive behavior in hyperactive children. The Tactile Sensitivity Behavioral Responses Checklist, developed by the author (Item No. 1795), was marked while the children took the Southern California Kinesthesia and Tactile Perception Tests. It was hypothesized that the hyperactive group would have greater tactile sensitivity which would be negatively correlated with tactile discrimination. The findings of the study support this hypothesis.

1795 ————. "Tactile sensitivity: development of a behavioral responses checklist." Am J Occup Ther 31(6): 357-61, July, 1977. (14 References).
Uses a group of ten hyperactive and ten normal five-year-old boys to test tactile defensiveness, i.e., sensitivity to being touched. The boys were administered the Southern California Kinesthesia and Tactile Perception Test battery to identify their behavioral reactions, which were videotaped during the test. These reactions were defined and categorized into a checklist of tactile-sensitive behavioral responses. The behavioral categories offer an objective guide to identifying those children who exhibit tactile defensiveness or sensitivity to tactile stimulation.

1796 Chisholm, R. C.; Milstein, V.; Small, J. G.; et al. "The electroencephalogram (EEG), evoked-response (ER), and contingent negative variation (CNV) in hyperkinetic children." Electroencephalogr Clin Neurol 43(2): 279, August, 1977. (0 References).
Abstract of a conference paper presented at the 1976 annual meeting of the Central Association of Electroencephalographers.

1797 Gabay, S. "Alteration in mono-aminergic functions in hyperkinetic syndromes." Dev Psychiatry 1: 33-46, 1979. (23 References).

Rosenfeld, Anne H., and Rosenfeld, Sam A.
see The roots of individuality: brain waves and perception. (Item No. 1805).

1798 Satterfield, James H. "Central and autonomic nervous system function in the hyperactive child syndrome: treatment and research implications." In: Child personality and psychopathology: current topics. Volume 3. Edited by Anthony Davids. New York, New York: Wiley, 1976. 237-58. (68 References).
Reviews studies that compare hyperactive children with normal control children on laboratory measures of autonomic and central nervous system functioning. Four studies of a subgroup of hyperactive children who obtained a good response to stimulant medication were used to develop a neurophysiological model to explain the pathological behavior of the "good responder" subgroup. Research and treatment implications are discussed.

1799 ————. "Discriminate function models of ERP data in hyperactive children." In: NATO Conference on Human Evoked Potentials, Constance, 1978. Human evoked potentials: applications and problems. Edited by Dietrich Lehmann and Enoch Callaway. New York, New York: Plenum, 1979. 472. (0 References). (NATO Conference Series 3: Human Factors, Volume 9).
Abstract.

1800 Satterfield, James H., and Braley, Brian W. "Evoked potentials and brain maturation in hyperactive and normal children." Electroencephalogr Clin Neurophysiol 43(1): 43-51, July, 1977. (24 References).
Studies evoked cortical potentials in two groups of children: thirty-nine hyperactive children and thirty-nine matched controls. Evidence is presented for two independent evoked potential components, both of which show abnormal changes with maturation in hyperactive children. It is suggested that changes in these two evoked potential components may reflect abnormal development of two quasi-independent neural substrates in hyperactive children.

1801 Shaywitz, Bennett A.; Cohen, Donald J.; Bowers, Malcolm B., Jr. "CSF amine metabolites in children with minimal brain dysfunction (MBD)--evidence for alteration of brain dopamine." Pediatr Res 9(4): 385, April, 1975. (0 References).
Abstract of research done at Yale University School of Medicine. Data suggest a reduced turnover of brain dopamine in children with MBD.

1802 Shetty, Taranath, and Chase, Thomas N. "Central monoamines and hyperkinesis of childhood." Neurology 26(10): 1000-1002, October, 1976. (20 References).
Attempts to determine whether hyperactive children have abnormalities in resting levels or amphetamine-induced alterations in the principal metabolites of dopamine and serotonin in lumbar spinal fluid. Twenty-three hyperactive children (nineteen boys and four girls, ages two to thirteen years) served as participants. An initial cerebrospinal fluid (CSF) sample was obtained. The major metabolites of dopamine and serotonin in the blood did not differ significantly between hyperactive children and controls. In the hyperactive children receiving dextroamphetamine, the amount of homovanillic acid decline correlated closely with the degree of clinical improvement. These results support the view that an alteration in central dopamine-mediated synoptic function may occur in children manifesting the hyperkinetic syndrome.

1803 ————. "Questions raised on monoamines in childhood hyperkinesis --reply." Neurology 27(8): 799-800, August, 1977. (3 References).
Letter to editor.

1804 Snead, O. Carter, III. "Questions raised on monoamines in childhood hyperkinesis." Neurology 27(8): 798-800, August, 1977. (10 References).
Letter to editor.

1805 U. S. National Institute of Mental Health. The roots of individuality: brain waves and perception. Prepared by Anne H. Rosenfeld and Sam A. Rosenfeld. Washington, D.C.: U.S. Government Printing Office, 1976. 29p. (DHEW Publication No. (ADM) 76-352). (ED 132 766).
Major findings are summarized from the use of computer techniques to study perceptual systems of the brain in schizophrenics, manic-depressives, pure depressives, hyperactive children, and normal persons. The use of the electroencephalograph in the early studies of A. Petrie, M. Buchsbaum, and J. Silverman to obtain average evoked response (AER) records are reviewed. Buchsbaum's works on the AER of hyperactive children indicate that those children showing the most abnormal AER patterns seem to respond best to drug therapy. It is predicted that 64 percent of the hyperactive children who will eventually respond to amphetamine treatment can be identified by their AER latency patterns before treatment.

1806 Ward, W. D. "The contingent negative variation (CNV) in hyperkinetic children." Electroencephalogr Clin Neurophysiol 41(6): 645, December, 1976. (0 References).
Abstract of a paper presented at the Western EEG Society, San Antonio, Texas, February 5-7, 1976.

M. SELF-CONCEPT

1. NONDRUG

1807 Charley, Michael J. "The relationship between self-esteem and learning disabilities: a comparative, cross-sectional, developmental study of white middle-class elementary school aged children." For a summary see: Diss Abstr Int 35B(6): 3009, December, 1974. (0 References).

1808 Glow, R. A., and Glow, P. H. "Children's perceptions of hyperkinetic impulse disorder (meeting)." Aust Psychol 14(2): 209, 1979. (0 References).
Abstract.

1809 Greer, Mescal E. "An investigation of influences of placement practices on the self-perception of hyperactive six-, seven-, and eight-year-old children." For a summary see: Diss Abstr Int 39A(2): 662, August, 1978. (0 References).

1810 Ribner, Sol. "The effects of special class placement on the self-concept of exceptional children." J Learn Disabil 11(5): 319-23, May, 1978. (16 References).
Compares the self-concept of minimally brain-damaged children in special classes to the self-concept of children with similar disabilities who

were attending regular classes in order to test the relationship between class placement and the dimensions of self-concept. There were 468 students (ages eight to sixteen years) in the study, some in special classes and others in regular classes. A twenty-nine-item self-concept questionnaire was administered and data factor analyzed. Interpretation of the data reveals: (1) children in regular grades had significantly lower self-concepts in school adequacy, but not in general competence; and (2) both groups of minimally brain-damaged children had significantly lower self-concepts in school adequacy, when compared with normal children, but only those in regular grades held significantly lower self-concepts than normal children in general competence.

1811 Wilson, William D. "A study of self-concept of hyperactive children." For a summary see: Diss Abstr Int 37B(1): 447-48, July, 1976. (0 References).

N. SKIN

1. NONDRUG

1812 Satterfield, James H.; Atoian, Grigor; Brashears, Gladys C.; et al. "Electrodermal studies in minimal brain dysfunction children." In: Clinical use of stimulant drugs in children. Edited by C. Keith Conners. Amsterdam: Excerpta Medica, 1974. 87-97. (11 References). (International Congress Series, No. 313).
Skin conductance levels (SCL) are examined in normal and MBD children to test the hypothesis that the latter group has abnormally high SCL. Eighteen MBD children were compared with eighteen normal matched control children on parent interview data, teacher rating scales, and SCL. It was found that MBD children had more behavioral pathology as reported by parents and teachers and significantly higher SCL. The role of the SCL as a diagnostic aid is discussed.

O. SLEEP

1. DRUG

1813 Conner, Alvin E. "Sleep disturbance in hyperkinetic children." Va Med 104(5): 316-18, May, 1977. (8 References).
Examines the effects of two drugs, methylphenidate and dextroamphetamine, on the sleep patterns of hyperkinetic children. Data are presented on six children (three boys and three girls) who were exhibiting a variety of sleep disturbances: delayed onset of sleep, frequent awakenings, marauding through the house, etc. Stimulant medication was administered to all children during the evening hours. It is concluded that, due to the small sample, firm findings cannot be drawn, but methylphenidate and dextroamphetamine may be effective when given to some hyperactive children with sleep problems.

1814 Feinberg, Irwin; Hibi, Satoshi; Braun, Madeleine; et al. "Sleep amphetamine effects in MBDS and normal subjects." Arch Gen Psychiatry 31(5): 723-31, November, 1974. (31 References).
Summarizes the effects of amphetamines on the electroencephalographic sleep patterns of a group of MBD children. Eight hyperactive boys and controls served as subjects and were given stimulant treatment. Findings indicate: (1) EEG sleep patterns were similar for both groups; (2) neither hyperactive nor normal young adults showed withdrawal elevations

of rapid eye movement (REM) sleep after drug treatment; and (3) stimulant drugs do not reduce eye movement activity during REM sleep, unlike sedative-hypnotics. It is concluded that the effects of amphetamines are not reflected in physiological sleep patterns.

1815 Haig, John R.; Schroeder, Carolyn, S.; Schroeder, Stephen R. "Effects of methylphenidate on hyperactive children's sleep." Psychopharmacologia 37(2): 185-88, 1974. (17 References).
Attempts to assess the chronic effects of methylphenidate and its withdrawal on the sleep of hyperactive children. Six hyperactive boys (ages eight to fourteen years) who had been taking methylphenidate for two to thirty-six months, and six normal boys (ages six to twelve years) served as subjects for the study. EEG sleep patterns were recorded for five consecutive nights in separate sound-attenuated rooms. For the hyperactive subjects, significant increases in latency to both sleep onset and the first rapid eye-movement period were obtained; other sleep measures were normal. Findings suggest that the use of methylphenidate affects the sleep of hyperactive children very little, even with large dosages and with administration close to bedtime.

1816 Matsumoto, Kazuo; Tsujimoto, Taro; Morishita, Hiroshi; et al. "A variation of acupuncture used in the sedation of hyperactive children." Am J Acupunct 3(1): 43-46, March, 1975. (11 References).
Documents a study designed to determine whether a modified acupuncture technique in combination with hypnotics would be effective to induce sleep in hyperactive children. Twenty boys and girls, previously diagnosed as hyperactive, were divided into two equal groups, acupuncture and control. They were administered 50 mg of monosodium trichlorethyl phosphate syrup per kg of body weight to induce sleep in preparation for an EEG recording. Tiny metal contacts about one square millimeter in size were used in place of needles and were affixed to prescribed points on the skin of the hyperactive group. Medication was also given. The control group received only medication. Results show that the time from administration of the drug until onset of sleep was 69.5 minutes (average) in the acupuncture group and 247.5 minutes (average) in the control group. The modified acupuncture technique failed to induce sleep without medication. It is concluded that the theory of Chinese medicine may be an effective adjunct for the sedation of hyperactive children.

1817 Nahas, Abbas D., and Krynicki, Victor. "Effect of methylphenidate on sleep stages and ultradian rhythms in hyperactive children." J Nerv Ment Dis 164(1): 66-69, January, 1977. (8 References).
Assesses the effects of two divided doses of methylphenidate on sleep patterns in a group of hyperactive children. Four boys (ages eight to nine years), who had been referred to the child psychiatry division of a hospital, served as subjects. Sleep was classified as to wake, movement time, REM, and stages I, II, III, and IV. All boys showed behavioral improvement during drug administration; however, no drug effect was seen when standard sleep variables such as sleep stages and sleep time were examined. Although the REM cycle was not affected by drug administration or withdrawal, a trend toward lengthening of the delta cycle was found on drug withdrawal.

2. NONDRUG

1818 White, J. C., and Tharp, B. R. "An arousal pattern in children with organic cerebral dysfunction." Electroencephalogr Clin Neurophysiol 37(3): 265-68, September, 1974. (6 References).

Examines EEG patterns occurring during arousal from sleep in a group of children with clinical evidence of organic cerebral disorder. Eight children (four boys and four girls, ages two to fourteen years) served as subjects and were given EEGs. The EEGs of the children awake and asleep were normal, but an unusual rhythm was produced in the frontal region from the spindle stage of sleep. Although these patterns emerged in only eight of the 4,780 children examined, the incidence of this type of rhythm was unknown in a normal population. It is suggested that the arousal state deserves study utilizing montages containing the frontal electrodes.

P. URINE

1. DRUG

1819 Rapoport, Judith L.; Mikkelsen, Edwin J.; Ebert, Michael H.; et al. "Urinary catecholamines and amphetamine excretion in hyperactive and normal boys." J Nerv Ment Dis 166(10): 731-37, October, 1978. (21 References).
Examines urinary catecholamines and metabolites and urinary amphetamine excretion in two groups of children following a single dose of dextroamphetamine (0.5 mg/kg) and placebo. Fifteen hyperactive boys and fourteen normal boys participated in the study. Tabulation reveals that: (1) hyperactive children had a faster rate of excretion of amphetamine; (2) urinary norepinephrine was significantly higher for the hyperactive group, but did not correlate with motor activity; and (3) normal children showed a significant rise in urinary epinephrine excretion. Further research is needed since these findings did not replicate those of earlier studies.

1820 Shekim, Walid O., and Chapel, James L. "The hyperactive child--effects of d-amphetamine." Hosp Pract 14(6): 18, June, 1979.
Letter to editor.

1821 Shekim, Walid O.; Dekirmenjian, Haroutune; Chapel, James L. "Norephinephrine metabolism and clinical response to dextroamphetamine in hyperactive boys." J Pediatr 95(3): 389-94, September, 1979. (40 References).
Measures the twenty-four-hour urinary catecholamine metabolites 3-methoxy-4-hydroxyphenylglycol (MHPG), normetanephrine (NM), and metanephrine in twenty-three hyperactive boys and thirteen matched healthy controls. The hyperactive children excreted lower MHPG and higher NM (low MHPG/NM ratio) than did controls. The administration of d-amphetamine in the dose of 0.5 mg/kg body weight divided over two doses daily for two weeks decreased MHPG excretion in the hyperactive children. When the hyperactive children were divided into drug responders and nonresponders according to their pre- and posttreatment scores on the Conners Teacher Questionnaire, d-amphetamine administration decreased MHPG excretion in the responders and did not change it in the nonresponders. Percent decrease in MHPG excretion correlated significantly with percent change in the hyperactivity factor of the questionnaire on the Spearman Rank Order Correlation Coefficient. Pretreatment urinary metabolites did not differentiate the responders from nonresponders. It is suggested that a relationship between CNS norepinephrine metabolism and hyperactivity exists and that d-amphetamine may achieve its therapeutic action in hyperactive children by altering CNS NF metabolism.

1822 ————. "Urinary catecholamine metabolites in hyperkinetic boys treated with d-amphetamine." Am J Psychiatry 134(11): 1276-79, November, 1977. (36 References).
Explores the relationship between central norepinephrine (NE) metabolism and hyperactivity and the effects of dextroamphetamine (DAMP) on catecholamine metabolism. Seven hyperactive boys and twelve control children participated in the experiment. Urinary excretion of 3-methoxy-4-hydroxyphenylglycol (MHPG) was lower in hyperactive children, while excretion of normetanephrine (NM) was higher. When the children were administered DAMP for a two-week period, MHPG, NM, and metanephine were significantly depressed. It is hypothesized that DAMP may exert its action on hyperactive children through feedback inhibition of brainstem NE neurons.

1823 ————. "Urinary catecholamines in hyperactive boys before and after treatment with d-amphetamine." Res Relat Child 41: 114-15, March, 1978-August, 1978. (0 References).
Abstracts a report of research in progress or recently completed research. Data are provided on: name of investigator(s), purpose of the study, number and kind of subjects used, methodology, principal findings, duration of research, cooperating group(s), and availability of publication(s). Research Relating to Children is compiled by the ERIC Clearinghouse on Early Childhood Education.

1824 ————. "Urinary MHPG excretion in minimal brain dysfunction and its modification by d-amphetamine." Am J Psychiatry 136(5): 667-71, May, 1979. (29 References).
Studies the excretion of 3-methoxy-4-hydroxyphenylglycol (MHPG) in fifteen hyperactive boys and thirteen controls. Also examined were soft neurologic signs and clinical drug response to d-amphetamine administration for two weeks in the hyperactive boys. MHPG excretion was significantly lower in the hyperactive boys than in the controls. d-Amphetamine decreased MHPG excretion significantly in the drug responders only. Pretreatment MHPG excretion did not predict clinical drug response. The responders had more soft neurologic signs than the nonresponders. Furthermore, soft neurologic signs were not related to pretreatment MHPG levels.

1825 ————. "Urinary MHPG excretion in the hyperactive child syndrome and the effects of dextroamphetamine." Psychopharmacol Bull 14(2): 42-44, April, 1978. (8 References).
Examines the correlation between the presence of hyperactivity in the natural fathers of hyperactive children with the urinary MHPG excretion of their children when they were in the drug-free state and during amphetamine intake. Ten hyperactive boys (ages seven to twelve years) and controls were given a battery of tests. After urine samples were collected, the children received dextroamphetamine for a two-week period. Urine was again tested. Results show: (1) there was a connection between CNS norepinephine metabolism and hyperactivity; (2) dextroamphetamine decreased norepinephrine cell activity; and (3) hyperactive children fall into two groups that can be identified biochemically.

Q. OTHER

1. DRUG

1826 Allen, Richard P.; Safer, Daniel; Covi, Lino. "Effects of psychostimulants on aggression." J Nerv Ment Dis 160(2): 138-45, February, 1975. (54 References).

Reviews the literature on the relation between psychostimulant drugs and aggression. From the accumulated evidence, the following conclusions are drawn: (1) high doses of the major stimulants increase aggression in most species of laboratory animals; (2) small and moderate acute doses reduce or have little effect on aggression; (3) in man, psychostimulants do not increase aggression; and (4) stimulant medications reduce aggression in hyperactive children and adolescents, although the effect of drugs on aggression may be separate from their effect on hyperactivity.

1827 Krippner, Stanley. "Hyperkinetic behavior, stimulant drugs, and creative behavior." Creat Child Adult Q 2(2): 75-81, Summer, 1977. (8 References).
Compares two groups of children (ages nine to eleven years) seen by the Foundation for Gifted and Creative Children. The children were seen because of school difficulties and were compared on tests for brain dysfunction, verbal intelligence, creativity, and mental health to determine differences between drug and nondrug groups. Research indicates that: (1) drug and nondrug groups did not differ significantly on tests for brain dysfunction, but did differ significantly on tests for mental ability, creativity, and mental health; (2) the nondrug group contained more pupils with above-average verbal intelligence and verbally creative scores than did the drug group; and (3) since most of the children in the drug group were not taking drugs at the time of testing, it cannot be claimed that their performance on the tests for brain dysfunction had been improved by medication.

1828 Lesnik-Oberstein, M.; van der Vlugt, Harry; Hoencamp, Eric; et al. "Stimulus-governance and the hyperkinetic syndrome." J Abnorm Child Psychol 6(3): 407-12, September, 1978. (12 References).
Reports on a study designed to test the hypothesis of the first author that hyperkinetic children are stimulus-governed in contrast to nonhyperkinetic children. Thirty-nine hyperactive boys, attending a Dutch special education primary school, served as subjects. The Kinesthetic Figural Aftereffects Test was carried out in two testing sessions. Results show that of the thirty-nine hyperkinetic children tested, twenty-six were stimulus-governed in contrast to twenty control children in which only six were stimulus-governed. The hypothesis is raised that response to methylphenidate is related to stimulus-governance.

1829 McManis, Donald L.; McCarthy, Mike; Koval, Randy. "Effects of a stimulant drug on extraversion level in hyperactive children." Percept Mot Skills 46(1): 88-90, February, 1978. (1 Reference)
Investigates three methods of assessing extraversion level: lemon juice stimulation, reactive inhibition on an audio-vigilance task, and visual-motor maze errors. Seven hyperactive children in a pilot study, and fifteen hyperactive and nonhyperactive control children in a later study served as subjects under varying drug and nondrug conditions. Findings indicate that hyperactive children under drug conditions are significantly less extraverted than without the drug, a finding which upholds Eysenck's procedures. Replication, with larger samples, is needed.

1830 Skinner, Richard G. "Effect of medication on the manual dexterity of hyperactive children." Clin Res 23(1): A65, 1975. (0 References).
Abstract of a conference paper presented at the annual meeting of the Southern Society for Pediatric Research.

1831 VanWyke, Paul E. "Dose effects of methylphenidate on behavioral inhibition and activation in hyperactive children." For a summary see: Diss Abstr Int 34B(11): 5696, May, 1974. (0 References).

1832 Wadeson, H., and Epstein, R. "Intra-psychic effect of amphetamine in hyperkinesis as revealed through art." In: Mental health in children. Volume 3. Edited by D. V. Siva Sankar. Westbury, New York: PJD Publications, 1977. 35-60. (7 References).

2. NONDRUG

1833 Copeland, Anne P. Types of private speech produced by hyperactive and non-hyperactive boys. 1978. 21p. (ED 161 197).
Reprints part of the author's doctoral dissertation which studies types and amount of private speech produced during the free play of sixteen hyperactive and sixteen nonhyperactive boys.

1834 ———. "Types of private speech produced by hyperactive and nonhyperactive boys." J Abnorm Child Psychol 7(2): 169-77, June, 1979. (24 References).
Types and amount of private speech (audible talking that is not addressed to another person) were assessed during the free play of sixteen hyperactive and sixteen nonhyperactive boys. Verbalizations were coded into nine categories that denoted the boys' level of use of verbal control of their own behavior (Luria, 1961; Kohlberg, Yeager, and Hjertholm, 1968). Differences in amount and type of private speech between hyperactive and nonhyperactive boys were found to indicate that hyperactive boys may be presenting a specific or general cognitive lag in development. Treatment ramifications are discussed.

1835 Fritz, Janet J. "Reversal-shift behavior in children with specific learning disabilities." Percept Mot Skills 38: 431-38, April, 1974. (15 References).
Examines response theory by comparing reversal- and intradimensional-shift discrimination tasks in LD and normal children. The three groups tested included twenty LD children not receiving drugs, ten LD children receiving drugs, and twenty normal controls. All groups given the intradimensional shift task performed better than those given the reversal shift task. Controls performed better than either LD group, but the drug group did not perform better than the nondrug groups. The article concludes with a discussion of the Zeaman and House attention theory.

1836 Horner, Gary C. "Hyperactive and non-hyperactive children's self-determined levels of stimulation." For a summary see: Diss Abstr Int 38A(6): 3287-88, December, 1977. (0 References).

1837 Lerner, Howard D. "Hypoactivity and hyperactivity in minimal brain dysfunction children: a comparative study of psycholinguistic abilities, visual-perceptual processes and social extraversion-introversion." For a summary see: Diss Abstr Int 35B(10): 5119-20, April, 1975. (0 References).

1838 Malyon, Alan K. "The effects of a rhythmic auditory stimulus on mentally retarded children." For a summary see: Diss Abstr Int 35B(4): 1919, October, 1974. (0 References).

1839 Miller-Jacobs, Sandra M. "The effects of increased and preferred auditory stimulation on hyperactive children." For a summary see: Diss Abstr Int 40A(3): 1407-8, September, 1979. (0 References).

1840 Morgan, Harry. Black children in American classrooms. 1977. 32p. (ED 139 901).
Presents evidence supporting the notion of advanced sensorimotor development in black children. Among other topics, the current use and abuse of medication for sensorimotor management and hyperactivity are discussed.

1841 Pearlman, Iris. "Relationships among hyperactivity, time of day, and test performance." For a summary see: Diss Abstr Int 40A(6): 3248, December, 1979. (0 References).

1842 Parr, Vincent E. "Auditory word discrimination in male children diagnosed as having minimal brain dysfunction." J Clin Psychol 33(4): 1064-69, October, 1977. (14 References).
Investigates auditory word discrimination in order to test the hypothesis that phonemic aural discriminations would be difficult to make for boys with MBD. Twenty-six boys, previously diagnosed as suffering from this syndrome, and twenty-six controls served as subjects and were tested with phonemically similar and dissimilar words. The MBD group proved to have a significantly higher error rate than the normal group. Further, these children were very susceptible to fatigue while performing the task.

1843 Peterson, Raymond M. "Neurological and sensory dysfunction." In: Peterson, Raymond M., and Cleveland, James O. Medical problems in the classroom: an educator's guide. Springfield, Illinois: Thomas, 1975. 247-58. (31 References).
Discusses some of the medical and psychological aspects of the MBD syndrome. Emphasis is on sensory modalities.

1844 Ramsey, Mary F. "The differential effects of auditory-visual stimuli, spoken-written responses, and task difficulty on activity levels of high and low activity children." For a summary see: Diss Abstr Int 36A(8): 5201-2, February, 1976. (0 References).

1845 Rees, R. J. "Key variables determining the acquisition of speech by autistic five year olds." Slow Learn Child 22(3): 159-72, November, 1975. (34 References).
Reports on a program designed to help two autistic-type five-year-old boys develop speech and language skills. Along with numerous other goals, the program attempted to reduce the boys' hyperactivity while taking the associated figure-ground problem into account. Only one of the boys acquired normal speech, possibly due to the variance in home environments.

1846 Satterfield, James H. "Psychophysiological studies in hyperactive children." Res Relat Child 40: 89, September, 1977-February, 1978. (0 References).
Abstracts a report of research in progress or recently completed research. Data are provided on: name of investigator(s), purpose of the study, number and kind of subjects used, methodology, principal findings, duration of research, cooperating group(s), and availability of publication(s). Research Relating to Children is compiled by the ERIC Clearinghouse on Early Childhood Education.

1847 Senior, Neil; Huessy, Hans; Towne, David. "Time estimation and hyperactivity: replication." Percept Mot Skills 49(1): 289-90, August, 1979. (1 Reference).

Tests the hypothesis that hyperactive children would show a longer estimation of time and a larger margin of error on an experimental task. Three groups of boys included: 135 of normal IQ and normal activity; six hyperactive boys with normal IQ; and six normal activity but low IQ boys. Each participant in each group was individually tested for his ability to estimate thirty-second intervals. Since the six normally active boys of low IQ had significantly different elapsed and estimated times, it is concluded that time estimation is not clinically useful for identifying hyperactive boys.

1848 Stern, John A. "Development of inhibitory controls in the child." Res Relat Child 35: 64, March, 1975-August, 1975. (0 References).

Abstracts a report of research in progress or recently completed research. Data are provided on: name of investigator(s), purpose of the study, number and kind of subjects used, methodology, principal findings, duration of research, cooperating group(s), and availability of publication(s). Research Relating to Children is compiled by the ERIC Clearinghouse on Early Childhood Education.

VII.
Animal Models

1849 Alpern, Herbert P., and Greer, Charles A. "A dopaminergic basis for the effects of amphetamine on a mouse 'preadolescent hyperkinetic' model." Life Sci 21(1): 93-98, July, 1977. (28 References).

Uses an animal model (mice) that might have utility and application for studying components of the hyperkinetic syndrome in children.

1850 Barcus, Robert A. "Food additives and hyperactivity in dogs: an animal model of the hyperactive child." For a summary see: Diss Abstr Int 39B(10): 5054, April, 1979. (0 References).

1851 Bareggi, S. R.; Becker, R. E.; Ginsburg, B. E.; et al. "Neurochemical investigation of an endogenous model of the hyperkinetic syndrome in a hybrid dog. Life Sci 24(6): 481-88, February, 1979. (25 References).

Proposes the use of a telomian-beagle hybrid as a possible model for the hyperkinetic child syndrome. Two groups of hybrids were tested with amphetamine for the study of the mechanism and therapy of this syndrome.

1852 Campbell, Byron A., and Randall, Patrick K. "Paradoxical effects of amphetamine on behavioral arousal in neonatal and adult rats: a possible animal model of the calming effect of amphetamine on hyperkinetic children." In: Aberrant development in infancy: human and animal studies. Edited by N. R. Ellis. Hillsdale, New York: Lawrence Erlbaum, 1975. 105-12. (20 References).

Reviews findings on the effects of amphetamine administration on hyperactivity in rats. Comparisons are made with the hyperkinetic syndrome in children, and it is suggested that amphetamine produces a different if not "paradoxical" effect on behavior in the neonatal animal and that the disappearance of this effect is dependent upon further maturation of the CNS.

1853 Egbe, Patrick C., and Wray, Samuel R. "Differential attenuation by atropine and d-amphetamine on hyperactivity: possible clinical implications." Psychopharmacology 54(1): 25-30, 1977. (41 References).

Reports on a study which uses female rats to measure the effects of physostigmine on motor activity. This animal model is used to discuss the relevance of the cholinergic system in mediating hyperactive behavior in children.

1854 Goldberg, Alan M., and Silbergeld, Ellen K. "Animal models of hyperactivity." In: Animal models in psychiatry and neurology.

Edited by I. Hanin and E. Usdin. Oxford, England: Pergamon Press, 1977. 371-84. (139 References).
Uses the characteristics of hyperactivity and motility to show the relevance, usefulness, and applicability of an animal model to a clinical situation. Some of the experimental paradigms producing hypermotility and some of the neuropharmacological and neurochemical characteristics are presented. The correlation of animal models to human disease is discussed.

1855 Grahame-Smith, D. G. "Animal hyperactivity syndromes: do they have any relevance to minimal brain dysfunction?" In: Minimal brain dysfunction: fact or fiction. Edited by A. F. Kalverboer, H. M. Van Praag, and J. Mendlewicz. Basel, New York: Karger, 1978. 84-95. (21 References). (Advances in Biological Psychiatry, Volume 1).
Considers the hyperactivity syndromes produced by pharmacological means in animals. The actions of amphetamine and methylphenidate are reported and relevance is shown to the minimal brain dysfunction syndrome in children.

1856 Kalat, James W. "Minimal brain dysfunction: dopamine depletion? I." Science 194(4263): 450-51, October, 1976. (13 References).
Comments on a study by Bennett A. Shaywitz, et al. (Item No. 1869).

1857 Lucas, L. A., and Scott, J. P. "Hyperactivity in two dog breeds and their hybrids." Behav Genet 7(1): 74-75, 1977. (0 References).
Reports on an experiment with two breeds of dogs in order to develop a model for hyperactivity in children. Inhibitory training and d-amphetamine were used in the study.

1858 McLean, Jack H.; Kostrezewa, Richard M.; May, James G. "Minimal brain dysfunction: dopamine depletion? II." Science 194(4263): 451, October, 1976. (6 References).
Comments on a study by Bennett A. Shaywitz, et al. (Item No. 1869).

1859 Michaelson, I. Arthur; Bornschein, Robert L.; Loch, Rita K.; et al. "Minimal brain dysfunction hyperkinesis: significance of nutritional status in animal models of hyperactivity." In: Animal models in psychiatry and neurology. Edited by I. Hanin and E. Usdin. Oxford, England: Pergamon Press, 1977. 37-50. (137 References).
Points out the importance of animal models in developmental research and how these models relate to the study of MBD. The role of nutrition and undernutrition in one such model using mice is detailed.

1860 Millichap, J. Gordon, and Johnson, Frederic H. "Methylphenidate in hyperkinetic behavior: relation of response to degree of activity and brain damage." In: Clinical use of stimulant drugs in children. Edited by C. Keith Conners. Amsterdam: Excerpta Medica, 1974. 130-40. (19 References). (International Congress Series, No. 313).
Details an experiment of laboratory-induced hyperactivity in animals and the effects of stimulants on their behavior. Discussion centers on the action of methylphenidate and the relevance of animal studies to hyperkinesis in children. General discussion follows.

1861 Pappas, Bruce A.; Ferguson, H. Bruce; Saari, Matti. "Minimal brain dysfunction: dopamine depletion? III." Science 194(4263): 451-52, October, 1976. (11 References).
Comments on a study by Bennett A. Shaywitz, et al. (Item No. 1869).

1862 Patton, Jim H. "The behavioral and physiological effects of administering lead to neonatal rats: a test of the model of childhood hyperactivity." For a summary see: Diss Abstr Int 39B(11): 5635, May, 1979. (0 References).

1863 "Protein and magnesium deficiency." Nutr Rev 32(3): 90-92, March, 1974. (6 References).
Investigates the acute and chronic changes which can occur in childhood malnutrition. The studies of J. L. Caddell and R. E. Olson using weanling rats show the clinical sequelae when rats are deprived of protein and magnesium in their diets. Abnormalities of behavior and electrocardiographic changes are noted, including hyperkinesis and convulsive states. Reference is made to work previously done by Dr. Caddell in Africa, where it was shown that diet deficiencies produced, among other symptoms, neurological disorders in children. It is stressed that in treatment of ill, malnourished children, attention must be paid not only to protein and calories, but also to the ions in which they are most likely deficient.

1864 Schechter, Martin D. "Caffeine potentiation of amphetamine implication for hyperkinesis therapy." Pharmacol Biochem Behav 6(3): 359-61, March, 1977. (15 References).
Reports on an experiment using an animal model to investigate caffeine potentiation of amphetamine. Results show that neither 0.05 mg/kg d-amphetamine nor 15 mg/kg caffeine alone produced amphetamine-like responding in rats trained in two-lever operant chambers to discriminate 0.8 mg/kg d-amphetamine from saline. The co-administration of the two drug doses produced responding similar to the 0.8 mg/kg d-amphetamine dose. The possible mechanism of action and a regimen for administration of caffeine in hyperkinetic children are discussed.

1865 Scott, John P. "Animal model for study of hyperkinesis and aggression." Psychopharmacol Bull 14(1): 68, January, 1978. (0 References).
Presents a resume of a research project using dogs as a model for the study of hyperactivity and the paradoxical effect of amphetamines.

1866 Sechzer, Jeri A.; Kessler, Pearl G.; Folstein, Susan F.; et al. "An animal model for the minimal brain dysfunction syndrome." In: Mental health in children. Volume II. Edited by D. V. Siva Sankar. Westbury, New York: PJD Publications, 1976. 411-28. (15 References).
Uses the neonatal split-brain cat as an animal model to show that hyperkinetic symptoms are present from birth; that they mimic those of MBD children; and that they can be altered by amphetamine. The cat is considered to be an appropriate model for the study of MBD. Experimental results suggest that: (1) MBD may be related to early brain injury; (2) MBD children have fewer neurons available for complex learning tasks; and (3) central catecholaminergic systems of MBD children may be injured at birth.

1867 ————. "A possible animal model for minimal brain dysfunction." Anat Rec 178(2): 522, February, 1974. (0 References).

Abstract of a conference paper presented at the 87th Annual Meeting of the American Association of Anatomists.

1868 Shaywitz, Bennett A. "Minimal brain dysfunction: dopamine depletion? IV." Science 194(4263): 452-53, October, 1976. (17 References).
Responds to the methodological criticisms of J. W. Kalat (Item No. 1856), J. H. McLean, et al (Item No. 1858), and B. A. Pappas, et al. (Item No. 1861). Further modifications of the animal model of MBD and certain criteria that would have to be fulfilled by it are specified.

1869 Shaywitz, Bennett A.; Yager, Robert D.; Klopper, Jeffrey, H. "Selective brain dopamine depletion in developing rats: an experimental model of minimal brain dysfunction." Science 191(4224): 305-8, January 23, 1976. (15 References).
Explores the relationship between deficiency of brain dopamine and MBD in children. Administration of 6-hydroxydopamine to neonatal rats produced a rapid and profound depletion of brain dopamine. Between twelve and twenty-two days of age, total activity of treated animals is significantly greater than that of controls, but then declines. This pattern is said to be characteristic of children with MBD and suggests a functional deficiency of brain dopamine in the pathogenesis of this disorder. For commentaries on the methodology used in this study refer to Item Nos. 1856, 1858, and 1861.

1870 Silbergeld, Ellen K., and Goldberg, Alan M. "Hyperactivity: a lead-induced behavior disorder." Environ Health Perspect 7: 227-32, May, 1974. (15 References).
Uses an animal model to demonstrate the influence of the ingestion of lead on hyperactive behavior. One hundred and fifty mice from more than thirty litters were exposed to lead from birth by substituting solutions of lead acetate for the drinking water of their mothers, thus exposing suckling mice to lead through their mother's milk, and after weaning, directly through the drinking water. Lead-treated mice were found to be more than three times as active as age-matched or size-matched controls. Lead-treated mice responded favorably when treated with CNS stimulants. The clinical relevance of this animal model to the hyperactive behavior disorder in children is discussed.

1871 ————. "Lead-induced behavioral dysfunction: an animal model of hyperactivity." Exp Neurol 42(1): 146-57, January, 1974. (42 References).
Uses an animal model to test the effects of lead poisoning. Mice exposed to lead acetate were found to be three times as active as a control group. Both l- and d-amphetamine and methylphenidate suppressed the activity level of the lead-treated mice, while phenobarbital increased motor activity. Implications for the hyperactive child are discussed.

1872 ————. "Lead-induced hyperactivity." Toxicol Appl Pharmacol 29(1): 118, July, 1974. (0 References).
Abstract of a conference paper presented at the 13th annual meeting of the Society of Toxicology.

1873 Sobotka, Thomas J., and Cook, Michelle P. "Postnatal lead acetate exposure in rats: possible relationship to minimal brain dysfunction." Am J Ment Defic 79(1): 5-9, July, 1974. (9 References).

Attempts to determine whether reports suggesting an association between lead and the minimal brain dysfunction syndrome in children could be supported by experimental studies. Characteristics of MBD were sought in male rats that were dosed orally with various amounts of lead acetate during their three-week postnatal period of development. No visible signs of neurointoxication were found in the animals. In the high-lead group there was an altered motor responsiveness to amphetamine seen as an attenuation of hypermotility. At 27 or 81 mg/kg, learning performance deteriorated; but it improved when the animals were pretreated with amphetamine. Data support the suggestion that perinatal exposure to lead could be related etiologically to some forms of MBD.

1874 Stinus, L.; Gaffori, O.; Simon, H.; et al. "Small doses of apomorphine and chronic administrations of d-amphetamine reduce locomotor hyperactivity produced by radiofrequency lesions of dopaminergic A10 neurons area." Biol Psychiatry 12(6): 719-32, December, 1977. (37 References).
Uses an animal model to investigate the DA hypothesis. Comments are made as to its relevance to the hyperkinetic syndrome in children.

1875 Wray, Samuel R., and Egbe, Patrick C. "The possible usefulness of anti-cholinergic drugs in the treatment of the hyperkinetic syndrome in children: part II." West Indian Med J 25(3): 155-57, September, 1976. (10 References).
Uses an animal model to determine the possible effectiveness of anticholinergic drugs in the treatment of hyperkinesis in children. Rats that were treated with physostigmine (0.05 mg/kg) showed marked hyperactive behavior. In a previous study, dexamphetamine (2.0 mg/kg) did not antagonize the physostigmine-induced locomotor hyperactivity. This study points to the effectiveness of atropine (10 mg/kg) on the rats' hyperactivity, and therefore suggests that anti-cholinergic agents may have a place in the therapeutic management of the child with MBD and hyperkinesis.

1876 ————. "Studies of the hyperkinetic syndrome--Part I: An experimental analysis." West Indian Med J 24(3): 160-64, September, 1975. (14 References).
Uses an animal model to suggest the effectiveness of anti-cholinergic drugs as a useful therapy in hyperactive children. Also tested was the hypothesis that the hyperkinetic syndrome may be due to transmitter disturbances in the neostriatum in the direction of cholinergic overactivity. Female albino rats received these drugs: carbachol; physostigmine sulphate (BDH); dl-methyl-para-tyrosine methyl ester (AMPT); and d-amphetamine sulphate. They were placed in the center of a Y maze where the number of entries into the arms of the maze was charted for a three-minute observational period. The effects of the various drugs on the locomotor behavior of the rats are detailed. The concept of a cholinomimetic dysfunction as a determinant of hyperactive behavior is also examined. It is felt that this approach would assist in delineating the nature of hyperkinesia, and that anti-cholinergics may represent useful therapy. Further research is needed for the validation of these concepts.

VIII. Follow-Up, Longitudinal, and Prognostic Studies

1877 Abbott, Ronald C., and Frank, Barbara E. "A follow-up of LD children in a private special school." Acad Ther 10(3): 291-98, Spring, 1975. (8 References).
Investigates the academic, social, and emotional progress of children who attended Pathway School, a day and residential facility for learning-disabled boys and girls (ages five to fifteen years). Although the sample was limited, it is suggested that the special school can have an important effect on the future of learning-disabled children. Other follow-up studies and government intervention are indicated.

1878 Ackerman, Peggy T.; Dykman, Roscoe; Peters, John E. "Teenage status of hyperactive and nonhyperactive learning disabled boys." Am J Orthopsychiatry 47(4): 577-96, October, 1977. (40 References).
Presents a follow-up study of sixty-two children first evaluated at age ten. Three groups of learning-disabled boys (twenty-three hyperactives, twenty-five normoactives, and fourteen hypoactives) were then reevaluated at age fourteen. Ratings were obtained from teachers, parents, and a psychiatrist. At follow-up, all three groups continued to lag behind normal controls on academic and cognitive measures and on complex reaction time; some of the teenagers presented varying behavior problems. Only the mental health of normoactives compared favorably with controls.

1879 Anderson, Camilla M. "Society pays for the learning disabled." J Am Med Wom Assoc 29(10): 458-62, October, 1974. (0 References).
Presents case studies from the author's files of nine delinquent young adults (six males and three females) previously diagnosed as having MBD. Many social ills--chronic welfare, divorce, child abuse, and violent crimes--are attributed to misdiagnosed and untreated MBD. Because of the heavy toll society ultimately pays for the learning disabled, the author calls for proper legislation, rehabilitation and educational programs, and limiting procreation to those families with necessary resources for successful management.

1880 Axelrod, Penny, and Haller, Jerome. "Questions about hyperkinesis study." Pediatrics 60(5): 770-72, November, 1977. (9 References).
Letter to editor.

1881 Barcai, Avner, and Rabkin, Leslie Y. "A precursor of delinquency: the hyperkinetic disorder of childhood." Psychiatr Q 48(3): 387-99, 1974. (37 References).
Investigates several behavior and personality variables as common both to theories of the etiology of delinquency and to the life histories of hyperkinetic children. One case history, representative of the link of hyperkinesis in childhood and later antisocial behavior, is cited. The

role of psychopharmacological agents in support of the hypothesized relationship is outlined.

1882 Beck, Mitchell A. "A follow-up study of adults who were clinically diagnosed as hyperkinetic in childhood." For a summary see: Diss Abstr Int 37A(11): 7066, May, 1977. (0 References).

1883 ————. "A follow-up study of adults who were clinically diagnosed as hyperkinetic in childhood." Paper presented at the 56th Annual International Convention, the Council for Exceptional Children, Kansas City, Missouri, May 2-5, 1978. 15p. (ED 153 384).
Examines the extent to which symptoms of hyperkinesis persist into adulthood. At follow-up young adults still showed signs of primary hyperkinesis: 58 percent had repeated at least one year of school, and 75 percent graduated from high school.

1884 ————. "A follow-up study of adults who were diagnosed as hyperkinetic in childhood." Coll Stud J 13(1): 44-50, Spring, 1979. (14 References).
Provides a follow-up assessment of the adult outcome of childhood hyperkinesis. Twenty-four subjects were located approximately thirteen years, seven months after being diagnosed as hyperactive. Tests were administered which would measure behavioral, emotional, social, and academic changes that occurred in this population over time. Because of the prevalence of "secondary symptoms," possible precursors of later psychopathology, the subjects are still considered to be at risk in adulthood.

1885 Bellak, Leopold. "Psychiatric aspects of minimal brain dysfunction in adults: their ego function assessment." In: Adult MBD Conference, Scottsdale, Arizona, 1978. Psychiatric aspects of minimal brain dysfunction in adults. Edited by Leopold Bellak. New York, New York: Grune & Stratton, 1979. 73-101. (41 References).
Reviews MBD characteristics present in children and studies the persistence of these characteristics in adults. Discussion centers on defining MBD in terms of ego functions.

1886 ————. "Psychiatric states in adults with minimal brain dysfunction." Psychiatr Ann 71(11): 58-76, November, 1977. (36 References).
Childhood MBD is designated as a recurring theme in adults presenting a variety of complaints: various neuroses, borderline states, affective disorders, and schizophrenia. Hyperkinesis is discussed as one of twelve ego functions characterizing and playing a role in most cases of MBD in adults. Cited and analyzed are various studies which have concluded that MBD is an etiologic factor in some of the most common but least understood psychiatric disorders.

1887 Bellak, Leopold, et al. "Schizophrenic syndrome related to minimal brain dysfunction: a possible neurologic subgroup." Schizophr Bull 5(3): 480-89, 1979. (32 References).
Studies the relationship between MBD in children and later schizophrenia. The hypothesis is tested that one subgroup of the schizophrenia syndrome is predicated upon some neurological deficit. A new diagnostic label is proposed for this subgroup: "schizophrenia syndrome related to MBD." Appropriate treatment is required.

1888 Berman, Allan, and Siegal, Andrew. "A neuropsychological approach to the etiology, prevention, and treatment of juvenile delinquency." In: Child personality and psychopathology: current topics. Volume 3. Edited by Anthony Davids. New York, New York: Wiley, 1976. 259-94. (89 References).
Focuses on the high incidence of hyperactivity, learning disabilities, and other neurological deficits among juvenile delinquents.

1889 Blouin, Arthur G.; Bornstein, Robert A.; Trites, Ronald L. "Teenage alcohol use among hyperactive children: a five-year follow-up study." J Pediatr Psychol 3(4): 188-94, 1978. (24 References).
Compares two groups of children at a five-year follow-up to determine alcohol use patterns. Twenty-three hyperactive children and twenty-two nonhyperactive children who were having other difficulties in school were matched for age, sex, and IQ. All children were eight to nine years old at first assessment. At follow-up five years later, hyperactives: (1) drank alcohol more frequently; (2) showed about the same achievement and intellectual ability; (3) tended to exhibit evidence of hyperactivity; and (4) were rated as having more conduct problems by their parents. It was also found that Ritalin-treated hyperactives showed no more behavioral or academic gains than untreated hyperactives at follow-up.

1890 Blythe, Peter. "Minimal brain dysfunction and treatment of psychoneuroses." J Psychosom Res 22(4): 247-55, 1978. (21 References).
Discusses the role of undetected MBD in the etiology of psychoneuroses. MBD children who reach chronological maturity without developing appropriate neurological organization become phobic and neurotic adults who cannot cope with life-stress situations. This perhaps explains why some patients are resistent to psychopharmacologic and psychotherapeutic treatment. It is suggested that with regression by both children and adults to a period where their development was arrested, neurological organization and vital perceptual changes become possible.

1891 Borland, Barry L. "Social adaptation in men who were hyperactive: a follow-up study of hyperactive boys and their brothers." In: Adult MBD Conference, Scottsdale, Arizona, 1978. Psychiatric aspects and minimal brain dysfunction in adults. Edited by Leopold Bellak. New York, New York: Grune & Stratton, 1979. 45-59. (8 References).
Examines the relationship between childhood hyperactivity and measures of adult social adaptation and self-concept by comparing men who were hyperactive in childhood with their unaffected brothers. Follow-up information was obtained through personal interviews of twenty men and eighteen brothers and two brothers-in-law of these men. Results show: (1) men who were hyperactive twenty to twenty-five years ago were all steadily employed and self-supporting; (2) more than half the men had entered military service, but had more problems and lower rank than their brothers; (3) nearly half the married probands had marital difficulties; (4) probands had little involvement in social groups and experienced difficulties in this area; and (5) symptoms of low self-esteem were most apparent in men who continued to have the greatest number of major symptoms of hyperactivity.

1892 Borland, Barry L., and Heckman, Harold K "Hyperactive boys and their brothers: a 25-year follow-up study." Arch Gen Psychiatry 33(6): 669-75, June, 1976. (18 References).
Reports on the results of a long-term follow-up study of a group of men who had previously conformed to the criteria for the hyperactive child

syndrome twenty to twenty-five years ago (1950-1951). Twenty men and their brothers were interviewed. The investigation shows: (1) a large majority of the hyperactive subjects had completed high school, and each was steadily employed and self-supporting; (2) half the men who were hyperactive continued to show signs of the syndrome; (3) nearly half had psychiatric problems; and (4) hyperactives had not achieved socioeconomic status equal to their fathers and brothers. Implications of these results are discussed.

1893 Butter, Hendrik J. "Attention, sensory reception, and autonomic reactivity of hyperkinetic adolescents: a follow-up study." Psychiatr J Univ Ottawa 2(3): 106-11, September, 1977.
Traces the persistence of the hyperkinetic syndrome into adolescence and adulthood. Fourteen hyperkinetic children participated in the study and were evaluated by various means (psychometrically, perceptually, and psychophysiologically). The psychometric and psychophysiological assessments indicated that some of the common hyperactive symptoms--short attention span, distractibility, and impulsivity--persisted in later life. A brief discussion of A. R. Luria's theory on inhibitory control completes the article.

1894 Campbell, Susan B.; Endman, Maxine W.; Bernfeld, Gary. "Three-year follow-up of hyperactive preschoolers into elementary school." J Child Psychol Psychiatry 18(3): 239-49, August, 1977. (15 References).
Presents the results of a follow-up study of a group of hyperactive and control children. Of fifty-four subjects who were originally observed in a research nursery at age four, only thirty-one (fifteen hyperactives and sixteen controls) participated in the study in their elementary school classroom at age seven-and-one-half. Observations were made in the regular classrooms by observers who were "blind" to group membership. Both child behaviors (out-of-seat, off-task, disruptive and attention-seeking behaviors) and teacher behaviors (negative feedback, directions) were rated. The hyperactive children tended to: (1) receive more negative feedback from teachers; (2) participate in more disruptive behavior; (3) be rated by teachers as more hyperactive; and (4) express lower self-esteem than controls. Discussion of the results is included.

1895 Campbell, Susan; Schleifer, Michael; Weiss, Gabrielle. "A two-year follow-up of hyperactive preschoolers." Am J Orthopsychiatry 47(1): 149-62, January, 1977. (21 References).
Twenty hyperactive children and twenty-one controls, studied in a research nursery at age four, were followed up at age six-and-one-half. The hyperactive children were still reported to have more behavior problems. Those rated extremely active in the nursery requested more feedback and made more comments in interactions with their mothers as well as more immature moral judgments. Children rated only moderately active did not differ from controls on these measures.

1896 Cantwell, Dennis P. "Hyperactivity and antisocial behavior." J Am Acad Child Psychiatry 17(2): 252-62, Spring, 1978. (40 References).
Reviews evidence that the hyperkinetic syndrome of childhood is strongly associated with the development of antisocial behavior in childhood, adolescence, and later life. Data were gathered from a number of sources: childhood histories of adults with antisocial disorders, post facto and prospective follow-up studies of hyperactive children, family studies,

and treatment studies. Discussion centers on the association between the hyperkinetic syndrome and antisocial disorders. The author concludes that: (1) this association exists; (2) although the mechanism of association is unknown, possibilities include the persistence of a physiological abnormality, genetic, familial, and environment factors, and educational failure; and (3) definitive studies have yet to be completed.

1897 ————. "Natural history and prognosis in the hyperactive child syndrome." In: Cantwell, Dennis P., ed. The hyperactive child: diagnosis, management, current research. New York, New York: Spectrum Publications, distributed by John Wiley and Sons, 1975. 51-64. (23 References). (Series on Child Behavior and Development, Volume I).
Reviews available research evidence pertaining to the natural history and ultimate prognosis of children with the hyperactive syndrome and gives consideration to prognostic factors and the effect of different treatment modalities. Follow-up studies (prospective and retrospective) indicate that: (1) hyperactive children are prone to develop significant psychiatric and social problems in adolescence and later life; (2) antisocial behavior, serious academic retardation, poor self-image, and depression seem to be the most common outcomes during the teenage years; (3) alcoholism, sociopathy, hysteria, and psychosis are possible outcomes in adulthood; (4) evidence for indicators of prognosis is limited and contradictory; and (5) research has not effectively demonstrated that treatment intervention really affects the long-term outcome of the hyperactive child.

1898 Casey, Patrick. "The hyperactive child: review and suggested management." Tex Med 73(6): 68-75, June, 1977. (35 References).
Compares chart reviews of the evaluation, treatment, and follow-up of a group of children seen in a university general outpatient department with an idealized management scheme for such problems. Thirty-seven hyperactive children participated in the study. Detailed tables display sources of data most frequently used and data on follow-up visits. Four recommendations are made concerning physicians' treatment of the hyperactive child.

1899 ————. "Minimal brain dysfunction in suicidal adolescents." J Pediatr 91(6): 1029, December, 1977. (3 References).
Letter to editor.

1900 Chazan, Maurice, and Jackson, Susan. "Behaviour problems in the infant school: changes over two years." J Child Psychol Psychiatry 15(1): 33-46, January, 1974. (4 References).
Compares the changes in behavior problems (including restlessness) in a sample of 602 children on two occasions: when they first entered nursery school and again two years later. Teachers' judgments were used to evaluate the behaviors on both occasions. Detailed information is given on incidence of behavior problems, distribution by socioeconomic area, sex differences, and persistence of behavior problems.

1901 Collis, P. "Does minimal brain dysfunction persist into adulthood?" S Afr Med J 53(13): 477, April 1, 1978. (3 References).
Letter to editor.

1902 Dykman, Roscoe A.; Peters, John E.; Ackerman, Peggy T. "Children with learning disabilities: a follow-up." Res Relat Child 34: 47-48, March, 1974-August, 1974. (0 References).

Abstracts a report of research in progress or recently completed research. Data are provided on: name of investigator(s), purpose of the study, number and kind of subjects used, methodology, principal findings, duration of research, cooperating group(s), and availability of publication(s). Research Relating to Children is compiled by the ERIC Clearinghouse on Early Childhood Education.

1903 Eaves, Linda C., and Crichton, John U. "A five-year follow-up of children with minimal brain dysfunction." Acad Ther 10(2): 173-80, Winter, 1974-75. (7 References).
Presents the results of a five-year follow-up study of a group of children previously diagnosed as showing unequivocal signs of brain dysfunction. Forty children (ages ten to thirteen years) were available from the original study. Data were collected on: (1) the relation between the original diagnosis and school placement; (2) parental evaluations of behavioral characteristics thought to be characteristic of MBD; (3) teacher evaluations of the presence of emotional disturbance; (4) general immaturity; (5) specific LD or mental retardation; and (6) parental involvement in organizations concerned with learning disabilities or special education. Findings show that 25 to 30 percent of the children at follow-up appeared to have specific learning disabilities or emotional disturbances, general immaturity, or slow learning. Almost 60 percent were performing below grade level, pointing to an unpromising prognosis for children with MBD.

1904 Goodwin, Donald W.; Schulsinger, Fini; Hermansen, Leif; et al. "Alcoholism and the hyperactive child syndrome." J Nerv Ment Dis 160(5): 349-53, May, 1975. (19 References).
Explores the relationship between hyperactive children and a predisposition to adult alcoholism. In a sample of 133 Danish male adoptees (ages twenty-three to forty-five years), comparisons were made between alcoholics and nonalcoholics. It was found that: (1) the alcoholics, as children, were frequently hyperactive, truant, antisocial, shy, aggressive, disobedient, and friendless; (2) ten of the fourteen alcoholics had biological parents who were alcoholics; (3) adoptive parents of the two groups did not differ with regard to socioeconomic class, psychopathology, or drinking histories; (4) there was no known alcoholism among the biological parents of the nonalcoholics; and (5) as adults, the alcoholics differed from the nonalcoholics only with regard to drinking history, use of drugs, and overt expression of anger.

1905 Hechtman, L.; Weiss, G.; Finklestein, J.; et al. "Hyperactives as young adults: preliminary report." Can Med Assoc J 115(7): 625-30, October 9, 1976. (17 References).
Consists of a preliminary report of a ten-year follow-up study of a group of hyperactive children. Thirty-five young adults (ages seventeen to twenty-four years) who had been diagnosed as hyperactive ten years earlier, served as the sample of the study. A control group was selected at the time of a five-year follow-up study. Interpretation of data shows: (1) the hyperactive group had a significantly higher mean pulse rate, but height, weight, and EEG were about the same as controls; (2) cognitive style tests indicated continued difficulty in reflection, but less impulsivity in the hyperactive group; (3) the hyperactive group still had more academic difficulties; (4) restlessness continued to be a problem in the hyperactive group; (5) general adjustment in work and living conditions was about equal for the two groups; (6) socialization skills were poorer than in controls; and (7) the hyperactive group did not show more antisocial behavior, drug use, or serious psychological disturbances than did controls.

1906 Hechtman, Lily; Weiss, Gabrielle; Metrakos, Kay. "Hyperactive individuals as young adults: current and longitudinal electroencephalographic evaluation and its relation to outcome." Can Med Assoc J 118(8): 919-21, 923, April 22, 1978. (14 References).
Compares EEG findings and global outcomes of a group of hyperactive children in a long-term study. Thirty-one hyperactive young adults (mean age 19.17 years) and twenty-seven matched controls (mean age 18.59 years) were assessed at follow-up ten years later. EEGs were recorded under various conditions. Tabulation reveals no significant differences between the two groups at the ten-year follow-up, although some differences were documented at a five-year follow-up. The hypothesis is supported that EEG abnormalities of hyperactive persons are those of an immature pattern that tends to normalize with age.

1907 Hopkins, J.; Perlman, T.; Hechtman, L.; et al. "Cognitive style in adults originally diagnosed as hyperactives." J Child Psychol Psychiatry 20(3): 209-16, July, 1979. (24 References).
Investigates several difficulties present in childhood and adolescence which persisted in the young adult age group. The cognitive styles of reflection-impulsivity, field-dependence-independence, and constricted-flexible control were studied in seventy hyperactive adults and forty-two matched controls as part of a follow-up study. Results indicated that the hyperactive adults were more field-dependent and more constricted than the controls. They were also less accurate, although they did not respond more quickly than the controls on a visual matching task. Educational implications are discussed.

1908 Hoy, Elizabeth; Weiss, Gabrielle; Minde, Klaus; et al. "The hyperactive child at adolescence: cognitive, emotional, and social functioning." J Abnorm Child Psychol 6(3): 311-24, September, 1978. (28 References).
Compares the performance of a group of adolescents diagnosed hyperactive five years previously to the performance of a control group matched in age, sex, intelligence, and social class. Fifteen adolescent boys and fifteen normal controls served as subjects; they were given eleven cognitive and three self-assessment tests. Hyperactive children performed significantly worse than controls on the sustained attention, visual-motor, and motor tasks, and on two of the four reading tests. Ratings on self-esteem were also lower. It is concluded that deficits suffered early in life are not transitory but often persist into adulthood.

1909 Huessy, Hans R. "The adult hyperkinetic." Am J Psychiatry 131(6): 724-25, June, 1974. (5 References).
Letter to editor.

1910 ————. "Questions about hyperkinesis study--reply." Pediatrics 60(5): 771-72, November, 1977. (1 Reference).
Letter to editor.

1911 Huessy, Hans R., and Cohen, Alan H. "Hyperkinetic behaviors and learning disabilities followed over seven years." Pediatrics 57(1): 4-10, January, 1976. (23 References).
Reports on a seven-year follow-up study of 501 children--all the second graders in a number of rural school districts in Vermont. The 1966 study was conducted by teacher questionnaire in the second, fourth, and fifth grades for the presence of behavior problems and learning disabilities usually associated with MBD. The same teacher questionnaire was again

filled out by the teachers in 1968, 1969, and 1973. Tabulated data from the 1973 study indicate that the 20 percent of children with the highest number of disabilities showed a rate of behavioral or academic maladjustment in the ninth grade of 35 percent. The 30 percent of children with the lowest number of disabilities showed no member performing poorly in the ninth grade. Of the group between the thirtieth and seventieth percentile, 5 percent were doing poorly and most of their scores placed them in the upper range. Figures in the text detail the classification and movement patterns within the group. For a commentary on this study refer to Item No. 1928.

1912 ————. "Vulnerability of a hyperkinetic (MBD) child to subsequent serious psychopathology: a controlled seven year follow-up." In: Child in his family, Volume 4: Vulnerable children. Edited by E. J. Anthony, C. Koupernik, and C. Chiland. New York, New York: Wiley, 1978. 491-504. (20 References). (A Wiley-Interscience Book). (International Association for Child Psychiatry and Allied Professions, Volume 4).

1913 Huessy, H. R.; Marshall, C. D.; Gendron, R. A. "Five hundred children followed from grade 2 through grade 5 for the prevalence of behavior disorder." In: Clinical use of stimulant drugs in children. Edited by C. Keith Conners. Amsterdam: Excerpta Medica, 1974. 79-86. (15 References). (International Congress Series, No. 313).

Reports on a study of both the prevalence and stability of hyperkinesis in a group of 500 second graders. The children were studied again one-and-one-half years later (at the beginning of the fourth grade) and once more in the fifth grade. All were rated by teachers and all were untreated. Results are given in detail.

1914 Huessy, H. R.; Metoyer, Marie; Townsend, Marjorie. "8-10 year follow-up of 84 children treated for behavioral disorder in rural Vermont." Acta Paedopsychiatr 40(6): 230-35, 1974. (11 References).

Eighty-four rural Vermont children, originally diagnosed as hyperkinetic and placed on psychopharmacologic therapy, were assessed eight to ten years later. The ages of the children and young adults ranged from nine to twenty-four years at the time of follow-up. Results show that hyperkinetic children were seriously at risk for later emotional, academic, and social problems. Contrary to some studies which show the symptoms of hyperactivity diminishing during adolescence, these statistics indicate that eighteen subjects were already institutionalized in either a mental hospital or a correctional facility, and the school dropout rate for this group was five times the usual rate for the State of Vermont. The hyperkinetic syndrome may appear to represent a lifetime disability requiring long-term therapeutic programming.

1915 "Hyperactives as teens: problems linger." Sci News 112(24): 389-90, December 10, 1977. (0 References).

Reports research by Dykman and Peters who conducted a follow-up study of sixty-two fourteen-year-old hyperactive boys. These children were found to have a variety of academic and social problems at the time of follow-up.

1916 Kohn, Martin. "From preschool to preadolescence: a longitudinal study." Res Relat Child 35: 60, March, 1975-August, 1975. (0 References).

Abstracts a report of research in progress or recently completed research. Data are provided on: name of investigator(s), purpose of the study, number and kind of subjects used, methodology, principal findings, duration of research, cooperating group(s), and availability of publication(s). Research Relating to Children is compiled by the ERIC Clearinghouse on Early Childhood Education.

1917 Kramer, John, and Loney, Jan. "Predicting adolescent antisocial behavior among hyperactive boys." Paper presented at the 86th Annual Meeting of the American Psychological Association, Toronto, Canada, August, 1978. 13p. (ED 169 723).
Presents the results of a follow-up study which was undertaken in an attempt to specify those factors which predict delinquent behavior. One hundred and thirty-five hyperactive boys (ages four to twelve years) participated in the study. Follow-up interviews examined norm-violating and delinquent behaviors. Results indicate the scores on the child aggression factor at referral were predictive of all drinking offenses, whereas scores on the child hyperactivity factor failed to predict any of the four categories tested.

1918 Milich, Richard, and Loney, Jan. "The role of hyperactive and aggressive symptomatology in predicting adolescent outcome among hyperactive children." Paper presented at the 86th Annual Meeting of the American Psychological Association, Toronto, Canada, August, 1978. 24p. (ED 169 728).
Reviews research regarding adolescent outcome for hyperactive children. It is generally concluded that, regardless of whether the child was successfully treated with medication, he is at risk for a variety of academic, emotional, and societal difficulties. Directions for future research are outlined.

1919 ————. "The role of hyperactive and aggressive symptomatology in predicting adolescent outcome among hyperactive children." J Pediatr Psychol 4(2): 93-112, June, 1979. (71 References).
A survey of the literature indicates that hyperactive adolescents are at risk for a variety of difficulties: academic, emotional, and societal. Further, these problems seem to persist whether or not the adolescent was successfully treated with medication. This finding is inconsistent with short-term studies which find stimulant medication to reduce the symptoms of hyperactivity. The authors present reasons for this seeming inconsistency.

1920 Miller, James S. "Hyperactive children: a ten-year study." Pediatrics 61(2): 217-23, February, 1978. (49 References).
Summarizes the observations of a physician's ten-year pediatric practice. Two hundred and ninety hyperactive children were examined during this period. Hyperactivity is seen as an emotional problem; thus, the child's inner state or family relationships should be central concerns. Family problems and disorders should be carefully considered in cases of hyperactivity, especially those in which there is insufficient evidence of neurological dysfunction. Additional studies of family dynamics and hyperactivity are needed. For a commentary on this study refer to Item No. 220.

1921 Milman, Doris H. "Minimal brain dysfunction in childhood: outcome in late adolescence and early adult years." J Clin Psychiatry 40(9): 371-80, September, 1979. (30 References).

Monitors the clinical course of a group of patients prospectively from childhood into adolescence and early adult life. Seventy-three patients, diagnosed in childhood as having minimal brain dysfunction syndrome and further classified as either developmental lag (38 percent) or organic brain syndrome (62 percent), were followed into late adolescence and early adult life. At follow-up 7 percent were free of psychiatric disorder, 80 percent had various types of personality disorder, and 14 percent were borderline psychotic. Global outcome was rated as satisfactory in 20 percent, unsatisfactory in 80 percent. Associated with an unsatisfactory outcome were low normal or borderline intelligence, multiplicity of behavioral and neuropsychological findings, learning disabilities, special class placement, and initial classification of organic brain syndrome.

1922 ————. "Minimal brain dysfunction in childhood: I. Outcome in late adolescence and early adult years. Final version." Paper presented at the Annual Meeting of the American Psychiatric Association. 1977. 33p. (ED 155 880).
Uses a group of seventy-three patients, diagnosed as having MBD in childhood, to study psychiatric status, educational attainment, social adjustment, and global adjustment of the patients in late adolescence and early adulthood. At the time of follow-up 6 percent had no psychiatric disorder, 80 percent had personality disorder, and 14 percent were borderline psychotic. In education, 84 percent had completed high school; and of 27 percent who had attempted higher education, 12 percent were still attending. In global ratings, 80 percent of the patients were marginal or poor.

1923 ————. "Minimal brain dysfunction in childhood: II. Late outcome in relation to initial presentation. III. Predictive factors in relation to late outcome." 1978. 38p. (ED 175 191).
Explores late outcome of MBD in seventy-three patients in relation to their initial presentation and predictive factors. This, as well as the earlier study, followed patients for ten to twenty years. Treatment did not have a differential effect on outcome, and poor prognosis for the MBD child is given.

1924 ————. "Minimal brain dysfunction syndrome in childhood: late outcome in relation to initial presentation and initial diagnostic categories." <u>Pediatr Res</u> 12(4, pt. 2): 374, April, 1978. (0 References).
An abstract of a conference paper presented at the annual meeting of the American Pediatric Society and the Society for Pediatric Research.

1925 Morrison, James R. "Diagnosis of adult psychiatric patients with childhood hyperactivity." <u>Am J Psychiatry</u> 136(7): 955-58, July, 1979. (16 References).
Studies the influence of childhood hyperkinesis on adult psychiatric status to determine if such children are at greater risk to become psychiatrically ill as adults. Forty-eight adult psychiatric patients (twenty-seven men and twenty-one women) who had been hyperactive as children were compared with two groups of patients who had not. Both comparison groups were matched for age and sex and the second was also matched for economic status. Although closer matching narrowed the gap somewhat, the formerly hyperactive subjects still showed significantly more personality disorder of all types than controls--more sociopathy, more alcoholism, and less affective disorder. Schizophrenia and drug

abuse occurred no more often in these subjects than in the comparison groups.

1926 Morrison, James R., and Minkoff, Kenneth. "Explosive personality as a sequel to the hyperactive-child syndrome." Compr Psychiatry 16(4): 343-48, July-August, 1975. (20 References).
Documents three case reports in which common background factors suggesting a possible etiology of the explosive personality are described. Results of the administration of tricyclic antidepressants in each case are discussed. Explosive personality has not met the criteria for diagnostic validity and is characterized by gross outbursts of rage or of verbal or physical aggressiveness not in keeping with the patient's usual personality.

1927 Murley, Harris D.; Milam, Donald R.; Gorman, Warren F. "The hyperactive child grows up." Ariz Med 34(11): 767-68, November, 1977. (20 References).
Reports on follow-up studies of treated and untreated hyperactive children. The untreated group was characterized by poor school performance, low self-esteem, emotional immaturity, and poor vocational development. Often proper diagnosis was made after the subject reached late adolescence or young adulthood. Hyperactive children who are diagnosed early and who receive multidisciplinary treatment show promising results.

1928 Myers, Gary J., and Pless, I. Barry. "Where's the hyperactive child going?" Pediatrics 57(1): 2-3, January, 1976. (4 References).
Comments on a study by Hans R. Huessy and Alan H. Cohen (Item No. 1911).

1929 Nichol, Hamish. "Children with learning disabilities referred to psychiatrists: a follow-up study." J Learn Disabil 7(2): 118-22, February, 1974. (15 References).
Examines how the findings of a psychiatric evaluation of LD children were utilized by school personnel. Data are presented on a random sample of 232 children under eighteen years old in the metropolitan area of Vancouver who were referred to psychiatric facilities in 1960 because of learning and behavioral problems. In 1966, thirty-four of these children were selected for follow-up from the original 232. School nurses, principals, and teachers were asked to complete a questionnaire which included information on the availability and utility of the psychiatric consultation to the school personnel and of the children's subsequent progress in school, including any remedial education which was provided. Results show that in only 40 percent of cases were the findings of psychiatric evaluation available to school personnel, and in less than half these cases were the psychiatrist's findings held by the teachers to be of assistance in their work with the children. Another follow-up study is planned to determine whether or not collaboration between psychiatrists and teachers has since improved.

1930 Offord, D. R.; Sullivan, K.; Allen, N.; et al. "Delinquency and hyperactivity." J Nerv Ment Dis 167(12): 734-41, December, 1979. (28 References).
Explores the relationship between two major psychiatric disorders: antisocial behavior and hyperactivity with delinquency. Thirty-one delinquent boys who were also hyperactive were compared with thirty-five delinquents who were not hyperactive on data gathered by parental interviews and record searches (primarily school, pregnancy, and birth rec-

ords). The finding that the families of the hyperactives were not disadvantaged compared to the families of the nonhyperactives provides support for the hypothesis that pregnancy and birth complications, primarily low birth weight, may be etiologically linked to hyperactivity. The data support the idea that the identification of a subgroup of delinquents on the basis of reported hyperactivity also identifies a subgroup with severe delinquency and a probable poor adult prognosis. An implication of the study is the need to define the hyperactive child syndrome by criteria that do not include antisocial behavior. If the original criteria allow the inclusion of antisocial children, then their adult prognosis may be relatively poor because antisocial children have a poor adult prognosis. More follow-up studies are required.

1931 Preis, Karen. "Minimal brain dysfunction and juvenile delinquency." Paper presented at Symposium on Minimal Brain Dysfunction, University of Vermont College of Medicine, April, 1976.

1932 Preis, Karen, and Huessy, Hans R. "Hyperactive children at risk." In: Drugs and the special child. Edited by Michael J. Cohen. New York, New York: Gardner Press, 1979. 129-87. (149 References).

Reviews literature supporting evidence that children diagnosed as hyperactive or MBD are at risk for future emotional, academic, and social difficulties. This evidence is gathered from six sources: (1) epidemiological studies of the natural history of children with hyperactive behaviors; (2) retrospective studies of adults whose histories have indicated hyperactivity or MBD in childhood; (3) prospective studies of children diagnosed as hyperactive or MBD: (4) identification of adolescents who manifest the symptoms of hyperactivity or MBD; (5) identification of adults who manifest the symptoms of hyperactivity or MBD; and (6) studies of the blood relatives of hyperactive children.

1933 Riddle, K. Duane, and Rapoport, Judith L. "A 2-year follow-up of 72 hyperactive boys." J Nerv Ment Dis 162(2): 126-34, February, 1976. (24 References).

Reports the results of a two-year follow-up study of hyperactive children and matched controls. Seventy-two boys (mean age 10.2 years at follow-up) were examined on classroom behavior, home behavior, academic achievement, peer status, and depressive symptomatology. Of the hyperactive subjects, 65 percent were still receiving medication at the time of follow-up. In spite of this drug therapy and ancillary educational and psychological treatment, the hyperactive subjects continued to show behavioral and academic difficulties, low peer status, and depressive symptoms--all exceeding those of the control group. It is concluded that although drug therapy may continue to have a suppressant effect on hyperactive behavior, peer status and academic achievement may not be improved. Subjects identified as "optimally medicated" had almost identical academic achievement and social acceptance as did a group of dropouts from drug treatment, or the sample as a whole.

1934 Robins, Lee N. Deviant children grown up: a sociological and psychiatric study of sociopathic personality. Huntington, New York: Krieger, 1974. 351p. (Bibliography).

Examines childhood factors that appear to predict adult sociopathic personality. Chapter VI details the deviant traits including twenty-six antisocial symptoms and thirty-three social symptoms. Restlessness, overactivity, and learning problems are classified as positive.

1935 Rohn, Reuben; Sarles, Richard M.; Kenny, Thomas J. "Minimal brain dysfunction in suicidal adolescents." J Pediatr 91(6): 1029-30, December, 1977. (1 Reference).
Letter to editor.

1936 Rohn, Reuben D.; Sarles, Richard M.; Kenny, Thomas J.; et al. "Adolescents who attempt suicide." J Pediatr 90(4): 636-38, April, 1977. (19 References).
Reports on data compiled from a two-year suicide prevention program for teenagers. Of a group of sixty-five adolescents who attempted suicide, three major characteristics emerged: family disruption, social isolation, and academic difficulties. A subgroup of twenty-five adolescents who attempted suicide had a significantly higher rate of minimal brain dysfunction when compared to a matched control group. The suicidal adolescents were seen to function poorly academically, have poor self-images, and possess a number of behavior and discipline problems.

1937 Satterfield, J. H. "The hyperactive child syndrome: a precursor of adult psychopathy?" Paper presented at the Advanced Study Institute on Psychopathic Behavior, Les Arcs, France, September, 1975.

1938 Satterfield, J. H., and Cantwell, D. P. "A one year follow-up study of treated hyperactive children." Paper presented at the Annual Meeting of the Psychiatric Research Society, Salt Lake City, Utah, 1977.

1939 ————. "Psychopharmacology in the prevention of antisocial and delinquent behavior." Int J Ment Health 4(1-2): 227-37, Spring-Summer, 1975. (45 References).
Explores the possible role of drugs in the prevention and treatment of delinquency and antisocial behavior. Because no other therapy has been effective, the use of stimulant medication in treating hyperactive children seems to be a promising area of research into the prevention of juvenile delinquency and subsequent adult sociopathy. Further long-term, clinical, and family studies are required. For a reprint of this study refer to Item No. 688.

1940 Shaffer, D. "Longitudinal research and the minimal brain damage syndrome." In: Minimal brain dysfunction: fact or fiction. Edited by A. F. Kalverboer, H. M. van Praag, and J. Mendlewicz. Basel, New York: Karger, 1978. 18-34. (56 References). (Advances in Biological Psychiatry, Volume 1).
Reviews literature examining long-term social and behavioral sequelae of four of the components of the MBD syndrome: (1) a history of perinatal complication; (2) early acute disturbances of the CNS, e.g., infection, trauma, or metabolic upset; (3) the presence of soft neurological signs; and (4) the so-called hyperkinetic behavior disorder. It is concluded that apparently transient disturbances of the CNS may be followed by adverse behavioral sequelae which persist in the absence of other hard neurological features. Further, some evidence suggests that soft neurological signs may determine later psychiatric disturbances.

1941 Siegel, Ernest. The exceptional child grows up: guidelines for understanding and helping the brain-injured adolescent and young adult. New York, New York: Dutton, 1974. 227p. (Bibliography). (A Sunrise Book).

Discusses four problem areas for the brain-damaged adolescent; psychological, social, educational, and vocational. Also discussed are secondary problems in adolescence, e.g., poor self-concept, anxiety, lack of motivation, social immaturity, and personality deficits. Two basic goals are increasing the suitability of the adolescent's behavior and performance and educating the public to respect those it perceives as different.

1942 Tarter, Ralph E.; McBride, Herbert; Buonpane, Nancy; et al. "Differentiation of alcoholics: childhood history of minimal brain dysfunction, family history, and drinking pattern." Arch Gen Psychiatry 34(7): 761-68, July, 1977. (26 References).
Attempts to establish a relationship between adult drinking patterns and childhood MBD. Severe drinkers (primary alcoholics) reported more symptoms of MBD, retrospectively, than did the less severe drinkers, psychiatric patients, and normals. MMPI and MacAndrew Alcoholism Scale scores are given. The findings are discussed in light of further delineating a specific subtype of alcoholism that may have a genetic-constitutional relationship with other pathological disorders.

1943 Virkkunen, Matti, and Nuutila, Arto. "Specific reading retardation, hyperactive child syndrome, and juvenile delinquency." Acta Psychiatr Scand 54(1): 25-28, July, 1976. (18 References).
Attempts to ascertain the extent to which a specific reading retardation or disability (dyslexia) leads to later behavioral disturbances and delinquency and to what factors such development is due in these cases. Subjects for the study were 224 adolescents with specific reading retardation. Results show that 12.1 percent of the children were prone to juvenile delinquency and criminality between ages fifteen and twenty. The severity of the specific reading retardation did not seem to contribute to this propensity, as did the symptoms of hyperactivity.

1944 Weiss, Gabrielle, and Hechtman, Lilly. "Hyperactive children as adults." Res Relat Child 36: 80-81, September, 1975-February, 1976. (0 References).
Abstracts a report of research in progress or recently completed research. Data are provided on: name of investigator(s), purpose of the study, number and kind of subjects used, methodology, principal findings, duration of research, cooperating group(s), and availability of publication(s). Research Relating to Children is compiled by the ERIC Clearinghouse on Early Childhood Education.

1945 Weiss, Gabrielle; Hechtman, Lilly; Perlman, Terrye; et al. "Hyperactives as young adults: a controlled prospective ten-year follow-up of 75 children." Arch Gen Psychiatry 36(6): 675-81, June, 1979. (19 References).
Reports on a variety of outcome variables from seventy-five hyperactive and forty-four matched control subjects ages seventeen to twenty-four years (mean ages, 19.5 and 19.0 years, respectively). All hyperactive subjects have been followed up for ten to twelve years; they were first evaluated at six to twelve years of age. None of the hyperactive subjects was treated with methylphenidate, although a subgroup received chlorpromazine or a mixture of drugs (excluding methylphenidate). Data reveal: (1) the hyperactive subjects had less education than the controls, a history of more car accidents, and more geographic moves; (2) only a minority were still engaged in continued antisocial behavior or had evidence of severe psychopathology; (3) no subjects were found to

be psychotic, but two were diagnosed as borderline psychotic; and (4) hyperactive subjects had some continued symptoms from the hyperkinetic child syndrome, including impulsive personality traits.

1946 ———. "Hyperactives as young adults: school, employer, and self-rating scales obtained during ten-year follow-up evaluation." Am J Orthopsychiatry 48(3): 438-45, July, 1978. (10 References).
This long-term follow-up study assessed the progress of a group of children previously diagnosed as hyperactive. Seventy-five hyperactive children and forty-four controls served as subjects of a comprehensive ten-to-thirteen-year study, of which this paper forms one part. It has been hypothesized that some of the typical behaviors of hyperactivity might be an asset in work situations. Rating scales were sent to employers, teachers, and to the subjects themselves. Analyzation shows: (1) hyperactives were rated as markedly inferior to normal controls by teachers; (2) hyperactive adults were seen by employers to function as competently at work as normal matched controls; and (3) hyperactive adults viewed themselves as inferior to controls on a personality test, but no different than controls on a psychopathology scale.

1947 Weiss, Gabrielle, and Minde, Klaus K. "Follow-up studies of children who present with symptoms of hyperactivity." In: Clinical use of stimulant drugs in children. Edited by C. Keith Conners. Amsterdam: Excerpta Medica, 1974. 67-78. (19 References). (International Congress Series, No. 313).
Presents findings from five investigations involving long-term follow-up studies of ninety-one hyperactive children referred to a psychiatric outpatient department of a children's hospital. Most of the follow-up studies indicate a lessening of the target symptoms of hyperactivity; however, in early adolescence the children can still be differentiated from normal control children in areas of school problems, attention and concentration, and psychopathology. General discussion follows.

1948 Wender, Paul H. "The concept of adult minimal brain dysfunction (MBD)." In: Adult MBD Conference, Scottsdale, Arizona, 1978. Psychiatric aspects of minimal brain dysfunction in adults. Edited by Leopold Bellak. New York, New York: Grune & Stratton, 1979. 1-15. (16 References).
Addresses the problem of syndromal definition and validation of MBD in childhood. It is concluded that the syndrome exists in adult life where it is commonly undiagnosed and infrequently treated. Validation for the notion of MBD in adulthood is given.

1949 White, James; Barratt, Ernest; Adams, Perrie. "The hyperactive child in adolescence: a comparative study of physiological and behavioral patterns." J Am Acad Child Psychiatry 18(1): 154-69, Winter, 1979. (10 References).
The purpose of this research was to search for differences among: (1) male adolescent psychiatric patients who were successfully treated for hyperactivity in childhood; (2) normal controls; and (3) adolescent psychiatric boys who were not formerly hyperactive. A variety of measures was used in the evaluation: cognitive, behavioral, and psychophysiological. The hypothesis that time perception would differentiate the three groups was also explored. The patients who were not formerly hyperactive did more poorly than the other two groups. Time perception significantly differentiated between controls and patients.

1950 Wood, David R.; Reimherr, Frederick W.; Wender, Paul H.; et al. "Diagnosis and treatment of minimal brain dysfunction in adults." Arch Gen Psychiatry 33(12): 1453-60, December, 1976. (44 References).

Monitors the continuation and persistence of MBD in adult life. Fifteen adults with MBD symptoms were given a trial with methylphenidate, pemoline, imipramine, or amitryptiline. Only five of the subjects were unresponsive to drug therapy. Relevance to children's MBD is discussed.

1951 Zambelli, Andrew J., and Stamm, John S. "Auditory evoked potentials and sustained attention in adolescents diagnosed as minimal brain dysfunctioned (MBD) in childhood." Electroencephalogr Clin Neurophysiol 39(2): 208-9, August, 1975. (0 References).

Abstract of a paper presented at a meeting of the Eastern Association of Electroencephalographers.

1952 Zambelli, Andrew J.; Stamm, John S.; Maitinsky, Steven; et al. "Auditory evoked potentials and selective attention in formerly hyperactive adolescent boys." Am J Psychiatry 134(7): 742-47, July, 1977. (28 References).

Investigates the persistence into adolescence of several prominent symptoms of MBD. Nine formerly hyperactive adolescent boys and nine matched controls served as subjects. The auditory average cortical evoked potentials and behavioral responses were studied as the groups performed a selective attention task. The experimental group continued to show a carry-over of impairments on both electrophysiological and behavioral measures of selective attention--a finding consistent with the generally recognized MBD neurodevelopmental lag.

1953 Zinkus, Peter W.; Gottlieb, Marvin I.; Zinkus, Cathleen B. "The learning-disabled juvenile delinquent: a case of early intervention of perceptually handicapped children." AJOT 33(3): 180-84, March, 1979. (33 References).

Examines the relationship between learning disabilities and juvenile delinquency. Studies are reviewed which support the contention that learning disabilities occur with significant frequency in delinquent populations. These children are at high risk for developing academic/behavioral problems. The role of the occupational therapist in intervention is highlighted.

IX.
Sociological Aspects

1954 Barkley, Russell A., and Cunningham, Charles E. "The effects of methylphenidate on the mother-child interactions of hyperactive children." Arch Gen Psychiatry 36(2): 201-8, February, 1979. (4 References).

Examines the effect of methylphenidate on rate and type of interaction between hyperactive children and their mothers. Twenty hyperactive boys (ages five to twelve years) previously diagnosed as hyperactive and their mothers were observed during free play and task period under three conditions: drug, placebo, and no-drug. Interactions were observed in a playroom equipped with microphones and a one-way observation mirror. Boys wore actometers on their wrists or ankles. Scores indicate that: (1) children were more compliant during drug treatment; (2) in response, mothers displayed increased attention to compliance while reducing their directiveness toward the boys; and (3) hyperactive boys receiving methylphenidate initiated fewer social interactions and exhibited reduced sociability.

1955 Campbell, Susan B. "Mother-child interaction: a comparison of hyperactive, learning-disabled, and normal boys." Am J Orthopsychiatry 45(1): 51-57, January, 1975. (11 References).

Reports on a study designed to measure mother-son interaction in groups of hyperactive, learning-disabled, and normal boys. Thirteen boys (mean age eight years) and their mothers were observed in a structured problem-solving situation. Subjects were given two tasks, block designs and anagrams, and mothers were instructed to help as much or as little as they liked. Maternal and child behavior were coded and the Behavior Problem Checklist was administered to the mothers. Data reveal that mothers of hyperactive boys showed a higher level of involvement in task solution and reported more behavior problems than did mothers in comparison groups. Hyperactive boys also interacted with mothers more than did the other two groups.

1956 Campbell, Susan B., and Paulauskas, Stana L. "Peer relations in hyperactive children." J Child Psychol Psychiatry 20(3): 233-46, July, 1979. (59 References).

This paper examines studies which bear on the peer relations of hyperactive children. Studies were reviewed and some new data reported under five headings: adult reports, self-reports, and peer reports of problems with social interaction, direct observational studies, and studies of social cognition. Few studies actually address issues of peer relations in hyperactive children, although available evidence suggests that this is an area of deficit which should be considered more carefully from both a research and a treatment perspective.

1957 Cunningham, Charles E., and Barkley, Russell A. "The effects of methylphenidate on the mother-child interactions of hyperactive identical twins." Dev Med Child Neurol 20(5): 634-42, October, 1978. (23 References).
Assesses the effects of methylphenidate on the behavioral interactions of identical hyperactive twins and their mother. Two extremely hyperactive five-and-one-half-year-old twin boys of low intelligence were placed on methylphenidate and were then examined in a triple-blind, drug-placebo, single-case, reversal design. Actometers were used to measure activity level in a specially designed room. Each child was observed interacting with his mother in a series of four thirty-minute sessions which included free play and structured tasks. Methylphenidate was found to reduce excessive activity, improve social behavior, increase compliance, and improve sustained attention in the two boys.

1958 ————. "The interactions of normal and hyperactive children with their mothers in free play and structured tasks." Child Dev 50(1): 217-24, March, 1979. (24 References).
Studies mother-child interaction in two groups of boys. Twenty normal and twenty hyperactive boys (ages six to twelve years) were observed interacting with their mothers in free play and structured task situations. Hyperactive boys were more active, less compliant, and less likely to remain on task than nonhyperactive peers. Mothers of hyperactive boys responded more negatively and imposed more structure and controls on their children than did mothers of the control group. Mothers of hyperactive boys were viewed as further contributing to their children's behavioral difficulties.

1959 Diamant, Daniel L. "The hyperactive syndrome as a function of object constancy in children and the use of denial and projection in mothers." For a summary see: Diss Abstr Int 38B(10): 5009, April, 1978. (0 References).

1960 Harris, Harold J. "Interactional patterns of hyperactive children." Res Relat Child 40: 88, September, 1977-February, 1978. (0 References).
Abstracts a report of research in progress or recently completed research. Data are provided on: name of investigator(s), purpose of the study, number and kind of subjects used, methodology, principal findings, duration of research, cooperating group(s), and availability of publication(s). Research Relating to Children is compiled by the ERIC Clearinghouse on Early Childhood Education.

1961 Humphries, Thomas; Kinsbourne, Marcel; Swanson, James. "Stimulant effects on cooperation and social interaction between hyperactive children and their mothers." J Child Psychol Psychiatry 19(1): 13-22, January, 1978. (16 References).
Investigates the relationship between hyperactive children, with and without stimulant medication, and their mothers. Twenty-six hyperactive children (mean age 10.2 years) and their mothers collaborated on a task. The children received methylphenidate or placebo in a double-blind design. Aspects of the quality and quantity of interaction were examined. It was found that a more favorable interaction occurred when the child was in the medicated state.

1962 Klein, Andrea R. "Hyperactive and active boys in the classroom: a naturalistic assessment of teacher ratings, classroom behaviors, peer interactions and perceptions, and subtypes of hyperactives." For a summary see: Diss Abstr Int 39A(9): 5413-14, March, 1979. (0 References).

1963 Klein, Andrea R., and Young, Richard D. "Hyperactive boys in their classroom: assessment of teacher and peer perceptions, interaction, and classroom behaviors." J Abnorm Child Psychol 7(4): 425-42, December, 1979. (25 References).
Compares seventeen hyperactive boys and seventeen normal boys by means of teacher ratings, peer perceptions, peer interactions, and classroom behaviors. Multivariate analyses were used to better describe and assess hyperactivity in the classroom setting. All data sources found the hyperactive boys to be significantly different from normals in that they were perceived and interacted more negatively. Four types of hyperactives were delineated: anxious, conduct problem, inattentive, and low-problem.

1964 Lundy, Nancy C. "Comparison of mother-child interactions in hyperactive and nonhyperactive groups under distraction conditions." For a summary see: Diss Abstr Int 39B(9): 4586, March, 1979. (0 References).

1965 Mainville, France, and Friedman, Ronald J. "Peer relations of hyperactive children." Ont Psychol 8(5): 17-20, December, 1976.
Attempts to study the sociality of a group of hyperactive children. Two hundred and fourteen third- and fourth-grade children were administered the Moreno Scale of Social Acceptance; their teachers were administered the Conners Abbreviated Symptom Questionnaire. Correlations between ratings of hyperactive and peer rejection were 0.74 for boys and 0.13 for girls. Pupils' conceptions of their undesirable behaviors were different from teachers' views of undesirable behavior. Implications for working with hyperactive children are discussed.

1966 Paulauskas, Stana L., and Campbell, Susan B. "Social perspective-taking and teacher ratings of peer interaction in hyperactive boys." J Abnorm Child Psychol 7(4): 483-93, December, 1979. (25 References).
Compares two groups of boys at two age levels on teacher ratings of peer interaction and three measures of social perspective-taking. Teachers' ratings of peer interaction successfully discriminated between hyperactive and control boys. Hyperactive children did not, however, differ from controls on the three measures of social perspective-taking. Implications for treatment are examined.

1967 Schleifer, Maxwell J., ed. "The 'hyperactive' child. Maybe he is emotionally disturbed, and maybe it's our fault." Except Parent 9(2): 22-26, April, 1979. (0 References).
The problems of a twelve-year-old hyperactive boy are related by the child's mother, father, and the child himself. It is pointed out that the boy's problems awakened painful childhood memories in both parents. Improvement in the boy and his mother is noted as a result of neurological evaluation, drug therapy, educational planning, and psychotherapy.

1968 Taichert, Louise C., and Harvin, Donya D. "Adoption of children with learning and behavior problems." West J Med 122(6): 464-70, June, 1975. (14 References).

Documents a case study of an adopted child with learning and behavior problems. This case, selected from a study of thirty-two adoptive families in conflict, shows the special and complicated problems which can exist between an adopted child and his parents. The main factors seen as contributing to dysfunction in this family structure are: (1) the presence of neurodevelopmental deviations in the adopted child, on the basis of which learning and behavior problems often develop; (2) failure of the adoptive parents to understand and cope with special adoption issues; and (3) the presence of serious personal and/or marital conflict, the solutions for which were sought by the adoption of a child.

1969 Warner, Barbara J. "Psychogenic hyperactivity: situational and relationship factors of the hyperactive couple." For a summary see: Diss Abstr Int 37B(9): 4710-11, March, 1977. (0 References).

1970 Whalen, Carol K.; Henker, Barbara; Collins, Barry E.; et al. "Peer interaction in a structured communication task: comparisons of normal and hyperactive boys and of methylphenidate (Ritalin) and placebo effects." Child Dev 50(2): 388-401, June, 1979. (52 References).

Assesses peer communication patterns in two groups of boys, hyperactive and controls. Some of the hyperactive boys were receiving methylphenidate; others received a placebo. All boys were observed and scored on a dyadic referential communication task. The results suggest that hyperactive children, regardless of medication status, are less likely than comparison peers to: (1) modulate ongoing or habitual behavior patterns in response to externally imposed shifts in role-appropriate behaviors; (2) maintain consistent, uninterrupted goal orientation; and (3) respond to subtle social learning opportunities. In this situation, methylphenidate appeared to have a greater impact on behavioral style than on competence, decreasing perceived intensity without influencing inefficiency A mild medication-induced dysphoria was also documented. Directions for future research and the need for caution in clinical interpretation are discussed.

1971 Wright, Eric R. "An investigation of hyperactivity and preschool experience." Res Relat Child 35: 90, March, 1975-August, 1975. (0 References).

Abstracts a report of research in progress or recently completed research. Data are provided on: name of investigator(s), purpose of the study, number and kind of subjects used, methodology, principal findings, duration of research, cooperating group(s), and availability of publication(s). Research Relating to Children is compiled by the ERIC Clearinghouse on Early Childhood Education.

X.
Ethical and Legal Issues

1972 Appleman, Michael A. "The legal issues involved in the use of stimulants on hyperactive school children." For a summary see: Diss Abstr Int 35A(8): 5161, February, 1975. (0 References).

1973 Bell, Joseph N. "The family that fought back." McCalls 104(8): 26ff., May, 1977. (0 References).
Presents an account of the controversy of Ritalin use in the Taft, California public schools. The parents of seventeen children treated with Ritalin filed a law suit against the school district because school attendance was contingent upon consent to the administration of the drug.

1974 Birch, E. L. "Symposium: Stimulant drugs and the schools: dimensions in remediation of social toxicity. IV. Development of a school system policy in the use of stimulant drugs for school children." Paper presented at the Annual Meeting of the Council for Exceptional Children, New York, New York, 1974.

1975 Broudy, Harry S. "Ideological, political, and moral considerations in the use of drugs in hyperkinetic therapy." Sch Rev 85(1): 43-60, November, 1976. (6 References).
Discusses the contexts in which the controversy over permitting schools to recommend treatment of hyperactivity occurs, and describes some popular positions. The issues involved in the controversy are scientific, practical, moral, and political. Until drug treatment is proven to enhance academic/behavioral performance, the controversy will remain a symptom of "the dissolution of the consensus" of the role of schools in a "hyperkinetic society." For a reprint of this study refer to Item No. 744.

1976 Brown, J. Larry, and Bing, Stephen R. "Drugging children: child abuse by professionals." In: Children's rights and the mental health professions." Edited by Gerald P. Koocher. New York, New York: Wiley, 1976. 219-28. (7 References). (Wiley Series on Personality Processes).
Views the use of psychotropic drugs on schoolchildren as a major public-policy decision that has been made without adequate public debate or scrutiny. The decision to drug children is seen as a decision arrived at by: (1) drug manufacturers; (2) researchers; (3) school managers; and (4) members of the medical community. Although this method of treatment represents a technologically easy response to medical and social problems, the underlying problems remain unsolved.

1977 Bruck, Connie. "Battle lines in the Ritalin war." Hum Behav 5(8): 24-33, August, 1976. (0 References).

Describes the development of a pending lawsuit in Taft, California. The lawsuit claims that the school system did not give parents the right of informed consent and due process before children were placed on Ritalin for alleged hyperactivity. Impressions gained through interviews with the families, the school physician, the school superintendent, and the school psychologist are summarized. It is concluded that the use of behavior-modifying drugs is a denial of individual differences and rights and a step toward social control through drugs.

1978 Conrad, Peter F. "The discovery of hyperkinesis: notes on the medicalization of deviant behavior." Soc Probl 23(1): 12-21, October, 1975. (31 References).
Presents a brief history of the diagnosis and treatment of hyperkinesis. Emphasis is placed on the social and clinical factors involved with the various aspects of this common syndrome. Also considered is the problem of expert control, medical social control, the individualization of social problems, and the depoliticization of deviant behavior. For a commentary on this study refer to Item No. 1993.

1979 ————. "Identifying hyperactive children: a study in the medicalization of deviant behavior." For a summary see: Diss Abstr Int 36A(9): 6317-18, March, 1976. (0 References).

1980 ————. Identifying hyperactive children: the medicalization of deviant behavior. Lexington, Massachusetts: D. C. Heath, 1976. 122p. (Bibliography).
Reports a sociological study of the process of identifying hyperactive children and an analysis of how deviant behavior comes to be defined as a medical problem. Chapter 1 gives a statement of the problem, an overview of the sociological literature, and a discussion of the conceptual framework. Chapter 2 describes the medical diagnosis of hyperkinesis and presents an analytical overview of how this diagnosis was discovered. Chapter 3 includes a statement of the method of studying this problem and a discussion of the issues of reliability, validity, and the limitations of this research. Chapter 4 is a description of the research setting and the sample. Chapter 5 analyzes how deviant behavior is identified and how it comes to be defined as a medical problem. The focus is on processes within and between the family, school, and physicians. Chapter 6 presents a phenomenological-type analysis of how physicians construct a diagnosis of hyperactivity at the HA-LD clinic. Chapter 7 is a theoretical discussion of the sociological ramifications of the medicalization of deviant behavior. Chapter 8 examines etiology, formulating a direction that a sociological theory of hyperactivity could take. Chapter 9 presents conclusions and suggests areas for further research. Chapter 10 offers elements of a theory of the medicalization of deviant behavior. Two appendixes and an index are included.

1981 Cottle, T. J. "Child control." Soc Policy 8(1): 49-51, May, 1977.

1982 Holder, Angela R. "The pediatrician and the schools." In: Holder, Angela R. Legal issues in pediatrics and adolescent medicine. New York, New York: Wiley, 1977. 189-210. (67 References). (A Wiley Medical Publication).
Examines four problems, in terms of their legal implications, that the pediatrician may encounter with the school-age child: (1) the pediatrician's role in the placement of children in special education; (2) the

pediatrician's role as a team physician; (3) the pediatrician and the child who is suspected of being hyperkinetic; and (4) questions of confidentiality that may arise in the school situation. The legal issues surrounding diagnosis, right to refuse medication, failure to discover another condition, and drug reactions are discussed in the section on the hyperkinetic child. It is concluded that the pediatrician should always place the child's interests first, even though they may be contrary to the requests of the school system. Pediatricians should be extremely cautious about attempting to resolve educational impasses in a misguided effort to help the child by dealing directly with school personnel without the knowledge of the child or his parents.

1983 Jackson, J. E. "The coerced use of Ritalin for behavior control in public schools: legal challenges." Clgh Rev 10(3): 181-93, July, 1976. (122 References and Footnotes).
Three main topics are covered: (1) the constitutional and statutory rights of the child; (2) coercion of the parent by the school system into drugging his child with Ritalin; and (3) the identifying and labeling of a child as hyperactive may be attacked as classification without due process, or possibly, as sexually discriminatory classification.

1984 Jones, Robert W. "Coercive behavior control in the schools: reconciling 'individually appropriate' education with damaging changes in educational status." Stanford Law Rev 29: 93-125, November, 1976. (190 References and Footnotes).
Delineates the role of the state and the parent in controlling misbehaving children and the part that the school system plays in the use of behavior control methods. Part I examines the two important types of "coercive" behavior control commonly practiced in the schools, behavior modification therapy and psychostimulant drugs, and the dangers associated with each. Part II evaluates current common procedures by which the decision is made to classify children as "behaviorally disordered" and subject them to "coercive" behavior control. Part III suggests legislative and judicial alternatives to existing procedures that will more adequately protect the interests of schoolchildren and their parents, while preserving the right of the school to control the truly disruptive child.

1985 McCoy, Rodman, and Koocher, Gerald P. "Needed: a public policy for psychotropic drug use with children." In: Children's rights and the mental health professions. Edited by Gerald P. Koocher. New York, New York: Wiley, 1976. 237-44. (13 References). (Wiley Series on Personality Processes).
Presents a set of antecedent criteria preceding the formulation of a specific policy to ensure that the final policy is safe, effective, considerate, consistent, and convenient. Discussed are the needs for: (1) well-conceived psychopharmacological research; (2) institutional reconciliation and communication; (3) a comprehensive assessment protocol; and (4) parental consciousness-raising and involvement.

1986 Padway, Larry. "Federal regulation of Ritalin in treatment of hyperactive children." Ecol Law Q 7(2): 457-95, 1978. (215 References and Footnotes).
Investigates the difficulty of identifying the hyperactive child, the resulting over-inclusiveness of the diagnostic criteria used in the drug label, and the issues thereby raised for federal drug regulators who must decide if Ritalin is safe and effective for use as a treatment for hyper-

active children. Also discussed are: (1) the federal regulation of Ritalin in situations where the patient's parents do not object to its use; (2) the complexity of the parental decision; (3) the subjective nature of the diagnosis of hyperactivity; (4) labeling problems; and (5) the type of clinical testing and evidence that should be required in order to secure FDA approval.

1987 Rosenberg, Irene M., and Rosenberg, Yale L. "Truancy, school phobia, and minimal brain dysfunction." Minn Law Rev 61: 543-600, 1977. (202 References).
Part IV of this lengthy article discusses school phobia and MBD as defenses of truancy. Arguments are given for and against the contention that school phobia and MBD afford defenses to PINS (Persons in Need of Supervision) truancy findings. Because an MBD child may be unable to learn in the traditional classroom setting, his or her avoidance of school is at least arguably justifiable or unintentional. The PINS statute is discussed in detail, and references are made to relevant court cases.

1988 Scoville, B. "Symposium: Stimulant drugs and the schools: Dimensions in remediation of social toxicity. III. Governmental perspectives in the evaluation and regulation of stimulant drugs for hyperkinetic children." Paper presented at the meeting of the Council for Exceptional Children, New York, New York, April, 1974.

1989 Sprague, R. L. "Research with preschool children and FDA regulations." In: Sprague, R. L. (chair). Hyperactivity: treatment for preschool children. Symposium presented at the meeting of the Council for Exceptional Children, Atlanta, Georgia, April, 1977.

1990 Stewart, Mark A. "Treating problem children with drugs: ethical issues." In: Children's rights and the mental health professions. Edited by Gerald P. Koocher. New York, New York: Wiley, 1976. 229-35. (6 References). (Wiley Series on Personality Processes).
Reviews some of the ethical issues surrounding the prescription of psychotropic drugs for children. Most issues revolve around the fact that a child's problem behavior is often subjectively assessed by a parent or a teacher and that children tend to be objects rather than active participants in a drug treatment program.

1991 U. S. National Commission for the Protection of Human Subjects of Biomedical and Behavioral Research. Research involving children. Washington, D.C.: Government Printing Office, 1977. 1 volume plus appendix. (Bibliography). (DHEW Publication No. [OS] 77-0004).
Discusses the ethical issues involved in using children in research. Questions include: (1) Under what conditions is the participation of children in research ethically acceptable?; and (2) Under what conditions may such participation be authorized by the subjects and their parents? Commission recommendations are set forth.

1992 Weithorn, Lois. "Drug therapy--children's rights." In: Drugs and the special child. Edited by Michael J. Cohen. New York, New York: Gardner Press, 1979. 203-37. (68 References).
Reviews the legal, psychological, social, and ethical issues raised by the administration of psychoactive medication to children. The presentation is designed to: (1) examine the basic rights of children with respect to this type of medical treatment; (2) explore relevant issues and questions; and (3) survey the pertinent trends in legal thinking.

1993 Whalen, C. K. "Pitfalls of politicization." Soc Probl 24(5): 590-95, June, 1977. (30 References).
Comments on a study by Peter F. Conrad (Item No. 1978).

XI.
Research and Methodology

1994 Arnold, L. Eugene. "A humanistic approach to neurochemical research in children." In: Anthony, E. James, ed. Exploratíons in child psychiatry. New York, New York: Plenum, 1975. 81-103. (25 References).
Discusses the problems, philosophy, ethics, and techniques of neurochemical research with children. Topics covered include selecting the research area, pilot studies, controlled studies, placebo, selection of samples, measuring instruments, analysis of results, and ethical issues relevant to the subject.

1995 Baxley, G. B., and Leblanc, J. "The hyperactive child: characteristics, treatment, and evaluation of research design." In: Advances in child development and behavior. Volume 11. Edited by Hayne W. Reese. New York, New York: Academic Press, 1976. 1-34. (118 References).

1996 Berler, E. S., and Romanczyk, R. G. "Assessment of the learning disabled and hyperactive child: therapeutic and research issues." Paper presented at the Meeting of the Association for the Advancement of Behavior Therapy, Atlanta, Georgia, December, 1977.

1997 Conners, C. Keith. "Methodological considerations in drug research with children." In: Psychopharmacology in childhood and adolescence. Edited by Jerry M. Wiener. New York, New York: Basic Books, 1977. 58-83. (61 References).
This chapter considers: (1) diagnosis and selection of subjects for drug treatment; (2) measurement of dependent variables; (3) research design; (4) ethical considerations; (5) nondrug variables; and (6) interactions with other treatments.

1998 Dalby, J. Thomas; Kapelus, Gary J.; Swanson, James M.; et al. "An examination of the double-blind design in drug research with hyperactive children." Prog Neuropharmacol 2(1): 123-27, 1978. (11 References).
Evaluates the utility of the double-blind design and examines the degree of naivety in both observers and hyperactive subjects in a double-blind drug-placebo research program. Although the double-blind design has become widely used in evaluating the effects of drugs on the behavior of hyperactive children, this study questions the extent to which the subjects are aware or unaware of their drug or placebo state. One hundred and seventy-seven hyperactive children participated in the study and they, along with their observers, were questioned on the identity of the substances they had received. Results indicate that children's predictions were not more accurate than that expected by chance, but experienced

observers could accurately predict the drug state of hyperactive children. Implications for further research are discussed.

1999 Douglas, Virginia I. "Research on hyperactivity: stage two." J Abnorm Child Psychol 4(4): 307-8, 1976. (0 References).
Presents an introductory statement by Dr. Virginia Douglas, guest editor of a special issue devoted to papers on hyperactivity. The author briefly discusses trends in research and treatment.

2000 Egan, Rosemary W. "Research variables in CNS studies." For a summary see: Diss Abstr Int 39A(10): 6061, April, 1979. (0 References).

2001 Eisenberg, Leon. "Future threats or clear and present dangers?" Sch Rev 85(1): 155-65, November, 1976. (23 References).
Discusses three broad areas: (1) the limitations as well as the promise of biological research for enhancing learning; (2) the problem of current inadequacy in public education; and (3) futurology as demonology rather than applied science in debates on public policy. For a reprint of this study refer to Item No. 744.

2002 First report of the preliminary findings and recommendations of the Interagency Collaborative Group on Hyperkinesis. Washington, D.C.: Interagency Collaborative Group on Hyperkinesis, 1976. 94p. (ED 122 467).
Presents the preliminary report of the Interagency Collaborative Group on Hyperkinesis. The functions of this group include exchanging information, coordinating expertise, evaluating existing data from ongoing research, and reviewing proposed research. The report contains sections on the definition of the syndrome; diagnostic procedures; prevalence rates; related factors; toxic reactions, safety testing of food additives; treatment programs; dietary intervention; research relevant to the Feingold hypothesis; minimum design requirements for a dietary study; and model research designs. Appended is a report on the use of stimulant drugs in school-age children who exhibit hyperactive behaviors.

2003 Greenberg, Lawrence M.; Deem, Michael A.; Yellin, Absalom M. "Psychopharmacotherapy of children: research design and methodology." In: Psychopharmacology of childhood. Edited by D. V. Siva Sankar. Westbury, New York: PJD Publications, 1976. 87-122. (43 References).
Studies factors which influence the design and methodology used in drug studies involving children. Some of these factors are: (1) the purpose of the study; (2) the setting; and (3) the target behavior or traits to be assessed. Problems of methodology are considered.

2004 Hoeffler, Dennis F. "The misuse of statistics." Pediatrics 53(4): 586-87, April, 1974. (7 References).
Letter to editor.

2005 Hudson, Russell E.; Allen, Richard P.; Safer, Daniel. "Reply to Hoeffler." Pediatrics 53(4): 587, April, 1974. (3 References).
Letter to editor.

2006 Keith, Kenneth D., and Erickson, Charles G. "Minimal brain dysfunction: a note on behavioral research." Clin Pediatr 17(3): 215-17, March, 1978. (17 References).

This short editorial stresses the point that although research into additional low-frequency, presumptive causes of MBD is important, emphasis should be placed on improved management techniques.

2007 Lipman, Ronald S. "Government policy on research with hyperactive children." Paper presented at the Annual Meeting of the Council for Exceptional Children, Atlanta, Georgia, 1977.

2008 ———. "NIMH-PRB support of research in minimal brain dysfunction in children." In: Clinical use of stimulant drugs in children. Edited by C. Keith Conners. Amsterdam: Excerpta Medica, 1974. 202-13. (33 References). (International Congress Series, No. 313).

The purpose of this paper is to summarize the role of the National Institute of Mental Health and the Psychopharmacology Research Branch in the stimulant drug treatment of hyperactive children. Also covered are a list of some of the PRB pediatric psychopharmacology grants, current needs in the field, and the social and political issues surrounding the use of stimulant drugs for hyperactive children. Future needs include: (1) retrospective studies to document the long-term effects of stimulant drug treatment; (2) legislation in the area of quality prenatal and postnatal care; and (3) specialized classes to deal with the multifaceted problems of the MBD child.

2009 McGaugh, James L. "Neurobiology and the future of education." Sch Rev 85(1): 166-75, November, 1976. (15 References).

Briefly reviews some of the recent evidence suggesting that progress in neurobiological research may lead to the development of treatments which can influence learning and memory. Also considered are several questions concerning the types of treatments which might be developed as well as their potential uses and abuses. For a reprint of this study refer to Item No. 744.

2010 McGlannan, Frances K. "Learning disabilities: the decade ahead." J Learn Disabil 8(2): 113-16, February, 1975. (0 References).

Summarizes papers presented at a conference on learning disabilities held in Ann Arbor, Michigan, November 20-22, 1974. The conference, hosted by Dr. William Cruickshank, reviewed the accomplishments in the LD field and discussed current trends. Additional issues to be explored by research in the decade ahead include: (1) the process of integrating intersensory information; (2) the role of structure; (3) the role of early stimulation and nutrition in perceptual development; (4) the unknown effects of medication during pregnancy; (5) biochemical imbalances; (6) proper training of professionals in the field; and (7) the need for continuing research into specific effects of medication.

2011 Nash, Ralph J. "Clinical research on psychotropic drugs and hyperactivity in children." Sch Psychol Dig 5(4): 22-33, Fall, 1976. (43 References).

Delineates and describes three phases in the development of psychotropic drugs for general population use: (1) information on the drugs' effects on humans is gathered; (2) clinical efficacy in design is studied; and (3) larger sample sizes are utilized to validate earlier data. Difficulties, such as classifying and categorizing emotional and mental disorders, are outlined.

2012 Pyck, K., and Baines P. "The influence of drugs on minimal brain dysfunction." In: Minimal brain dysfunction: fact or fiction. Edited by A. F. Kalverboer, H. M. van Praag, and J. Mendlewicz. Basel, New York: Karger, 1978. 68-83. (48 References). (Advances in Biological Psychiatry, Volume 1).

Appraises the importance of pharmacological research as part of the psychopathological and psychiatric investigation of MBD and reviews the various drugs used to treat the symptoms of MBD. Also considered is the contribution pharmacological research can make to the knowledge of the MBD syndrome. Some practical suggestions for clinical use of drugs complete the chapter.

2013 Salkind, Neil J., and Poggio, John P. "The measurement of hyperactivity: trends and issues." In: Principles and techniques of intervention with hyperactive children. Edited by Marvin J. Fine. Springfield, Illinois: Thomas, 1977. 244-68. (60 References).

Surveys the pertinent issues involved in the assessment of hyperactivity, reviews some of the existing methods employed in the measurement and evaluation of activity level, and outlines a model which synthesizes the methodological concerns and limitations inherent in existing research. Regardless of the theoretical definition of hyperactivity, the researcher should strive to use an instrument which is nonobtrusive, inconspicuous, relatively inexpensive and portable, reliable across the situations for which it was designed, and valid within the context for which it was intended.

2014 Sheinbein, M. L., and Wiggins, K. M. "An operant counting scale for children: a preliminary methodological psychoactive drug case study." Child Psychiatry Hum Dev 5(3): 142-49, Spring, 1975. (34 References).

This pilot study is the first attempt at objective measurement of well-defined molecular behaviors through covert field observation. Though the main thrust is the development of a methodology for the clinical investigation of drug effects on children, a method that minimizes or overcomes many of the special problems that have plagued child drug research in the past, some preliminary data on the behavioral effects of haloperidol and imipramine were obtained. The technique developed is called an operant counting scale, and it promises to be useful in future full-drug studies.

2015 Smithsonian Science Information Exchange. Notice of research projects. Title of this Search: D110, Hyperkinetic children. Washington, D.C., April, 1975.

2016 Sprague, Robert L. "Assessment of intervention." In: Hyperactivity in children: etiology, measurement, and treatment implications. Edited by Ronald L. Trites. Baltimore, Maryland: University Park Press, 1979. 217-29. (45 References).

Point out the importance of assessment methodology. Many current studies are seen as methodologically weak, unsophisticated, and biased; they contribute to an already existing mass of confusing, contradictory, and misleading literature. Hyperactivity, a complex constellation of a number of behavioral symptoms, will best be treated by the use of the multitrait-multimethod technique.

2017 Sulzbacher, Stephen I. "Psychotropic medication with children: an evaluation of procedural biases in results of reported studies." In: Behavior therapy with hyperactive and learning disabled chil-

dren. Edited by Benjamin B. Lahey. New York, New York: Oxford University Press, 1979. 61-65. (21 References).
Reprints an article from Pediatrics 51(3): 513-17, March, 1973.

2018 Weakland, John H. "The double-blind theory: some current implications for child psychiatry." J Am Acad Child Psychiatry 18(1): 54-66, Winter, 1979. (13 References).
The behavioral-interactional view of problems in the original statement of the double-blind theory is outlined, and the broad significance of this viewpoint for treatment is discussed. Recent emphasis on the cybernetic causal model is noted, and its implications for family therapy in general and for child-centered problems in particular are reviewed. A case example of brief treatment of hyperactivity based on this approach is described.

XII. Miscellaneous and Addendum

Miscellaneous

2019 Attwood, E. J. "Hyperactivity Association of South Australia." Med J Aust 2(1): 34, 1979. (1 Reference).
Letter to editor.

2020 Jampolsky, Gerald G., and Haight, Maryellen J. A study of ESP in hyperkinetic children. 1974. 16p. (ED 104 113).
Studies the frequency of ESP in ten hyperactive and normal children. Results did not support the hypothesis that hyperactive children have more ESP than normal children.

2021 Mitchell, Reg; Hodgson, Barbara; Bernstein, Lead. "National Hyperactivity Association." Med J Aust 2(12): 568, December 2, 1978. (0 References).
Letter to editor.

2022 Thompson, Ann R., and Wade, M. G. "Real play and fantasy play as modified by social and environmental complexity in normal and hyperactive children." Ther Recreat J 8(4): 160-67, 1974. (15 References).
Studies the interrelationship of real and fantasy play in normal and hyperactive children. The subjects were four hyperactive boys and four normal boys (ages four to eight years). The content of the play activities in response to various stimuli was compared in order to test the Linford and Jeanrenaud four-stage theory of play, i.e., preplay, exploration, conditioned responding, and creative play. It is concluded that: (1) the study provided only weak support for the Linford-Jeanrenaud play model; (2) normal children did not indulge in fantasy play in the monad condition, but did engage actively in real play; and (3) hyperactive children showed higher levels of fantasy play than did normal subjects.

2023 "Time goes slowly for hyperactive children." Brain/Mind Bull 2(20): 3, September 5, 1977.

Addendum*

2024 "Additives at fault in hyperactivity." Sci News 117: 199ff., March 29, 1980.

2025 Aman, M. G., and Singh, N. N. "The usefulness of thioridazine for treating childhood disorders--fact or folklore?" Am J Ment Defic 84(4): 331-38, January, 1980. (32 References).

*References in the Addendum have not been included in the Indexes.

2026 Anderson, J. "Methylphenidate and hyperactivity." S Afr Med J 57(6): 181-82, February 9, 1980. (16 References).

2027 Arnold, L. Eugene. "Parents of hyperactive and aggressive children." In: Helping parents help their children. Edited by L. Eugene Arnold. New York, New York: Brunner/Mazel, 1978. 192-207. (5 References).

2028 Arnold, L. Eugene, and Sheridan, Katherine. "Hyperactivity with tactile defensiveness as a phobia." J Sch Health 50(9): 531-33, November, 1980. (8 References).

2029 Barkley, R. A. "A review of stimulant drug research with hyperactive children." In: Annual progress in child psychiatry and child development, 1978. Edited by Stella Chess and Alexander Thomas. New York, New York: Brunner/Mazel, 1978. 345-81. (100+ References).

2030 Barkley, R. A., et al. "Self-control classroom for hyperactive children." J Autism Dev Disabil 10(1): 75-89, March, 1980. (22 References).

2031 Brown, G. L.; Ebert, M. H.; Hunt, R. D.; et al. "Behavior and motor activity response in hyperactive children and plasma amphetamine levels following a sustained-release preparation." J Am Acad Child Psychiatry 19(2): 225-39, Spring, 1980. (References).

2032 Brown, R. T. "Impulsivity and psychoeducational intervention in hyperactive children." J Learn Disabil 13(5): 249-54, May, 1980. (22 References).

2033 Brumback, Roger A. "Use of operational criteria in an office practice for diagnosis of children referred for evaluation of learning or behavior disorders." Percept Mot Skills 49(1): 299-311, August, 1979. (15 References).

2034 Cannon, I. P., and Compton, Carolyn L. "School dysfunction in the adolescent." Pediatr Clin North Am 27(1): 79-96, February, 1980. (128 References).

2035 Carter, Edwin N., and Shostak, David A. "Imitation in the treatment of the hyperkinetic behavior syndrome." J Clin Child Psychol 9(1): 63-66, Spring, 1980. (6 References).

2036 Conners, C. Keith, and Taylor, Eric. "Pemoline, methylphenidate, and placebo in children with MBD." Arch Gen Psychiatry 37(8): 922-30, August, 1980. (9 References).

2037 Copeland, Anne P., and Moll, Nadine W. Relationships among cognitive measures in learning disabled and non-learning disabled children. 1979. 12p. (ED 182 906).

2038 Crook, W. G. "Can what a child eats make him dull, stupid or hyperactive?" J Learn Disabil 13(5): 281-86, May, 1980. (22 References).

2039 Dickerson, J. W., et al. "Diet and hyperactivity." J Hum Nutr 34(3): 167-74, June, 1980. (31 References).

2040 Dunn, Freeman M. "Relaxation training and its relationship to hyperactivity in boys." For a summary see: Diss Abstr Int 41B(1): 348, July, 1980. (0 References).

2041 Evans, Ronald G. "Reduction of hyperactive behavior in three profoundly retarded adolescents through increased stimulation." AAESPH Rev 4(3): 259-63, Fall, 1979.

2042 Feingold, B. E. "Feingold diet: letter." Aust Fam Physician 9(1): 60-61, January, 1980.

2043 "Food dye furor." Sci Quest 53: 5, May-June, 1980.

2044 Freeman, D. F., and Cornwall, T. P. "Hyperactivity and neurosis." Am J Orthopsychiatry 50(4): 704-11, October, 1980. (19 References).

2045 Furneaux, Barbara. "The diary of Henry." Spec Educ: Forward Trends 6(4): 25-27, December, 1979.

2046 Golden, G. S. "Nonstandard therapies in the developmental disabilities." Am J Dis Child 134(5): 487-91, May, 1980. (32 References).

2047 Green, R. G. "Hyperactivity and the learning-disabled child." J Orthomol Psychiatry 9(2): 93- , 1980.

2048 Haavik, S., et al. "Effects of the Feingold diet on seizures and hyperactivity: a single-subject analysis." J Behav Med 2(4): 365-74, December, 1979.

2049 Hobbs, S. A.; Moguin, L. E.; Tyroler, M.; et al. "Cognitive behavior therapy with children: has clinical utility been demonstrated?" Psychol Bull 87(1): 147-65, January, 1980. (95 References).

2050 Lambert, N. M., and Sandoval, J. "The prevalence of learning disabilities in a sample of children considered hyperactive." J Abnorm Child Psychol 8(1): 33-50, March, 1980. (24 References).

2051 Levine, M. D., and Oberklaid, F. "Hyperactivity. Symptom complex or complex symptom?" Am J Dis Child 134(4): 409-14, April, 1980. (59 References).

2052 "Living and coping with a hyperactive child." Aust Fam Physician 9(4): 285-86, April, 1980.

2053 Loiselle, D. L.; Stamm, J. S.; Maitinsky, S.; et al. "Evoked potential and behavioral signs of attentive dysfunctions in hyperactive boys." Psychophysiology 17(2): 193-201, March, 1980. (33 References).

2054 Loney, Jan. "Hyperkinesis comes of age: what do we know and where should we go?" Am J Orthopsychiatry 50(1): 28-42, January, 1980. (76 References).

2055 McLennand, W. "Hyperactive children." Am Psychol 35(4): 392-93, April, 1980.

2056 McMahon, Robert C. "Genetic etiology in the hyperactive child syndrome: a critical review." Am J Orthopsychiatry 50(1): 145-50, January, 1980. (23 References).

2057 McMahon, R. J., et al. "Relaxation training as an adjunct to treatment in a hyperactive boy." Clin Pediatr 19(7): 497-98, July, 1980.

2058 Madle, Ronald A.; Neisworth, John T.; Kurtz, P. David. "Biasing of hyperkinetic behavior ratings by diagnostic reports: effects of observer training and assessment method." J Learn Disabil 13(1): 30-33, January, 1980. (9 References).

2059 Mailman, R. B.; Ferris, Robert M.; Tang, F. L.; et al. "Erythrosine (Red No. 3) and its nonspecific biochemical actions: what relation to behavioral changes?" Science 207(4430): 535-37, February 1, 1980. (19 References).

2060 Majovski, Lawrence C., and Oettinger, Leon, Jr. "Neuropsychological and treatment aspects of learning and behavior disorders in children." Behav Disord 5(1): 30-40, November, 1979.

2061 Mattes, J. A. "The role of frontal lobe dysfunction in childhood hyperkinesis." Compr Psychiatry 21(5): 358-69, September-October, 1980. (75 References).

2062 Maurer, R. G., and Stewart, M. A. "Attention deficit without hyperactivity in a child psychiatry clinic." J Clin Psychiatry 41(7): 232-33, July, 1980. (1 Reference).

2063 Minde, K. K. "Some thoughts on the social ecology of present day psychopharmacology." Can J Psychiatry 25(3): 201-12, April, 1980. (24 References).

2064 Morrison, J. R. "Adult psychiatric disorders in parents of hyperactive children." Am J Psychiatry 137(7): 825-27, July, 1980. (11 References).

2065 ———. "Childhood hyperactivity in an adult psychiatric population: social factors." J Clin Psychiatry 41(2): 40-43, February, 1980. (9 References).

2066 Naylor, H.; Hardyck, C.; Lambert, N. M.; et al. "Lateral asymmetry in perceptual judgments of reading disabled, hyperactive and control children." Int J Neurosci 10(2-3): 135-43, 1980.

2067 Oberklaid, Frank, et al. "Developmental-behavioral dysfunction in preschool children." Am J Dis Child 133(11): 1126-31, November, 1979.

2068 O'Leary, K. D. "Pills or skills for hyperactive children." J Appl Behav Anal 13(1): 191-204, Spring, 1980. (67 References).

2069 Omizo, M. M. "The effects of biofeedback-induced relaxation training in hyperactive adolescent boys." J Psychol 105(1st half): 131-38, May, 1980. (24 References).

2070 ————. "Effects of relaxation and biofeedback training on dimensions of self-concept (DOSC) among hyperactive male children." Educ Res Q 5(1): 22-30, Spring, 1980. (20 References).

2071 Ozolins, D. A., and Anderson, R. P. "Effects of feedback on the vigilance task performance of hyperactive and hypoactive children." Percept Mot Skills 50(2): 415-24, April, 1980. (11 References).

2072 Pelham, W. E.; Schnedler, Robert W.; Bologna, N. C.; et al. "Behavioral and stimulant treatment of hyperactive children: a therapy study with methylphenidate probes in a within-subject design." J Appl Behav Anal 13(2): 221-36, Summer, 1980. (43 References).

2073 Prior, M. R., et al. "Classification of hyperactive children." Med J Aust 1(8): 375-76, April 19, 1980. (11 References).

2074 Prout, H. T. "Behavioral intervention with hyperactive children: a review." In: Annual progress in child psychiatry and child development, 1978. Edited by Stella Chess and Alexander Thomas, 1978. 382-91. (39 References).

2075 Quay, Lorene C., and Brown, Ronald T. "Hyperactive and normal children and the error, latency, and double median split scoring procedures of the Matching Familiar Figures test." J Sch Psychol 18(1): 12-16, Spring, 1980. (11 References).

2076 Rapoport, J. L., et al. "Decreased motor activity of hyperactive children on dextroamphetamine during active gym program." Psychiatry Res 2(3): 225- , 1980.

2077 Rapoport, J. L.; Bucksbaum, M. S.; Weingartner, H.; et al. "Dextroamphetamine: cognitive and behavioral effects in normal and hyperactive boys and normal adult males." Psychopharmacol Bull 16(1): 21-23, January, 1980. (9 References).

2078 ————. "Dextroamphetamine: its cognitive and behavioral effects in normal and hyperactive boys and normal men." Arch Gen Psychiatry 37(8): 933-43, August, 1980. (55 References).

2079 Roberts, Bruce. "A computerized diagnostic evaluation of a psychiatric problem." Am J Psychiatry 137(1): 12-15, January, 1980. (13 References).

2080 Satterfield, J. H.; Satterfield, B. T.; Cantwell, D. P. "Multimodality treatment: a two-year evaluation of 61 hyperactive boys." Arch Gen Psychiatry 37(8): 915-19, August, 1980. (16 References).

2081 Schofield, Leon J. Hyperkinesis: recent diagnostic and treatment trends. 1979. 22p. (ED 182 884).

2082 Simpson, Richard L., et al. "Stimulant medications and the classroom attention-to-task and deviant social behaviors of twelve hyperactive males." Learn Disabil Q 3(1): 19-27, Winter, 1980.

2083 Singh, V., et al. "Amphetamines in the management of children's hyperkinesis." Bull Narc 31(3-4): 87-94, July-December, 1979.

2084 Sleator, E. K. "Deleterious effects of drugs used for hyperactivity on patients with Gilles de la Tourette syndrome." Clin Pediatr 19(7): 453-54, July, 1980. (8 References).

2085 Stare, F. J.; Whelan, E. M.; Sheridan, M. "Diet and hyperactivity: is there a relationship?" Pediatrics 66(4): 521-25, October, 1980. (12 References).

2086 Swanson, J. M., and Kinsbourne, M. "Food dyes impair performance of hyperactive children on a laboratory learning test." Science 207(4438): 1485-87, March 28, 1980. (25 References).

2087 Thompson, L. M. "The effects of methylphenidate on self-concept and locus of control of hyperactive children." For a summary see: Diss Abstr Int 40B(10): 5026-27, April, 1980. (0 References).

2088 Weingartner, H., et al. "Cognitive processes in normal and hyperactive children and their response to amphetamine treatment." J Abnorm Psychol 89(1): 25-37, February, 1980. (37 References).

2089 Weiss, B., et al. "Behavioral responses to artificial food colors." Science 207(4438): 1487-89, March 28, 1980. (16 References).

2090 Werry, J. S.; Aman, M. G.; Diamond, E. "Imipramine and methylphenidate in hyperactive children." J Child Psychol Psychiatry 21(1): 27-35, January, 1980. (24 References).

2091 Whalen, C. K.; Henker, B.; Dotemoto, S. "Methylphenidate and hyperactivity: effects on teacher behaviors." Science 208(4449): 1280-82, June 13, 1980. (11 References).

2092 Winsberg, B. G.; Kupietz, S. S.; Yepes, L. E.; et al. "Ineffectiveness of imipramine in children who fail to respond to methylphenidate." J Autism Dev Disord 10(2): 129-37, June, 1980. (22 References).

2093 Zelman, J. B., and Arbogast, R. C. "Doctor, is my child hyperactive?" Am Fam Physician 21(5): 105-11, May, 1980.

2094 Zentall, S. S. "Behavioral comparisons of hyperactive and normally active children in natural settings." J Abnorm Child Psychol 8(1): 93-109, March, 1980. (29 References).

Appendix A: Nomenclature

Activity level

Aggressive behavior disorder

Aphasoid syndrome

Association deficit pathology

Attention deficit disorder (ADD)

Attention disorder

Behavior disorder

Brain damaged

Brain dysfunction

Brain injured

Central nervous system deviation

Cerebral damage

Cerebral dysfunction

Cerebral dys-synchronization syndrome

Character impulse disorder

Child behavior disorder

Choreiform syndrome

Clumsy child syndrome

Conceptually handicapped

Developmental dyslexia

Developmental imbalance

Diffuse brain damage

Dyslexia

Educationally handicapped

Emotionally disturbed

Exceptional child

Hyperactive

Hyperexcitability syndrome

Hyperkinesis

Hyperkinetic behavior syndrome

Hyperkinetic impulse disorder

Hyperkinetic syndrome

Hypokinetic syndrome

Impulse disorder

Interjacent child

Learning disability

Learning disabled

Learning disorder

Learning impaired

Minimal brain damage

Minimal brain dysfunction

Minimal brain injured

Minimal cerebral damage

Minimal cerebral dysfunction

Minimal cerebral injury

Minimal cerebral palsy

Minimal chronic brain syndrome

Minor brain damage

Motor activity

Movement disorder

Nervous

Neurologically handicapped

Neurophrenia

Non-attending behavior

Organic behavior problem

Organic brain disorder

Organic brain damage

Organic brain disease

Organic brain driveness

Organic brain dysfunction

Organic driveness

Organic hyperkinetic syndrome

Overactive

Perceptual cripple

Perceptually handicapped

Performance deviation

Performance disability

Performance handicapped

Post-encephalitic behavior disorder

Primary reading retardation

Problem children

Problem learner

Problem reader

Psychoneurological learning disorder

Restless

Slow learner

Special learning disability

Specific learning disability

Specific reading disability

Strauss Syndrome

Tension discharge syndrome

Underachiever

Appendix B: Drug Table

GENERIC NAME	TRADE NAME	THERAPEUTIC CLASS	CHEMICAL CLASS	MANUFACTURER
Amitriptyline (1961)*	Elavil	Antidepressant	Dibenzocycloheptene	Merck Sharp & Dohme
Amphetamine (Before 1950)	Benzedrine	Stimulant	Phenethylamine	Smith Kline & French and others
Caffeine (Before 1950)	No-Doz	Stimulant	Xanthine	Bristol-Myers
Carisoprodol (1959)	Soma Rela	Muscle Relaxant	Carbamate	Wallace Schering
Chlordiazepoxide (1960)	Librium	Antianxiety	Benzodiazepine	Roche
Chlorpromazine (1954)	Thorazine Largactil	Antipsychotic	Phenothiazine	Smith Kline & French Rhome-Poulenc
Chlorprothixene (1962)	Taractan	Antipsychotic	Thiothixene	Roche
Deanol (1958)	Deaner	Stimulant	Tertiary Amine	Riker
Desipramine (1964)	Pertofrane Norpramin	Antidepressant	Dibenzazepine	Geigy Lakeside
Dextroamphetamine (Before 1950)	Dexedrine	Stimulant	Phenethylamine	Smith Kline & French and others
Diazepam (1963)	Valium	Antianxiety	Benzodiazepine	Roche
Diphenhydramine (1946)	Benadryl	Antihistamine	Ethanolamine	Parke, Davis
Fluphenazine (1959 & 1966)	Prolixin Permitil	Antipsychotic	Phenothiazine	Squibb White

*Denotes Year of Introduction

GENERIC NAME	TRADE NAME	THERAPEUTIC CLASS	CHEMICAL CLASS	MANUFACTURER
Haloperidol (1967)	Haldol Serenace	Antipsychotic	Butyrophenone	McNeil
Hydroxyzine Pamoate / Hcl (1958 & 1956)	Atarax Vistaril	Antihistamine	Piperazine	Roerig Pfizer
Imipramine Hcl / Pamoate (1959 & 1973)	Tofranil	Antidepressant	Dibenzazepine	Smith Kline & French
Lithium (1970)	Lithicarb Priadel	Antimanic	Lithium	Various
Meprobamate (1955)	Miltown Equanil	Sedative	Carbamate	Wallace Wyeth
Methamphetamine (Before 1950)	Methedrine Desoxyn	Stimulant	Phenethylamine	Burroughs Wellcome Abbott and others
Methocarbamol (1957)	Robaxin	Muscle Relaxant	Carbamate	Robins
Methylphenidate (1956)	Ritalin	Stimulant	Piperidine	CIBA
Nortriptyline (1965)	Aventyl	Antidepressant	Dibenzcycloheptene	Lilly
Opipramol (1964)	Ensidon	Antidepressant	Benzodiazepine	Geigy
Oxazepam (1965)	Serax	Antianxiety	Benzodiazepine	Wyeth
Pemoline (1975)	Cylert	Stimulant	Oxazolindone Derivative	Abbott
Perphenazine (1957)	Trilafon	Tranquilizer	Phenothiazine	Schering
Phenobarbital (Before 1950)	Luminal (many others)	Sedative/ Anticonvulsant	Barbiturate	Various
Pipradrol (1955)	Meratran	Stimulant	Piperidine	Merrell

GENERIC NAME	TRADE NAME	THERAPEUTIC CLASS	CHEMICAL CLASS	MANUFACTURER
Prochlorperazine (1956)	Compazine	Antipsychotic	Phenothiazine	Smith Kline & French
Promazine (1955)	Sparine	Tranquilizer	Phenothiazine	Wyeth
Promethazine (1951)	Phenergan	Antihistamine	Phenothiazine	Wyeth
Reserpine (1953)	Serpasil	Antihypertensive	Rauwolfia Alkaloid	CIBA
Thioridazine (1959)	Mellaril	Antipsychotic	Phenothiazine	Sandoz
Thiothixene (1967)	Navane	Antipsychotic	Thioxanthene	Roerig
Trifluoperazine (1959)	Stelazine	Antipsychotic	Phenothiazine	Smith Kline & French
Triflupromazine (1957)	Vesprin	Tranquilizer	Phenothiazine	Squibb
Trihexyphenidyl (1949)	Artane	Antispasmodic	Piperidine	Lederle
Tybamate (1965)	Solacen Tybatran	Sedative	Carbamate	Wallace

Appendix C: Glossary

ACHIEVEMENT LEVEL - Expected grade level minus actual achievement grade level; the distance in months and years a child is behind his average peers in the same grade.

ADAPTIVE BEHAVIOR - Refers to the degree to which an individual meets standards for independence and responsibility for his age and social group.

ACTING-OUT BEHAVIOR - Inappropriate behavior of an aggressive type.

ANOMALY - A growth, development, or formation that differs from the usual.

ANOXIA - A severe reduction in the normal concentration of oxygen within the body.

ANTICONVULSANT - A drug utilized to treat and prevent convulsions.

ANTIDEPRESSANT - A drug used to evaluate the mood of a depressed individual.

ANTISOCIAL BEHAVIOR - Offensive behavior characterized by deliberateness, an understanding of the consequences of the behavior, and lack of remorse.

ANXIETY - A feeling of uneasiness or dread without specific cause, usually accompanied by physical symptoms such as increased heart rate, dryness of the mouth, body tremors, etc.

AROUSAL - Cortical readiness in response to sensory stimulation.

ASSESSMENT - A term used for psychological testing or measurement; an evaluation.

ATTENTION SPAN - The number of briefly presented objects that can be recalled immediately.

BASELINE DATA - Data that are collected before behavioral intervention begins.

BEHAVIOR MODIFICATION - The use of learning theory principles to bring about changes in specified target behaviors.

BEHAVIOR RATING SCALE - An instrument that allows the observer to record the estimated magnitude of a behavior.

BEHAVIORAL ANALYSIS - The diagnostic methodology used in conjunction with behavior modification.

BIOFEEDBACK - Provision of information to the subject based on one or more of his physiologic processes (such as brainwave activity or blood pressure).

BRAIN DYSFUNCTION - A medical designation for abnormalities of behavior and/or intellectual functioning which results from a central nervous system and/or developmental dysfunction.

BRAIN-INJURED CHILD - A child who before, during, or after birth has received an injury to, or suffered an infection of, the brain. As a result of such organic impairment, there may be disturbances that prevent or impede the normal learning process.

BRAIN STEM - That section of the brain which includes the vital centers for heart and respiratory rate as well as the control of consciousness.

BRAIN SYNDROMES - A generic term for a system of acute and chronic conditions, variously reversible and irreversible, resulting from physiological impairment and intoxication of the brain.

CENTRAL NERVOUS SYSTEM (CNS) - The CNS is composed of the brain and the spinal cord.

CHRONOLOGIC AGE - The actual age of the individual.

COGNITION - Refers to the mental process of comprehension, judgment, memory, and reasoning.

CONCEPTUAL TEMPO - The speed of information processing.

CONDITIONING - A type of learning in which there is a pairing based on repeated simultaneous association in time or place or other similarity of objects, persons, or situations.

CONDUCT DISORDER: CONDUCT PROBLEM - Disorder characterized by acting out, aggressive, or disruptive behavior.

CONGENITAL - Existing at or dating from birth.

CONTINGENCY - The conditions under which a response is followed by a positive or negative reinforcing stimulus or the removal of the stimulus.

CONTROL GROUP - A group which is equivalent to the experimental group in every respect except for the independent variable to which the experimental group is treated and the control group is not.

CORRELATION - The extent to which two variables co-relate or go together.

CORTEX - The outer or external layer of the brain; gray matter.

CRISIS INTERVENTION - Intervention which takes place during a crisis in a child's behavior, with the emphasis placed on the crisis situation.

DEVELOPMENTAL DEVIATION - A generic term referring to expressions of adjustment or coping problems beyond the normal range of difficulty.

DEVELOPMENTAL DISORDERS - Behavior disorders apparently caused by failure of the child to develop at a normal rate or according to the usual sequence.

DIAGNOSIS - The act of finding out what problem a person has, i.e., the symptoms and causes.

DIFFERENTIAL DIAGNOSIS - A diagnosis which distinguishes between two similar diseases or disorders on the basis of their compared characteristics.

DIRECTIONALITY - A child's perception of an object's relationship to another object or point in space. Left-right confusion may result from difficulty with this skill.

DISTRACTIBILITY - Refers to the inability to direct and sustain attention to the appropriate or relevant stimuli in a given situation.

DOMINANCE - The tendency for one side of the body and related organ systems to assume direction and control over those of the other side.

DOUBLE-BLIND - A study in which one or more drugs and/or a placebo are compared in such a way that neither the patient nor the administrator know which preparation is being administered.

DSM-II - Diagnostic and Statistical Manual, 2nd ed.; the 1968 revision of the nomenclature of mental disorders by the American Psychiatric Association.

DYSLEXIA - A term for an impairment of the ability to attain reading skills.

ELECTROCARDIOGRAM (EKG) - A graphic record of the electrical activity accompanying the heartbeat.

ELECTROENCEPHALOGRAM (EEG) - A tracing showing the pattern of electrical activity in the cortical areas of the brain.

ELECTROMYOGRAM (EMG) - A recording of muscle potentials showing the amount and nature of muscle activity.

EMOTIONALLY DISTURBED - A term that refers to a child's unexplained inability to learn, to act as mature as his peers, to achieve adequate social relationships, to display confidence, and to cope with stress.

ENCOPRESIS - Incontinence of feces, which may consist of passing feces into the clothing or bed at regular intervals or leaking mucus and feces into the clothing or bed almost continuously.

ENURESIS - Incontinence of urine, which may be diurnal (wetting during the day) or nocturnal (bedwetting).

ENVIRONMENTAL ALTERATION - An approach in which the child is removed from present family or environment and placed in a totally new situation, such as a residential school.

ENVIRONMENTAL MODIFICATION - An approach in which the child continues to live with his family but there is some rearrangement of the surroundings.

EPIDEMIOLOGIC - Pertaining to the incidence, distribution, and control of disease.

ETIOLOGY - The cause of a disorder or condition.

EVOKED POTENTIAL - The electrical response recorded from the cerebral cortex after stimulation of a peripheral sense organ.

EXPERIMENTAL GROUP - The subjects in an experiment who are exposed to the independent or experimental variable and whose performance is thought to reflect the influence of that condition.

EXTINCTION - Refers to the reduction of a conditioned response to its preconditioned level by a discontinuation of reinforcement for that response.

FACTOR ANALYSIS - A statistical method to identify the minimum number of factors responsible for the relationship among characteristics.

FAMILIAL - Tending to manifest itself in family lines; thus, hereditary.

FAMILY THERAPY - A generic term for a class of therapies based on the proposition that disordered behavior is a function of the entire family rather than only one of its members.

FEEDBACK - Information presented to the subject on his performance.

FETUS - A developing organism; in the human, the period after the third month of intrauterine development.

FOLLOW-UP STUDY - A reevaluation of deviant individuals after a period of time has elapsed.

FOOD ADDITIVES - A substance added to foodstuffs to improve color, flavor, texture, or keeping qualities.

GILLES DE LA TOURETTE - This childhood disease is characterized by repetitive tics, movement disorders, and uncontrollable sounds.

GLOBAL - Universal, comprehensive.

HALLUCINOGENS - Psychoactive drugs that increase arousal and activity while impairing inhibitory control, perception, and information processing.

HEREDITARY - Genetically transmitted from parent to offspring.

HYPERACTIVITY - A pattern of behavior characterized by a high degree of mobility and motor restlessness, distractibility, short attention span, and socially inappropriate behavior.

HYPOACTIVE - Underactivity; diminished activity level.

IMPULSIVITY - Refers to the tendency to react quickly and inappropriately to a situation rather than to take the time to consider alternatives and choose carefully.

INCIDENCE - The number of cases of disease which come into being during a specific period of time.

INTERVENTION - The method or strategy used in the treatment of a behavior disorder.

INVENTORY - A device used to assess personality and interests.

LABELING THEORY - A theory which holds that labeling alone is a powerful inducement toward deviance or conformity.

LATERALITY - The preferential use of one side of the body, especially in tasks demanding the use of only one hand, one eye, or one foot.

LEARNING DISABILITY - An educationally significant discrepancy between a child's apparent capacity for language behavior and his actual level of functioning, resulting from cerebral dysfunction and/or emotional behavioral disturbances.

LESION - A change in tissue due to injury, disease, or surgical procedure.

LOCUS OF CONTROL - The belief that one's behavior is under internal or external control; an individual has an internal locus to the extent that he believes he is responsible for his actions, an external locus to the extent that he believes chance or others' actions determine his behavior.

LONGITUDINAL STUDIES - Studies which focus on the change in a person or a group of people over an extended period of time.

MAINSTREAMING - The inclusion of special education students into regular classrooms with nonhandicapped students.

MALADAPTATION - Inability to adapt one's behavior to the conditions of his environment; it is sometimes referred to as maladjustment.

MATURATIONAL LAG - A delay in attaining a recognized stage or point in development sequence, such as ability to walk alone.

MEGAVITAMIN THERAPY - The administration of extremely large doses of vitamins in the hope of improving or curing behavior disorders.

MILIEU THERAPY - A method of therapy based on consideration of the total environment in which a child lives.

MINIMAL BRAIN DYSFUNCTION; MINIMAL BRAIN DAMAGE - A term applied to children who exhibit behavioral characteristics (e.g., hyperactivity, distractibility) thought to be associated with brain damage, in the absence of other evidence that their brains have been damaged.

MIXED DOMINANCE - The failure of one side of the brain to be clearly dominant over the other in motor control. The resulting conflict is held to be the cause of speech and perceptual deficits.

MODELING - Learning through imitation and observation of the behavior of others (imitation).

MULTIDISCIPLINARY - A term pertaining to the cooperative participation by several professional groups.

MULTISENSORY APPROACHES - Educational techniques which require the use of several sensory modalities used simultaneously or individually to facilitate learning.

NARCOTICS - Psychoactive drugs that reduce arousal, activity, biosocial drives, and responses to stimuli.

NEGATIVISM - A pattern of adjustment consisting of uncooperative and disagreeable behavior.

NEONATAL - Pertaining to the initial month of life.

NEUROLOGICAL IMPAIRMENT - Damage to or some deficiency in the nervous system of the body.

NEUROTIC - Pertaining to a functional nervous disorder without demonstrable physical lesion; or an emotionally unstable individual.

OPERANT CONDITIONING - Management of the consequences of behavior in order to increase or decrease the frequency of a response.

ORGANIC BRAIN SYNDROME; ORGANIC PSYCHOSIS - A behavior disorder caused by damage to the brain.

ORGANICITY - A dysfunction due to structural changes in the central nervous system.

ORTHOMOLECULAR THERAPY - The administration of chemical substances, vitamins, or drugs under the assumption that a basic chemical or molecular error which causes behavior disorders will be corrected.

PARADOXICAL EFFECT - Refers to the surprisingly calming effect that CNS stimulants have on hyperactive children.

PERCEPTION - The interpretation of sensory information, association of stimulus with meaning.

PERINATAL - Occurring at about the time of birth.

PERSEVERATION - The tendency to continue with a task or activity without the ability to shift or change easily to another task.

PERSONALITY DISORDER; PERSONALITY PROBLEM - A disorder characterized by neurotic behavior, depression, and withdrawal.

PETIT MAL SEIZURE - A form of epilepsy in which there is a brief lapse of consciousness; it is sometimes referred to as an absence attack. It is usually seen in children and may occur many times daily.

PLACEBO - An inactive treatment not designed specifically to bring about changes in behavior.

POSITIVE REINFORCEMENT - The process in which the presentation of a stimulus increases the frequency of the behavior it follows.

POSTNATAL - Pertaining to the time following birth.

PRENATAL - Pertaining to the period existing before birth.

PROGNOSIS - The projected outcome or course for a given condition.

PSYCHOACTIVE DRUGS - Drugs capable of manipulating psychological and behavioral characteristics.

PSYCHOANALYSIS - The Freudian theory of personality and technique for treating personality disturbances.

PSYCHOEDUCATIONAL APPROACH - The application of psychological and psychodynamic approaches in the school by school staff.

PSYCHOGENIC - Disorders originating psychologically as opposed to disorders originating from an organic basis.

PSYCHOPATHOLOGY - Mental illness; in psychiatry, the study of significant causes and development of mental illness; more generally, behavior disorder.

PSYCHOPHARMACOLOGY - The study of the mental and behavioral effects of certain drugs.

PSYCHOPHYSIOLOGICAL - Physical disorders thought to be caused by psychological (emotional) conflict.

PSYCHOTHERAPY - The use of psychological methods in the treatment of emotional and behavior disorders; any type of treatment relying primarily on verbal and nonverbal communication between patient and therapist rather than medical procedures.

PSYCHOTROPIC - Drugs which have a special action or effect on psychic function, behavior, or experience.

RANDOM SAMPLE - A group of subjects selected in such way that each member of the group from which the sample is derived has an equal chance of being chosen for the sample.

RATING SCALE - A type of test used in evaluating personality and other factors.

REACTION TIME - The interval between the beginning of a stimulus and the initiating of a response.

REFLECTION - A type of thinking characterized by introspection, deliberation, or contemplation.

REINFORCEMENT - Refers to a process that increases the strength of a behavior by the delivery of a particular consequence for that behavior.

RELIABILITY - Replicability or the extent to which the same test will yield the same results on repetition.

RESIDENTIAL TREATMENT - A general term referring to treatment approaches carried out in an institutional setting.

RETROSPECTIVE STUDY - A research technique involving selection of subjects on the basis of certain deviant characteristics and the subsequent reconstruction of their childhoods.

SALICYLATE - A salt or ester of salicylic acid which may be etiological in hyperkinesis.

SCREENING - The process of selecting a small group of children from a much larger group for a specific purpose.

SELF-CONCEPT - An individual's thoughts about his physical, cognitive, social, and emotional capacities.

SELF-CONTROL - The undertaking, by the subject, of certain behaviors in order to achieve self-selected goals.

SELF-ESTEEM - A positive and favorable concept of oneself.

SEQUELAE - The permanent consequences of an injury or disease.

SEROTONIN - A hormone-like substance in the brain, blood, and smooth tissues. Abnormal serotonin metabolism may cause some psychoses.

SIDE EFFECT - A result of drug or other form of therapy in addition to the desired therapeutic effect. Usually connotes an undesirable effect.

SOCIAL REINFORCEMENT - A reinforcement resulting from interpersonal interaction such as attention, praise, smiling, physical contact.

SOFT NEUROLOGICAL SIGNS - A term applied to the subtle and minimal deficiencies in fine-gross motor coordination and perceptual-motor integration.

STANFORD-BINET INTELLIGENCE SCALE (BINET SCALE) - A widely used scale for assessing school learning ability in individual examination of persons aged 2 through approximately 16 years.

STATE-DEPENDENT LEARNING - The reduction or lack of transfer of a habit learned under a drug state to a nondrug state, or vice-versa.

STIGMATA - A physical mark(s) or pecularity(ies) which aids in identification or in the diagnosis of a condition.

STIMULANT - Psychoactive drugs that increase arousal, activity, inhibitory control, and wakefulness.

STRAUSS SYNDROME - The cluster of symptoms characterizing the "brain-injured" child; includes hyperactivity, distractibility, and impulsivity.

TANGIBLE REINFORCER - A material reward, such as candy or tokens, for desired behavior.

TARGET BEHAVIOR - The specific behavior to be changed in conjunction with a behavior modification program.

THERAPEUTIC MILIEU - A total treatment setting that is therapeutic; a therapeutic environment including attention to the therapeutic value of both physical and social surroundings.

THERAPEUTIC TEAM - A team of individuals who work together cooperatively to plan for and service an individual child who has special needs. The team can include the classroom teacher, school psychologist, nurse, social worker, physician, and psychiatrist.

TIC - A spasmodic or sudden twitch, usually of one of the face or head muscles, which results from excessive anxiety.

TIME OUT - A punishment procedure in which positive reinforcement is denied.

TOKEN - A tangible reinforcer, such as poker chips, stars, tickets, etc. that may be exchanged for back-up reinforcers.

TOKEN ECONOMY - This term refers to a reinforcement system in which tokens are earned by specific behaviors.

TRANQUILIZERS - Psychoactive drugs, classified into major and minor varieties, that generally reduce arousal, inhibitory control, responses to stimuli, fighting behavior, and passive avoidence to varying degrees.

TRAUMA - A sudden negative experience and/or shock, producing sustained and lasting emotional or psychological effects for the individual.

UNDERACHIEVER - A student whose academic performance is significantly lower than his measured ability.

VALIDITY - The degree to which a measure gives an indication of a particular quality or attribute that it claims to measure.

VIGILANCE - Readiness or alertness in response to stimuli.

WECHSLER INTELLIGENCE SCALE FOR CHILDREN (WISC), REVISED - A widely used scale for individual assessment of learning ability of persons aged 6 through 16 years.

Appendix D: Audiovisual Materials

ABCs of behavioral education. [Motion Picture]. Baltimore, Maryland: Hallmark Films (1511 East North Avenue, Baltimore, Maryland 21213), 1972. 16 mm/color/20 min.

Describes a behavioral education program for twelve- to seventeen-year-old students who had been ejected from other schools. The Arundel Learning Center's program demonstrates the use of behavioral procedures within the special education setting.

Additives and hyperactivity. [Sound Recording]. New York, New York: Huxley Institute for Biosocial Research, 1978. 1 cassette/2 track/mono.

Aggressive child. [Motion Picture]. New York, New York: McGraw-Hill Films (330 West Hill Films, New York, New York 10036), b&w/28 min.

This film focuses on an intelligent six-year-old boy, Philip, whose disruptive behavior causes authorities to suggest psychiatric help to the parents.

Behavioral analysis classroom. [Motion Picture]. Lawrence, Kansas: Audio-Visual Center (746 Massachusetts Street, University of Kansas, Lawrence, Kansas 66044). 16 mm/color/20 min.

Focuses on classrooms that use behavior analysis techniques and token reinforcement systems. In this setting parents are used to supplement the regular teaching staff.

Behavioral modification in the classroom. [Motion Picture]. Berkeley, California: Extension Media Center, University of California, 1970. 16 mm/color/or b&w/24 min.

Illustrates the use of operant conditioning and modeling to strengthen task-oriented behavior in elementary schoolchildren. Behavior is contrasted before and after the application of behavioral principles. Methods of training teachers in the use of behavior modification strategies are included.

Brain-damaged child. [Motion Picture]. University Park, Pennsylvania: Pennsylvania State University, Psychological Cinema Register, 1978. 1 reel/16 mm/b&w/31 min./sound.

Presents the case of a seven-year-old boy with a diagnosis of chronic brain syndrome in order to observe aspects of communication related to this disorder. This objective is achieved in an interview with the child and his psychiatrist. The characteristics of the syndrome are noted in the film.

Children's rights: the legal aspects of drugs and the hyperactive child (Joseph Fleming) and Whose problem: school, family, or child? (Priscilla Watson). [Audio Cassette]. New York, New York: New York Institute for Child Development (205 Lexington Avenue, New York, New York 10016), 1976. 4 cassettes.

This cassette is of a presentation at the Reaching Children Conferences on Hyperactivity and Learning Disabilities. Two topics are covered: The New York Institute's approach to treating drug abuse, and the problems involved when using drug therapy for hyperactive children.

The diagnostic interview in child psychiatry. [Motion Picture]. Oklahoma City, Oklahoma: Fernando Tapia, 1972. 1 reel/16 mm/b&w/35 min./ sound.

Presents the principles of an interview designed to clarify and confirm the biological and social facts which provide a longitudinal view of an individual's life. Suggestions are given for conducting an interview and brief excerpts of interviews with four children are provided to illustrate these principles. One case study involves a hyperactive boy.

Discipline and self-control. [Motion Picture]. New York, New York: Duart Film Laboratories (245 West 55th Street, New York, New York 10019). b&w/25 min.

Discusses the problems of discipline and how teachers can develop control in a friendly atmosphere.

Food additives and the hyperactive child. [Slide]. Buffalo, New York: Communications in Learning, 1975. 13 slides/color/2x2 in. & cassette (2 track/mono/30 min.) and handout.

How to use tokens in teaching. [Motion Picture]. Lawrence, Kansas: Audio Visual Center (746 Massachusetts Street, University of Kansas, Lawrence, Kansas 66044). 16 mm/color/8 min.

A teacher demonstrates the proper way to use tokens in preschool education.

Hyperactive child: film for health professionals. Produced by CIBA Pharmaceutical Company and distributed by Association-Sterling Films (600 Grand Avenue, Ridgefield, New Jersey 07656). 30 min.

Hyperactive child: finding the cause. Produced by CIBA Pharmaceutical Company and distributed by Association-Sterling Films (600 Grand Avenue, Ridgefield, New Jersey 07656). 25 min.

Hyperactive child. [Filmstrip]. Garden Grove, California: Trainex Corporation, 1973. 56 fr/color/35 mm & cassette (2 track/mono/15 min.) and study guide.

This program presents an overview of the characteristics and management of the hyperactive child. Parental guidance is also covered.

Descriptions of typical characteristics, evaluative measures, and medical and behavioral management are included.

Hyperactive child. [Sound Recording]. Buffalo, New York: Communications in Learning, 1975. 1 cassette/2 track/mono/guide.

If a boy can't learn. [Motion Picture]. Burlingame, California: Lawren Productions (P. O. Box 1542, Burlingame, California 94010).

Is allergy related to hyperactivity and learning problems? (Doris Rapp). [Audio Cassette]. New York, New York: New York Institute for Child Development (205 Lexington Avenue, New York, New York 10016), 1976. 4 cassettes.

This cassette is of a presentation at the Reaching Children Conferences on Hyperactivity and Learning Disabilities, and presents the views of a pediatrician on the relationship between additives, allergy, and hyperactivity.

Jamie: a behavioral approach to family intervention. [Motion Picture]. Los Angeles, California: Neuropsychiatric Institute (760 Westwood Plaza, Los Angeles, California 90024). b&w/15 min.

This film shows how parents of a disturbed child can receive help from a behavioral approach. Behavior therapy is used with one five-year-old child. Discussions with the parents are shown.

Johnny. [Motion Picture]. Boston, Massachusetts: Guidance Camps, Inc. (for loan and sale by Harvard Medical School), 1971. 1 reel/16 mm/ b&w/32 min./sound and guide.

The purpose of this program is to acquaint teachers with the behavior of an emotionally disturbed child. The experiences of a hyperactive and aggressive nine-year-old boy at a therapeutic camp are related. Camp Wediko, a camp for emotionally disturbed boys aged 9 to 15, is the setting. A counselor uses various techniques to help Johnny control his temper tantrums.

Like any child or more so. [Motion Picture]. [Videotape]. Berkeley, California: Lifelong Learning, University Extension, University of California, 1978. 16 mm/color/29 min./sound.

Profiled are three families with children labeled hyperactive. The complex physiological, emotional, and environmental influences on a child's behavior are explored. Also covered are: (1) the lawsuit filed by parents against the school district in Taft, California; (2) the use and side effects of drugs used in treating hyperactivity; and (3) an experimental preschool for hyperactive children in Escondido, California.

Low blood surgar and learning (Roberts) and Nutritional analysis of the learning disabled child (Agree). [Audio Cassette]. New York, New York: New York Institute for Child Development (205 Lexington Avenue, New York, New York 10016), 1976. 4 cassettes.

This cassette is of a presentation at the Reaching Children Conferences on Hyperactivity and Learning Disabilities. A physician explains the problems of low blood sugar and its effects on behavior and learning. A nutritionist discusses diagnosis and treatment of dietary disorders in learning disabled and hyperactive children.

Managing the hyperactive child. [Motion Picture]. New York, New York: Network for Continuing Medical Education (NCME) (15 Columbus Circle, New York, New York 10023). 35 min.

Medical diagnosis of the hyperactive and learning disabled child (Sydney Walker). [Audio Cassette]. New York, New York: New York Institute for Child Development (205 Lexington Avenue, New York, New York 10016), 1976. 4 cassettes.

This cassette is of a presentation at the Reaching Children Conferences on Hyperactivity and Learning Disabilities. It provides a physician's analysis of the nature and treatment of hyperactivity in learning disabled children.

Nutritional management and the school system (Jordan) and A critical review of behavior modification and the hyperactive child (Kazaoka). [Audio Cassette]. New York, New York: New York Institute for Child Development (205 Lexington Avenue, New York, New York 10016), 1976. 4 cassettes.

This cassette is of a presentation at the Reaching Children Conferences on Hyperactivity and Learning Disabilities. The role of nutrition in human learning is reviewed. Also discussed are the aims and limitations of behavior modification with hyperactive children.

Peer conducted behavior modification. [Motion Picture]. Los Angeles, California: Neuropsychiatric Institute (760 Westwood Plaza, Los Angeles, California 90024), 1976. 16 mm/color/20 min.

A child's parents are taught to use behavior management procedures in modifying maladaptive behaviors. Peer influence is explored. Emphasis is given to the effects of both positive and negative reinforcement.

PREP (Preparation through responsive educational program). [Motion Picture]. Silver Springs, Maryland: Institute for Behavioral Research (2429 Linden Lane, Silver Springs, Maryland 20910). 16 mm/color/27 min.

Describes a highly individualized junior high school program for adolescents with social and academic problems.

The program at number twenty-three. [Videotape Cassette]. Norristown, Pennsylvania: Montgomery County Intermediate Unit (Special Education Center, 1605-B West Main Street, Norristown, Pennsylvania 19403). color/45 min./sound/1/2 inch reel to reel; 3/4 inch videotape cassette.

This series of five videotapes and booklets describes the program for the emotionally disturbed and brain injured children (grades k-12) of Intermediate Unit #23 in Montgomery County, Pennsylvania. Covered in the series are the following: an overview (philosophy, administration, supervision, and operation of the program); the mental health professional in the school (weekly group therapy sessions and training teachers in therapeutic techniques); the teacher in the classroom (psychodynamic and behavior modification techniques in classroom management); the teacher and the therapeutic group; and the child and the program (admission, continuation, and withdrawal).

A psychiatrist looks at the hyperactive, learning disabled child (Michael B. Schachter). [Audio Cassette]. New York, New York: New York Institute for Child Development (205 Lexington Avenue, New York, New York 10016), 1976. 4 cassettes.

This cassette is of a presentation at the Reaching Children Conferences on Hyperactivity and Learning Disabilities. An orthomolecular psychiatrist describes the body's biochemistry and discusses new treatment methods for such imbalances as hyperactivity.

Psychotropic drugs and the hyperkinetic syndrome. [Motion Picture]. Lawrence, Kansas: University of Kansas, Audiovisual Center (746 Massachusetts Street, Lawrence, Kansas 66044), 1974. 16 mm/b&w/ 24 min./sound.

Shows an experiment on the effects of methylphenidate (Ritalin) on the performance of mentally retarded children. Included are comments from drug researchers on the considerations involved in administering drugs to normal and retarded children.

Randy. [Motion Picture]. Boston, Massachusetts: Guidance Camps, Inc. (for sale by Harvard Medical School), 1970. 16 mm/b&w/27 min./ guide.

Offers suggestions for managing a seriously disturbed child, such as Randy. The various forms of treatment observed in the program serve only as an example and are intended to illustrate their use in Camp Wediko. Randy, an eleven-year-old hyperactive, anxious, and fearful child, is shown as he manifests various behavior patterns. The types of therapy illustrated in this program include suggestions of verbalizing anger rather than physically hitting, and the "holding" technique which is used to calm Randy. Candy is used to reward good behavior.

Rewards and reinforcements. [Motion Picture]. Bloomington, Indiana: Audio-Visual Center, Indiana University. b&w/26 min.

This film demonstrates the principles of operant conditioning in teaching economically underprivileged children. Reinforcers include candy, money, clothes, and other material objects.

The role of the pediatrician: testing and therapy (Alexander Horowitz). [Audio Cassette]. New York, New York: New York Institute for Child Development (205 Lexington Avenue, New York, New York 10016), 1976. 4 cassettes.

The cassette is of a presentation at the Reaching Children Conferences on Hyperactivity and Learning Disabilities. A physician's views are presented on the medical aspects of learning disability and hyperactivity.

Speech, hearing and hyperactivity (Harvey Gardner) and Biochemistry and learning (Levin). [Audio Cassette]. New York, New York: New York Institute for Child Development (205 Lexington Avenue, New York, New York 10016), 1976. 4 cassettes.

The cassette is of a presentation at the Reaching Children Conferences on Hyperactivity and Learning Disabilities. Two topics are covered: the role of audition in learning disabilities and hyperactivity, and the effects of body chemistry on the central nervous system and the learning process.

Who did what to whom. [Motion Picture]. Champaign, Illinois: Research Press Company (2612 North Mattis Avenue, Champaign, Illinois 61820). 16 mm/color/17 min.

This film is designed to provide an opportunity to practice behavior analysis in everyday interactions. Each of forty short scenes is followed by five seconds of black leader so that projector may be stopped and the scene discussed. The behavior principles of positive and negative reinforcement, punishment, and extinction are shown in scenes in home, school, and office.

Appendix E: Service Organizations

American Academy of Allergy
611 East Wells Street
Milwaukee, Wisconsin 53202

American Academy of Child Psychiatry
Suite 201A - 1424 16th Street, N.W.
Washington, D.C. 20009

American Academy of Neurology
4015 West 65th Street
Minneapolis, Minnesota 55435

American Academy of Pediatrics
1801 Hinman Avenue
Evanston, Illinois 60204

American Association of Opthalmology
1100 17th Street, N.W.
Washington, D.C. 20036

American Education Association
663 5th Avenue
New York, New York 10022

American Educational Research Association
1230 17th Street, N.W.
Washington, D.C. 20036

American Electroencephalographic Society
38238 Glenn Avenue
Willoughby Hills, Ohio 44094

American Foundation for Learning Disabilities
P. O. Box 196
Convent Station, New Jersey 07961

American Neurological Association
P. O. Box 520875 Biscayne Annex
Miami, Florida 33152

American Optometric Association
7000 Chippew Street
St. Louis, Missouri 63119

American Psychiatric Association
1700 18th Street, N.W.
Washington, D.C. 20009

American Psychological Association
1200 17th Street, N.W.
Washington, D.C. 20036

American Society for Adolescent Psychiatry
24 Green Valley Road
Wallingford, Pennsylvania 19086

American Speech and Hearing Association
10801 Rockville Pike
Rockville, Maryland 20852

Association for the Advancement of Behavior Therapy
420 Lexington Avenue
New York, New York 10017

Association for Children with Learning Disabilities
4156 Library Road
Pittsburgh, Pennsylvania 15234

Asthma and Allergy Foundation of America
801 Second Avenue
New York, New York 10017

California Association for Neurologically Handicapped Children
Literature Distribution Division
P. O. Box 1526
Vista, California 92083

Canadian Association for Children with Learning Disabilities
Suite 316 - 88 Eglinton Avenue
East Toronto 12, Ontario, Canada

Child Neurology Program
Box 403
University of Virginia Hospital
Charlottesville, Virginia 22901

Child Study Association of America
50 Madison Avenue
New York, New York 10010

Child Welfare League of America
1346 Connecticut Avenue, N.W.
Washington, D.C. 20036

Coalition for Children and Youth
815 15th Street, N.W.
Washington, D.C. 20005

Council for Children with
Behavioral Disorders
1920 Association Drive
Reston, Virginia 22091

Council for Exceptional Children
1920 Association Drive
Reston, Virginia 22091

Council of National Organizations
for Children and Youth
c/o National Committee for
Children and Youth
#132, 1401 K Street, N.W.
Washington, D.C. 20005

Foundation for Child Development
345 East 46th Street
New York, New York 10017

Foundation for Children with
Learning Disabilities
99 Park Avenue, South
New York, New York 10016

International Federation of
Learning Disabilities
4934 East 21st Street
Indianapolis, Indiana 46218

International Reading Association
P. O. Box 8139
800 Barksdale Road
Newark, Delaware 19711

Jean Piaget Society
College of Education
University of Delaware
Newark, Delaware 19711

Kiwanis International
101 East Erie Street
Chicago, Illinois 60611

Mental Health Association
1800 North Kent Street
Rosslyn, Virginia 22209

National Association of Private
Schools for Exceptional Children
130 East Orange Avenue
Lake Wales, Florida 33853

National Catholic Educational
Association
1 DuPont Circle, N.W.
Washington, D.C. 20036

National Center on Educational
Media and Materials for the
Handicapped
829 Eastwind Drive
Westerville, Ohio 43081

National Easter Seal Society for
Crippled Children and Adults
2023 West Ogden Avenue
Chicago, Illinois 60612

National Foundation - March of
Dimes
1275 Mamaroneck Avenue
White Plains, New York 10602

National Health Council
1740 Broadway
New York, New York 10019

National PTA
700 North Rush Street
Chicago, Illinois 60611

Orton Society
8415 Bellona Lane
Towson, Maryland 21204

Research and Demonstration Center
for the Education of Handicapped
Children and Youth
Box 51
Teachers College
Columbia University
New York, New York 10027

Society for Adolescent Medicine
P. O. Box 3462
Granada Hills, California 91344

Society for Pediatric Research
Department of Pediatrics
Stanford University
School of Medicine
Stanford, California 94305

U.S. Department of Health,
Education and Welfare
200 Independence Avenue, S.W.
Washington, D.C. 20201

U.S. National Institute of Child
Health and Human Development
9000 Rockville Pike
Bethesda, Maryland 20205

U.S. National Institute of
Mental Health
Citizens Participation Branch
5600 Fishers Lane
Rockville, Maryland 20857

U.S. Office of Education
400 Maryland Avenue, S.W.
Washington, D.C. 20202

U.S. Office of Human Development
Services
Developmental Disabilities Office
330 C Street, S.W.
Washington, D.C. 20201

Appendix F: Basic Bibliographical Sources

1. Abstracts of Popular Culture
2. Access
3. Arts and Humanities Citation Index
4. Bibliographic Index
5. Books in Print
6. British Education Index
7. Canadian Education Index
8. Canadian Periodical Index
9. Child Development Abstracts
10. Cumulative Book Index
11. Cumulative Index to Nursing and Allied Health Literature
12. Current Contents/Social and Behavioral Sciences
13. Current Index to Journals in Education (CIJE)
14. Developmental Disabilities Abstracts
15. Developmental Medicine and Child Neurology Bibliography
16. Digest of Neurology and Psychiatry
17. Dissertation Abstracts International
18. DSH Abstracts
19. Education Index
20. Exceptional Child Education Abstracts (now Exceptional Child Education Resources)
21. Excerpta Medica
22. Feelings and their Medical Significance

23. Hospital Literature Index
24. Index Medicus
25. Index to Dental Literature
26. Index to Legal Periodicals
27. International Nursing Index
28. International Pharmaceutical Abstracts
29. Mental Retardation Abstracts
30. Mental Retardation and Developmental Disabilities Abstracts
31. Monthly Catalog of U.S. Government Publications
32. National Library of Medicine Current Catalog
33. National Union Catalog
34. New Periodicals Index
35. Nutrition Abstracts and Reviews
36. Popular Periodicals Index
37. Psychological Abstracts
38. Psychopharmacology Abstracts
39. Readers' Guide to Periodical Literature
40. Rehabilitation Literature
41. Research Relating to Children
42. Resources in Education (ERIC)
43. Science Citation Index
44. Social Sciences Citation Index
45. Social Sciences Index
46. Social Work Research and Abstracts
47. Sociological Abstracts
48. Subject Guide to Books in Print
49. Subject Guide to Forthcoming Books
50. Vision Index

Author Index

In the list below, the numbers after each name

refer to item numbers in the Bibliography

D

H

I

J

K

XYZ

Selective Key Word Subject Index

In the list below, the numbers after each word

refer to item numbers in the Bibliography

C

D

E

F

G

N

O

Q

R

S

U

V

List of Journal Abbreviations

Abbreviation	Title
A	A
Acad Ther	Academic Therapy
Act Nerv Super	Activitas Nervosa Superior
Acta Paedopsychiatr	Acta Paedopsychiatrica
Acta Psychiatr Scand	Acta Psychiatrica Scandinavica
Adolescence	Adolescence
Adv Biochem Psychopharmacol	Advances in Biochemical Psychopharmacology
AJOT	AJOT: The American Journal of Occupational Therapy
Am Baby	American Baby
Am Correct Ther J	American Corrective Therapy Journal
Am Educ	American Education
Am Fam Physician	American Family Physician
Am J Acupunct	American Journal of Acupuncture
Am J Dis Child	American Journal of Diseases of Children
Am J Epidemiol	American Journal of Epidemiology
Am J Hosp Pharm	American Journal of Hospital Pharmacy
Am J Ment Defic	American Journal of Mental Deficiency
Am J Nurs	American Journal of Nursing
Am J Occup Ther	American Journal of Occupational Therapy
Am J Orthopsychiatry	American Journal of Orthopsychiatry
Am J Psychiatry	American Journal of Psychiatry
Am Pharm	American Pharmacy
Am Psychol	American Psychologist
Am Sch Board J	American School Board Journal
Anat Rec	Anatomical Record
Ann Allergy	Annals of Allergy
Ann Neurol	Annals of Neurology
Annu Rev Med	Annual Review of Medicine
AORN J	American Operating Room Nurses Journal
Arch Dis Child	Archives of Disease in Childhood
Arch Gen Psychiatry	Archives of General Psychiatry
Ariz Med	Arizona Medicine
ASHA	ASHA: Journal of the American Speech and Hearing Association
Aust Fam Physician	Australian Family Physician
Aust Nurses Journal	Australian Nurses Journal
Aust NZ J Psychiatry	Australian and New Zealand Journal of Psychiatry
Aust Paediatr J	Australian Paediatric Journal

Abbreviation	Title
Aust Psychol	Australian Psychologist
AV Commun Rev	AV Communication Review
AVISO	Assocazione Volontari Italiani del Sangue
B	B
Behav Eng	Behavioral Engineering
Behav Genet	Behavior Genetics
Behav Modif	Behavior Modification
Behav Neuropsychiatry	Behavioral Neuropsychiatry
Behav Ther	Behavior Therapy
Biochem Med	Biochemical Medicine
Biofeedback Self Regul	Biofeedback and Self-Regulation
Biol Psychiatry	Biological Psychiatry
Biol Psychol	Biological Psychology
Biomed Mass Spectrom	Biomedical Mass Spectrometry
Br J Clin Pharmacol	British Journal of Clinical Pharmacology
Br J Psychiatry	British Journal of Psychiatry
Br Med J	British Medical Journal
Brain/Mind Bull	Brain/Mind Bulletin; Frontiers of Research, Theory and Practice
Bull Eleventh Dist Dent Soc	Bulletin of the Eleventh District Dental Society (Jamaica, New York)
Bull NY Acad Med	Bulletin of the New York Academy of Medicine
Bull Psychon Soc	Bulletin of the Psychonomic Society
Bur Memo	Bureau Memorandum
C	C
Can Consum	Canadian Consumer
Can Couns	Canadian Counsellor/Conseille Canadien
Can Fam Physician	Canadian Family Physician/Medecin de Famille Canadien
Can J Neurol Sci	Canadian Journal of Neurological Sciences
Can Med Assoc J	Canadian Medical Association Journal
Can Ment Health	Canada's Mental Health
Can Nurse	Canadian Nurse
Can Pharm J	Canadian Pharmaceutical Journal
Can Psychiatr Assoc J	Canadian Psychiatric Association Journal
Canadian	The Canadian
Cat Sel Doc Psychol	Catalog of Selected Documents in Psychology
Cereal Foods World	Cereal Foods World
Chatelaine	Chatelaine
Child Care Health Dev	Child: Care, Health and Development
Child Dev	Child Development

Abbreviation	Title
Child House	Children's House Magazine
Child Psychiatry Hum Dev	Child Psychiatry and Human Development
Child Psychiatry Q	Child Psychiatry Quarterly
Child Study J Monogr	Child Study Journal Monographs
Child Welfare	Child Welfare
Clgh Rev	Clearinghouse Review
Clin Electroencephalogr	Clinical Electroencephalography
Clin Pediatr	Clinical Pediatrics
Clin Pharmacol Ther	Clinical Pharmacology and Therapeutics
Clin Proc Child Hosp	Clinical Proceedings of the Children's Hospital
Clin Res	Clinical Research
Coll Stud J	College Student Journal
Compr Psychiatry	Comprehensive Psychiatry
Compr Ther	Comprehensive Therapy
Connecticut	Connecticut
Consultant	Consultant
Consum Res Mag	Consumers' Research Magazine
Contemp Nutr	Contemporary Nutrition
Coronet	Coronet
Cortex	Cortex; a Journal Devoted to the Study of the Nervous System and Behavior
Creat Child Adult Q	Creative Child and Adult Quarterly
Curr Dev Psychopharmacol	Current Developments in Psychopharmacology
Curr Ther Res	Current Therapeutic Research
D	D
Day Care Early Educ	Day Care and Early Education
Del Med J	Delaware Medical Journal
Dev Med Child Neurol	Developmental Medicine and Child Neurology
Dev Psychiatry	Developments in Psychiatry
Dev Psychol	Developmental Psychology
Devereux Forum	Devereux Forum
Dis Nerv Syst	Diseases of the Nervous System
Diss Abstr Int	Dissertation Abstracts International
Drug Forum	Drug Forum; the Journal of Human Issues
Drug Ther	Drug Therapy
Drug Ther Bull	Drug and Therapeutics Bulletin
Drugs	Drugs
E	E
Early Years	Early Years
East Afr Med J	East African Medical Journal
Ecol Law Q	Ecology Law Quarterly
Edcentric	Edcentric
Educ Dig	Education Digest
Educ Horiz	Educational Horizons

Abbreviation	Title
Educ Leadership	Educational Leadership
Educ Psychol Meas	Educational and Psychological Measurement
Educ Res (U.K.)	Educational Research (U.K.)
Educ Treat Child	Education and Treatment of Children
Educ Urban Soc	Education and Urban Society
Electroencephalogr Clin Neurophysiol	Electroencephalography and Clinical Neurophysiology
Elem Sch Guid Couns	Elementary School Guidance and Counseling
Elem Sch J	Elementary School Journal
Environ Health Perspect	Environmental Health Perspectives
Essence	Essence
Ethics Sci Med	Ethics in Science and Medicine
Except Child	Exceptional Children
Except Parent	Exceptional Parent
Exp Neurol	Experimental Neurology
Eye Ear Nose Throat Mon	Eye, Ear, Nose, and Throat Monthly
F	F
Fam Community Health	Family and Community Health
Fam Health	Family Health
FDA By-lines	FDA By-lines
FDA Consum	FDA Consumer
Film News	Film News
Food Cosmet Toxicol	Food and Cosmetics Toxicology
Front Psychiatry	Frontiers in Psychiatry
G	G
Genet Psychol Monogr	Genetic Psychology Monographs
Good Housekeeping	Good Housekeeping
H	H
Harpers Wkly	Harper's Weekly
Hastings Cent Rep	Hastings Center Report
Health Soc Work	Health and Social Work
Hosp Formul	Hospital Formulary
Hosp Pract	Hospital Practice
Hum Behav	Human Behavior
I	I
Ill Med J	Illinois Medical Journal
Int J Addict	International Journal of the Addictions
Int J Clin Exp Hypn	International Journal of Clinical and Experimental Hypnosis
Int J Clin Pharmacol Biopharm	International Journal of Clinical Pharmacology and Biopharmacy
Int J Dermatol	International Journal of Dermatology
Int J Early Child	International Journal of Early Childhood

Abbreviation	Title
Int J Ment Health	International Journal of Mental Health
Int J Neurol	International Journal of Neurology
Int Pharmacopsychiatry	International Pharmacopsychiatry
Intellect	Intellect
Isr Ann Psychiatry	Israel Annals of Psychiatry and Related Disciplines
Isr J Med Sci	Israel Journal of Medical Sciences
J	J
J Abnorm Child Psychol	Journal of Abnormal Child Psychology
J Abnorm Psychol	Journal of Abnormal Psychology
J Am Acad Child Psychiatry	Journal of the American Academy of Child Psychiatry
J Am Diet Assoc	Journal of the American Dietetic Association
J Am Med Wom Assoc	Journal of the American Medical Women's Association
J Am Optom Assoc	Journal of the American Optometric Association
J Am Pharm Assoc	Journal of the American Pharmaceutical Association
J Appl Behav Anal	Journal of Applied Behavior Analysis
J Appl Nutr	Journal of Applied Nutrition
J Autism Child Schizophr	Journal of Autism and Childhood Schizophrenia
J Behav Ther Exp Psychiatry	Journal of Behavior Therapy and Experimental Psychiatry
J Bone Joint Surg	Journal of Bone and Joint Surgery
J Child Psychol Psychiatry	Journal of Child Psychology and Psychiatry and Allied Disciplines
J Clin Child Psychol	Journal of Clinical Child Psychology
J Clin Psychiatry	Journal of Clinical Psychiatry
J Clin Psychol	Journal of Clinical Psychology
J Commun	Journal of Communication
J Consult Clin Psychol	Journal of Consulting and Clinical Psychology
J Drug Educ	Journal of Drug Education
J Educ Psychol	Journal of Educational Psychology
J Educ Res	Journal of Educational Research
J Exp Child Psychol	Journal of Experimental Child Psychology
J Fam Pract	Journal of Family Practice
J Fla Med Assoc	Journal of the Florida Medical Association
J Genet Psychol	Journal of Genetic Psychology
J Int Assoc Pupil Pers Work	Journal of the International Association of Pupil Personnel Workers
J Iowa Med Soc	Journal of the Iowa Medical Society
J Labelled Compo Radiopharm	Journal of Labelled Compounds and Radiopharmaceuticals

Abbreviation	Title
J Learn Disabil	Journal of Learning Disabilities
J Music Ther	Journal of Music Therapy
J Natl Med Assoc	Journal of the National Medical Association
J Negro Educ	Journal of Negro Education
J Nerv Ment Dis	Journal of Nervous and Mental Disease
J Oper Psychiatry	Journal of Operational Psychiatry
J Orthomol Psychiatry	Journal of Orthomolecular Psychiatry
J Pediatr	Journal of Pediatrics
J Pediatr Psychol	Journal of Pediatric Psychology
J Pract Nurs	Journal of Practical Nursing
J Psychiatr Nurs	Journal of Psychiatric Nursing and Mental Health Services
J Psychosom Res	Journal of Psychosomatic Research
J Rehabil Asia	Journal of Rehabilitation in Asia
J Res Dev Educ	Journal of Research and Development in Education
J Sch Health	Journal of School Health
J Spec Educ	Journal of Special Education
J Spec Educ Ment Retarded	Journal for Special Educators of the Mentally Retarded
J Thought	Journal of Thought
JAMA	JAMA: Journal of the American Medical Association
Jpn J Hum Genet	Japanese Journal of Human Genetics/ Jinrui Idengaku
Jpn Psychol Res	Japanese Psychological Research
L	L
Lancet	Lancet
Learn Disabil Q	Learning Disabilities Quarterly
Learning	Learning
Lets Live	Let's Live
Life Sci	Life Sciences
Lutheran Educ	Lutheran Education
M	M
McCalls	McCalls
Med Dig	Medical Digest
Med Hypotheses	Medical Hypotheses
Med J Aust	Medical Journal of Australia
Med Lett Drugs Ther	Medical Letter on Drugs and Therapeutics
Med Times	Medical Times
Ment Hyg	Mental Hygiene
Ment Retard	Mental Retardation
Ment Retard Bull	Mental Retardation Bulletin
MH	MH: Mental Hygiene
Midwife Health Visit	Midwife and Health Visitor
Minn Law Rev	Minnesota Law Review
Mo Med	Missouri Medicine
Mod Med	Modern Medicine
Monogr Neural Sci	Monographs in Neural Sciences

Abbreviation	Title
N	N
N Engl J Med	New England Journal of Medicine
Nation	Nation
Nations Sch Coll	Nation's Schools and Colleges
Nebr Med J	Nebraska Medical Journal
Neurology	Neurology
Neuropaediatrie	Neuropaediatrie: Journal of Pediatric Neurobiology, Neurology and Neurosurgery
Neuropharmacology	Neuropharmacology
Neuropsychobiology	Neuropsychobiology
New Sci	New Scientist
New Soc	New Society
Newsweek	Newsweek
Nurs Care	Nursing Care
Nurs Clin North Am	Nursing Clinics of North America
Nurs Mirror	Nursing Mirror
Nurs Times	Nursing Times
Nurse Pract	Nurse Practitioner: a Journal of Primary Nursing Care
Nutr Rev	Nutrition Reviews
NYSSNTA	New York State School Nurse Teachers Association
NZ Med J	New Zealand Medical Journal
O	O
Ohio J Sci	Ohio Journal of Science
Ohio Pharm	Ohio Pharmacist
Ont Med Rev	Ontario Medical Review
Ont Psychol	Ontario Psychologist
Optom Wkly	Optometric Weekly
P	P
PA J	P. A. Journal
Paediatrician	Paediatrician; International Journal for Postgraduate Education in General Pediatrics and Allied Disciplines
Parents Mag	Parents' Magazine and Better Homemaking
Patient Care	Patient Care
PDM	PDM: Physicians' Drug Manual
Peabody J Educ	Peabody Journal of Education
Pediatr Ann	Pediatric Annals
Pediatr Clin North Am	Pediatric Clinics of North America
Pediatr Nurs	Pediatric Nursing
Pediatr Res	Pediatric Research
Pediatrics	Pediatrics
People	People
Percept Mot Skills	Perceptual and Motor Skills
Perspect Psychiatr Care	Perspectives in Psychiatric Care
Pharmacol Biochem Behav	Pharmacology, Biochemistry and Behavior

Abbreviation	Title
Phi Delta Kappan	Phi Delta Kappan
Phoenix J	Die Phoenix Journal
Physiologie	Physiologie
Physiotherapy	Physiotherapy
Plain Truth	Plain Truth
Postgrad Med	Postgraduate Medicine
Practitioner	Practitioner
Prevention	Prevention
Prime Areas	Prime Areas (British Columbia Primary Teachers' Association)
Prog Neuropharmacol	Progress in Neuropharmacology
Progressive	Progressive
Psychiatr Ann	Psychiatric Annals
Psychiatr Forum	Psychiatric Forum
Psychiatr J Univ Ottawa	Psychiatric Journal of the University of Ottawa
Psychiatr Neurol Japonica	Psychiatria et Neurologia Japonica
Psychiatr Q	Psychiatric Quarterly
Psychol Bull	Psychological Bulletin
Psychol Med	Psychological Medicine
Psychol Rep	Psychological Reports
Psychol Sch	Psychology in the Schools
Psychol Today	Psychology Today
Psychopharmacol Bull	Psychopharmacology Bulletin
Psychopharmacologia	Psychopharmacologia
Psychopharmacology	Psychopharmacology
Psychophysiology	Psychophysiology
Psychosomatics	Psychosomatics
Psychother Theory Res Pract	Psychotherapy: Theory, Research and Practice
Q	Q
QRB	QRB: Quality Review Bulletin
R	R
Read Dig	Reader's Digest (Can)
Read Teach	Reading Teacher
Read World	Reading World
Redbook	Redbook
Rehabil Lit	Rehabilitation Literature
Rem Educ	Remedial Education
Res Commun Psychol Psychiatry Behav	Research Communications in Psychology, Psychiatry, and Behavior
Res Q Am Assoc Health Phys Educ	Research Quarterly: American Association for Health, Physical Education and Recreation
Res Rel Child	Research Relating to Children
Rev Educ Res	Review of Educational Research
Rev Mex Anal Conducta	Revista Mexicana de Analisis de la Conducta/Mexican Journal of Behavior Analysis
RI Med J	Rhode Island Medical Journal

Abbreviation	Title
S	S
S Afr Med J	South African Medical Journal
SALT	SALT: School Applications of Learning Theory
Sask J Educ Res Dev	Saskatchewan Journal of Educational Research and Development
Sch Psychol Dig	School Psychology Digest
Sch Rev	School Review
Schizophr Bull	Schizophrenia Bulletin
Sci Am	Scientific American
Sci Dig	Science Digest
Sci News	Science News
Science	Science
Slow Learn Child	Slow Learning Child: The Australian Journal on the Education of Backward Children
Soc Policy	Social Policy
Soc Probl	Social Problems
Spec Child	Special Children
Spec Educ Can	Special Education in Canada
Spec Educ Forward Trends	Special Education: Forward Trends
Stanford Law Rev	Stanford Law Review
T	T
Teach Coll Rec	Teachers College Record
Teacher	Teacher
Tex Key	Texas Key
Tex Med	Texas Medicine
Ther Recreat J	Therapeutic Recreation Journal
This Mag	This Magazine
Thrust Educ Leadership	Thrust for Educational Leadership
Times Educ Suppl	Times Educational Supplement
Todays Educ	Today's Education
Toxicol Appl Pharmacol	Toxicology and Applied Pharmacology
Town Ctry	Town and Country
Trans Anal J	Transactional Analysis Journal
U	U
Univ NC Sch Med Bull	University of North Carolina School of Medicine Bulletin
Urban Health	Urban Health
Urban League Rev	Urban League Review
US News World Rep	U. S. News and World Report
V	V
Va Med	Virginia Medical
W	W
W Va Med J	West Virginia Medical Journal
West Indian Med J	West Indian Medical Journal
West J Med	Western Journal of Medicine